Handbook of Nutrition and Diet in Palliative Care

Second Edition

Handbook of Nutrition and Diet in Palliative Care

Second Edition

Edited by

Victor R. Preedy

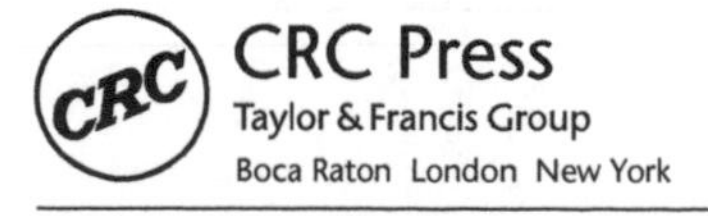

CRC Press is an imprint of the
Taylor & Francis Group, an **informa** business

CRC Press
Taylor & Francis Group
6000 Broken Sound Parkway NW, Suite 300
Boca Raton, FL 33487-2742

First issued in paperback 2020

ISBN 13: 978-0-367-72716-1 (pbk)
ISBN 13: 978-1-138-06407-2 (hbk)

Library of Congress Cataloging-in-Publication Data

Names: Preedy, Victor R., editor.
Title: Handbook of nutrition and diet in palliative care / editor, Victor R. Preedy.
Other titles: Diet and nutrition in palliative care | Nutrition and diet in palliative care
Description: Second edition. | Boca Raton : Taylor & Francis, 2019. | Preceded by Diet and nutrition in palliative care / edited by Victor R. Preedy. c2011. | Includes bibliographical references and index.
Identifiers: LCCN 2018060916| ISBN 9781138064072 (hardback : alk. paper) | ISBN 9781315160627 (general) | ISBN 9781351662970 (pdf) | ISBN 9781351662963 (epub) | ISBN 9781351662956 (mobi/kindle)
Subjects: | MESH: Palliative Care | Nutrition Therapy | Terminal Care
Classification: LCC RT87.T45 | NLM WB 310 | DDC 616.02/9--dc23
LC record available at https://lccn.loc.gov/2018060916

Visit the Taylor & Francis Web site at
http://www.taylorandfrancis.com

and the CRC Press Web site at
http://www.crcpress.com

Contents

SECTION I Setting the Scene

SECTION II Cultural Aspects

SECTION III General Aspects

SECTION IV Cancer

Preface

Optimal terminal and palliative care requires consideration of the patient and family unit as well as cultural and religious sensitivities. The patient's well-being in terms of mobility, anxiety, stress, social interaction and pain control needs expert focus and attention. However, there is an increasing awareness that diet and nutritional support play an integral part of the patient's holistic well-being. Many books on nutrition will have material aimed at prolonging life, preventing disease, or alleviating symptoms with a long-term view of complete rehabilitation. Occasionally, such books are directed toward subgroups, for example, infants or the elderly. However, there are no comprehensive books on nutrition in terminal or palliative care that simultaneously cover physical, cultural and ethical aspects. Nor are there many nutrition books that bridge the intellectual divide and are suitable for novices and experts alike. This book is aimed at addressing such deficiencies.

The *Handbook of Nutrition and Diet in Palliative Care*, second edition, is divided into six sections:

1. Setting the scene
2. Cultural aspects
3. General aspects
4. Cancer
5. Non-cancer conditions and pharmacologic aspects
6. Case study and resources

Coverage in the *Handbook of Nutrition and Diet in Palliative Care*, second edition, combines palliative care and nutrition in relation to numerous areas. Briefly, the material includes the following: Section I: needs in palliative care, features of palliative care, religion and culture, quality of life, cancer cachexia, sedation, pain control and communications; Section II: cultural aspects of enteral feeding, Indian and Italian perspectives; Section III: stents in the gastrointestinal tract, artificial nutrition, support for hydration, dysphagia, olfaction and appetite; Section IV: preoperative assessments, gastrojejunostomy, upper gastrointestinal symptoms, head and neck cancer, appetite and nausea, vitamin deficiency, childhood leukemia and eating-related distress; Section V: end-stage renal failure, HIV, gastroparesis, severe and enduring eating disorders, neurodevelopmental disorders, appetite stimulants and cannabinoids; and Section VI: a case study on refractory cancer cachexia and recommended resources. There are, of course, other areas too numerous to mention here.

Unique features of each chapter include relevant sections on

- Applications to other areas of terminal or palliative care
- Practical methods, techniques or guidelines
- Key facts that highlight important areas within chapters
- Ethical issues
- Summary points

The *Handbook of Nutrition and Diet in Palliative Care*, second edition, is for doctors, nurses and carers and those interested in or working within the palliative or end-of-life domain. This will include nutritionists and dietitians, health workers and practitioners, hospice or palliative centre managers, college and university teachers and lecturers and undergraduates and graduates. The chapters are written by national or international experts or specialists in their field. The material is well illustrated with numerous figures and tables.

Professor Victor R. Preedy

Editor

Victor R. Preedy BSc, PhD, DSc, FRSB, FRSPH, FRCPath, FRSC, is a senior staff member of the Faculty of Life Sciences and Medicine within King's College London. He is a member of the Division of Diabetes and Nutritional Sciences (research) and the Department of Nutrition and Dietetics (teaching). He is Director of the Genomics Centre of King's College London.

Preedy graduated in 1974 with an Honours Degree in Biology and Physiology with Pharmacology. He gained his PhD at the University of London in 1981. In 1992, he received his Membership of the Royal College of Pathologists, and in 1993 he gained his second doctorate (DSc) for his outstanding contribution to protein metabolism in health and disease. Preedy was elected as a Fellow to the Institute of Biology in 1995 and to the Royal College of Pathologists in 2000. Since then he has been elected as a Fellow to the Royal Society for the Promotion of Health (2004) and the Royal Institute of Public Health. In 2009, Preedy became a Fellow of the Royal Society for Public Health and, in 2012, a Fellow of the Royal Society of Chemistry. Preedy has carried out research at the National Heart Hospital (part of Imperial College London), The School of Pharmacy (now part of University College London) and the MRC Centre at Northwick Park Hospital. He has collaborated with research groups in Finland, Japan, Australia, the United States and Germany. Preedy is a leading expert on the science of health and has a long-standing interest in diet, nutrition and disease. He has lectured nationally and internationally. To his credit, Preedy has published over 600 articles, including peer-reviewed manuscripts based on original research, abstracts and symposium presentations, reviews and numerous books and volumes.

Contributors

Maria Ida Amabile
Department of Clinical Medicine
Sapienza University of Rome
Rome, Italy

Koji Amano
Department of Palliative Medicine
Osaka City General Hospital
Osaka, Japan

N. Ananthakrishnan
Department of Surgery
Mahatma Gandhi Medical College and Research Institute
Pondicherry, India

María Salome Anaya-Florez
Servicio de Nutrición Parenteral
UMAE Hospital de Pediatría "Dr. Silvestre Frenk Freund"
Centro Medico Nacional Siglo XXI, IMSS
Mexico City, Mexico

Keiron A. Audain
Department of Food Science and Nutrition
School of Agricultural Sciences
University of Zambia
Lusaka, Zambia

David Blum
Department of Oncology, Hematology and Bone Marrow Transplant
Palliative Care Unit
University Medical Center Hamburg
Hamburg, Germany

Giacomo Bovio
Metabolic–Nutritional Unit and Palliative Care Unit
Salvatore Maugeri Foundation
IRCCS, Rehabilitation Institute of Pavia
Pavia, Italy

Allison Bruff
Temple University Hospital
Department of Surgery
Philadelphia, Pennsylvania

Hans-Henrik Bülow
Intensive Care Unit
Holbaek Hospital, Region Zealand
University of Copenhagen
Copenhagen, Denmark

Riccardo Caccialanza
Clinical Nutrition and Dietetics Unit
Fondazione IRCCS Policlinico San Matteo
Pavia, Italy

Roberto Cavagnola
Disability Department, Fondazione Sospiro Onlus
Amico Di (Association on Contestualistic Model of Intervention Association in Intellectual Disabilities)
Sospiro, Italy

Emanuele Cereda
Fondazione IRCCS Policlinico San Matteo
Pavia, Italy

Helen Yue-lai Chan
Nethersole School of Nursing
Chinese University of Hong Kong
Hong Kong, People's Republic of China

Edward Chow
Department of Radiation Oncology
Odette Cancer Centre
Sunnybrook Health Sciences Centre
Toronto, Ontario, Canada

Selina Chow
Department of Radiation Oncology
Odette Cancer Centre
Sunnybrook Health Sciences Centre
Toronto, Ontario, Canada

Giuseppe Chiodelli
Disability Department
Fondazione Sospiro Onlus
Amico Di (Association on Contestualistic Model of Intervention Association in Intellectual Disabilities)
Italy

Marcin Chwistek
Department of Hematology and Oncology
Fox Chase Cancer Center
and
Department of Hematology and Oncology
Lewis Katz School of Medicine
Temple University
Philadelphia, Pennsylvania

Serafino Corti
Disability Department
Fondazione Sospiro Onlus
Amico Di (Association on Contestualistic Model of Intervention Association in Intellectual Disabilities)
Italy

Carlo DeAngelis
Department of Radiation Oncology
Odette Cancer Centre
Sunnybrook Health Sciences Centre
Toronto, Ontario, Canada

Jörg Dötsch
Department of Pediatrics
Head of Department
University of University of Cologne, Medical Faculty
Cologne, Germany

Robin L. Fainsinger
Division of Palliative Care Medicine
Grey Nuns Hospital
Edmonton, Alberta, Canada

Jeffrey M. Farma
Fox Chase Cancer Center
Department of Surgical Oncology
Philadelphia, Pennsylvania

Francesco Fioriti
Disability Department
Fondazione Sospiro Onlus
Amico Di (Association on Contestualistic Model of Intervention Association in Intellectual Disabilities)
Italy

Mick Fleming
Learning Education and Development (LEaD)
Cabinet Office, Isle of Man Government
Education and Training Centre
Keyll Darree
Strang, Isle of Man

Maria Luisa Fonte
Clinical Nutrition Specialist
Travacò Siccomario (PV), Italy

Maria Laura Galli
Disability Department
Fondazione Sospiro Onlus
Amico Di (Association on Contestualistic Model of Intervention Association in Intellectual Disabilities)
Italy

Vithusha Ganesh
Department of Radiation Oncology
Odette Cancer Centre
Sunnybrook Health Sciences Centre
Toronto, Ontario, Canada

Renata Gorska
Human Nutristasis Unit
Guy's and St. Thomas' Hospital
London, United Kingdom

Dominic J. Harrington
King's College London
Guy's and St. Thomas' Hospital
London, United Kingdom

Jeroen H. Hasselaar
Anesthesiology, Pain and Palliative Medicine
Radboud University Medical Centre
Nijmegen, The Netherlands

Blair Henry
Ethics Centre
Sunnybrook Health Sciences Centre
Toronto, Ontario, Canada

Elva Jiménez-Hernández
Coordinación de Investigación en Salud, Instituto Mexicano del Seguro Social (IMSS)
and
Servicio de Hematología Pediátrica
UMAE Hospital General "Dr. Gaudencio González Garza"
Centro Medico Nacional "La Raza", IMSS
Mexico City, Mexico

Vikram Kate
Department of Surgery
Jawaharlal Institute of Postgraduate Medical Education and Research
Pondicherry, India

Michelle Koh
Paediatric Palliative Care
Department of Child Health
University Hospital Southampton NHS Foundation Trust
Southampton, United Kingdom

Akanksha Kulshreshtha
Department of Radiation Oncology
Odette Cancer Centre, Sunnybrook Health Sciences Centre
Toronto, Ontario, Canada

Sofia Lakhdar
Department of Gastroenterology
Cleveland Clinic Florida
Weston, Florida

Henry Lam
Department of Radiation Oncology
Odette Cancer Centre
Sunnybrook Health Sciences Centre
Toronto, Ontario, Canada

Derek Larkin
Department of Psychology
Edge Hill University
Ormskirk, Lancashire, United Kingdom

Alessandro Laviano
Department of Clinical Medicine
Sapienza University of Rome
Rome, Italy

Mauro Leoni
Disability Department
Fondazione Sospiro Onlus
Amico Di (Association on Contestualistic Model of Intervention Association in Intellectual Disabilities)
Italy

Iruru Maetani
Division of Gastroenterology and Hepatology
Department of Internal Medicine
Toho University Ohashi Medical Center
Tokyo, Japan

Nanda Kishore Maroju
Department of Surgery
Jawaharlal Institute of Postgraduate Medical Education and Research
Pondicherry, India

Caroline J. Hollins Martin
Theme Lead for Women and Children's Health and Wellbeing (WACHAW)
School of Health and Social Care
Edinburgh Napier University (Sighthill Campus)
Midlothian, United Kingdom

Colin R. Martin
Faculty of Society and Health
Buckinghamshire New University
Uxbridge Campus
Uxbridge, Middlesex, United Kingdom

Philip S. Mehler
ACUTE, Denver Health
and
Department of Internal Medicine
University of Colorado School of Medicine
Denver, Colorado

Juan Manuel Mejía-Aranguré
Coordinación de Investigación en Salud
Instituto Mexicano del Seguro Social (IMSS)
Mexico City, Mexico

Giovanni Michelini
Disability Department
Fondazione Sospiro Onlus
Amicó Di (Association on Contestualistic Model of Intervention Association in Intellectual Disabilities)
Italy

Giovanni Miselli
Disability Department
Fondazione Sospiro Onlus
Amico Di (Association on Contestualistic Model of Intervention Association in Intellectual Disabilities)
Italy

Alessio Molfino
Department of Clinical Medicine
Sapienza University of Rome
Rome, Italy

Cheryl Ann Monturo
John A. Hartford Foundation Claire M. Fagin Fellow
Department of Nursing
College of Health Sciences
West Chester University of Pennsylvania
Exton, Pennsylvania

Tatsuya Morita
Palliative and Supportive Care Division
Seirei Mikatahara General Hospital
Shizuoka, Japan

Dorotea Mutabdzic
Complex General Surgical Oncology Fellow
Fox Chase Cancer Center
Philadelphia, Pennsylvania

Samya Z. Nasr
Department of Pediatric Pulmonology
University of Michigan Health System
Ann Arbor, Michigan

Juan Carlos Núñez-Enríquez
Unidad de Investigación Médica en Epidemiologia Clinica
UMAE Hospital de Pediatría "Dr. Silvestre Frenk Freund"
Centro Medico Nacional Siglo XXI, IMSS
Mexico City, Mexico

Kai-Dietrich Nüsken
Department of Pediatrics
Section of Pediatric Nephrology
University of University of Cologne, Medical Faculty
Cologne, Germany

Shalana O'Brien
Fox Chase Cancer Center
Department of Surgical Oncology
Philadelphia, Pennsylvania

Vinood B. Patel
University of Westminister
School of Life Sciences
London, United Kingdom

Paolo Pedrazzoli
Fondazione IRCCS Policlinico San Matteo
Pavia, Italy

Victor R. Preedy
Diabetes and Nutritional Sciences Research Division
Faculty of Life Science and Medicine
King's College London
London, United Kingdom

Rajkumar Rajendram
Department of Medicine
King Abdulaziz Medical City
Ministry of National Guard Health Affairs
Riyadh, Saudi Arabia

and

Diabetes and Nutritional Sciences Research Division
Faculty of Life Science and Medicine
King's College London
London, United Kingdom

Poornima B. Rao
Division of Surgical Oncology
Department of Surgery
South Pasadena, California

Christian P. Selinger
Department of Gastroenterology
Leeds Teaching Hospitals NHS Trust
St. James University Hospital
Beckett Street
Leeds, United Kingdom

Aarti Shakkottai
Department of Pediatric Pulmonology
University of Michigan Health System
Ann Arbor, Michigan

Takeshi Shinozaki
Department of Head and Neck Surgery
National Cancer Center Hospital East
Kashiwa, Japan

Sagit Shushan
Department of Otolaryngology-Head and Neck Surgery
Edith Wolfson Medical Center
Holon, Israel

and

Sackler School of Medicine
Tel Aviv University
Tel Aviv, Israel

Florian Strasser
Clinic Oncology and Hematology
Department of Internal Medicine and Palliative Center
Cantonal Hospital St. Gallen
St. Gallen, Switzerland

Kelay E. Trentham
MultiCare Regional Cancer Center
Tacoma, Washington

Eleni Tsiompanou
Woking and Sam Beare Hospices
Surrey, United Kingdom

Michela Uberti
Disability Department
Fondazione Sospiro Onlus
Amico Di (Association on Contestualistic Model of Intervention Association in Intellectual Disabilities)
Italy

Andrew Ukleja
Department of Gastroenterology and Hepatology
Beth Israel Deaconess Medical Center
Boston, Massachusetts

Carel M. M. Veldhoven
Anesthesiology, Pain and Palliative Medicine
Radboud University Medical Centre
Nijmegen, The Netherlands

Constans A. V. H. H. M. Verhagen
Anesthesiology, Pain and Palliative Medicine
Radboud University Medical Centre
Nijmegen, The Netherlands

Kris C. P. Vissers
Anesthesiology, Pain and Palliative Medicine
Radboud University Medical Centre
Nijmegen, The Netherlands

Catherine Walshe
Division of Health Research
Lancaster University, Bailrigg
Lancaster, United Kingdom

Patricia Westmoreland
Eating Recovery Center
and
Department of Psychiatry
University of Colorado School of Medicine
Denver, Colorado

Kitty Ka Yee Wong
Alice Ho Miu Ling Nethersole Hospital
Hong Kong, People's Republic of China

Arkadi Yakirevitch
Department of Otolaryngology-Head and Neck Surgery
Sheba Medical Center
Tel-Hashomer, Israel

Caitlin Yee
Department of Radiation Oncology
Odette Cancer Centre
Sunnybrook Health Sciences Centre
Toronto, Ontario, Canada

Section I

Setting the Scene

1 Need for Specialized Interest in Food and Nutrition in Palliative Care

Eleni Tsiompanou

CONTENTS

INTRODUCTION

Since antiquity, it has been known that food, exercise and lifestyle, as well as our external environment, influence our health. Hippocrates, the father of medicine, advocated the treatment of illnesses through modification of diet (δίαιτα), which in ancient Greek meant "way of life" and encompassed food, exercise and massage, baths and other aspects of everyday life. Food was a subject of interest for laypeople, writers and philosophers. In the *Deipnosophists* (*The Banquet of the Philosophers*), written by Athenaeus in the early third century AD, we read the story of Democritus of Abdera, the "Laughing Philosopher" (Athenaeus, 1927–41). At the age of 104, Democritus, approaching the end of his life, had gradually reduced his food intake and was expecting to die. It was the time of the important Thesmophorian festival (a women's festival in honor of goddesses Demeter and Persephone), and his centenarian sister, who looked after him at his home, asked him not to die during the festivities so that she could take part in them. Wanting to grant her request, he asked for a pot of honey to be brought to him. He was kept alive for three days by inhaling the fumes from the honey. When the festival finished, the pot of honey was taken away, and he passed away without any suffering. This story from Ancient Greece graphically depicts many elements of nutritional care we categorize as physical, cultural, social, ethical and emotional, which we encounter in our modern palliative care practice.

NUTRITION: AN IMPORTANT SUBJECT FOR PATIENTS AND CARERS

Every healthcare professional would agree that our duty is to take an active interest in what matters most to patients. Primarily this is about relieving suffering, pain and other debilitating symptoms.

In palliative care there is a critical interlinking of nutrition, symptoms and patient experience. Symptoms can not only adversely affect food and fluid intake, but also, importantly, a patient's nutritional intake can influence their symptoms and general state of being. Research has again confirmed that appetite and the ability to eat are very important physical aspects of a patient's quality of life. These are affected as the disease progresses and the patient experiences a series of losses: loss of weight and the desire to eat; loss of the ability to smell, taste, chew and swallow food; and loss of the ability to digest, absorb nutrients and eliminate waste products independently.

Good nutrition can enhance recovery, when healing is possible. Conversely, poor nutrition can result in poor resistance to infections, impaired wound healing, increased susceptibility to pressure ulcers and fatigue. Good, nutritious food contributes to the patient's overall sense of well-being. A drop in essential amino acids, glucose or vitamins and minerals in the body tends to affect the nervous system and behaviour adversely (Table 1.1).

Nutrition is also important as it is an avenue of empowerment for patients; it offers them the possibility to do something for themselves. Once a patient has been diagnosed with a serious illness, they become more aware of the impact their lifestyle has on their body. So they often initiate changes hoping this will help relieve their suffering and increase their chances of survival. They seek to improve their diet, physical activity and daily routine in general. Their carers want to show their love and care by providing good food and drink. Patients and carers alike often turn to healthcare professionals for information and advice. We need to assist them to appreciate the importance and relevance of nutrition and discuss with them what can help and what can harm them.

As we meet people at different stages of their illnesses we can help them understand how their nutritional needs may change as their disease progresses. We can support them, and those caring for them, to acknowledge the inevitable changes in their body and the nutritional decline prior to death.

Nutrition as a Safety Issue

When caring for people, one always has to consider safety matters around nutrition (National Patient Safety Agency, 2009) (Table 1.2). This becomes especially critical when these are vulnerable patients with advanced illness. In modern palliative care, understanding of the most important safety issues around oral nutrition and artificial nutrition and hydration (ANH) will help professionals provide better care for an increasing variety of conditions, minimising risk for patients.

TABLE 1.1
Key Nutrients Needed for the Optimal Functioning of the Nervous System

- Glucose
- Fatty acids
- Amino acids
- B-vitamins (vitamin B12, thiamine, niacin, pyridoxine)
- Folic acid
- Vitamins A, D and E
- Iron
- Copper

TABLE 1.2
Safety Issues Around Nutrition

1. Lack of nutrition screening and assessment
2. Inappropriate diet
3. Inappropriate fluid provision: dehydration, overhydration
4. Food allergies and intolerances
5. Choking
6. Nil by mouth
7. Artificial nutrition
8. Re-feeding syndrome
9. Missed meals
10. Lack of assistance with eating and drinking
11. Catering issues

RECENT ADVANCES IN SCIENCE OF NUTRITION: EPIGENETICS, MICROBES AND THE ENVIRONMENT

Knowledge of nutrition has progressed from simple data about macronutrients (fat, proteins and carbohydrates), micronutrients (minerals and vitamins) and calories, to the more complex world of phytochemicals and bioactive food components which can alter our cells' phenotype and, ultimately, influence how a disease progresses. More recently, an exciting research frontier has emerged with the discoveries of the effect of gut microbiota on human health. This may have relevance to treatments for palliative care patients.

Macronutrients, Micronutrients and Calories

The complexity and importance of nutritional care become apparent when we consider the powerful effects of macronutrients and micronutrients.

A steady supply of a combination of nutrients determines the functioning of various organs and systems in the body. The hypothesis is that during a chronic illness, if the nutrients missing in a particular case are identified and then replenished, the healing effect can be dramatic and function can improve. However, in actual practice, the situation is much more complex. For example, people who have advanced cancer quite often develop *anorexia-cachexia syndrome* (ACS) which is characterised by protein and weight loss. According to traditional dietary advice, ACS is treated with high caloric and protein foods and supplements. But when systematic reviews looked at existing trials, the conclusion was that increasing food intake and/or oral nutritional supplements does not change clinical outcomes, that is, disease status and survival, and they have a debatable effect on quality of life (Brown, 2002; Baldwin et al., 2012). This lack of evidence calls for new ways of approaching the complex issue of nutrition in advanced illness (Arends et al., 2017), which includes nutritional assessment of palliative care patients and nutritional training of all healthcare professionals. The first step to improving nutritional care is acknowledging that nutrition is everybody's responsibility.

Nutrigenomics and Epigenetics

A key number of nutrients working in combination can alter our cells' protein expression and metabolite production and, in some cases, switch certain of our genes on or off. Following these discoveries, a new branch of science, *nutrigenomics*, has emerged which studies the relationship between nutrition, genetics and health (Table 1.3). Our developing understanding of the effect environmental factors have at a cellular level has led to *epigenetics*, another new field of research

TABLE 1.3
New Definitions in Science

Nutrigenomics: a new science looking at the relationship between nutrition, genetics and health
Epigenetics: the study of mechanisms that cause changes in gene activity, without modifying the DNA sequence, which are maintained during cell division
Telomere: the end region of the chromosome that protects it from alteration during replication; its length controls how long cells live
Telomerase: the enzyme that sustains the length of telomere

which looks at the mechanisms that cause changes in gene activity, without modifying the DNA sequence, which are maintained after cell division. Epigenetics is attracting intense research activity around the world. Different environmental factors, such as a poor diet can initiate epigenetic changes: DNA methylation and histone modification. In turn, these translate into abnormal gene expression, which encourages the initiation and progression of cancer (Tollefsbol, 2009). Further research will help us understand better the impact of diet and behaviour on the development and progression of chronic diseases.

What makes the study of epigenetic changes so important and exciting is that they can be reversed with even simple lifestyle changes, including the right diet (Feinberg, 2008). For example, garlic, turmeric, broccoli, tomatoes and green tea contain a variety of active dietary photochemicals that influence the release of Nrf2 (nuclear factor erythroid-derived 2-related factor 2). Nrf2 is a "master gene" product that co-ordinates the activation of a number of antioxidant genes that maintain or restore the activity of normal cells and promote apoptosis of malignant cells (Gopalakrishnan and Tony Kong, 2008). The activation of Nrf2 by these nutrients promises to result in powerful beneficial effects that invite further study. This limited description, hopefully, provides an indication as to why some investigators think that epigenetics may, in the future, play a greater role in health and disease than genetics currently does. How this knowledge can help patients with advanced disease, needs to be tested.

The Gut Microbiome Revolution

The influence of gut microbes on various aspects of human health is the subject of many revolutionary research projects around the world. Clinicians are asked to find ways to support gut health, as it has become apparent that the trillions of gastrointestinal (GI) bacteria can interfere with the effectiveness of oncological treatments. Furthermore, gut bacteria have an effect on our immunity and have been linked to mood disorders such as anxiety and depression (Anderson et al., 2017). Palliative care patients can suffer from a variety of GI problems, including gut toxicity, as a consequence of cancer treatments. Healthcare professionals need to develop effective ways of diagnosing and managing these conditions, using nutritional and other therapeutic approaches (Andreyev, 2016).

CANCER SURVIVORS

Cancer survivors is a term encompassing all people who have had a diagnosis of cancer and have recovered from it following treatment or continue to live with residual or recurrent disease. In this group are included patients with metastatic and terminal cancer.

Cancer survivors have a number of medical and psychosocial needs that can benefit from palliative care. Studies have shown a survival benefit in people with cancer who are referred to palliative care services early in their disease trajectory (Temel et al., 2010) and, an improvement in their quality of life (Vanbutsele et al., 2018). Subsequently, it is increasingly common that cancer survivors are followed up by palliative care professionals who then need to be able to treat them if they present with symptoms due to the long-term and late effects of cancer treatment (Economou, 2014).

TABLE 1.4
World Cancer Research Fund/American Institute for Cancer Research Recommendations for Cancer Survivors

1. Avoid smoking and exposure to tobacco
2. Aim to be slim without being underweight
3. Maintain regular physical activity
4. Avoid drinks full of sugar
5. Include in your diet a variety of vegetables, fruits, whole grains and legumes
6. Reduce red meats and processed meats in your diet
7. Limit consumption of alcohol
8. Limit consumption of salt
9. Avoid use of supplements for protection against cancer

Source: Adapted from World Cancer Research Fund/American Institute for Cancer Research (AICR). 2007. *Food, Nutrition, and Physical Activity, and the Prevention of Cancer: A Global Perspective*. Washington, DC: AICR.

A number of programmes are being developed to assist cancer survivors in making the right lifestyle choices, as it is increasingly obvious that these can influence morbidity and mortality (Demark-Wahnefried and Jones, 2008). The World Cancer Research Fund (WCRF) and American Institute for Cancer Research (AICR) in their report on "Food, Nutrition, Physical Activity and the Prevention of Cancer" make a number of recommendations, based on current evidence, to promote cancer prevention through changes in diet (WCRF/AICR, 2007). They recommend cancer survivors also observe the same advice (Table 1.4). A further report by World Cancer Research Fund International (WCRFI) published recommendations for diet, nutrition and physical activity for breast cancer survivors (WCRFI/AICR, 2014). Cancer survivors and their carers would welcome advice from healthcare professionals about diet and physical activity (Beeken et al., 2016).

MULTI-STEP APPROACH TO NUTRITIONAL CARE

Patients who are referred to palliative care services have a range of cancer and non-cancer diagnoses and are at different stages along their disease trajectory. Some of them present with a longer prognosis of many months to a few years while others are at the end of their lives. This means that patients can have a wide spectrum of nutritional needs that change throughout the different stages of their illness.

Nutritional care is complex because of its many aspects: physical, emotional, social and cultural. This has been captured in the well-known phrase: "we are what we eat". A multi-step approach is required to recognize the patient's needs and what is needed to help them (Table 1.5).

Step 1: Assessment of nutritional status

Patients with palliative care needs are nutritionally "at-risk" for many reasons: disease factors, medication side effects, socio-economic reasons and other causes. The first step in the provision of nutritional care is to assess the patient's nutritional status and the factors that can influence nutrition, whether they are reversible and treatable or not. The nutrition

TABLE 1.5
Multi-Step Approach to Nutritional Care of Palliative Care Patients

- Step 1: Assessment of nutritional status
- Step 2: Development of a care plan
- Step 3: Recognition of changes in nutritional needs

TABLE 1.6
Professional Consensus Statement on Nutritional Care in Palliative Care Patients

1. Nutritional care
   - Is an essential aspect of palliative care
   - Needs to be individualized
   - May change for people at the end of life
   - Needs to be delivered safely and with compassion and dignity
   - Can have physical, social, cultural and emotional aspects
   - Is a matter for all palliative care professionals
2. All staff and volunteers should receive regular training on nutrition
3. Healthcare organisations are responsible for delivering nutritional care

Source: Adapted from the Food and Nutrition Group at Hospice UK. 2009. Professional consensus statement of nutritional care in palliative care patients. https://www.hospiceuk.org/what-we-offer/clinical-and-care-support/clinical-resources.

assessment should lead to an individualised nutritional care plan (Food and Nutrition Group at Hospice UK, 2009) (Table 1.6). As Lennard-Jones said two decades ago: "only when the assessment of every patient's nutritional status has become routine will the full benefits of nutrition treatment be realised" (Lennard-Jones, 1992).

A nutrition assessment tool called the Palliative Life-State and Nutrition Tool (PLANT) has been developed and piloted in the United Kingdom (Tsiompanou, 2017). The PLANT tool has been designed to take into account aspects of life-state, food and nutrition that are significant for palliative care patients. It highlights specific food and nutritional needs that can be translated into care plans.

Step 2: Development of a care plan

Nutritional treatment will vary considerably from patient to patient. A cachectic patient with oesophageal cancer and dysphagia needs a nutrition intervention, food consistency and diet distinct from that of a cachectic patient with lung cancer and no swallowing difficulties. An overweight patient with metastatic breast carcinoma and prognosis of months to years requires a different dietary approach to that of an overweight bedridden patient with a brain tumour and a prognosis of a few weeks. Furthermore, the needs of patients with end-stage dementia, amyotrophic lateral sclerosis, congestive heart failure, chronic obstructive pulmonary disease, chronic renal failure and chronic hepatic failure are also quite variable and complex.

Step 3: Recognition of changes in nutritional needs

Nutritional needs often change when the patient approaches the last days of their life. The primary focus of nutritional intervention can shift at this point towards maintenance of optimal quality of life and general support of patients and carers to help them recognise and accept this transition. Carers often say: "food and love" are the last precious gifts we can offer our loved one at the end of their life. Who are we to argue? Perhaps one could say that, at the end of life, food is not the only important aspect of care. The total comfort and peace of mind of the patient at this time is paramount and we can support carers to help "nourish" the dying person in holistic ways.

DIET OF PEOPLE IN ILLNESS SHOULD BE DIFFERENT TO THEIR DIET IN HEALTH

In his book *Ancient Medicine* (Αρχαία Ιητρική), Hippocrates traces the origins of dietetics and explains how cooking methods influenced human evolution (Tsiompanou and Marketos, 2013). Approximately 2,500 years ago he wrote how primitive people suffered many illnesses as a result of eating unprocessed raw foods, which led them to seek and discover cooking methods. It is remarkable that there was an appreciation, even millennia ago, that certain foods had harmful constituents (which we now call nutrients), which needed to be avoided or modified. The search/re-search for the impact of diet and lifestyle modification on people's health is what the ancients first called *medicine*. The practice of medicine developed as doctors observed that men in illness benefited from a diet that was different from that of healthy men.

Alteration of Diet in Palliative Care Patients

It is important for the public to recognize that dietary guidelines followed by healthy people could be inappropriate for ill people. This is equally applicable to palliative care patients. For example:

- The advice to have three meals a day and to consume a certain number of calories when healthy, would need to be modified to meet the needs of a cancer patient with anorexia-cachexia syndrome.
- Patients with advanced heart failure often need to follow fluid restrictions.
- Inability to digest certain foods secondary to gut problems can contribute to a multitude of symptoms. For example, people belonging to certain ethnic groups (Chinese, Japanese, Africans, Southern Europeans, Jewish) often become lactose intolerant as they grow older (Johnson, 1981). Others (up to 70% of the population) can develop temporary hypolactasia due to a variety of reasons (Matthews et al., 2005), while a few can become lactose intolerant after radiotherapy (Wedlake et al., 2008), GI infection or complex antibiotic treatment (Noble et al., 2002). Taking into account the underlying condition and temporarily (until the gut problems improve) changing the patient's diet and pharmacologic treatment to avoid foods, drugs and supplements that contain lactose, can make a huge difference to quality of life (Vaillancourt et al., 2009).
- A number of dietary challenges are common in patients with other advanced non-cancer diseases, such as dementia. This is particularly relevant to palliative care services, as in the last few years they have been looking after more patients with advanced dementia. People with dementia often need changes to their diet as their appetite changes, their ability to feed themselves is diminished and they experience swallowing difficulties. Such patients may benefit from increasing meal frequency, a texture-modified diet, assistance with feeding, flexibility with mealtimes and the use of nutritional supplements.

Nutritional Care at the End of Life

Nutritional care at the end of life calls for a sensible, informed and sensitive personalised approach. There is a prevailing opinion that it is too late to employ meaningful changes in diet when a person is approaching the end of their life. While this certainly is a time when the priority is in comfort and quality of life, it is also a time when we need to minimise any harm to the patient so that they are allowed to face their approaching end in peace. In a case review study (Tsiompanou et al., 2013), withdrawal of ANH in elderly patients who appeared to be dying and who were put on the Liverpool Care Pathway for the care of the dying (Ellershaw and Wilkinson, 2003) was followed by unexpected improvement in their symptoms and, in one case, survival of 10 months. Their improvement was thought to be a positive effect of the withdrawal of ANH which had contributed to the deterioration in the first place of these patients through overhydration and a degree of re-feeding syndrome.

In conclusion, giving the right nutrition and removing anxieties about food and fluid intake may not only give valuable relief and increased comfort for patients but may also provide some precious time. Healthcare professionals working in palliative care, when asked to express an opinion on a variety of complex psychosocial and ethical issues in relation to nutritional care and support at the end of life, need to use a flexible and compassionate approach to be reassuring and supportive for the patient and the relatives.

DEVELOPMENT OF SPECIALISTS: NEED FOR NUTRITION EDUCATION

In the United Kingdom, the Royal College of Nursing launched the Nutrition Now campaign in 2007 which stated that: "Nutrition and hydration are essential to care, as vital as medication and other types of treatment… it is the responsibility of the multidisciplinary team to ensure that patients have the right type of nutrition and hydration at the right time." This message is slowly spreading to reach all healthcare disciplines. As a result, there is a growth in interest from healthcare professionals who want to acquire a sufficient scientific and research background to appreciate the enormous advances in nutritional knowledge and be able to translate them into clinical practice.

Our current education system urgently needs to incorporate the new findings and include upgraded and expanded nutrition education for healthcare professionals. Palliative care centres need to become aware of the importance of providing advanced nutrition education and be encouraged to participate in research projects that will increase the understanding of numerous nutritional issues. A training programme is needed to provide palliative care professionals with the nutritional knowledge to help patients and carers. This will lead to a better experience for patients, as doctors, nurses, dieticians and other palliative care professionals who have an advanced understanding of nutrition will then care for them.

The vast amount of new data in nutrition means that it is difficult for the individual healthcare professional to find, assimilate and interpret all the information. Professionals would benefit from guidelines and recommendations to help them in their practice. We need specialists within palliative care with a particular interest and expertise on nutrition, capable of translating scientific findings into practical help and advice for patients and carers.

CONCLUSION

In the last few years the subject of nutrition has increasingly come to the forefront of patient care and media interest. Public, healthcare professionals and organisations are beginning to acknowledge the contribution of appropriate nutritional care and treatment in the therapeutic process. Research findings are beginning to influence our clinical practice. Nutritional medicine is becoming increasingly important in almost all areas of medicine driven largely by media doctors such as Michael Mosley and Rangan Chatterjee. In palliative care multidisciplinary teams, now we all need to give greater prominence in learning about nutrition research, lay aside professional prejudices and take an active approach in our practice to provide better patient care.

KEY FACTS

- Nutrition is a priority for patients and carers and needs to be individualized
- Nutrition is an important safety issue
- The field of nutrition is changing rapidly with new exciting knowledge needing to inform healthcare
- Palliative care patients have a multitude of reasons for poor nutrition
- Nutritional assessment is the first step to recognising the patient's needs
- Nutritional needs may change at the end of life
- All staff and volunteers should receive regular training on nutrition

SUMMARY POINTS

- Recent advances in scientific and nutritional knowledge have paved the way to a deeper understanding of the interaction between nutrition, health and disease.

- Diet affects our "internal environment" in profound ways.
- The study of the effect of micronutrients on cell and organ function has revealed their importance in improving symptom control.
- Cancer survivors have special nutritional considerations that palliative care professionals are often asked to address.
- Every palliative care patient needs a nutritional assessment and a nutritional care plan.
- The diet of people in illness should be different to their diet in health.
- The incorporation of advanced nutritional knowledge in palliative care practice will result in better patient care and experience.

LIST OF ABBREVIATIONS

ACS	Anorexia-Cachexia Syndrome
AICR	American Institute for Cancer Research
ANH	Artificial Nutrition and Hydration
GI	Gastrointestinal
Nrf2	Nuclear Factor (Erythroid-Derived 2)-Related Factor 2
PLANT	Palliative Life-State and Nutrition Tool
WCRF	World Cancer Research Fund
WCRFI	World Cancer Research Fund International

REFERENCES

Anderson, S.C., Cryan, J.F. and Dinan, T. 2017. The Psychobiotic Revolution: Mood, Food, and the New Science of the Gut. *National Geographic.*

Andreyev, H.J. 2016. GI consequences of cancer treatment. *Radiation Research* 185:341–8.

Arends, J., Baracos, V., Bertz, H., Bozzetti, F., Calder, P. C., Deutz, N.E.P., Erickson, N. et al. 2017. ESPEN expert group recommendations for action against cancer-related malnutrition. *Clinical Nutrition* 36:1187–96.

Athenaeus 1927–41. *The Deipnosophists* ed. and tr. C. B. Gulick. Cambridge, MA: Harvard University Press, 7 vols.

Baldwin, C., Spiro, A., Ahern, R. and Emery, P.W. 2012. Oral nutritional interventions in malnourished patients with cancer: A systematic review and meta-analysis. *Journal of the National Cancer Institute* 104:371–85.

Beeken, R.J., Williams, K., Wardle, J. and Croker, H. 2016. "What about diet?" A qualitative study of cancer survivors' views on diet and cancer and their sources of information. *European Journal of Cancer Care* 25:774–83.

Brown, J.K. 2002. A systematic review of the evidence on symptom management of cancer-related anorexia and cachexia. *Oncology Nursing Forum* 29:517–32.

Demark-Wahnefried, W. and Jones, L.W. 2008. Promoting a healthy lifestyle among cancer survivors. *Hematology/Oncology Clinics of North America* 22:319–42.

Economou, D. 2014. Palliative care needs of cancer survivors. *Seminars in Oncology Nursing* 30:262–7.

Ellershaw, J.E. and Wilkinson, S. (eds) 2003. *Care of the Dying: A Pathway to Excellence.* Oxford: Oxford University Press.

Feinberg, A.P. 2008. Epigenetics as the epicenter of modern medicine. *Journal of the American Medical Association* 299:1345–50.

Food and Nutrition Group at Hospice UK 2009. Professional consensus statement of nutritional care in palliative care patients. https://www.hospiceuk.org/what-we-offer/clinical-and-care-support/clinical-resources

Gopalakrishnan, A. and Tony Kong, A.N. 2008. Anticarcinogenesis by dietary photochemical: Cytoprotection by Nrf2 in normal cells and cytotoxicity by modulation of transcription factors NF-κB and AP-1 in abnormal cancer cells. *Food and Chemical Toxicology* 46:1257–70.

Johnson, J.D. 1981. The regional and ethnic distribution of lactose malabsorption. Adaptive and genetic hypotheses. In *Lactose digestion. Clinical and nutritional implications*, eds. D.M. Paige, and T.M. Bayless, 11–22. Baltimore, MD: John Hopkins University Press.

Lennard-Jones, J.E. (ed.) 1992. *A Positive Approach to Nutrition as Treatment*. London: King's Fund Centre.

Matthews, S.B., Wad, J.P., Roberts, A.G. and Campbell, A.K. 2005. Systemic lactose intolerance: A new perspective of an old problem. *Postgraduate Medical Journal* 81:167–73.

National Patient Safety Agency: Nutrition Factsheets 2009. 10 key characteristics of good nutritional care 01– Food and nutritional care is delivered safely. http://www.nrls.npsa.nhs.uk/resources/?entryid45=59865

Noble, S., Rawlinson, F. and Byrne, A. 2002. Acquired lactose intolerance: A seldom considered cause of diarrhoea in the palliative care setting. *Journal of Pain and Symptom Management* 23:449–50.

Temel, J.S., Greer J.A., Muzikansky, A., Gallagher, E.R., Admane, S., Jackson, V.A., Dahlin, C.M. et al. 2010. Early palliative care for patients with metastatic non-small cell lung cancer. *New England Journal of Medicine* 363:733–42.

Tollefsbol, T.O. 2009. Role of epigenetics in cancer. In *Cancer Epigenetics*, ed. O. Tollefsbol Trygve, 1–4. Boca Raton, FL: CRC Press.

Tsiompanou, E. 2017. P-117 PLANT: Palliative Life-State and Nutrition Tool© – A prototype tool. *BMJ Supportive and Palliative Care* 7:A51.

Tsiompanou, E., Lucas, C. and Stroud, M. 2013. Over-feeding and over-hydration in elderly medical patients – Lessons from the Liverpool Care Pathway. *Clinical Medicine* 13:248–51.

Tsiompanou, E. and Marketos, S.G. 2013. Hippocrates: Timeless still. *Journal of the Royal Society of Medicine* 106:288–92.

Vaillancourt, R., Siddiqui, R., Vadeboncoeur, C., Rattrap, M. and Lariviere, D. 2009. Treatment of medication intolerance with lactase in a complex palliative care patient. *Journal of Palliative Care* 25:142–4.

Vanbutsele, G., Pardon, K., Van Belle, S., Surmont, V., De Laat, M., Colan, R., Eecloo, K., Cocquyt, V., Geboes, K. and Delines, L. 2018. Effect of early and systematic integration of palliative care in patients with advanced cancer: A randomised controlled trial. *Lancet Oncology* 19(3):394–404.

Wedlake, L., Thomas, K., Cough, C. and Andreyev, H.J. 2008. Small bowel bacterial overgrowth and lactose intolerance during radical pelvic radiotherapy: An observational study. *European Journal of Cancer* 44:2212–7.

World Cancer Research Fund/American Institute for Cancer Research. 2007. *Food, Nutrition, and Physical Activity, and the Prevention of Cancer: A Global Perspective*. Washington, DC: AICR.

World Cancer Research Fund International/American Institute for Cancer Research Continuous Update Project Report. 2014. *Diet, Nutrition, Physical Activity, and Breast Cancer Survivors*. www.wcrf.org/sites/default/les/Breast-Cancer-Survivors-2014-Report.pdf

2 What Do We Mean by Palliative Care?

Catherine Walshe

CONTENTS

INTRODUCTION: WHY IS IT IMPORTANT TO DEFINE PALLIATIVE CARE?

Defining what we mean by a term is important. This enables clarity on issues such as the practice of palliative care, by whom, and to whom. However, defining terms in the area of palliative care seems challenging. There are three broad reasons for these difficulties:

1. The terms used have changed over time.
2. Our interpretations are value laden.
3. Defining palliative care itself seems difficult.

CHANGING TERMS AND THEIR USAGE

There is a plethora of terms in current and past usage used to refer to the care of people before and around the time of an anticipatable death. Terms such as *hospice care*, *palliative care*, *end-of-life care* and *supportive care* are in current usage, whereas terms such as *continuing care* and *terminal care* seem to have fallen out of favour.

Chronologically, hospice appears to be one of the earliest terms used. It is derived from the words "hospes" and "hospitium", which denoted not only a relationship between individuals, but also the place in which the relationship developed. Later, hospice, derived from these words, described a place of refuge for weary or sick travellers seeking rest on life's journey (Hawthorne and Yurkovich, 2004). Those building the earliest physical spaces for the provision of palliative care, primarily to cancer patients whose curative treatment was ended, adopted the term. The first "modern" hospice is identified as St. Christopher's Hospice, opened in the United Kingdom in 1967 (Clark, 2007). While in some countries, the term *hospice* is still used primarily to denote a building or physical space within which care is delivered, in other countries it describes more of an approach to care, such as home hospice provision in the United States.

The term *terminal care* was also in wide usage at the time the first "modern" hospices were being built, describing much of the care they provided. Terms started to change when the philosophies of care promoted by these hospices started to move into other settings. For example, the team at St. Thomas' hospital established in 1976 was called the "hospital support team for terminal care" (Clark, 2007), and the unit at the Royal Marsden Hospital (opened in 1964) was called the "Continuing Care Unit" (Hanks, 2008).

The term *palliative care* was coined by Balfour Mount around 1973 to describe a new programme in Canada, based on St. Christopher's hospice (Billings, 1998). In French the term *hospice* had negative connotations, and so he wished to use a different term when embracing the hospice philosophy of care and bringing the approach to a wider group of patients (Meghani, 2004). Palliative care rapidly became a widely adopted term, especially as it became the chosen term to describe medical care with the recognition of palliative medicine as a medical speciality in the United Kingdom and elsewhere (Doyle, 2005).

The literal, dictionary definition of palliation does not easily assist a clinical definition of care. *Palliate* is normally described as derived from the Latin palla (garment) and pallium, meaning "to cloak", seen as "covering up problems" (Billings, 1998). It is also suggested that the understanding could be from an Indo-European linguistic tradition, derived from "pelte" that means to shield. This has been related to palliative care as the shielding of patients from the assault of symptoms. Palliate has been described as a transitory verb, "to make disease less severe, without removing its cause" (Meghani, 2004).

End-of-life care started to be used in some areas in the 2000s, perhaps because palliative care had become associated for some with cancer care. In the United Kingdom particularly, it has become widely used, particularly strategically, as in the eponymous End-of-Life Care Strategy (Department of Health, 2008).

A term that appears to be increasing in popularity is *supportive care*. Supportive care definitions have focused more on treatment, and less on interdisciplinary care (Hui et al., 2013). However, as discussed in the following text, it is also increasingly used to avoid other terms that may be negatively perceived.

A major problem with definitions therefore seems to be the varied terms used to describe care around the time of an anticipatable death, and the way that the use of such terms has changed over time.

Value-Laden Interpretations

One possible explanation for the many terms used to describe care around the time of an anticipatable death is that some terms have or have acquired value-laden interpretations. While there are many identified barriers to referral to specialist palliative care, some appear to relate to concerns about maintaining hope, the communication challenges of discussing dying, and a reluctance to stop or change treatment (Fadul et al., 2009; Horlait et al., 2016). Participants in one trial identified initial perceptions of palliative care of death, hopelessness and dependency that provoked fear and avoidance. While understandings developed during the trial to incorporate ongoing care focused on quality of living, they still felt a different name was required to avoid stigma (Zimmermann et al., 2016). People exposed to palliative care services value prompt attention to concerns, and although in one study some were ambivalent about their current need for palliative care, no distress was reported as a consequence of the intervention (Hannon et al., 2017).

Studies identify that patients and professionals would prefer the name *supportive care* to *palliative care*, and that professionals would be more likely to refer patients (Boldt et al., 2006; Maciasz et al.,

2013; Rhondali et al., 2013; Hui et al., 2015). One service that tested a name change to *supportive care*, found a 41% increase in in-patient referrals, and a shorter duration to palliative or supportive care consultations in outpatient settings (Dalal et al., 2011).

Cherny (2009) argues that this is because there is dissonance between the defined meanings of terms such as *palliative care* (i.e., to improve quality of life of patients and families at all stages of a life-threatening illness) and the meaning derived from common association (i.e., care in the last days of life). Supportive care is more acceptable because although it is often used as a euphemism for palliative care it also has a wider, acceptable definition that includes toxicity minimisation and survivorship (Cherny, 2009).

It seems therefore that people are keen to use terms, which are interpreted by patients in more positive ways, which seems to explain some of the changes in terminology from, for example, *hospice care* to *palliative care*, and from *palliative care* to *supportive care*.

Defining Palliative Care Is Difficult

Defining what we mean by palliative care, or indeed any other term referring to care around the time of an anticipatable death, appears to be difficult because it is not a "neat" definition.

- Palliative care is not neatly delineated, as other specialities are, by reference to organs (such as the kidney and renal services), by reference to systems (such as the gastrointestinal system and gastroenterologists), or by reference to age (such as children and paediatricians) (Billings, 1998). While the term was initially associated with cancer services, developments in the definition have widened this focus (Sepúlveda et al., 2002).
- Palliative care is not limited to a particular healthcare setting. Palliative care's reference point is the patient, not the setting (Pastrana et al., 2008).
- Palliative care can be seen as a function (the direct provision of care to patients), a structure (such as a specialist palliative care service) or a philosophy of care (an underlying approach to care) (Pastrana et al., 2008; Van Mechelen et al., 2013).

These complexities mean that agreeing on a definition of palliative care is especially important so that confusion is avoided between healthcare professionals and patients about when, how, why and by whom such care should and could be provided.

CURRENT DEFINITIONS OF PALLIATIVE CARE AND ITS ASSOCIATED TERMS

Because of these complexities in definition, there are, and have been, a multiplicity of definitions. The first widely cited is the World Health Organisation's (WHO) constructed definition of palliative care:

> Palliative care is the active total care of patients whose disease is not responsive to curative treatment. Control of pain, of other symptoms, and of psychological, social and spiritual problems is paramount. The goal of palliative care is achievement of the best possible quality of life for patients and their families. Many aspects of palliative care are also applicable earlier in the course of the illness, in conjunction with anti-cancer treatment. (World Health Organisation Expert Committee, 1990)

This definition was not without its critics. Criticisms centred on some of the terms such as "active" and "total" (and whether this means other care is inactive or partial), and the use of euphemisms such as "not responsive to curative treatment" rather than a focus on death and dying. It was also argued that palliative care does not have a special claim on particular virtues such as quality of care, compassion etc. (Billings, 1998).

Following on from this, many definitions of palliative care and associated terms have been developed (Pastrana et al., 2008; Cramp and Bennett, 2013; Hui et al., 2013, 2014; Sigurdardottir et al., 2013; Van Mechelen et al., 2013; Hui, 2014; Mitchell et al., 2015). Some examples of current definitions of palliative care, supportive care and end-of-life care are displayed in Box 2.1, including the updated WHO definition of palliative care. These definitions appear to be most widely used, or represent definitions used in major policies or from significant national associations. It seems that many different international and national organisations have developed definitions of supportive and palliative care. These different definitions may lead to different interpretations of terms in different situations and settings, and mean that it is important to clarify meanings when communicating with others.

It appears from these definitions that they range from the broadest (supportive care) to the narrowest (terminal care), such that it could be argued that all terminal care is palliative care, but not all palliative care is terminal care. All palliative care could be described as supportive care, but

BOX 2.1 SELECTED CURRENT DEFINITIONS OF PALLIATIVE CARE, END-OF-LIFE CARE AND SUPPORTIVE CARE

World Health Organisation Definition of Palliative Care

Palliative care is an approach that improves the quality of life of patients and their families facing the problem associated with life-threatening illness, through the prevention and relief of suffering by means of early identification and impeccable assessment and treatment of pain and other problems, physical, psychosocial and spiritual. Palliative care:

- Provides relief from pain and other distressing symptoms
- Affirms life and regards dying as a normal process
- Intends neither to hasten or postpone death
- Integrates the psychological and spiritual aspects of patient care
- Offers a support system to help patients live as actively as possible until death
- Offers a support system to help the family cope during the patient's illness and in their own bereavement
- Uses a team approach to address the needs of patients and their families, including bereavement counselling, if indicated
- Will enhance quality of life, and may also positively influence the course of illness
- Is applicable early in the course of illness, in conjunction with other therapies that are intended to prolong life, such as chemotherapy or radiation therapy, and includes those investigations needed to better understand and manage distressing clinical complications

(Sepúlveda et al., 2002). Also available at http://www.who.int/cancer/palliative/definition/en/

European Association of Palliative Care Definition of Palliative Care

Palliative care is the active, total care of the patients whose disease is not responsive to curative treatment. Control of pain, of other symptoms, and of social, psychological and spiritual problems is paramount.

Palliative care is interdisciplinary in its approach and encompasses the patient, the family and the community in its scope. In a sense, palliative care is to offer the most basic concept of care – that of providing for the needs of the patient wherever he or she is cared for, either at home or in the hospital.

Palliative care affirms life and regards dying as a normal process; it neither hastens nor postpones death. It sets out to preserve the best possible quality of life until death.

Available at: http://www.eapcnet.eu/Themes/AbouttheEAPC/DefinitionandAims.aspx

New Zealand Definition of Palliative Care

Care for people of all ages with a life-limiting illness which aims to

1. Optimise an individual's quality of life until death by addressing the person's physical, psychosocial, spiritual and cultural need.
2. Support the individual's family, whānau, and other caregivers where needed, through the illness and after death.

Palliative care is provided according to an individual's need, and may be suitable whether death is days, weeks, months or occasionally even years away. It may be suitable sometimes when treatments are being given aimed at improving quantity of life. It should be available wherever the person may be. It should be provided by all heathcare professionals, supported where necessary, by specialist palliative care services. Palliative care should be provided in such a way as to meet the unique needs of individuals from particular communities or groups. These include Maori, children and young people, immigrants, refugees, and those in isolated communities.

New Zealand Ministry of Health, Cancer treatment working party (2007). Available at: http://www.health.govt.nz/our-work/life-stages/palliative-care/about-palliative-care

A U.S. Definition of Palliative Care

Palliative care means patient and family-centered care that optimizes quality of life by anticipating, preventing and treating suffering. Palliative care throughout the continuum of illness involves addressing physical, intellectual, emotional, social and spiritual needs and to facilitate patient autonomy, access to information and choice.

The following features characterise palliative care philosophy and delivery:

- Care is provided and services are coordinated by an interdisciplinary team.
- Patients, families, palliative and non-palliative healthcare providers collaborate and communicate about care needs.
- Services are available concurrently with or independent of curative or life-prolonging care.
- Patient's and family's hopes for peace and dignity are supported throughout the course of illness, during the dying process, and after death.

National Consensus Project for Quality Palliative Care (3rd Edition) (2013). Available at: https://www.nationalcoalitionhpc.org/wp-content/uploads/2017/04/NCP_Clinical_Practice_Guidelines_3rd_Edition.pdf

Terminal Care Definition

Terminal care is an important part of palliative care and usually refers to the management of patients during the last few days or weeks or even months of life from a point at which it becomes clear that the patient is in a progressive state of decline.

Source: National Council for Hospice and Specialist Palliative Care Services, 1995. Occasional paper 8. *Specialist Palliative care: A statement of definitions.* NCHSPC. London.

A Working Definition of End-of-Life Care

End-of-life care is care that: Helps all those with advanced, progressive, incurable illness to live as well as possible until they die. It enables the supportive and palliative care needs of both patient and family to be identified and met throughout the last phase of life and into bereavement. It includes management of pain and other symptoms and provision of psychological, social, spiritual and practical support.

Source: The End of Life Care Strategy (2008). Available at: https://www.gov.uk/government/publications/end-of-life-care-strategy-promoting-high-quality-care-for-adults-at-the-end-of-their-life

Definition of Supportive Care

Supportive care is the multi-disciplinary holistic care of patients with malignant and non-malignant chronic diseases and serious illness, and those that matter to them, to ensure the best possible quality of life. It extends as a right and necessity for all patients, is available throughout the course of the condition, concurrent to condition management and is given equal priority alongside diagnosis and treatment. It should be individualised, taking into account the patient's past life experiences, their current situation and personal goals.

Supportive care aims to

- Control the symptoms that occur as a result of the condition or its treatment and prevent complications thus allowing the individual to tolerate and benefit from active therapy more easily.
- Meet a patient's spiritual, practical, physical, social, psychological, sexual and cultural needs.
- Inform patient decision-making and optimise patient understanding in relation to the illness and its treatment.
- Enhance health professional–patient communication.
- Improve general physical and mental health.
- Optimise patient comfort and ease the physical burden of the condition thus in turn improving the ability to function and reducing the impact of disability.
- Help the patient and their family cope with their illness and the treatment of it.
- Empower the patient and their family as well as promoting self-help and user involvement thus enabling the individuals to draw upon their own strengths.

Supportive care may include the following, as needed:

- Issues of survivorship, palliation and bereavement
- Support groups
- Professional counselling and psychotherapy
- Rehabilitation
- Practical help
- Benefits advice
- Pharmacological and non-pharmacological interventions
- Nutritional support

Cramp, F. and M. I. Bennett. 2013. Development of a generic working definition of "supportive care." *BMJ Supportive and Palliative Care* 3:53–60.

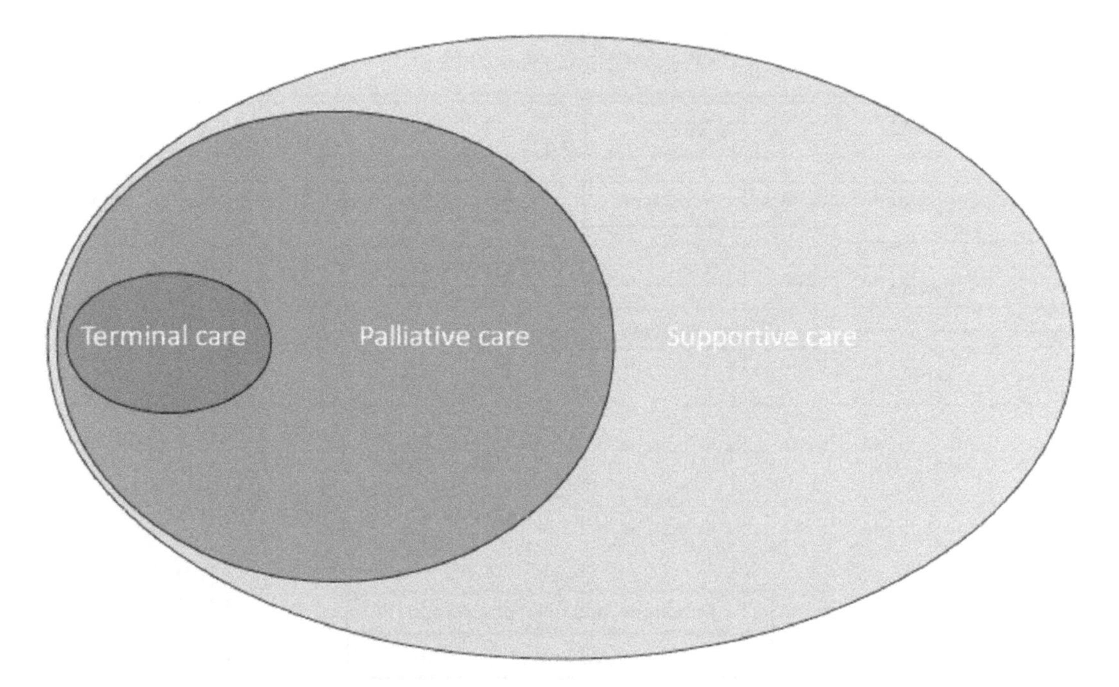

FIGURE 2.1 The interrelationship of supportive, palliative and terminal care.

not all supportive care is palliative care. The relationships between these definitions are represented in Figure 2.1.

KEY ELEMENTS OF DEFINITIONS

Even with the wide range of definitions of palliative, supportive, end-of-life and terminal care in Figure 2.1, it can be seen that there are certain key features common to many definitions. There have been attempts to capture the key elements of palliative care from these definitions and Figures 2.2 and 2.3 display two different, but clearly related, approaches to this work (Meghani, 2004; Pastrana et al., 2008). The major elements of the definitions identified in Figures 2.2 and 2.3 are explored in turn.

Patient Population

Palliative care was originally a disease-specific approach, associated very clearly with cancer care in the original WHO definition (World Health Organisation Expert Committee, 1990). Developments in the definition have widened this approach. Most definitions include reference to the target population for palliative care, with reference to issues such as "life-threatening illness" (Sepúlveda et al., 2002) or "disease not responsive to curative treatment" (EAPC). These mainly refer to attributes of the illness, such as its progressive, far-advanced, life-threatening and active nature (Pastrana et al., 2008). The widening of these definitions is argued to reflect demographic and technological advances such as an ageing population, longer life expectancies, changing illness trajectories, and advances in pharmacologic and surgical techniques (Meghani, 2004).

Timing

The timing of the provision of palliative care has always been problematic. This is related to the difficulties in defining the patient population, in prognostication and in generating referrals. While

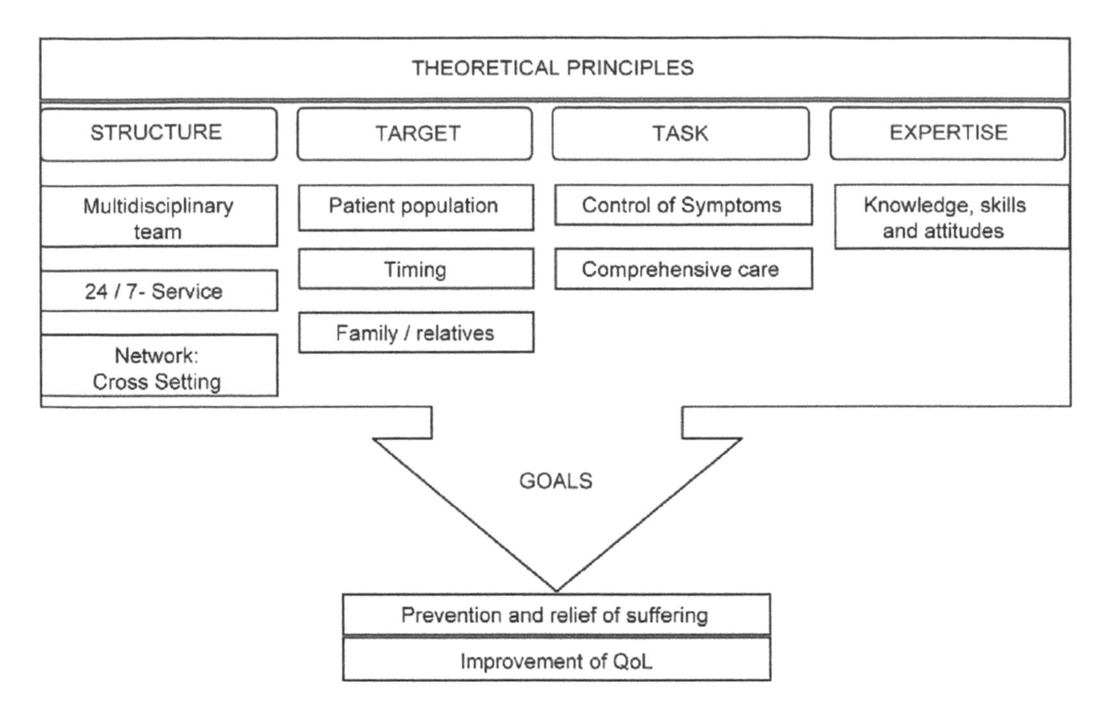

FIGURE 2.2 Key elements of palliative care. (From Pastrana, T. et al. 2008. *Palliative Medicine* 22(3):222–232.)

it is apparent that palliative care should be provided in the last days and weeks of life, there is now wide recognition that the principles of palliative care should be applied as early as possible in the course of any chronic, ultimately fatal illness (Sepúlveda et al., 2002).

Evidence is mounting that "early" palliative care can have benefits for patients and family carers. Reviews of trials of early palliative care have found evidence of benefit in areas such as quality

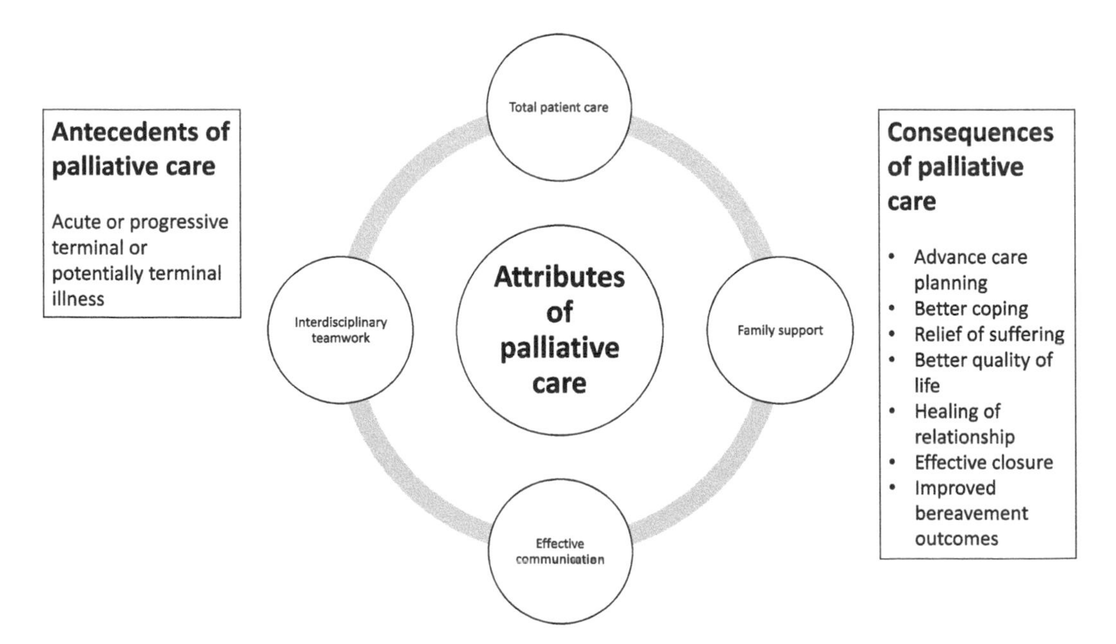

FIGURE 2.3 The antecedents, attributes and consequences of palliative care. (After Meghani, S. H. 2004. *Journal of Advanced Nursing* 46(2):152–161.)

of life, symptom control, care quality, hospital length of stay, cost and survival (Dalgaard et al., 2014; Davis et al., 2015; Tassinari et al., 2016; Haun et al., 2017). However, caution is needed as the effect sizes are small, and results are not consistent (Kavalieratos et al., 2016; Gaertner et al., 2017). Challenges include the difficulties of understanding what is meant by early palliative care in the context of diagnosis, disease progression, need and treatment, and for researchers and practitioners in determining models of care, and what "usual care" means in this context (Davis et al., 2015). Most studies investigate early palliative care for people with cancer, although trials in other diseases are underway (e.g., Weber et al., 2014).

Complex and extended disease courses also affect decisions on when palliative care could or should be offered. People with cancer were traditionally considered to follow a typical trajectory including a short decline before death, a trajectory considered to map well onto traditional models of palliative care provision (Lynn and Adamson, 2003; Murray et al., 2005). Those with organ failure or frailty had different trajectories described, which could be characterised by gradual decline, punctuated by episodes of acute deterioration and some recovery (Lynn and Adamson, 2003). A number of factors mean that such trajectories may have less utility in assisting understanding timing of referral to palliative care.

First, the trajectory for many with advanced disease is changing. Survival rates are improving for some cancers, associated with new and improved therapies (Siegel et al., 2012). This means increasing periods where people consider themselves to be living well with advanced disease (Lobb et al., 2015; Walshe et al., 2017). Referral to palliative care services may not be wanted or possible for all due to service limitations.

Second, the prevalence of multi-morbidity is increasing. The prevalence of multi-morbidity increases substantially with age, and is associated with a higher risk of death (Barnett et al., 2012; Nunes et al., 2016). These data challenge a single disease framework around which much healthcare is currently oriented.

Phase of illness or needs-based approaches to palliative care are gaining traction, which address these challenges. These imply a dynamic and responsive palliative care approach, depending on current need or phase of illness (Waller et al., 2008; Waller et al., 2013; Masso et al., 2015; Mather et al., 2017).

Holistic Care (Total, Active and Individualised Patient Care)

The "care" part of the definitions of palliative care is of fundamental significance to those who provide palliative care. The physical, emotional, social, cultural and spiritual needs of the patient are all considered important concerns in palliative care (Sepúlveda et al., 2002), and these emerge as a central attribute of the concept of palliative care (Meghani, 2004; Pastrana et al., 2008). Caring and compassionate attributes of health and social care professionals are recognised as important in the provision of excellent palliative care, and skills that require nurture and support (Grothe et al., 2015; Mills et al., 2017). Care and compassion is not necessarily seen as time consuming, requiring previous knowledge of the person, nor delivered by health and social care professionals (Hill et al., 2014; Jors et al., 2017).

Patient, Family and Carers (Support for the Family) and Bereavement Care

It is clear from the definitions of palliative care that both the patient and the family/informal carers are seen as recipients of care. Family are seen as part of the patient's social context, as decision makers, as part of the team, as team partners, and as part of the "unit of care" (Pastrana et al., 2008). Family/informal carers therefore have a double role; they are both recipients of care given by the palliative care team, but also frequently givers of care. This has the potential to lead to tension, but most agree that the primary focus of the palliative care team should be on the patient.

It is argued that the need for family support becomes more critical as patients progress towards the end of their lives on the palliative care continuum. It is at this stage that families can encounter many problems, and the provision of palliative care can offer opportunities to reconcile conflicts, heal relationships, provide counselling and commence bereavement support (Meghani, 2004).

Bereavement support is an integral part of palliative care, and it is argued that this should start early, assessing family/informal carers for the likelihood of adverse grief reactions, and then assessing and providing bereavement support after the death of the patient (Walshe, 1997).

Multi-Disciplinary/Multi-Professional Team

While it is argued that anyone can subscribe to the palliative philosophy of care, the organisation of specific palliative care services is often multi-disciplinary and multi-professional. The integration of palliative care at different levels of service provision, and as a framework for organising services is increasingly suggested, with some evidence of benefit (Higginson et al., 2014; Ewert et al., 2016; Siouta et al., 2016). Teams also need to consider how to work in new ways and new settings, given the demographic shifts to death out of hospital and into domestic and nursing home settings (Kalseth and Theisen, 2017; Bone et al., 2018). Teamwork can be challenging, however, with evidence that referrals, collaboration and care outcomes are influenced by issues with team functioning (Walshe et al., 2008; Firn et al., 2017).

Palliative care provision is, however, not restricted to health and social care professionals or family carers. The contribution of communities, the wider public and volunteers is increasingly recognised (Sallnow et al., 2016). Community networks are suggested as important, and requiring development attention (Abel et al., 2013; Burns et al., 2013; Leonard et al., 2013), and volunteers having an effect on care outcomes (Candy et al., 2015; Walshe et al., 2016).

KEY FACTS: DEFINITIONS

- *Patient population*: The target population for palliative care is wide, and not constrained by diagnosis.
- *Timing*: Palliative care should be provided as early as possible.
- *Holistic care*: Palliative care should encompass physical, psychological and social aspects.
- *Patient, family and carers*: Palliative care is not just focused on the patient, but on their family and informal carers and through to bereavement care.
- *Multi-disciplinary and multi-professional teams*: All professionals should provide palliative care, but some may have particular expertise in this area. Effective communication between professionals, patient and carer is essential.

SUMMARY POINTS

- It appears that palliative care is not straightforward to define because terms associated with care at the time of an anticipatable death have had a complex history, are value laden, and are not straightforward to define.
- This has led to multiple definitions of palliative care, although many have similar, core features.
- The key issue for most healthcare professionals is to be clear and unambiguous to those with whom we work about the definition of palliative care (or supportive, or end-of-life care, etc.) that is subscribed to.
- These definitions should be explicitly shared so that all those working with particular patients or within or across organizations are working with the same definition so there is clarity about role and function.
- Such clarity should both allow excellence in current care to those at the end of their lives, and stimulate debate about how to improve care in the future.

REFERENCES

Abel, J., T. Walter, L. B. Carey, J. Rosenberg, K. Noonan, D. Horsfall, R. Leonard, B. Rumbold, and D. Morris. 2013. Circles of care: Should community development redefine the practice of palliative care? *BMJ Supportive and Palliative Care* 3(4):383–388.

Barnett, K., S. W. Mercer, M. Norbury, G. Watt, S. Wyke, and B. Guthrie. 2012. Epidemiology of multimorbidity and implications for health care, research, and medical education: A cross-sectional study. *Lancet* 380(9836):37–43.

Billings, J. A. 1998. What is palliative care? *Journal of Palliative Medicine* 1(1):73–81.

Boldt, A. M., F. Yusuf, and B. P. Himelstein. 2006. Perceptions of the term palliative care. *Journal of Palliative Medicine* 9(5):1128–1136.

Bone, A. E., B. Gomes, S. N. Etkind, J. Verne, F. E. M. Murtagh, C. J. Evans, and I. J. Higginson. 2018. What is the impact of population ageing on the future provision of end-of-life care? Population-based projections of place of death. *Palliative Medicine* 36.

Burns, C. M., A. P. Abernethy, E. Dal Grande, and D. C. Currow. 2013. Uncovering an invisible network of direct caregivers at the end of life: A population study. *Palliative Medicine* 27(7):608–615.

Candy, B., R. France, J. Low, and L. Sampson. 2015. Does involving volunteers in the provision of palliative care make a difference to patient and family wellbeing? A systematic review of quantitative and qualitative evidence. *International Journal of Nursing Studies* 52(3):756–768.

Cherny, N. 2009. Stigma associated with "palliative care." Getting around it or getting over it. *Cancer* 115(1808):1812.

Clark, D. 2007. From margins to centre: A review of the history of palliative care in cancer. *Lancet Oncology* 8(5):430–438.

Cramp, F., and M. I. Bennett. 2013. Development of a generic working definition of "supportive care." *BMJ Supportive and Palliative Care* 3(1):53–60.

Dalal, S., S. Palla, D. Hui, L. Nguyen, R. Chacko, Z. Li, N. Fadul et al. 2011. Association between a name change from palliative to supportive care and the timing of patient referrals at a comprehensive cancer center. *Oncologist* 16(1):105–111.

Dalgaard, K. M., H. Bergenholtz, M. E. Nielsen, and H. Timm. 2014. Early integration of palliative care in hospitals: A systematic review on methods, barriers, and outcome. *Palliative and Supportive Care* 12(6):495–513.

Davis, M. P., J. S. Temel, T. Balboni, and P. Glare. 2015. A review of the trials which examine early integration of outpatient and home palliative care for patients with serious illnesses. *Annals of Palliative Medicine* 4(3):99–121.

Department of Health. 2008. End of life care strategy. Promoting high quality care for all adults at the end of life. Gov.UK.

Doyle, D. 2005. Palliative medicine: The first 18 years of a new sub-speciality of General Medicine. *Journal of the Royal College of Physicians of Edinburgh* 35:199–205.

Ewert, B., F. Hodiamont, J. van Wijngaarden, S. Payne, M. Groot, J. Hasselaar, J. Menten, and L. Radbruch. 2016. Building a taxonomy of integrated palliative care initiatives: Results from a focus group. *BMJ Supportive and Palliative Care* 6(1):14–20.

Fadul, N., A. Elasayem, L. Palmer, E. Del Fabbro, K. Swint, Z. Li, V. Poulter, and E. Bruera. 2009. Supportive versus palliative care: What's in a name. *Cancer* May 1:2013–2021.

Firn, J., N. Preston, and C. Walshe. 2017. Ward social workers' views of what facilitates or hinders collaboration with specialist palliative care team social workers: A grounded theory. *BMC Palliative Care* 17(1):7.

Gaertner, J., W. Siemens, J. J. Meerpohl, G. Antes, C. Meffert, C. Xander, S. Stock, D. Mueller, G. Schwarzer, and G. Becker. 2017. Effect of specialist palliative care services on quality of life in adults with advanced incurable illness in hospital, hospice, or community settings: systematic review and meta-analysis. *BMJ* 357:j2925.

Grothe, A., S. Biong, and E. K. Grov. 2015. Acting with dedication and expertise: Relatives' experience of nurses' provision of care in a palliative unit. *Palliative and Supportive Care* 13(6):1547–1558.

Hanks, G. 2008. Palliative care: Careless use of language undermines our identity. *Palliative Medicine* 22:109–110.

Hannon, B., N. Swami, G. Rodin, A. Pope, and C. Zimmermann. 2017. Experiences of patients and caregivers with early palliative care: A qualitative study. *Palliative Medicine* 31(1):72–81.

Haun, M. W., S. Estel, G. Rucker, H. C. Friederich, M. Villalobos, M. Thomas, and M. Hartmann. 2017. Early palliative care for adults with advanced cancer. *Cochrane Database of Systematic Reviews* 6:CD011129.

Hawthorne, D. L. and N. J. Yurkovich. 2004. Hope at the end of life: Making a case for hospice. *Palliative and Supportive Care* 2(4):415–417.

Higginson, I. J., C. Bausewein, C. C. Reilly, W. Gao, M. Gysels, M. Dzingina, P. McCrone, S. Booth, C. J. Jolley, and J. Moxham. 2014. An integrated palliative and respiratory care service for patients with advanced disease and refractory breathlessness: A randomised controlled trial. *Lancet Respiratory Medicine* 2(12):979–987.

Hill, H. C., J. Paley, and L. Forbat. 2014. Observations of professional–patient relationships: A mixed-methods study exploring whether familiarity is a condition for nurses' provision of psychosocial support. *Palliative Medicine* 28(3):256–263.

Horlait, M., K. Chambaere, K. Pardon, L. Deliens, and S. Van Belle. 2016. What are the barriers faced by medical oncologists in initiating discussion of palliative care? A qualitative study in Flanders, Belgium. *Supportive Care in Cancer* 24(9):3873–3881.

Hui, D. 2014. Definition of supportive care: Does the semantic matter? *Current Opinion in Oncology* 26(4):372–379.

Hui, D., M. De La Cruz, M. Mori, H. A. Parsons, J. H. Kwon, I. Torres-Vigil, S. H. Kim et al. 2013. Concepts and definitions for "supportive care," "best supportive care," "palliative care," and "hospice care" in the published literature, dictionaries, and textbooks. *Supportive Care in Cancer* 21(3):659–685.

Hui, D., Z. Nooruddin, N. Didwaniya, R. Dev, M. De La Cruz, S. H. Kim, J. H. Kwon, R. Hutchins, C. Liem, and E. Bruera. 2014. Concepts and definitions for "actively dying," "end of life," "terminally ill," "terminal care," and "transition of care": A systematic review. *Journal of Pain and Symptom Management* 47(1):77–89.

Hui, D., M. Park, D. Liu, A. Reddy, S. Dalal, and E. Bruera. 2015. Attitudes and beliefs toward supportive and palliative care referral among hematologic and solid tumor oncology specialists. *Oncologist* 20(11):1326–1332.

Jors, K., S. Tietgen, C. Xander, F. Momm, and G. Becker. 2017. Tidying rooms and tending hearts: An explorative, mixed-methods study of hospital cleaning staff's experiences with seriously ill and dying patients. *Palliative Medicine* 31(1):63–71.

Kalseth, J. and O. M. Theisen. 2017. Trends in place of death: The role of demographic and epidemiological shifts in end-of-life care policy. *Palliative Medicine* 31(10):964–974.

Kavalieratos, D., J. Corbelli, D. Zhang, J. N. Dionne-Odom, N. C. Ernecoff, J. Hanmer, Z. P. Hoydich et al. 2016. Association between palliative care and patient and caregiver outcomes: A systematic review and meta-analysis. *JAMA* 316(20):2104–2114.

Leonard, R., D. Horsfall, and K. Noonan. 2013. Identifying changes in the support networks of end-of-life carers using social network analysis. *BMJ Supportive and Palliative Care* 5(2):153–159.

Lobb, E. A., J. Lacey, J. Kearsley, W. Liauw, L. White, and A. Hosie. 2015. Living with advanced cancer and an uncertain disease trajectory: An emerging patient population in palliative care? *BMJ Supportive and Palliative Care* 5(4):352–357.

Lynn, J. and D. M. Adamson. 2003. *Living Well at the End of Life. Adapting Healthcare to Serious Chronic Illness in Old Age*. Santa Monica, CA: Rand.

Maciasz, R. M., R. M. Arnold, E. Chu, S. Y. Park, D. B. White, L. B. Vater, and Y. Schenker. 2013. Does it matter what you call it? A randomized trial of language used to describe palliative care services. *Supportive Care in Cancer* 21(12):3411–3419.

Masso, M., S. F. Allingham, M. Banfield, C. E. Johnson, T. Pidgeon, P. Yates, and K. Eagar. 2015. Palliative care phase: Inter-rater reliability and acceptability in a national study. *Palliative Medicine* 29(1):22–30.

Mather, H., P. Guo, A. Firth, J. M. Davies, N. Sykes, A. Landon, and F. E. Murtagh. 2017. Phase of illness in palliative care: Cross-sectional analysis of clinical data from community, hospital and hospice patients. *Palliative Medicine* 32(2):404–412.

Meghani, S. H. 2004. A concept analysis of palliative care in the United States. *Journal of Advanced Nursing* 46(2):152–161.

Mills, J., T. Wand, and J. A. Fraser. 2017. Palliative care professionals' care and compassion for self and others: A narrative review. *International Journal of Palliative Nursing* 23(5):219–229.

Mitchell, H., S. Noble, I. Finlay, and A. Nelson. 2015. Defining the palliative care patient: Its challenges and implications for service delivery. *BMJ Supportive and Palliative Care* 5(4):328–334.

Murray, S. A., M. Kendall, K. Boyd, and F. Sheldon. 2005. Illness trajectories and palliative care. *British Medical Journal* 330:1107–1111.

Nunes, B. P., T. R. Flores, G. I. Mielke, E. Thume, and L. A. Facchini. 2016. Multimorbidity and mortality in older adults: A systematic review and meta-analysis. *Archives of Gerontology and Geriatrics* 67:130–138.

Pastrana, T., S. Junger, C. Ostgathe, F. Elsner, and L. Radbruch. 2008. A matter of definition—Key elements identified in a discourse analysis of definitions of palliative care. *Palliative Medicine* 22(3):222–232.

Rhondali, W., S. Burt, E. Wittenberg-Lyles, E. Bruera, and S. Dalal. 2013. Medical oncologists' perception of palliative care programs and the impact of name change to supportive care on communication with patients during the referral process. A qualitative study. *Palliative and Supportive Care* 11(5):397–404.

Sallnow, L., F. Khan, N. Uddin, and A. Kellehear. 2016. The impact of a new public health approach to end-of-life care: A systematic review. *Palliative Medicine* 30(3):200–211.

Sepúlveda, C., A. Marlin, T. Yoshida, and A. Ullrich. 2002. Palliative care: The World Health Organisation's global perspective. *Journal of Pain and Symptom Management* 24(2):91.

Siegel, R., C. DeSantis, K. Virgo, K. Stein, A. Mariotto, T. Smith, D. Cooper et al. 2012. Cancer treatment and survivorship statistics, 2012. *CA: A Cancer Journal for Clinicians* 62(4):220–241.

Sigurdardottir, K. R., L. Oldervoll, M. J. Hjermstad, S. Kaasa, A. K. Knudsen, E. T. Løhre, J. H. Loge, and D. F. Haugen. 2013. How are palliative care cancer populations characterized in randomized controlled trials? A literature review. *Journal of Pain and Symptom Management* 47(5):906–914.e17.

Siouta, N., K. Van Beek, M. E. van der Eerden, N. Preston, J. G. Hasselaar, S. Hughes, E. Garralda et al. 2016. Integrated palliative care in Europe: A qualitative systematic literature review of empirically-tested models in cancer and chronic disease. *BMC Palliative Care* 15:56.

Tassinari, D., F. Drudi, M. C. Monterubbianesi, L. Stocchi, I. Ferioli, A. Marzaloni, E. Tamburini, and S. Sartori. 2016. Early palliative care in advanced oncologic and non-oncologic chronic diseases: A systematic review of literature. *Reviews on Recent Clinical Trials* 11(1):63–71.

Van Mechelen, W., B. Aertgeerts, K. De Ceulaer, B. Thoonsen, M. Vermandere, F. Warmenhoven, E. Van Rijswijk, and J. De Lepeleire. 2013. Defining the palliative care patient: A systematic review. *Palliative Medicine* 27(3):197–208.

Waller, A., A. Girgis, D. Currow, and C. Lecathelinais. 2008. Development of the palliative care needs assessment tool (PC-NAT) for use by multi-disciplinary health professionals. *Palliative Medicine* 22(8):956–964.

Waller, A., A. Girgis, P. M. Davidson, P. J. Newton, C. Lecathelinais, P. S. Macdonald, C. S. Hayward, and D. C. Currow. 2013. Facilitating needs-based support and palliative care for people with chronic heart failure: Preliminary evidence for the acceptability, inter-rater reliability, and validity of a needs assessment tool. *Journal of Pain and Symptom Management* 45(5):912–925.

Walshe, C. 1997. Whom to help? An exploration of the assessment of grief. *International Journal of Palliative Nursing* 3:132–137.

Walshe, C., C. Chew-Graham, C. Todd, and A. Caress. 2008. What influences referrals within community palliative care services? A qualitative case study. *Social Science and Medicine* 67(1):137–146.

Walshe, C., D. Roberts, L. Appleton, L. Calman, P. Large, M. Lloyd Williams, and G. Grande. 2017. Coping well with advanced cancer: A serial qualitative interview study with patients and family carers. *PLOS ONE* 12(1):e0169071.

Walshe, C., S. Dodd, M. Hill, N. Ockenden, S. Payne, N. Preston, and G. P. Algorta. 2016. How effective are volunteers at supporting people in their last year of life? A pragmatic randomised wait-list trial in palliative care (ELSA). *BMC Medicine* 14(1):203.

Weber, C., J. Stirnemann, F. R. Herrmann, S. Pautex, and J. P. Janssens. 2014. Can early introduction of specialized palliative care limit intensive care, emergency and hospital admissions in patients with severe and very severe COPD? A randomized study. *BMC Palliative Care* 13:47.

World Health Organisation Expert Committee. 1990. Cancer Pain Relief and Palliative Care Technical Report Series. No. 804. Geneva, Switzerland.

Zimmermann, C., N. Swami, M. Krzyzanowska, N. Leighl, A. Rydall, G. Rodin, I. Tannock, and B. Hannon. 2016. Perceptions of palliative care among patients with advanced cancer and their caregivers. *CMAJ* 188(10):E217–E227.

3 Religion, Culture and End-of-Life Issues

Hans-Henrik Bülow

CONTENTS

INTRODUCTION

This chapter presents the rules and points of view of the major religions in the world regarding end-of-life decisions. Many of the references are from intensive care unit (ICU) studies, because that branch of medical science, frequently deals with the ethics of withholding or withdrawing life-sustaining therapy, alleviation of pain, treatment of patients in a persistent vegetative state and whether further therapy will be futile.

This review is an update of a paper from intensive care medicine with a considerably larger list of references than those given here (Bülow et al. 2008). Table 3.1 summarizes the various religions' attitudes and rulings with regard to end-of-life decisions, but not all religions have a ruling/point of view on all of the above-mentioned issues.

DEMOGRAPHIC CHALLENGES

Key facts of major demographic changes in the Western world

- The three major religions of the world are Christianity 2.4 billion, Muslims 1.8 billion and Hinduism 1.15 billion.
- Islam (Muslims) is the religion that presently is expanding most from its original areas into a worldwide presence, constituting a constantly growing, larger proportion in many countries.

TABLE 3.1
The Various Religions' View on End-of-Life Decisions

	Withhold	Withdraw	Withdraw Artificial Nutrition	Double Effect[a]	Euthanasia
Catholics	Yes	Yes	No	Yes	No
Protestants	Yes	Yes	Yes	Yes	Some
Greek Orthodox	No	No	No	No[b]	No
Muslims	Yes	Yes	No	Yes	No
Orthodox Judiasm	Yes	No	No	Yes	No
Buddhism	Yes	Yes	Yes	Yes	No
Hinduism and Sikhism	Yes	Yes	?	?	Some
Taoism	Most	Most	?	?	?
Confucianism	No	No	?	?	No

Source: With kind permission from **Springer Science+Business Media**: *Intensive Care Med*, The world's major religions' point of view on end-of-life decisions in the intensive care unit, 34, 2008, 423–30, Bülow HH, Sprung CL, Reinhart K, Prayag S, Du B, Armaganidis A, Abroug F, Levy MM.

Note: Shows which end-of-life decisions and acts are allowed by the world's major religions. Question marks show that the religion has no of.cial stance on that question.

[a] Double effect. (See Table 3.2.)

[b] Alleviation of pain is allowable, if it will in no way lead to the patient's death.

Healthcare systems have to acknowledge and cope with patients and physicians from many ethnic and religious groups, because the globalization of the world has meant that few countries now consist of homogeneous religious and cultural entities. The challenge in the forthcoming years is that patients and medical teams with different religious, cultural and ethical backgrounds adopt different approaches, even within the same religion (Daar and Khitamy 2001; Pauls and Hutchinson 2002; Sprung et al. 2007).

Islam is *the* example of a worldwide expanding religion with 1.8 billion Muslims (24% of the world's population). About 31% of all Muslims are of South Asian origin – the rest is worldwide (Wikepidea 2017). There are approximately 44 million Muslims in Europe and the prediction is that by 2050, one in five Europeans will likely be Muslim. Likewise, North America is changing. In the United States Hispanics in 2015 represented 17.6% of the population, compared to 6% in 1980 (http://www.pewresearch.org 2017). In Ontario, Canada, the number of Muslims increased 142% from 1991 to 2001 and the number of Sikh increased 110% while the Christian community only increased 3%.

Only one religious group is not expanding globally. At the end of World War II there were 800,000 Jews living in the Arabic countries – where they have been present for more than 2000 years. Today they are still in small numbers present in Tunisia and Morocco, but they have been expelled from most other countries on the Arabic peninsula – constituting a few thousand Jews among 280 million Arabs. This is in striking contrast to Israel, where in 1948 lived less than 200,000 Arabs – a population who has now grown to 1 million (20% of the Israel population) (Ziadeh 2017).

THE VARIOUS RELIGIONS

Key religious facts on eight major religions of the world

- Christian, Muslim, Greek orthodox and Hebrew points of view are based on holy scriptures, whereas universal scriptures in Far Eastern religions are not available.
- Almost all religions take the point of view, that patients should not suffer and that physicians should alleviate suffering if possible.

TABLE 3.2
The Doctrine of Double Effect

- Definition: Nothing hinders one act from having two effects, only one of which is intended, while the other is beside the intention.
- In this context: to relieve pain and suffering with the unintended side effect, that the medication can lead to death.

A variety of substantive medical and ethical judgments provide the justification:

- The patient is terminally ill
- There is an urgent need to relieve pain and suffering
- Death is imminent
- The patient and/or the patient's proxy consents

Source: McIntyre A, 2009. Doctrine of Double Effect. In *The Stanford Encyclopedia of Philosophy*. ed. Edward N. Zalta.
Note: Explains the term "double effect" where provision of pain relief may lead to a somewhat hastened death and the table also explains under which circumstances such an act is acceptable/allowed.

- There are important differences in patient autonomy among the various religions – but these differences are more based on culture than religious rulings.

Christianity

Christianity encompasses such diverse groups as Mormons, Jehovah's Witnesses, Lutherans, Roman Catholics, and Orthodox Christians.

Roman Catholic Perspective

The Roman Catholic Church's official attitude was published in 1997 during the reign of Pope John Paul II (Cathechismus Catholicae Ecclesia 1997). If futile therapy is burdensome or disproportionate to the expected outcome, then withholding or withdrawing is allowed. Despite allowing withdrawal of futile therapy, Pope John Paul II shortly before his death, expressed a firm stand against withdrawing artificial nutrition from patients in a persistent vegetative state – a statement that has raised controversy (Shannon 2006).

In 1980 "Declaration on Euthanasia" allowed alleviation of pain in the dying, even with life shortening as a non-intended side effect, also known as "the double effect" (McIntyre 2009) (Table 3.2), but active euthanasia is never allowed and palliative care is to be offered (Cathechismus Catholicae Ecclesia 1997).

Protestantism

Most Protestants will, if there is little hope of recovery, understand and accept the withholding or withdrawal of therapy (Pauls and Hutchinson 2002). However, there is diversity within Protestantism on the question of euthanasia. The Evangelical Lutheran church in Germany has developed advance directives for end-of-life choices but rejects active euthanasia (May 2003), whereas theologians in the reformed tradition, for example, in the Netherlands defend active euthanasia.

Greek Orthodox

The Greek Orthodox Church has no position on end-of-life decisions, since the task of Christians is to pray and not to decide about life and death. The Greek Orthodox Church does not allow human decisions on such matters, and condemns as unethical every medical act, which does not contribute to the prolongation of life. The bioethics committee of the Church of Greece has stated: "There is always the possibility of an erroneous medical appraisal or of an unforeseen outcome of the disease, or even a miracle" (The Holy Synod 2000). Therefore, it is not surprising that the withholding or withdrawing of artificial nutrition is not allowable even if there is no prospect of recovery.

The church also states that should a fully conscious patient request an omission of treatment (that might save him/her) it is the moral obligation of the physician to try persuading him/her to consent to that treatment.

Alleviation of pain is allowable only if the medication with certainty does not to lead to death. This is somewhat surprising, since "euthanasia" is actually the Greek word for "good death" which is defined as "a peaceful death with dignity and without pain."

The actual international meaning of "active euthanasia" is perceived as "mercy killing" and is under no circumstances allowed by the Greek Church.

Judaism

There are three Jewish denominations: reform, conservative and religious orthodox.

The Jewish legal system (*Halacha)* was developed from the Bible (Tanach), Talmud and rabbinic responsa (Steinberg and Sprung 2006). Israeli law was updated in 2006 in order to balance between the sanctity of life and the principle of autonomy. Withdrawing a continuous life-sustaining therapy is still not allowed, but withholding further treatment is allowed as part of the dying process, if it is an intermittent life-sustaining treatment – and if it was the clear wish of the patient (Steinberg and Sprung 2006). This is based on the assumption that each unit of treatment is an independent and new decision; hence it is permissible to withhold it. Thereby you can withhold chemotherapy or dialysis, even after initiation, because such treatment is viewed as omitting the next treatment rather than committing an act of withdrawal.

Food and fluid are regarded as basic needs and not treatment. Withholding food and fluid from a dying patient (or patients with other disorders) is therefore prohibited and regarded as a form of euthanasia. If a dying patient is competent and refuses treatment, including food and fluids, he/she should be encouraged to change his/her mind regarding food and fluid, but should not be forced against his/her wishes (Steinberg and Sprung 2006). The situation changes however, when the patient approaches the final days of life, when food and even fluids may cause suffering and complications. In such an event, it is permissible to withhold food and fluid if this was the patient's expressed wish.

Based on the moral requirement to alleviate pain and suffering, the law and *Halacha* require providing palliative care to the patient and to his/her family. Treatments include palliative therapy that might unintentionally shorten life, based on the principle of double effect (Steinberg and Sprung 2006; McIntyre 2009).

However, active euthanasia or physician-assisted suicide is prohibited even at the patients' request (Steinberg and Sprung 2006).

Islam

Islamic bioethic is an extension of Shariah (Islamic law) based on the Qur'an (the holy book of all Muslims) and the Sunna (Islamic law based on the Prophet Muhammad's words and acts) (Daar and Khitamy 2001), and the primary goal is: "*la darar wa la dirar*" (no harm and no harassment).

For Muslims, premature death should be prevented, but not at any cost, and treatments can be withheld or withdrawn in terminally ill Muslim patients when the physicians are certain about the inevitability of death, and that treatment *in no way* will improve the condition or quality of life (Ebrahim 2000). The intention must never be to hasten death, only to abstain from overzealous treatment.

According to Islamic faith, it would be a crime to withdraw basic nutrition (Ebrahim 2000; da Costa et al. 2002) because such a withdrawal would in effect starve the patient to death.

The Qur'an states that "Allah does not tax any soul beyond that which he can bear" and pain and suffering is a "*kaffarah*" (expiation) for one's sins. However, relieving a patient with painkillers or a sedative drug is allowed even if death is hastened (double effect) (McIntyre 2009), if death was definitely not intended by the physician (da Costa et al. 2002).

The two major branches of Islamic faith, the Shia and the Sunni branches, may differ somewhat, but not fundamentally in bioethical rulings. Nevertheless, the majority of Islamic communities will seek advice from their own religious scholars because the Islamic faith is not monolithic but rather a diversity of opinions (Daar and Khitamy 2001).

The Qur'an emphasizes that "it is the sole prerogative of Allah to bestow life and to cause death" and consequently euthanasia is not allowable (Ebrahim 2000).

Hindu and Sikh

Hindu and Sikh religions are different, but both are duty based rather than rights based, and they both believe in *karma*, a causal law where all acts and human thoughts have consequences, good *karma* leads to a good rebirth and vice versa. Since Hindu religion does not have a single central authority to secure enforcement in Hinduism (Desai 1988), diverse interpretations, opinions and followings are possible.

Hindus and Sikhs do not die – death is merely a passage to a new life, but untimely death is seriously mourned (Desai 1988). The way you die is important. A good death is when you are old, have said your goodbyes and all duties are settled. Bad death is violent, premature and in the wrong place (not at home or at the river of Ganges).

A do-not-resuscitate order is usually accepted or desired because death should be peaceful (Desai 1988).

There is almost no teaching in Indian medical schools on palliative care and management of death.

The Indian Penal Code from 1860 British India prohibits euthanasia, but there is a long-standing tradition for suicide in certain defined circumstances – exemplified by the rule, that a terminally ill person may hasten death – as a spiritual purification and to ensure no signs of bad death (faeces, vomit or urine).

Confucianism and Taoism

Bioethics does not formally exist within traditional Chinese culture. The predominant religion in the elderly Chinese population is Buddhism/Taoism, whereas almost 60% of the younger generation claims having no religion, because, Confucianism is not generally considered as a religion by most Chinese people. The moral perspective is primarily Confucianism but also Taoism and Buddhism (Bowman and Hui 2000). Consequently, with this mixture of different religions and philosophies in one population, very diverse opinions and dilemmas can be encountered.

According to Confucian teaching, death is good if one has fulfilled one's moral duties in life, and resistance to accept terminal illness or insisting on futile treatment may reflect the patient's perception of unfinished business (Bowman and Hui 2000).

Taoism is both philosophical and religious. In philosophical Taoism acceptance is the only appropriate response when facing death and artificial measures contradict the natural events. In religious Taoism death may lead to an afterlife in torture in endless hell – where a Taoist might cling to any means of extending life to postpone that possibility (Bowman and Hui 2000).

One thing is common in Chinese culture: The maintenance of hope is very important in the care of the dying, as hope prevents suffering by avoiding despair. Face-to-face interviews with 40 Chinese seniors 65 years of age or older showed that all respondents rejected advance directives (Bowman and Singer 2001). This is problematic seen from a Western (autonomous) point of view because it prohibits the physicians from discussing death in much detail with the patient.

The Chinese are more likely to prefer family-centred decision-making than other racial or ethnic groups. For example, do-not-resuscitate orders in dying Chinese cancer patients were seldom signed by the patient personally (Liu et al. 1999). Moreover, even if a Chinese patient is resigned to death, the children may strongly advocate for (even) futile therapy, because filial piety can only be shown when a parent is alive – and accepting impending death is equalled with removing the opportunity to show piety (Bowman and Hui 2000). Some Chinese patients may think differently. A study in Taiwan showed that cancer patients strongly proclaimed their superior rights to be informed about their disease before their family was informed (Tang et al. 2006).

Euthanasia is illegal in Hong Kong and on mainland China. The first reported case of euthanasia in China caused great debate because the Supreme Court announced the accused physician innocent of a crime, but the topic is seldom discussed in medicine and the law.

Buddhism

As with Hinduism, there is no central authority to pronounce on doctrine and ethics. Buddhism is a flexible and moderate religion, and in practice, local customs will often be more important in the relationship between physician and patient than Buddhist doctrine (Keown 2005).

Classically, attitudes towards illness and death may be different for Tibetan, Indian, Thai, Japanese and Western Buddhists, because they are more culturally than religiously based.

Nevertheless, there are basic values shared by most Buddhists. The primary point is that there is no mandate or moral obligation to preserve life at all costs in Buddhism – this would be a denial of human mortality. There are no specific Buddhist teachings on patients in a persistent vegetative state, but maintaining artificial nutrition is a way to keep the patient alive artificially – which is not mandatory in Buddhism. Alleviation of pain, and the principle of double effect (McIntyre 2009), is accepted, but Buddhists strive to meet death with mental clarity. Therefore, some may abstain from analgesia or sedation. Hence, it is extremely important to inquire about specific attitudes that may be deeply held by a Buddhist patient and family who come from a particular culture.

Terminal care should be available and Buddhism supports the hospice movement (Keown 2005).

Euthanasia or mercy killing is not acceptable (Keown 2005).

GUIDELINES

Key facts of how to cope with religious/cultural challenges

- There are major differences between the religions' view on palliation, information and end-of-life decisions, but almost universally euthanasia is not allowed.
- Medical teams should early on determine if there is a religious/cultural agenda as well as a medical one.
- Do not guess or suppose that you understand the patient's religious or cultural background. The only way to understand the situation correctly is to ask specifically about the areas you want to know about.
- Independently from the patients' religion and/or pressure from the patients' culture, you must of course adhere to the judicial and ethical rules that you usually work under.

There are five inevitable palliative care questions: What level of life-sustaining therapies? Alleviation of pain? What level of information to patient and relatives? Is euthanasia an issue? What are the final wishes with regard to death and burial?

Medical teams should early on establish their patients' and relatives' cultural background and religious affiliations, before deciding on these five issues.

Many authors (e.g., Daar and Khitamy 2001; Pauls and Hutchinson 2002) have recommended that the clergy of the patient's religion should be involved. If you identify and name differences between the frame of the patient and that of the medical team, you will most likely minimize the potential religious conflicts and discussions (Hendriks 2012). Never promise beforehand unconditionally to follow religious rulings or advice though, as these may contradict local standards of ethics or care (e.g., keeping a brain-dead patient on a ventilator) or contradict secular law (e.g., abstaining from blood transfusion to a minor patient). Also, be aware, that people who classify themselves as belonging to a religion, do not necessarily attend their church or follow any of the religion's rulings.

Alleviation of pain is almost universally accepted (Table 3.1).

When it comes to information, protestant Reformation which celebrated its 500-year anniversary in 2017 put emphasis on personal freedom and the patients' right to be truthfully informed. In Western countries, this concept is no longer considered a unique feature of Protestant (religious) bioethics (Pauls and Hutchinson 2002). Greece, however, is an example of a Western country with a different view on patient autonomy. Approximately 96% of Greek orthodox believes that communication is important in the final stage of a disease, but only 23% agree that the patient should be informed of the prognosis (Mystakidou et al. 2005). This must be due to culture, because the Orthodox Church has not issued such a statement.

In many Asian cultures, patient autonomy is not an agenda (Bowman and Hui 2000), and death and dying is often viewed as a taboo subject. Discomfort with end-of-life conversations among physicians, the ignorance of patient wishes, no widespread tradition for advance directives and traditional Asian values of filial piety mean that in Asia you may meet a more aggressive stance by default than in the West (Koh and Hwee 2015).

The question of euthanasia is the least complicated religious issue. In Table 3.1, it is evident that euthanasia is almost universally not accepted.

When death is imminent, the question of tending to the dead and burial arrangements will arise. Again, it is important to adhere to the wishes of the patient and the family, because each person may have specific rules based on culture and religion (Cheraghi et al. 2005).

Reaching consensus is a key to success but is not always possible. In those (hopefully few) instances where consensus cannot be accomplished, you must act according to the local rules and ethics of your workplace. You will cause confusion and uncertainty and ruin the work climate within the medical team, if you change your way of dealing with end-of-life issues for each new patient (Brierly et al. 2012).

ETHICAL ISSUES

Key facts of ethical challenges in modern medicine

- Religions and cultures have since the 1980s had to adhere to a new reality where advances in medical technology have forced society, religious leaders and people to understand that end-of-life decisions must be dealt with.
- There are presently large differences in the world as to how this issue is dealt with.
- Second- or third-generation immigrants may be very different from their original background and their parents on this issue – as they may have assimilated and adopted the point of view of their new homeland.

The bioethics committee of the Church of Greece has stated: "Modern medical technology has produced unprecedented forms of death or conditions of painful survival incompatible with life; leading to new dilemmas and bringing forth unanswered questions" (The Holy Synod 2000). This highlights the problem that religious leaders have faced during the last 25 years. They have had to contemplate and agree on epoch-making decisions concerning end-of-life decisions. The Pope has issued statements, there have been Islamic international conferences, the Jewish legal system has issued rulings so that cessation of therapy becomes legally possible within the framework of Jewish religious law and Western Buddhists accept organ donation.

Until now, critical care medicine, including other advanced medical measures to keep patients alive, has essentially been a discipline of Western medicine because it demands a highly developed medical and economic system. Far Eastern countries have no established head of the various Far Eastern religions who can adjust and express the religious rulings on these issues during the twenty-first century. Nevertheless, with increasing economic growth, these countries will also have to develop local guidelines covering advanced medical therapy. In fact, India in 2012 issued guidelines for end of life with among other issues a modern approach to informed consent: "The physician has a moral and legal obligation to disclose to the capable patient/family, with honesty and clarity, any dismal prognostic status when further aggressive support appears non-beneficial" (Mani 2012).

Nevertheless, even when there is a clear-cut statement from church leaders, it may be difficult to incorporate the religious perspectives into modern medical decision-making. The Catholic Church allows withholding or withdrawing "extraordinary" therapy, but what is extraordinary? Mechanical ventilation could be ordinary at one stage in an illness, and extraordinary at a later stage of the same illness.

Strict ethnic and religious background is not the only factor that one must take into account, when dealing with end-of-life decisions. Recent immigrants will generally adhere rather strictly to the rules of the religion and culture in their native country (Bowman and Hui 2000), whereas second- or third-generation immigrants will often have adopted the dominant bioethics of their new country (this is known as acculturation) (Matsumura et al. 2002). However, when facing death, many individuals tend to fall back on their traditional cultural or religious background (Klessig 1992).

Not only are patients changing their behavioural patterns when they move to other parts of the world, so are physicians. Although religion is an important part of decision-making, regional differences among physicians of the same religion have been documented too, and these differences are most probably due to acculturation (Matsumura et al. 2002; Sprung et al. 2007). Even a straight religious statement is not necessarily adopted. According to Islamic law one is allowed to abstain from futile treatment, but in Tunisia withdrawing of treatment (Ouanes et al. 2012) or do-not-resuscitate orders (da Costa et al. 2002) is less frequent than in Western Europe – and in both papers this difference is mainly explained by cultural differences.

KEY MAIN CONCLUSIONS

- Due to globalization medical staff must cope with many ethnic and cultural groups.
- The key to working with these different groups is to ask about and explore attitudes and beliefs, never to assume that you know beforehand.
- If conflicting views make consensus impossible, then the staff must apply local ruling laws and guidelines as their frame for work.

TABLE 3.3
Checklist to Establish Religious Beliefs, Cultural Affiliation and Family Background When End-of-Life Decisions Are Necessary

- What do they think of the sanctity of life?
- What is their definition of death?
- What is their religious background, and how active are they presently?
- What do they believe are the causal agents in illness, and how do these relate to the dying process?
- What is the patient's social support system?
- Who makes decisions about matters of importance in the family?

Source: Klessig J. 1992. *West J Med* 157: 316–22.
Note: Examples of questions that are suitable to ask when trying to explore patients' and relatives' cultural and religious background.

SUMMARY POINTS

- Globalization changes many parts of the world, diminishing homogeneous religious and cultural entities. Consequently, the medical staff has to acknowledge and cope with religious attitudes, beliefs and wishes of patients from many ethnic and religious groups.
- In a globalised world, religion and culture also have an impact on how physicians and nursing staff from different parts of the world interact and reach decisions.
- Worldwide patient autonomy often plays less of a role than in Western countries. Here family interactions can play a prominent role regarding treatment and information, very different from the usual Western context.
- Both religion and culture play an important role in end-of-life issues, but most physicians do not know their patients' religious affiliation, which can lead to a complete breakdown in communication.
- To avoid pitfalls, using the checklist in Table 3.3 is one way to explore culture and religion.
- Identify and name differences between the frame of reference of the patient and that of the medical team.
- It has been widely recommended early on to involve the clergy of the patient's religion. However, do not ever promise unconditionally to follow the clergy's advice or rulings, if you seek information, as this may clash directly with local legislation or the usual ethical framework in your workplace.
- By exploring these issues, it is usually possible to reach consensus, but if that is impossible, then the staff must apply the local ruling laws and ethical guidelines.
- In the context of a globalized world the statement of the ethics committee at Stanford University is important: "the key to resolving ethical problems lies in clarifying the patient's interests."

REFERENCES

Bowman KW, Hui EC. 2000. Bioethics for clinicians: Chinese bioethics. *CMAJ* 163: 1481–85.

Bowman KW, Singer PA. 2001. Chinese seniors' perspectives on end-of-life decisions. *Soc Sci Med* 53: 455–64.

Brierly J, Linthicum J, Petros A. 2012. Should religious beliefs be allowed to stonewall a secular approach to treatment in children? *J Med Ethics* 39:573–7.

Bülow HH, Sprung CL, Reinhart K, Prayag S, Du B, Armaganidis A, Abroug F, Levy MM. 2008. The world's major religions' point of view on end-of-life decisions in the intensive care unit. *Intensive Care Med* 34: 423–30.

Catechismus Catholicae Ecclesiae. 1997. Section 2278 and 2279, *Libreria Editrice Vaticana.*

Cheraghi MA, Payne S, Salsali M. 2005. Spiritual aspects of end-of-life care for Muslim patients: Experiences from Iran. *Int J Palliat Nurse* 11: 468–74.

Daar SA, Khitamy BA. 2001. Bioethics for clinicians: 21. Islamic bioethics. *CMAJ* 164: 60–3.

da Costa DE, Ghazal H, Khusaiby SA, Gatrad AR 2002. Do Not Resuscitate orders in a neonatal ICU in a Muslim community. *Arch Dis Child Fetal Neonatal Ed* 86: F115–9.

Desai PN. 1988. Medical ethics in India. *J Med Phil* 13: 231–255.

Ebrahim AFH. 2000. The living will (Wasiyat Al-Hayy): A study of its legality in the light of Islamic jurisprudence. *Med Law* 19: 147–60.

Flores A. 2017. How the US Hispanic population is changing. http://www.pewresearch.org. Accessed 13 November 2017.

Hendriks MP 2012. Palliative care for an Islamic patient. *J Palliat Med* 15:1053–55.

Keown D. 2005. End-of-life: The Buddhist view. *Lancet* 366: 952–55.

Klessig J. 1992. Cross-cultural medicine. The effect of values and culture on life support decisions. *West J Med* 157: 316–22.

Koh M, Hwee PC. 2015. End-of-life care in the intensive care unit. How Asia differs from the West. *JAMA Intern Med* 175:371–2.

Liu JM, Lin WC, Chen YM, Wu HW, Yao NS, Chen LT, Whang-Peng J. 1999. The status of the do-not-resuscitate order in Chinese clinical trial patients in a cancer centre. *J Med Ethics* 25: 309–14.
Mani RK, Amin P, Chavla R et al. 2012. Guidelines for end-of-life and palliative care in Indian intensive care units. *Indian J Crit Care Med* 16:166–81.
Matsumura S, Bito S, Liu H, Kahn K, Fukuhara S, Kagawa-Singer ML. 2002. Acculturation of attitudes toward end-of-life care. *J Gen Intern Med* 17: 531–9.
May AT 2003. Physician assisted suicide, euthanasia, and Christian bioethics: moral controversy in Germany. *Christ Bioeth* 9: 273–83.
McIntyre A, Doctrine of double effect. 2009. In *The Stanford Encyclopedia of Philosophy.* ed. Edward N. Zalta.
Mystakidou K, Parpa E, Tsilika E, Katsouda E, Vlahos L. 2005. The evolution of euthanasia and its perceptions in Greek culture and civilization. *Perspect Biol Med* 48: 95–104.
Ouanes I, Stambouli N, Dachraoui F et al. 2012. Pattern of end-of-life decisoons in two Tunisian ICU's: The role of culture and intensivists' training. *ICM* 38:710–7.
Pauls M, Hutchinson RC 2002. Bioethics for clinicians: Protestant bioethics. *CMAJ* 166: 339–44.
Shannon TA. 2006. Nutrition and hydration: An analysis of the recent Papal statement in the light of the Roman Catholic bioethical tradition. *Christ Bioeth* 12: 29–41.
Sprung CL, Maia P, Bülow HH et al. and The Ethicus Study Group. 2007. The impact of religion on end-of-life decisions in European intensive care units. *Intensive Care Med* 33: 1732–9.
Steinberg A, Sprung CL. 2006. The dying patient: New Israeli legislation. *Intensive Care Med* 32: 1234–7.
Tang ST, Liu TW, Lai MS, Liu LN, Chen CH, Koong SL. 2006. Congruence of knowledge, experiences, and preferences for disclosure of diagnosis and prognosis between terminally-ill cancer patients and their family caregivers in Taiwan. *Cancer Invest* 24: 360–6.
The Holy Synod of the Church of Greece Bioethics Committee. 2000. Press Release on 17 August. Basic positions on the ethics of transplantation and euthanasia. http://www.bioethics.org.gr
www.wikepedia.org Islam by country. Accessed 2 November 2017.
Ziadeh H. 2017. *"They went away" (Danish).* 3 November. Weekend Avisen. Berlingske, Copenhagen.

4 Nutrition and Quality of Life in Children Receiving Palliative Care

Michelle Koh

CONTENTS

INTRODUCTION

The Royal College of Paediatrics and Child Health (RCPCH) defines palliative care for children as the care of children suffering from conditions that will limit their life span, particularly those who are not expected to survive beyond childhood. This encompasses "an active and total approach to care, from the point of diagnosis, embracing physical, emotional, social and spiritual elements." It focuses on enhancing the quality of life (QOL) for the child and support for the family (TfSL 2018).

Children with a diagnosis of a life-limiting or life-threatening condition should gain access to palliative care services at the time of diagnosis. When considering nutrition in paediatric palliative care, we have to address not only the issues during the end-of-life phase of the child's illness, but also in the early stages of their disease, when they may have many months or years of life ahead (Table 4.1).

Nutrition in children has an important role in a child's normal development and learning. In a child with life-limiting/life-threatening disease, it impacts the child's QOL, ability to recover from crises and overall prognosis. Samson-Fang et al. (2002) demonstrated that poor nutritional status in

TABLE 4.1
Key Facts on the Categories of Life-Limiting and Life-Threatening Conditions

The four categories can be defined as follows:

1. Life-threatening conditions for which curative treatment may be feasible but can fail.
   Access to palliative care services may be necessary when treatment fails or during an acute crisis.
   Examples: Cancer, irreversible organ failure, for example, complex congenital heart disease.
2. Conditions where premature death is inevitable.
   There may be long periods of intensive treatment aimed at prolonging life and allowing participation in normal activities.
   Examples: Cystic fibrosis, Duchenne muscular dystrophy.
3. Progressive conditions without curative treatment options.
   Treatment is exclusively palliative and may commonly extend over many years.
   Examples: Adrenoleukodystrophy, mucopolysaccharidoses.
4. Irreversible but non-progressive conditions causing severe disability, leading to susceptibility to health.
   Children can have complex healthcare needs, a high risk of an unpredictable life-threatening event or episode, health complications and an increased likelihood of premature death.
   Examples: Severe cerebral palsy, acquired brain or spinal cord injury.

Source: Together for Short Lives. 2018. Introduction to children's palliative care: Categories of life-limiting conditions. http://www.togetherforshortlives.org.uk

Note: Children's palliative care services are set up to manage children with life-limiting and life-threatening conditions as defined.

children with cerebral palsy (CP) correlated with increased hospitalizations, increased number of doctor visits and decreased participation in usual activities.

An unsafe swallow, gastro-oesophageal reflux (GOR), feed intolerance, abdominal pain, and constipation are frequently encountered in children with developmental disabilities. Schwarz et al. (2001) showed that in these children, successful management of feeding problems results in significantly improved energy consumption, nutritional status and decreased morbidity.

However, obesity can also be a problem, for example in children with Duchenne's muscular dystrophy (DMD) and CP. This may be exacerbated in children requiring high-dose or long-term steroids as part of their treatment, for example boys with DMD where the early introduction of steroids has an important role in preserving the child's mobility.

Feeding also affects the emotional and social bonds between a child and his or her parents. Feeding and nourishing one's child is a fundamental instinct for every parent. Problems and decisions surrounding feeding and nutrition can be emotive and potentially distressing for families.

NUTRITIONAL ASSESSMENT

Growth measurements and the use of growth percentile charts are fundamental to the examination of the paediatric patient. Mascarenhas et al. (1998) recommend that patients with chronic complex needs should have appropriate nutritional assessments including the following:

- Medical and nutritional history including dietary intake.
- Physical examination.
- Anthropometrics (weight, length or stature, head circumference, mid-arm circumference, triceps skinfold thickness) and use of appropriate anthropometric charts.
- Pubertal staging.
- Skeletal maturity staging.
- Biochemical tests of nutritional status: micronutrients, protein and fat profiles.
- For patients at risk of fractures, bone density scans can be used to assess bone mineralization and the risk of fracture.

Closely working with the wider multi-disciplinary team is essential for a comprehensive assessment. Speech and language therapists are expert in assessing the safety of a child's swallow and aspiration risk. They can recommend if the child will benefit from having the consistency of their food modified or if further investigations such as video fluoroscopy will be helpful.

Dieticians will often take a detailed dietary history from families, including the child's past dietary preferences as well as the child's current intake. They also assess the child's energy requirements according to age, size and diagnosis. Dieticians then work closely with families to recommend appropriate interventions (calorie supplements, feed, volume, regimen, etc.) and to monitor the effects of their recommendations.

Further investigations should be tailored to the specific feeding or dietary issues that are identified and will be considered in the corresponding sections.

FEEDING AND NUTRITIONAL DIFFICULTIES IN CHILDREN WITH LIFE-LIMITING/LIFE-THREATENING DISEASE

Mechanical Difficulties: Unsafe Swallow, Gastro-Oesophageal Reflux

A significant proportion of children with life-limiting diagnoses have mechanical difficulties with feeding and GOR. For example, children with neurodevelopmental or metabolic disorders may have feeding difficulties from birth or early infancy. Other children with progressive disorders such as DMD may establish normal feeding before losing their ability to feed orally. As the child's oro-pharyngeal control diminishes, he or she will be unable to suck, chew and swallow and to co-ordinate the sequence of actions. Ultimately, this not only leads to under-nutrition but also poses significant risk for the child aspirating food into his or her lungs (Morton et al. 1999).

Difficulties with feeding also prolong the time it takes to feed the child, and feeding becomes a stressful and distressing experience instead of an enjoyable and nurturing time.

Sullivan (2008) demonstrated that children with neurodevelopmental disabilities commonly have foregut dysmotility causing dysphagia from oesophageal dysmotility, GOR and delayed gastric emptying.

GOR is a clinical diagnosis. Further investigations are only required if the reflux is severe or complications are suspected: a pH or impedance study to identify degree of acid and non-acid reflux, and a chest X-ray if pulmonary aspiration is suspected.

Gut Dysfunction (Dysmotility and Hypersensitivity)

It is increasingly recognized that children with severe neurological disorders may develop gut dysfunction as their neurological disease progresses. Their underlying diagnoses include progressive, neurodegenerative disorders as well as static neurological disorders. The gut dysfunction is characterized by dysmotility and hypersensitivity to milk feeds.

The underlying mechanisms and pathophysiology are not clearly known. Altaf and Sood (2008) summarized that the enteric nervous system modulates motility, secretions, microcirculation and immune and inflammatory responses of the gastrointestinal tract. A primary defect in the enteric neurons or central modulation in children with developmental disabilities could adversely affect intestinal motility, neurogastric reflexes and brain perception of visceral hyperalgesia.

It is also postulated that antral dysmotility exacerbated after fundoplication and sympathetic over-activity may contribute to the gut dysfunction (Carachi et al. 2009). In addition, these children are often on proton pump inhibitors and H_2-receptor antagonists, resulting in gastric hypochlorhydria and small bowel bacterial overgrowth.

The prime symptoms of gut dysfunction in these children are abdominal pain when being fed, and vomiting. If the child has a gastrostomy or nasogastric tube (NGT) left on free drainage, large volumes of aspirate (either bile-stained or non-bile-stained) reflux back.

Typically, these symptoms gradually resolve when the milk feeds are stopped, and recur when the feeds are re-started. Once the gut dysfunction is established, a notable feature is the degree of pain and distress even a small amount, either in volume or concentration, of milk feed can trigger.

Over time, the child not only fails to thrive, but also steadily loses weight and subcutaneous fat stores, eventually resulting in muscle wasting. The child inevitably develops pressure sores and is at high risk of infection and respiratory failure.

Investigating these children is difficult as the gut dysfunction generally occurs at the end stages of their underlying illness and they are unlikely to tolerate any invasive procedure such as an endoscopy or impedance study. The few children who have undergone an endoscopy and biopsy have shown an eosinophilic infiltration of their intestinal mucosa; however, the significance of this is unclear. In addition, as the investigations make little difference to their overall management, it is difficult to justify the burden of putting the child through the invasive procedures.

There has been no successful management strategy reported. The pain is refractory to opioid and neuropathic analgesia and only resolves when the child's feed is stopped. Treatment for GOR and anti-emetics are used empirically. The child eventually ends up in a cycle of having his feed stopped and substituted with an oral rehydration solution, such as Dioralyte, when the symptoms are too distressing, and then being re-started on milk feeds when he is more comfortable. The distress induced by the feeds and the malabsorption result in an inadequate caloric intake and drastic weight loss, and this ultimately contributes to the child's end-of-life event.

Physiological and Other Contributory Factors

Anorexia and weight loss are common symptoms in the paediatric palliative care population.

In the children with cancer, poor appetite and cachexia are frequent at presentation, through their treatment and during disease progression. Their carbohydrate, protein and fat metabolism is altered via cytokine-mediated pathways. In addition to the catabolic effects of their disease, their therapy frequently induces mucositis, alters taste sensation and causes nausea, further depressing their appetite (Ward et al. 2009). Malnutrition is an adverse risk factor for compliance to the chemotherapy and radiotherapy treatment regimen, and for disease-free outcome (Gómez-Almaguer et al. 1998; Sala et al. 2004).

It is also important to address any other symptoms such as pain, dry mouth and constipation, which may contribute to the child's lack of appetite and inability to eat.

NUTRITION AND FEEDING CARE AT THE END OF LIFE

It is well recognised that loss of appetite and loss of interest in food are common in children who are dying (Hechler et al. 2008; Theunissen et al. 2007). Fluid and caloric requirements decrease as their underlying illness deteriorates and activity levels decrease (Thompson et al. 2013).

It is important to establish the aims of feeding and nutrition at this stage. Goals will usually shift from providing adequate nourishment for the child to thrive and grow, to providing enough food or fluid to satisfy hunger and thirst without causing fluid overload.

Artificial hydration and feeds need to be given judiciously. If the child is already on artificial hydration, it is essential to re-assess the child's likely fluid requirement and reduce the amount being given appropriately. If the child had previously been orally feeding, it is not usually beneficial to start artificial hydration.

At the end of life, artificial hydration could alleviate signs of dehydration, but worsen peripheral oedema, ascites, pleural effusions (Morita et al. 2005), respiratory distress and frequent urination (Thompson et al. 2013). The intended benefits of artificial hydration therapy need to be considered against prolonging or increasing the morbidity of the dying process.

The focus should be on allowing the child to have some control over his or her eating and drinking so they provide comfort and enjoyment. Often small amounts of food or sips of fluid taken frequently is a good approach. Palliative measures such as oral hygiene, care of pressure areas and appropriate sedation must be provided as necessary (Larcher et al. 2015).

MANAGEMENT

The management of feeding problems and optimizing a child's nutrition begins with an open discussion with the family and if appropriate, the child. It is important to establish the family's and child's priorities and for them to feel that their concerns are recognized.

An individualized, rather than "blanket policy" approach in addressing the issues is essential. Moreover, decision-making about feeding is a dynamic process, with changing needs at different stages of illness.

This care and attention from an early stage help the family build a relationship of trust and mutual respect with the professional team, making discussions and decision-making easier when the child is deteriorating and the difficult issues surrounding limiting or withholding feeds and fluids arise.

If at all possible and safe, oral feeding should be encouraged and preserved. The expertise of the speech and language therapist (SALT) and dietician should be sought to determine if the child's food should be modified, such as having softened or pureed solids or thickened fluids. The dietician may suggest fortifying the child's normal diet to make it more calorific (e.g., by the addition of cream, butter, oil, etc.) or additional supplementation (e.g., high-energy milkshakes, etc.). They are also best placed to advise when oral feeding alone is no longer adequate or safe and artificial feeding should be considered.

The impact of introducing artificial feeding should not be underestimated. While for health professionals tube feeding is a common intervention, it represents a significant change in the child's everyday reality: in the physical care, in the psychological impact on the child (and the child's body image) and family, and in the social impact of planning life around a feeding regimen.

Artificial feeding is emotive and conflicting for families. It often represents deterioration in the child's condition, a progression into the "next stage" of the disease. Parents may feel a sense of failure, as nourishing their child was primarily their responsibility, and guilt over depriving their child of the pleasure of orally feeding (Craig 2013).

Petersen et al. (2006) examined the perceptions of gastrostomy tube feeding by caregivers of children with CP. They found that most caregivers had an initial negative response when the gastrostomy was recommended, perceiving gastrostomy feeding as "unnatural." Some parents persisted in orally feeding their child even though meals were an unpleasant experience or despite advice against oral feeding. Although the children received a complete formula through the gastrostomy, some families gave other foods through the gastrostomy (juice, cereal, soup or table food).

Resistance to tube feeding is also common from the children themselves. Younger children often resist NGT placements and older children are concerned about their body image: having a visible tube as well as with potential weight gain. Home adaptations may be required to accommodate the increased care and the paraphernalia of equipment that comes with artificial feeding, reinforcing the perception of disability that they may resist.

Care planning for the child also becomes more difficult and needs to take into consideration a variety of settings such as school and respite care. The child's carers will need to be trained in giving the artificial feed and in managing any difficulties that may arise, such as the child "vomiting up" his or her NGT.

TUBE FEEDING

Several studies have supported the benefits of tube feeding. Sullivan et al. (2005) reported that after the introduction of gastrostomy feeding in children with CP, increase in weight and subcutaneous fat deposition were noted. Almost all parents reported a significant improvement in their child's health

TABLE 4.2
Key Indications for Consideration of Tube Feeding

- Unsafe swallow and aspiration.
- Inability to consume at least 60% of energy needs by mouth.
- Total feeding time is greater than four hours a day.
- Oral feeding is unpleasant.
- Weight loss or no weight gain for a period of three months (or sooner for younger children or infants).
- Weight-for-height less than second percentile for age and sex.

Source: Thompson A, MacDonald A, Holden C. Feeding in palliative care. In *Oxford Textbook of Palliative Care for Children*. eds. A Goldman, R Hain and S Liben, Chapter 25. 2013, by permission of Oxford University Press. The authors recommend that tube feeding should be considered if one or more of these indications are present.

and a significant reduction in time spent feeding. In the study period, complications were rare, with no evidence of an increase in respiratory complications (Table 4.2).

TYPES OF FEEDING TUBES

Nasogastric Tubes

As the child's oral feeding begins to falter, the use of a NGT is usually the first intervention. For children who still retain some ability to orally feed, NGT feeding can be used as complementary or "top-up" feeding in addition to their oral intake. In children whose swallow is deemed unsafe for any oral intake, oral-motor and taste stimulation should be encouraged, and they should be included during mealtimes with the family.

There are two types of NGT commonly used. A long-term tube is made from silicone elastomer (known as "silk tubes") and can be left in for four to six weeks. A short-term tube is made of polyvinyl chloride and needs to be changed every five to seven days. Both tubes are easy to insert and can be changed by community nurses at the child's home or school.

Gastrostomy Tubes

For these reasons, when children require long-term tube feeding, a gastrostomy tube should be considered. These are now usually inserted by the percutaneous endoscopic route, or less commonly, by a formal surgical procedure. Both techniques can combine a gastrostomy tube insertion with a fundoplication should the child require this for management of GOR.

Once the gastrostomy tract is established, the gastrostomy tube can subsequently be changed for a skin-level gastrostomy device. These devices (commonly called gastrostomy "buttons") sit flush with the skin and can be left in place for several months. They are easy to change and can be done in the outpatient setting, or if community nurses are trained, can be done in the child's home.

Gastrostomy tubes can be used to administer medications but the feeds are special formulations, which are recommended and monitored by a dietician and prescribed by the child's general practitioner (GP).

Nasojejunal and Jejunostomy Tubes

Jejunal feeding is helpful with the management of severe GOR and the prevention of aspiration events. Jejunal tubes can be placed nasojejunally or as a jejunostomy. A nasojejunal tube (NJT) is difficult to accurately place and requires an X-ray to confirm its position. They are especially prone to displacement secondary to vomiting (as the main indication for their placement is GOR) and often require multiple, distressing re-insertions. If the child is able to tolerate an anaesthetic, the NJT should be regarded as a holding measure to protect the child from aspiration pneumonia, until a jejunostomy tube can be arranged.

A jejunostomy tube is inserted into the jejunum, either from the abdominal wall directly into the jejunum with a surgical procedure, or trans-gastrically via a previous gastrostomy.

BOLUS AND CONTINUOUS TUBE FEEDS

Tube feeding can be administered as multiple bolus feeds through the day, as a continuous feed, or most commonly, as a combination of both.

With bolus feeding, a relatively large volume of feed (typically 100–200 mL depending on the size of the child and what the child will tolerate) is given over 15–30 minutes. Bolus feeding is a more physiological pattern of feeding, more convenient and allows the family more freedom in planning the feeds with their activities.

The disadvantages of bolus feeding are that the child is at higher risk of aspiration compared to continuous feeding and is more likely to have abdominal distension, nausea and diarrhoea.

For children unable to tolerate the larger bolus volumes, continuous feeding can be delivered via an infusion feed pump. It is generally given over an 8–10 hour period overnight in addition to smaller bolus feeds or oral feeding during the daytime. Uninterrupted, longer periods of continuous feeding, for example, over 16–24 hours, are possible and can be considered for the child in whom any bolus feed induces GOR or pain. However, the child is attached to the feeding pump continuously, and this may cause metabolic changes such as elevated insulin levels.

BLENDERISED FOOD FOR TUBE FEEDING

There is a growing demand from parents for delivering food blended with liquid (usually water) through feeding tubes, rather than using commercial formula feeds. Parents perceive blended food as being a more natural option, and with variable reports of improved absorption with fewer symptoms of feed-related discomfort, reflux and improvement in both symptoms of constipation and diarrhoea. There is currently no objective evidence demonstrating either the benefits or risks of blenderised food.

The main concerns are tube blockage, inadequate nutrition (as the food has to be blended with a large proportion of water to reduce the viscosity enough to avoid tube blockage) and infection risk (Armstrong et al. 2017).

Although giving blenderised food via feeding tubes is currently not recommended practice in the United Kingdom due to the risk of inadequate nutrition, the British Dietetic Association (BDA) has produced guidance for dieticians on the advice, risk assessment and framework for support that should be provided for families (BDA 2013), working alongside the multi-disciplinary team.

TOTAL PARENTERAL NUTRITION

Total parenteral nutrition (TPN) in the context of a child's palliative care, may be indicated as a short-term nutritional measure to support the child through times of crises or acute complications, for example, during post-operative recovery, chemotherapy-induced mucositis, etc. It is well recognised that in children with cancer, optimising nutrition reduces acute complications, treatment delays and drug dose alterations; improves tumor response, time to first event (relapse or death) and survival (Bozzetti et al. 2009).

TPN may also be considered if the child has a malabsorption enteropathy or gut dysfunction. In this situation, TPN would be long-term management and will require homecare support. The decision to start TPN would need a multi-disciplinary and ethical discussion. Gut dysfunction usually develops in the end stages of the child's illness and the ethics of commencing TPN in this

TABLE 4.3
Benefits and Complications of the Different Feeding Methods

Feeding Method	Benefits	Complications
Nasogastric tube (NGT)	Complements oral feeding in children with a faltering swallow or who have a prolonged feeding time.	Misplacement or migration of tube. Exacerbation of gastro-oesophageal reflux (GOR) as the NGT keeps the gastro-oesophageal sphincter open. Trauma during insertion of the NGT. Local mucosal ulceration with long-term use. Displacement of the NGT with vomiting and requiring repeated re-insertion. Psychological impact of an NGT (child's refusing the tube insertion, or body image issues).
Gastrostomy tube	In children requiring long-term tube feeding, a gastrostomy tube avoids regular NGT re-insertion. A skin-level gastrostomy device is easily hidden under clothing and cosmetically more acceptable for the child.	Infection or over-granulation of the gastrostomy stoma. Leakage of the site. Tube displacement. Tube occlusion.
Jejunostomy tube	Similar advantages to gastrostomy tubes. As the feed is administered distal to the stomach, there is a reduced risk of GOR and pulmonary aspiration.	Similar complications to gastrostomy tubes. Jejunal feeds must be given as a continuous feed, not as a bolus feed. As the feed is administered distally, there is an increased incidence of diarrhoea and feed intolerance.
Total parenteral nutrition	Provides nutrition and calories to children who are unable to receive tube feeding or who are unable to absorb adequate nutrition enterally.	Requires central venous access; line displacement or occlusion. Line sepsis: in vulnerable, immuno-compromised patients potentially fatal. Cholestatic liver disease. Metabolic disturbances. Requires intensive support from a multi-disciplinary nutrition team.

setting will need to be clearly discussed, taking into account the burdens of TPN versus benefits and the family's priorities (Tables 4.3 and 4.4).

MULTIDISCIPLINARY TEAM WORKING

A large number of professionals need to work together with the child and family to address the changing feeding and nutritional challenges for each child. It involves the SALT, dietician, GP, paediatrician, tertiary specialist, play therapist and the palliative care, gastroenterology, surgical and psychology teams.

It is vital that these professionals are co-ordinated by the child's key worker. The community nurse usually fulfils this role and is the point of contact for the family and professionals, ensures that communication is cascaded to everyone involved in the child's care. This is especially important as the child is often cared for in multiple settings (e.g., home, school, hospital, respite care). It also facilitates an efficient response by professionals to changes in the child's condition.

ETHICAL ISSUES

The RCPCH has published a framework for practice in decision-making in children with palliative care conditions (RCPCH 2015). It emphasises that parents "should be fully involved in the decision

TABLE 4.4
Symptom Management Guidelines

1. Gastro-oesophageal reflux
   The medical management of gastro-oesophageal reflux includes:
   a. Anti-secretory drugs (proton pump inhibitors and H_2-receptor antagonists).
   b. Pro-motility agents (Metoclopramide or Domperidone).
   c. Jejunal feeding.
   If symptoms persist, a surgical referral can be considered for:
   a. Nissen fundoplication, the fundus of the stomach is wrapped around the lower oesophagus, forming a valve at the junction of the oesophagus and stomach.
      As the gastric fundus is used to fashion the anti-reflux valve, the stomach volume is reduced, the child may have some retching after the procedure. Small volume, more frequent feeds are needed, and the retching usually, but not always, resolves after a few weeks or months. Some children may eventually vomit past the valve or the fundoplication wrap fails and needs to be revised.
2. Appropriate management of contributory symptoms:
   a. Pain
      i. Simple analgesia (Paracetamol).
      ii. Opiates (Morphine) need to be used judiciously as it will further exacerbate poor gut motility.
      iii. Neuropathic agents as adjuncts (Gabapentin, Carbamazepine or Amitriptyline).
      Non-steroidal anti-inflammatory drugs should be avoided as they have significant gastro-intestinal side effects.
   b. Nausea
      The choice of anti-emetics is guided by the probable cause of the nausea and vomiting and drug's mechanism of action:
      i. Vomiting centre (Cyclizine, Hyoscine hydrobromide, Levomepromazine).
      ii. Chemoreceptor trigger zone (Ondansetron, Haloperidol).
      iii. Cerebral cortex (Dexamethasone).
      iv. Gastrointestinal tract (Metoclopramide, Hyoscine butylbromide).
   c. Depression
      The pharmacological treatment of depression and other psychological symptoms should be managed by a specialist. Non-medical interventions, such as counselling or cognitive behavioural therapy, are also important.
3. Steroids as an appetite stimulant are rarely used in children as they have a high tendency to develop cushingoid, behavioural and psychological side effects.
4. Temporary cessation of feeding may have to be considered for children who have severe gut dysfunction. As previously described, these children have extremely distressing gastro-intestinal symptoms, from which they may only obtain relief when their feed is stopped. A gradual re-introduction of feed and fluid can then be tried; feeds are upgraded and increased to an amount that the child is able to reasonably tolerate. The nutrition of these children is always balanced against the symptoms that their feed induces.

making and should support the decision to withhold or withdraw clinically assisted nutrition." It highlights that artificial hydration/nutrition is a medical treatment and decisions to provide it "should be based on whether it provides overall benefit to the child." Like other forms of treatment, it may be withheld or withdrawn if it is futile and burdensome and if continuation is not in their best interests.

The use of TPN in supporting the nutrition of children with life-limiting disease is an ethical challenge. TPN may be initiated with the intention of a short-term intervention to support an acute intercurrent illness, but there may be no assurance that the child's absorption of enteral feeds will recover enough for the TPN to be stopped. The family and healthcare team are then confronted by the choices of either withdrawing the TPN and leaving the child on sub-optimal nutrition; or committing to the burdens and risks of long-term TPN in the context of a child with chronic complex needs or a progressive, deteriorating condition.

Another ethical dilemma we encounter is in managing gut dysfunction. Optimising the child's nutrition and weight gain has to be balanced with the day-to-day palliation of distressing symptoms, which often requires the reduction or cessation of feeds. In these situations, decisions should be made in discussion with the wider multi-professional team, the child and the child's parents and regularly reviewed.

In conclusion, the family of Frances, a girl who died at age 13 years of a neurodegenerative disorder, reflected: "Because a medical intervention is available, it does not always make it right and they need to consider the burden and benefit of any treatment they are recommending. That burden and benefit needs to take into account the whole family and extended carers (Marcovitch 2005)."

SUMMARY POINTS

- Nutritional problems in children with life-limiting and life-threatening illnesses are common and adversely impact their development, QOL and clinical outcome.
- The causes of poor nutrition in children with palliative care needs are often multi-factorial and dynamic. They need to be re-assessed regularly and interventions modified appropriately.
- Supplemental and tube feeding should be considered early and approached in a family-centred manner. In particular, the social, psychological and emotional impacts of tube feeding need to be considered.
- Assessing and supporting the child and family require an active, co-ordinated, multi-disciplinary approach. The burdens and benefits of artificial feeding and nutritional interventions need to be taken into account and decisions individualised for each child and family.
- The decision-making about hydration and nutrition of the dying child should be shared jointly with the family and with reference to national guidance if necessary.

LIST OF ABBREVIATIONS

CP	Cerebral Palsy
DMD	Duchenne's Muscular Dystrophy
GOR	Gastro-oesophageal Reflux
GP	General Practitioner
NGT	Nasogastric Tube
NJT	Nasojejunal Tube
QOL	Quality of Life
RCPCH	Royal College of Paediatrics and Child Health
SALT	Speech and Language Therapy
TfSL	Together for Short Lives (UK charity for children's palliative care)
TPN	Total Parenteral Nutrition

REFERENCES

Altaf MA, Sood MR. 2008. The nervous system and gastrointestinal function. *Developmental Disabilities Research Reviews*. 14:87–95.

Armstrong J, Buchanan E, Duncan H et al. 2017. Dietitians' perceptions and experience of blenderised feeds for paediatric tube-feeding. *Archives of Disease in Childhood*. 102:152–6.

Bozzetti F, Arends J, Lundholm K, Micklewright A, Zurcher G, Muscaritoli M; ESPEN. 2009. ESPEN Guidelines on Parenteral Nutrition: Non-surgical oncology. *Clinical Nutrition (Edinburgh, Scotland)*. 28:445–54.

British Dietetic Association. 2013. Policy statement use of liquidised food with enteral feeding tubes.

Carachi R, Currie JM, Steven M. 2009. New tools in the treatment of motility disorders in children. *Seminars in Pediatric Surgery*. 18:274–7.

Craig G. 2013. Psychosocial aspects of feeding children with neurodisability. *European Journal of Clinical Nutrition* 67:s17–20.

Gómez-Almaguer D, Ruiz-Argüelles GJ, Ponce-de-León S. 1998. Nutritional status and socio-economic conditions as prognostic factors in the outcome of therapy in childhood acute lymphoblastic leukemia. *International Journal of Cancer.* Supplement. 11:52–5.

Hechler T, Blankenburg M, Friedrichsdorf SJ, Garske D, Hübner B, Menke A, Wamsler C, Wolfe J, Zernikow B. 2008. Parents' perspective on symptoms, QOL, characteristics of death and end-of-life decisions for children dying from cancer. *Klinische Padiatrie.* 220:166–74.

Larcher V, Craig F, Bhogal K, Wilkinson D, Brierley J, on behalf of the Royal College of Pediatrics and Child Health. 2015. Making decisions to limit treatment in life-limiting and life-threatening conditions in children: A framework for practice. *Archives of Disease in Childhood.* 100(Supp. 2):s1–23.

Marcovitch H, 2005. Artificial feeding for a child with a degenerative disorder: A family's view. The mother and grandmother of Frances. *Archives of Disease in Childhood.* 90:979.

Mascarenhas MR, Zemel B, Stallings VA. 1998. Nutritional assessment in pediatrics. *Nutrition.* 14:105–15.

Morita T, Hyodo I, Yoshimi T, Ikenaga M, Tamura Y, Yoshizawa A, Shimada A, Akechi T, Miyashita M, Adachi I; Japan Palliative Oncology Study Group. 2005. Association between hydration volume and symptoms in terminally ill cancer patients with abdominal malignancies. *Annals of Oncology.* 16:640–7.

Morton RE, Wheatley R, Minford J. 1999. Respiratory tract infections due to direct and reflux aspiration in children with severe neurodisability. *Developmental Medicine and Child Neurology.* 41:329–34.

Petersen MC, Kedia S, Davis P, Newman L, Temple C. 2006. Eating and feeding are not the same: Caregivers' perceptions of gastrostomy feeding for children with cerebral palsy. *Developmental Medicine and Child Neurology.* 48(9):713–7.

Sala A, Pencharz P, Barr RD. 2004. Children, cancer, and nutrition—A dynamic triangle in review. *Cancer* 15;100:677–87.

Samson-Fang L, Fung E, Stallings VA et al. 2002. Relationship of nutritional status to health and societal participation in children with cerebral palsy. *Journal of Pediatrics.* 141:637–43.

Schwarz SM, Corredor J, Fisher-Medina J, Cohen J, Rabinowitz S. 2001. Diagnosis and treatment of feeding disorders in children with developmental disabilities. *Pediatrics.* 108:671–6.

Sullivan PB. 2008. Gastrointestinal disorders in children with neurodevelopmental disabilities. *Developmental Disabilities Research Reviews.* 14:128–36.

Sullivan PB, Juszczak E, Bachlet AM, Lambert B, Vernon-Roberts A, Grant HW, Eltumi M, McLean L, Alder N, Thomas AG. 2005. Gastrostomy tube feeding in children with cerebral palsy: A prospective, longitudinal study. *Developmental Disabilities Research Reviews.* 47:77–85.

Theunissen JM, Hoogerbrugge PM, van Achterberg T, Prins JB, Vernooij-Dassen MJ, van den Ende CH. 2007. Symptoms in the palliative phase of children with cancer. *Pediatric Blood and Cancer.* 49:160–5.

Thompson A, MacDonald A, Holden C. 2013. Feeding in palliative care. In *Oxford Textbook of Palliative Care for Children.* eds. A Goldman, R Hain and S Liben, Chapter 25. Oxford University Press.

Together for Short Lives. 2018. Introduction to children's palliative care; Categories of life-limiting conditions. http://www.togetherforshortlives.org.uk

Ward E, Hopkins M, Arbuckle L, Williams N, Forsythe L, Bujkiewicz S, Pizer B, Estlin E, Picton S. 2009. Nutritional problems in children treated for medulloblastoma: Implications for enteral nutrition support. *Pediatric Blood and Cancer.* 53:570–5.

5 Nutrition and Quality of Life in Adults Receiving Palliative Care

Mick Fleming, Caroline J. Hollins Martin, Derek Larkin, and Colin R. Martin

CONTENTS

INTRODUCTION: IMPORTANCE OF NUTRITION DURING PALLIATIVE CARE

Palliative care refers to treatment and care delivered where the disease/illness is not responsive to curative treatment. The World Health Organisation defines palliative care as: "an approach that improves the quality of life of patients and their families facing the problems associated with life threatening illness, through the prevention and relief of suffering by means of an early identification and impeccable assessment and treatment of pain and other problems, physical, psychosocial and spiritual" (WHO, 2004). It has been proposed by Etkind et al. (2017) that by 2040 there will be a 25% projected rise in those requiring palliative care. This rise would see an increase from 375,398 in 2014 to 469,305 people per year in England and Wales. These figures are at the low end; if figures of the upward trend shown from 2006 to 2014 are realised, the percentage increase could be in the order of 42%, which amounts to 537,240 individuals per year requiring palliative care, mainly as a consequence of dementia and cancer (Etkind et al., 2017).

Palliative care and treatment strategies can also be used to manage the side effects of intrusive treatments within curative treatment. Often associated in the mind as being related to oncology and cancer, palliative care can be delivered to people experiencing any form of life-threatening illness, such as chronic heart failure, respiratory disease, neurological disorders such as motor neurone disease and multiple sclerosis. Palliative care can also be distinguished from end-of-life care. Within the United Kingdom, end-of-life care is written into clinical pathways concerned with the final days and hours of a person's life (Department of Health, 2008; LCP, 2008). The key aims of these care pathways are to improve quality of care of the dying in the last hours and days of life and to improve the knowledge related to the process of dying.

Since 2008, the Liverpool Care Pathway (LCP) fell under the spotlight, and a review was commissioned that questioned the LCP approach (Neuberger et al., 2013). The review acknowledged that when the LCP was implemented correctly, it facilitated good care of the dying, but there were occasions when it was associated with poor care experiences; consequently, the LCP was phased out. In June 2014, a response document to the independent review was published, which outlined five priorities for care in the last few hours of life (Harrison, 2014). One of the five priorities is that an individual plan of care, which includes food and drink, symptom control and psychological, social and spiritual support, is agreed, co-ordinated and delivered with compassion.

Nutritional support is a recognised element of palliative care; it provides a useful strategy for the achievement of clinical outcomes, and there are other comfort and ethical reasons for the justification of the use of nutrition during the provision of palliative care and end-of-life treatment. Effects of the health condition such as dysphagia, metabolic responses to the health condition and treatment and mood/thinking changes all contribute to a reduced inability for people who are receiving palliative care and treatment to maintain an adequate nutritional intake to satisfy their physical, psychological and social functioning needs (Harrison, 2014; Hickson & Frost, 2004; Sobotka et al., 2009). Inadequate hydration and malnutrition and the effects of this, such as muscle waste and strength, vulnerability to infection, delirium and respiratory problems, are common potential risks for people receiving palliative care and treatment, particularly when people are near the end of life (Kutner, 2005). The essential skills clusters for nutrition and fluids management impact on care professionals who must be able to assess and monitor nutritional and fluid status and, in partnership with patients and their carers, formulate an effective plan of care to ensure patients receive adequate nutrition and hydration (Harrison, 2014; Nursing Midwifery Council, 2010).

The criteria for malnourishment and providing nutritional support are defined as follows:

- Body mass index (BMI) units kg/m^2 = Weight (kg)/Height^2 (m).
- BMI of less than 18.5 kg/m^2.
- Unintentional weight loss greater than 10% within the last three to six months.
- A BMI of less than 20 kg/m^2 and unintentional weight loss greater than 5% within the last three to six months (National Institute of Health and Clinical Excellence [NICE], 2006, updated 2017).
- A BMI of less than 20 is indicative of mild undernutrition.
- A BMI of less than 18 is indicative of moderate undernutrition.
- A BMI of less than 16 is indicative of severe undernutrition (Hanks et al., 2011).

Many patients who are terminally ill generally experience weight loss, loss of energy and loss of appetite (Hanks et al., 2011). The definition for the risk of malnutrition includes not eating or eating very little for the previous five days or longer and the capacity for absorption and/or the need for increased nutritional need (NICE, 2006, updated 2017). Nutrition screening is a process of identifying patients who are at risk of malnutrition although they may already be malnourished, in order to determine if a detailed nutrition assessment is indicated. The screening process may involve anthropometric, dietary, clinical and/or biochemical parameters, and can be general in nature or focus on a specific aspect of nutritional status (Wenhold, 2017). Generic nutritional screening tools such as the Malnutrition Universal Screening Tool (Todorovic et al., 2003) are commonly used in clinical practice. This specific screening tool has five steps that start with the measurement of BMI, unplanned weight loss, acute illness effects, risk for malnutrition and formulation of care plan.

Cachexia is a complex metabolic syndrome associated with underlying illness and characterized by loss of muscle with or without loss of fat mass (Evans et al., 2008). The condition is seen as irreversible because of its association with progressive and terminal health conditions such as advanced cancer. Although a co-morbid condition, it is a metabolic response to the health condition. Catabolic processes have been found in certain cancer conditions; the development of cachexia has been associated with the growth of tumours and increasing competition for nutrients as the tumour develops (Argilés et al., 2005; Evans et al., 2008; Kir & Spiegelman, 2016). Consequently, cachexia can occur even when the person has adequate nutritional intake. It has been found significantly in people who experience deteriorating health conditions such as cancer, neurologic disorders, chronic cardiac failure and conditions relating to older age (Davidson et al., 2004; Kutner, 2005).

CATEGORIES OF NUTRITIONAL SUPPORT

Three categories of strategies for nutritional support can be found in the literature, and a combination of these three nutritional strategies can also be used.

1. *Support of natural nutritional intake*: Wherever possible, the health practitioners will seek to support and maintain natural routes of nutritional intake especially in cases where use of the normal digestive system is not compromised. The aim of this type of intervention strategy is to ensure the correct amount and balance of the required nutrients are consumed, digested and metabolised. The most common strategy would be through the provision of oral supplements. A range of prescribed oral nutritional supplements (ONSs) in the forms of tablet, drink and concentrated droplet can be administered in addition to a manageable diet. Mechanical aids to eating for people who can manage to chew, swallow and digest food have been recommended as an intervention strategy (Hanks et al., 2011; NICE, 2006, updated 2017).
2. *Artificial methods of nutritional intake and hydration*: There are two routes for the administration of artificial nutrition. Nutritional support using both routes is provided both in hospital and in the person's home:
   a. *Enteral route*: Considered a short-term nutritional intervention (four weeks or less), this route is usually the first choice for nutritional support (Sobotka et al., 2009) essentially for people who do not have problems with the functioning of their gastrointestinal tract but are unable to swallow or feed orally. Nutrition is administered in two ways: 1) into the stomach via a nasogastric tube or; 2) directly into the stomach via a percutaneous endoscopic gastrostomy, which is passed into the stomach through an incision into the abdominal wall (Hanks et al., 2011).
   b. *Parenteral route*: Where the gastrointestinal tract is not functioning because of obstruction or the digestive system is not able to function or where preventing enteral feeding, nutrition is delivered into the body through a non-alimentary route via central or peripheral veins. Total nutritional requirements that satisfy fully the energy requirements can be delivered through this parenteral route (total parenteral nutrition) and partial nutritional requirements can also be delivered by this route. The amount and type of nutritional mixture delivered are individualised and dependent on the nutritional needs of the person. A range of nutritional products such as amino acids, essential fatty acids, vitamins and other nutrients can be delivered. Peripheral veins are used where the need for the parenteral route is required for less than 14 days (NICE, 2006, updated 2017).
   c. Where parenteral feeding is required for longer than 14 days, a central vein is used to deliver the nutrients through a larger-diameter intravenous catheter which is placed directly into the superior vena cava or right atrium. Risk of infection and condition of the person are also considered when making clinical decisions about which parenteral route to use (Gavin et al., 2017; Pittiruti et al., 2009).
   d. Hyperacidity, hyperglycaemia and refeeding syndrome can be consequences of the use of parenteral nutrition. Refeeding syndrome occurs within the first three to four days of reintroducing nutritional support and can be fatal. It is more likely to occur when high-calorie nutrition is rapidly re-introduced to malnourished people. The effects of the syndrome include low amounts of phosphate in the blood, electrolyte imbalances, the metabolism of fats, protein and glucose, thiamine deficiency and hypokalaemia

(Mehanna et al., 2009). The effects are metabolic and can lead to cardiac, skeletal, respiratory and gastrointestinal disorders. The gradual re-introduction of nutritional support up to 50% of requirement over the first two days and then further gradual re-introduction up to optimal nutritional support with full biochemical monitoring are recommended as preventative measures (NICE, 2006, updated 2017).

3. *Dietary advice/counselling*: Health practitioners can offer advice to both the person receiving palliative care and his or her carers or relatives. The aim of this strategy would be to increase encouragement of positive eating habits such as the inclusion of high-protein, carbohydrate and energy nutrition into diets. Often this strategy would not be used as a stand-alone intervention and would be delivered in conjunction with oral supplements (Baldwin & Weekes, 2009). Clinical guidelines recommend that alongside all forms of nutritional support, tailored information should be given about physical, psychological and social issues. In order to support the use of artificial feeding in people's homes and away from hospital, people and their carer's/relatives should be trained to manage, recognise the risks and problem-solve the process of artificial nutrition (NICE, 2006, updated 2017).

ISSUES REGARDING NUTRITIONAL STATE AND PALLIATIVE CARE AND TREATMENT

1. *Clinical rationale*: For many people receiving palliative care and treatment, sub-optimal nourishment and malnutrition are co-morbid complications of the health condition that they are experiencing. Nutritional support is often an indispensable part of their overall care and treatment (Sobotka et al., 2009). The aim of nutritional support may not be curative, but it is nevertheless an integral strategy for maintaining QOL for a period of time. The maintenance of a person's physical, psychological and social functioning requires adequate nutrition and hydration (Marin Caro et al., 2007). Optimization of nutritional support may help patients improve their tolerance to oncological treatments and health-related QOL (Vigano et al., 2017). Clinical outcomes need to consider the specific nutritional needs of those receiving palliative care and treatment. If there is a need to feed a patient, it is recommended that enteral nutrition is first considered; if oral nutrition remains insufficient despite other interventions such as counselling or oral nutritional supplement, then parenteral nutrition, may be considered if enteral nutrition is not sufficient or feasible (Arends et al., 2017). Chronic obstruction caused by tumour growth prevents the digestion of adequate nutrition, and starvation may be prevented by the administration of parenteral nutrition (Arends et al., 2017; Bozzetti et al., 2002).
2. *Disease process*: The disease process of pancreatic cancer is associated with pain, nausea, anorexia, early satiety and pancreatic insufficiency. Alteration in metabolic responses leads to weight loss, insufficient nutritional intake and cachexia (Davidson et al., 2004). There is a further acknowledgement within the literature that weight loss from cancer is different from simpler forms of starvation (Marin Caro et al., 2007). Details regarding the metabolic abnormalities and changes that lead to weight loss and cachexia are given. These metabolic changes render normal re-feeding ineffective in restoring nutritional status. Marin Caro et al. (2007) suggest cachexia accounts for 10%–22% of all cancer deaths and summarise the range of clinical benefits of nutritional support for people with cancer as controlling cancer-related symptoms, reducing post-operative complications and improving tolerance to treatment. These are sound justifications for the use of nutritional support and artificial feeding based on non-curative clinical outcomes regardless of the ethical issues associated with comfort and QOL.

3. *Ethical and cultural rationale*: Decisions about the use of nutritional support that does not have a curative/life-sustaining outcome are embedded within social, ethical and cultural belief systems about death for health practitioners, the person receiving palliative care and treatment and relatives (Hughes & Neal, 2000). However, all three groups would aim to maintain comfort and QOL. Hughes and Neal (2000) point out that the effects of malnutrition are uncomfortable, and nutritional support can be justified on the grounds that it maintains the comfort and QOL of the person. This is based on the assumption that nutritional support itself does not cause discomfort. A number of secondary causes of reduced nutritional intake include oral ulceration, xerostomia, poor dentition, intestinal obstruction, malabsorption, constipation, diarrhoea, nausea, vomiting, reduced intestinal motility, chemosensory alteration, uncontrolled pain and side effects of drugs (Arends et al., 2017).
4. *Side effects and outcomes*: Some artificial feeding can have uncomfortable side effects and fatal outcomes. Comfort care rather than life-sustaining treatments were preferred by 70% of a sample of 1,266 aged 80 years or older who were admitted to intensive coronary care units in the United States (Somogyi-Zalud et al., 2002). The literature suggests the perceived importance of nutritional support, particularly artificial feeding and hydration, decreases as people reach the end of life. From a sample of 104, 97.1%–99% of house officers believed that people who were seen as having the capacity to make the decision to end artificial feeding and hydration should be able to refuse (Schildmann ett al., 2006). Tube feeding was considered as inappropriate for 20.5% of people experiencing dementia in the last 48 hours of life (Di Giulio et al., 2008). In comparison to other life-sustaining treatments, artificial nutrition is considered to be indispensable by health practitioners (Aita et al., 2008). This view is shared by the general population and bereaved family members; 33%–50% believed that artificial hydration should be continued as the minimal standard until death. Ethical and cultural beliefs may well mediate these beliefs, but 15%–31% also believed that artificial hydration relieved symptoms (Morita et al., 2006). The withdrawal of artificial nutrition and hydration when they do not cause pain and discomfort has been questioned (Hildebrand, 2000). The arguments within the literature are based on moral codes of ethics and do not explicitly consider QOL issues. Although some may point out that as nutrition and hydration are required to sustain life, withdrawal resulting in death extinguishes QOL. Arends et al. (2017) argue that there are many benefits of artificial feeding in patients with prolonged inability to consume oral food, but they would recommend against using the cancer diagnosis per se as an indication for supplying artificial nutrition.

QUALITY OF LIFE

A number of factors have contributed to QOL becoming a standard health outcome. Ideological shifts in health concepts, such as the emergence of person-centred health provision, have led to a focus on health and well-being rather than illness (Pais-Ribeiro, 2004). Holism and consumerism place the person at the centre of health provision, and from this there has been recognition of the multi-dimensional nature of the impact of illness on all parts of a person's life and functioning. Within palliative care treatment, choices are of great importance to the person (Mystakidou et al., 2004). Health conditions affect psychological and social well-being as well as physical well-being (Arends et al., 2017). The individualised and personal nature of health and illness has also become more prevalent in modern health systems. Each person responds to a health condition in his or her own individual way. Two people at the same stage of the same illness will respond and react differently. Their behaviours in relation to their health condition will be determined by a number of non-physical factors such as previous experiences, health attributions, emotional response and emotional environment. This is further indication of the multi-dimensional nature of the health concept. Definitions of health reflect this recognition and include physical, mental and social well-being within their scope (Marin Caro et al., 2007). Developments in health technologies have led to populations living longer, and it is the quality of that existence rather than the quantity of that existence that is important to people. This is particularly apparent for those people who are living longer with ongoing and chronic health conditions. The debilitating nature of the health condition and the side effects of ongoing treatment will have an adverse impact on several domains of that person's life (Mystakidou et al., 2004). Pols and Limburg (2016) suggest that offering artificial nutrition and hydration has to be understood as a process rather than as an outcome. This process becomes a different idea as patients move from one phase of their illness to the next, and may change according to living circumstances, concerns and values.

Although developed for mental health services, Oliver et al. (1996) provide a taxonomy of the justification for the use of QOL in (mental) health services: comfort, not cure, is important; complex health programmes require complex outcome measures; better QOL keeps the customer happy; the holistic perspective is re-emerging; QOL is good politics (the emergence of the feel-good factor); it is accepted by patients and carers; it serves as a common basis for multi-disciplinary work; it is an effective economic measurement; achievability is used for studies of communities; it is useful for evaluating community-delivered services; empirical measures are linked to theory; and satisfaction with role performance is central to recovery.

DEFINITIONS OF QUALITY OF LIFE

While QOL is a multi-dimensional but general concept that can be applied to a wide range of health conditions, it is distinct from the health condition itself (Oliver et al., 1996). Health-related QOL is a multi-dimensional concept that focuses specifically on the impact of health, health treatments and illness on a person's physical, psychological and social functioning and well-being and an essential element of healthcare evaluation (Coons et al., 2000). Common terms and themes such as multi-dimensional, well-being, satisfaction, expectations and functioning are prevalent in the QOL literature. Definitions of QOL and health-related QOL do vary, and this variation is determined by the philosophical and theoretical stance of the researcher. Subjective versus objective are the two dominant theoretical models of QOL. The subjective model is individualised and places the person and his or her internal or perceived satisfaction with well-being and life at the heart of the investigation of QOL. External factors such as culture, value systems and the person's environment are seen as factors that influence the person's QOL, because it is these that determine their goals. Subjective measures of QOL are concerned with the person's own view of his or her QOL and are more likely to be self-report measures. The objective model does not see QOL as being individually determined. There is an acceptance that QOL is an external phenomenon; observable, shared across communities/populations, measurable and associated with factors such as social contact, housing, role performance, functional ability and income (Gellrich et al., 2015; Oliver et al., 1996). There is an agreement that subjective and objective views of QOL apply to two different dimensions of the concept of QOL (Ruggeri et al., 2001).

ASSESSMENT OF QUALITY OF LIFE IN PEOPLE RECEIVING PALLIATIVE CARE

There is a consensus about the domains within QOL measures. Mobility, self-care, usual activities, pain/discomfort and anxiety/depression are domains measured by the EQ-5D (EuroQoL Group, 1990). Physical functioning, role limitation due to physical problems, bodily pain, general health, vitality, social functioning, role limitation due to emotional problems and mental health are domains measured by the Medical Outcomes Short Form Health Survey 36 (SF-36) (Ware et al., 1993). This similarity between these two commonly used QOL measures is reflected within other

QOL measures. Other health-related generic QOL measures commonly used in the literature include the Nottingham Health profile, the Sickness Impact Profile, the Dartmouth Primary Care Co-operative Intervention Project Charts, the Quality of Well Being Scale and the Health Utilities Index (Coons et al., 2000). Within cancer treatment, tumour growth has been linked to functioning ability, and studies compare measures of QOL with measures of functioning ability, such as the Karnofsky Performance Status Scale (Bozzetti et al., 2002; Karnofsky & Burchenal, 1949). Specific palliative care QOL measures incorporate physical functioning into the domains of the measure (Figures 5.1 and 5.2).

It has been argued that specific elements or domains relate to palliative and end-of-life care. Spirituality, existential issues (purpose and meaning of life), family members' perceptions of QOC, symptom control and family support have been identified as specific to palliative and end-of-life care (Kaasa & Loge, 2003). In their review of generic QOL instruments, Coons et al. (2000) suggested choice of measure should be determined by the purpose of measurement, characteristics of client population and environment. The recommendation to clinicians and researchers working with people who are receiving palliative care is that while multi-dimensional measures should be used, these should have a limited number of items, and these should be based on the clinical outcomes and research question (Kaasa & Loge, 2003).

Three specific QOL measures for people receiving palliative care were found within the literature. The "Palliative Care Quality of Life Instrument" (Mystakidou et al., 2004) is a 28-item measure composed of six multi-item scales: two functional, one symptom, one choice of treatment and one psychological. There is a final single-item overall QOL scale. The measure takes approximately eight minutes to complete, and when people who have advanced-stage cancer were tested, test-retest reliability ($p < 0.05$ Spearman-rho) and Cronbach's alpha co-efficient greater than 0.70 showed

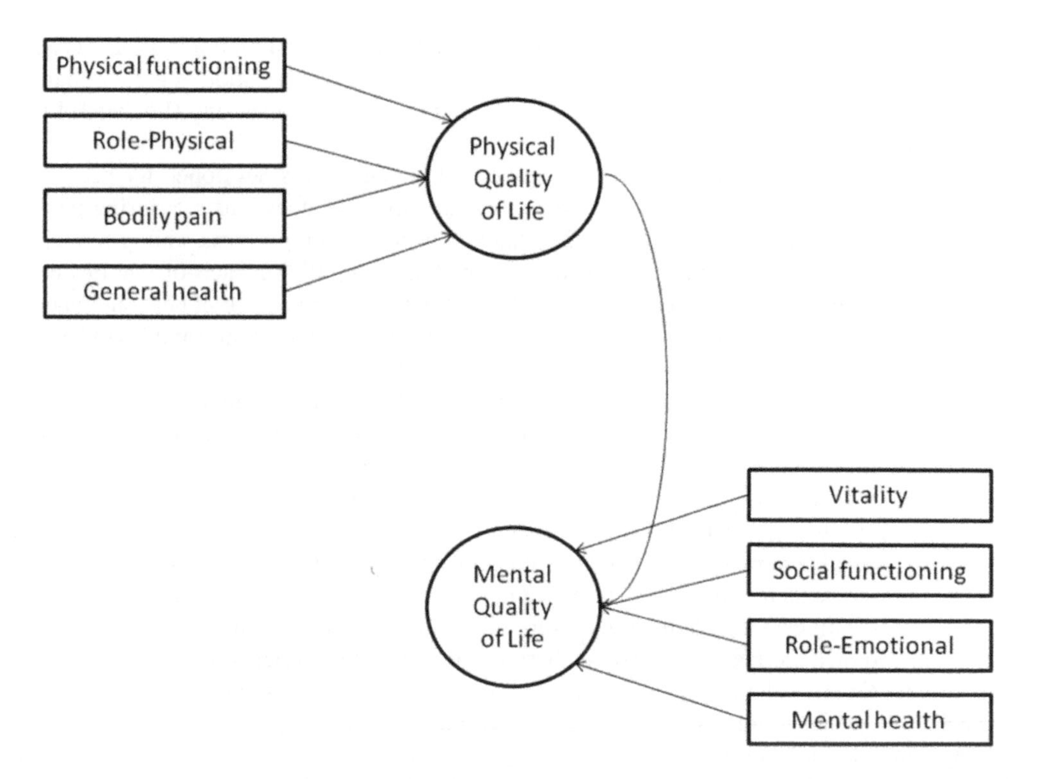

FIGURE 5.1 This figure illustrates the sub-scale and higher order domains of the popular SF-36 quality-of-life assessment tool. This instrument allows the measurement of not only the eight sub-scale dimensions described, but also physical health and mental health component scores based on combination of sub-scales results.

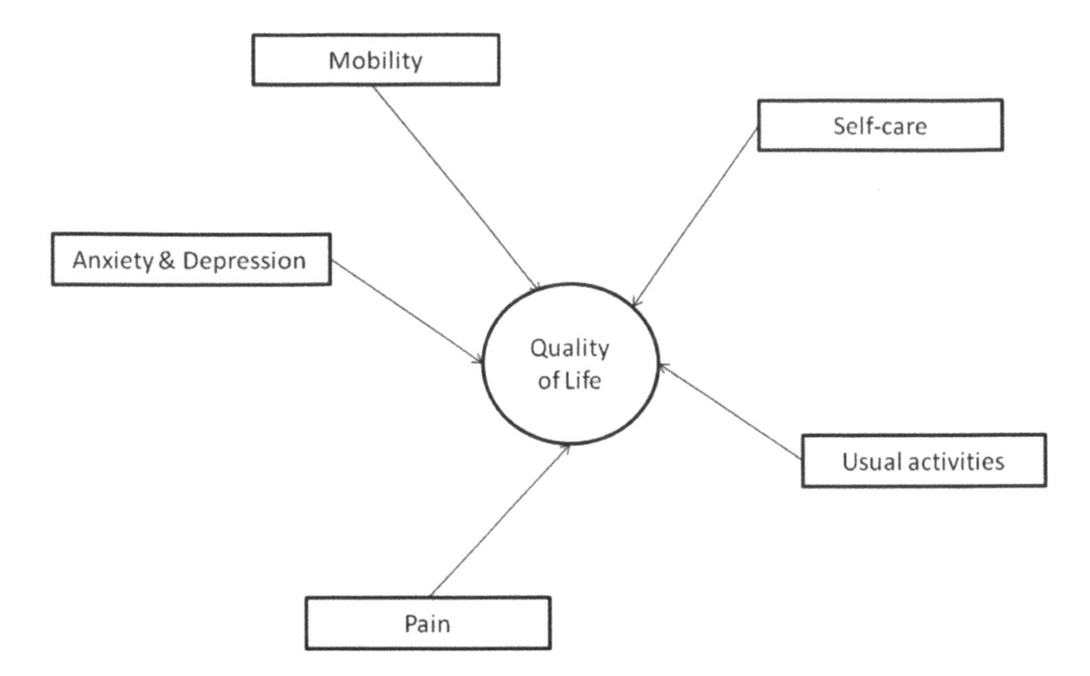

FIGURE 5.2 This figure illustrates the sub-scale domains of the EuroQol EQ-5D quality-of-life assessment tool. This is a quick, accurate and easy to administer quality-of-life assessment tool, covering key dimensions which are of important relevance to palliative care patients.

minimal reliability standards. Validity was also assessed using inter-item correlations, criterion validity and factor analysis. When comparing 14 of the 17 factors, a correlation of greater than 0.70 was shown. The measure showed acceptable to very good reliability and validity (Locker & Lübbe, 2015; Mystakidou et al., 2004).

The Assessment of Quality of Life at the End of Life (AQEL) was developed for people who had cancer and were receiving palliative care. It is made up of 19 questions measuring physical, psychological, social, existential (ability to do what you want, meaningfulness, ability to feel joy), medical/care and global domains of QOL (Axelsson & Sjödén, 1998). Each of the 19 items is measured using a linear analogue scale from 0 to 10. It is considered to be a brief but comprehensive specific measure (Henoch et al., 2010). Two studies were conducted with small samples (37 and 71). The existential domain was seen as strongly related to global QOL, and QOL ratings became lower during the final six weeks of life (Axelsson & Sjödén, 1998). While the measure was described as valid and reliable, the domains within the measure were not supported by factor analysis; the social domain did not correlate well with similar domains from comparable measures, and it was recommended that the measure should be viewed as 19 single items. A further recommendation was for further trials with larger sample sizes (Axelsson & Sjödén, 1998; Henoch et al., 2010). A further validation study, with a sample of 106 people, found low internal consistency with the social domain within the 20-item version of the scale (dyspnoea item included for the study). The study confirmed that correlations with comparable measures were found for all domains, but that healthcare issues and physical and medical/healthcare worked best as individual items (Henoch et al., 2010).

The Spitzer Quality of Life Index (SQLI) is made up of five items scored on a 0–2 scale and was specifically designed for assessing clinical programmes within palliative care. The scale takes on average one minute to complete. Activity, daily living, health, support from family/friends and outlook make up the five items on the scale (Spitzer et al., 1981). In subsequent studies, the scale has demonstrated higher than acceptable levels of reliability and good content and convergent validity (Addington-Hall et al., 1990).

The European Organisation for Research and Treatment of Cancer Quality of Life (EORTC QLQ-C30) questionnaire has been used, but this measure is not specifically designed for people receiving palliative care (Scott et al., 2008).

NUTRITION, NUTRITIONAL INTERVENTIONS AND QUALITY OF LIFE

A search was conducted of the electronic databases CINAHL, MEDLINE, PsycINFO and the British Nursing Index using the following search terms: 'nutrition AND palliative care AND quality of life'. This search strategy identified 24 sources. A hand search found a further three sources relating to nutrition and quality of care. Only four of the sources accessed related directly to nutritional intake, palliative care and QOL effects. The sources not directly relating to nutritional intake, palliative care and QOL effects included people within samples who were diagnosed as having cancer, but it was not clearly identified if or how many people within the sample were receiving or went on to receive palliative care. There also appears to be a crossover within the literature that palliative care is also end-of-life care. The literature suggests that end-of-life care occurs anywhere between two months and 48 hours prior to death (DoH, 2008), and although end-of-life care may be part of palliative care, these two concepts are distinctly different; this is reflected in their definitions. These sources, for the most part, were not included within this section; where they have been included, uncertainty about the numbers of the sample receiving palliative care is indicated. The confounding effect of survival time on QOL is potentially significant, as indicated in the two studies that follow, and so including studies where clients may be receiving curative treatment is likely to influence the conclusions drawn regarding the findings from studies measuring nutritional and QOL outcomes.

Since this original search was conducted, 51 further studies have been published that meet the search terms of 'nutrition AND palliative care AND quality of life'. Of these, seven studies directly explore the issue of nutrition, palliative care and QOL as interconnected features. A small number of studies explored neonatal intensive care and the withdrawal of artificial nutrition and hydration (Hellmann et al., 2013; Larcher, 2013). These studies discuss nutrition, palliative care and QOL from a much different perspective than nutrition, palliative care and QOL in an adult population. Neonatal clinicians sometimes need to have conversations regarding withdrawing or withholding nutrients to provide comfort and relieve pain and suffering (Larcher, 2013), whereas much of the conversation facing clinicians in an adult population is to promote consumption of nutrients to optimize QOL and comfort (Mailhot Vega et al., 2016; Pazart et al., 2014; Saiki et al., 2016).

The distinction between end-of-life care and palliative care has not been resolved in the intervening years since this chapter was first published; the term *end of life* remains ambiguous, and patients can survive for a period ranging from a few months to a few days, with little ability by the caregivers and clinical professionals to predict the length of survival (Orrevall, 2015), making the distinction between end-of-life care and palliative care difficult. Sources in which the distinction was not clear were not included within this section.

There is an assumed link between weight loss, weight stability and QOL; this association has been confirmed in studies. In samples where nutritional status and weight loss have been stabilised, resulting in an increase in length of time of survival, there have been consequent comparative increases in QOL. Home parenteral nutrition was found to maintain the nutritional status of 69 people with advanced cancer. Survival ranged from 1 to 14 months, and a third of people in the sample survived for more than seven months (Bozzetti et al., 2002). QOL was measured using the Rotterdam Symptom Checklist Questionnaire at the start of the home parenteral nutrition intervention, then after the first month and then monthly. Fluctuations in scores showed that QOL scores stabilised at the first month and continued until two months prior to death. Only those people who survived more than three months benefitted from the stabilisation of nutritional status and QOL (Bozzetti et al., 2002). A similar association was found by Davidson et al. (2004). They divided a sample of 107 people with unresectable pancreatic cancer into two independent groups depending on the amount of weight loss after completing a nutritional intervention of oral supplements, food diaries and support for eight weeks. From post hoc scores from the European Organisation for Research and Treatment of Cancer Quality of Life questionnaire, comparison between the two groups showed an association between weight stabilisation, longer survival and higher QOL scores. Self-monitoring of nutritional intake for people with the digestive complications of pancreatic cancer was seen as being of limited value in this study.

The nutritional impact of dietary advice/counselling and dietary advice plus protein supplements was compared to usual nutritional intake in a group of people with colo-rectal cancer. The group of 111 was randomly assigned to one of the three groups, and QOL was measured using the European Organisation for Research and Treatment of Cancer Quality of Life questionnaire. Energy uptake and nutritional status improved in the first two groups; there was proportionate improvement in QOL scores for the people in these two groups. Benefits to nutritional intake, energy levels and QOL were maintained for a period of three months in the dietary advice/counselling group compared to the other two groups (Ravasco et al., 2005). This pattern of findings was only partially confirmed in a meta-analysis reviewing the results of five trials of dietary counselling with a pooled sample of 388 people (Halfdanarson et al., 2008). An overall statistically significant benefit on QOL was not found in all five studies. Three studies showed benefits and two showed no benefit from dietary advice/counselling. The authors concluded that dietary intake did have positive clinical outcomes and is a justifiable intervention, but that the findings of the review could not confirm any significant relationship between dietary advice/counselling and improvements in QOL.

Specific N-3 polyunsaturated fatty acids nutritional supplements have been found to stabilize weight and lead to improvements in QOL (Marin Caro et al., 2007). These benefits have been found in people in cachexic states. Stabilisation and/or improvements in QOL were proportionate to weight gain. The immunomodulating effects of these supplements were seen to produce benefits of improved immune function and mediate the metabolic effects and processes associated with tumour growth and development. These benefits required three weeks of oral supplementation at adequate levels to ensure sufficient concentrations are achieved (Marin Caro et al., 2007). Calorie intake, protein, calcium, iron, zinc, selenium, thiamine, riboflavin and niacin were all positively correlated with QOL in 285 people with stomach cancer. The study also confirmed that better nutritional status was associated with improved QOL (Tian & Chen, 2005).

Enteral and parenteral nutrition was found to be beneficial in maintaining or improving nutritional status, leading to increases in body composition and mass and providing consequent improvements in QOL (Bozzetti et al., 2002), particularly in people with advanced incurable cancer with associated nutrition malnutrition (Marin Caro et al., 2007). Those on home enteral nutrition report lower QOL than the general population during treatment, especially those who have cancer and are over the age of 45 years (Schneider et al., 2000). Survival time has been linked to the level of QOL within people who receive palliative care; many of the studies do not include assumed or real survival time as a potential influential variable in the assessment of QOL. Similarly, the characteristics of people within the studies were heterogeneous in terms of cancer, goals of treatment received and tumour stage. The lack of homogeneity within the people and stage of cancer in these studies means that this review provides only limited and general clues as to the effects of nutritional status on QOL and its relationship to people receiving palliative care.

APPLICATION TO OTHER AREAS OF HEALTH AND DISEASE

There are two key findings from the studies included within this chapter that are applicable to other areas of health and disease. First, nutritional support stabilises and sometimes increases weight. This, in turn, provides people with the energy to help them fulfil their physical, social and psychological functioning and goals, which have a proportionate positive effect on QOL. These findings have particular relevance in other conditions, not necessarily where palliative care is being delivered, but where there is a risk of under-nourishment and/or gastric tract compromise, such as recovery from complex surgery, injury, neurological conditions and cognitive functioning problems such as dementia. Second, QOL is the only indicator that encompasses a range of physical, social and psychological domains. In twenty-first century healthcare, where the emphasis is on person-centred and individualised healthcare, and in communities where people are living with long-term health conditions that would have previously resulted in death, QOL provides health organisations with an ideally suited outcome measure for planning, targeting and evaluating health interventions.

Issues regarding QOL for children and adolescents receiving palliative care have not been considered within this chapter. Issues regarding the complex effects of the disease process and treatment, nutritional support and the physical, psychological and social functioning needs of the child are similar to those of adults. There are added complexities such as parental support, the goals of treatment and parental decision-making. These issues render the findings from studies included here only partially relevant.

KEY FACTS: DEFINITIONS

Body mass index (BMI): A recognised measure of total body mass and body fat. The calculation involves dividing weight in kilogrammes by the square of height in metres. There is a criterion against which people can compare their final BMI to see if they are underweight, normal weight, overweight, obese or morbidly obese.

Cachexia: A condition of severe debilitation and loss of body mass. Characterised by significant weight loss, muscle atrophy and loss of energy the process also includes a metabolic abnormality where the body breaks down its own tissues. The condition is often linked to metabolic processes arising from specific disease conditions such as "cancer cachexia."

Digestive tract: The alimentary canal is the tract that passes from the mouth to the anus and traverses through the major organs that break down the foods into a form that can be absorbed as nutrients or waste products by the body.

Enteral nutrition: The process of providing shorter-term nutritional support for people who have a functioning gastric tract but are unable to swallow. Nutrition is delivered directly into the stomach either through a nasogastric tube or through a tube that is inserted directly into the stomach via an incision in the abdominal wall.

Nutrition: The provision of essential nutrients and chemicals usually in the form of food or food supplements in digestible form for use by the body for its effective functioning.

Nutritional advice/counselling: Any form of intervention that includes the provision of information directly to the person or carer with the purpose of altering/improving suitable nutritional intake.

Parenteral nutrition: The process of providing longer-term nutritional support for people who do not have a functioning gastric tract and who require nutrition to be delivered through a non-alimentary route. Nutrition is delivered via central and/or peripheral veins depending on the length of time required to provide nutrition through this route.

SUMMARY POINTS

- Palliative care is concerned with treatments other than non-curative treatment. Treatments within the sphere of palliative care have the aims of optimising comfort, reducing the side effects of treatment and maintaining quality of life. People experiencing chronic cardiac failure, renal disease, neurological conditions and cancer receive palliative care.

- End-of-life care refers to treatment that is provided during the last two months to hours of life and can be part of palliative care but is not the same as palliative care.
- The metabolic processes associated with specific disease processes and the direct physical effects of both the disease process and side effects of treatment can lead to malnutrition; other serious wasting conditions such as cachexia are common in people who receive palliative care.
- There is a sound clinical rationale for maintaining weight and nutritional intake. These are important elements of palliative care and can help to alleviate some of the metabolic and other physical effects of the disease process and treatment.
- QOL is a concept that when applied to people receiving palliative care covers all aspects of a person's physical, mental, spiritual and psychological functioning. It is a suitable measure for planning and evaluating outcomes for people receiving palliative care.
- A number of general and specific QOL measures have been developed for measuring the QOL of people receiving palliative care. The specific measures include spiritual, existential and family/friend support – three domains considered to be important and specific to palliative care.
- Weight stabilisation achieved through nutrition is key to maintaining physical, social and psychological well-being, and these outcomes have a proportional effect on improvements in QOL.
- Many studies include people with cancer and do not specifically include only those receiving palliative care so the findings of these studies do not provide definitive ideas about how nutritional intervention influences the QOL of people receiving palliative care. In the small number of studies including only people receiving palliative care, perceived or real length of survival influences QOL outcomes. This is a key factor, and its influence can only be understood from studies where people are receiving palliative care.

LIST OF ABBREVIATIONS

BMI Body Mass Index
DoH Department of Health
EN Enteral Nutrition
HPN Home Parenteral Nutrition
NICE National Institute of Health and Clinical Excellence
ONS Oral Nutritional Supplements
TPN Total Parenteral Nutrition
WHO World Health Organisation

REFERENCES

Addington-Hall, J., MacDonald, L., & Anderson, H. 1990. Can the Spitzer Quality of Life Index help to reduce prognostic uncertainty in terminal care? *British Journal of Cancer*, 62(4): 695–699.

Aita, K., Miyata, H., Takahashi, M., & Kai, I. 2008. Japanese physicians' practice of withholding and withdrawing mechanical ventilation and artificial nutrition and hydration from older adults with very severe stroke. *Archives of Gerontology and Geriatrics*, 46(3): 263–272.

Arends, J., Bachmann, P., Baracos, V., Barthelemy, N., Bertz, H., Bozzetti, F., … Preiser, J.-C. 2017. ESPEN guidelines on nutrition in cancer patients. *Clinical Nutrition*, 36(1): 11–48.

Argilés, J. M., Busquets, S., García-Martínez, C., & López-Soriano, F. J. 2005. Mediators involved in the cancer anorexia cachexia syndrome: Past, present, and future. *Nutrition*, 21(9): 977–985.

Axelsson, B. & Sjödén, P.-O. 1998. Quality of life of cancer patients and their spouses in palliative home care. *Palliative Medicine*, 12(1): 29–39.

Baldwin, C. & Weekes, C. E. 2009. Dietary advice for illness-related malnutrition in adults (Review). *The Cochrane Library*, Issue 1.

Bozzetti, F., Cozzaglio, L., Biganzoli, E., Chiavenna, G., De Cicco, M., Donati, D., ... Pironi, L. 2002. Quality of life and length of survival in advanced cancer patients on home parenteral nutrition. *Clinical Nutrition*, 21(4): 281–288.

Coons, S. J., Rao, S., Keininger, D. L., & Hays, R. D. 2000. A comparative review of generic quality-of-life instruments. *Pharmacoeconomics*, 17(1): 13–35.

Davidson, W., Ash, S., Capra, S., & Bauer, J. 2004. Weight stabilisation is associated with improved survival duration and quality of life in unresectable pancreatic cancer. *Clinical Nutrition*, 23(2): 239–247.

Department of Health. 2008. *End of Life Care Strategy—Promoting High-Quality Care for All Adults at the End of Life*. London: Department of Health.

Di Giulio, P., Toscani, F., Villani, D., Brunelli, C., Gentile, S., & Spadin, P. 2008. Dying with advanced dementia in long-term care geriatric institutions: A retrospective study. *Journal of Palliative Medicine*, 11(7): 1023–1028.

Etkind, S., Bone, A., Gomes, B., Lovell, N., Evans, C., Higginson, I., & Murtagh, F. 2017. How many people will need palliative care in 2040? Past trends, future projections and implications for services. *BMC Medicine*, 15(1): 102.

EuroQoL Group. 1990. EuroQoL—A new facility for the measurement of health-related quality of life. *Health Policy*, 16(3): 199–208.

Evans, W. J., Morley, J. E., Argilés, J., Bales, C., Baracos, V., Guttridge, D., ... Mantovani, G. 2008. Cachexia: A new definition. *Clinical Nutrition*, 27(6): 793–799.

Gavin, N. C., Button, E., Keogh, S., McMillan, D., & Rickard, C. 2017. Does parenteral nutrition increase the risk of catheter-related bloodstream infection? A systematic literature review. *Journal of Parenteral and Enteral Nutrition*, 41(6): 918–928.

Gellrich, N.-C., Handschel, J., Holtmann, H., & Krüskemper, G. 2015. Oral cancer malnutrition impacts weight and quality of life. *Nutrients*, 7(4): 2145–2160.

Halfdanarson, T. R., Thordardottir, E. O., West, C. P., & Jatoi, A. 2008. Does dietary counseling improve quality of life in cancer patients? A systematic review and meta-analysis. *Journal of Supportive Oncology*, 6: 234–237.

Hanks, G., Cherny, N., Christakas, N., Fallon, M., Kaasa, S., & Portenoy, R. 2011. *Oxford Textbook of Palliative Medicine*, 4th ed. University Press Oxford, Oxford.

Harrison, S. 2014. Leadership Alliance for the Care of Dying People, One Chance to Get It Right: Improving People's Experience of Care in the Last Few Days and Hours of Life. London: LACDP, 2014, Publications Gateway Reference 01509. *Health and Social Care Chaplaincy*, 2(1): 146–148.

Hellmann, J., Williams, C., Ives-Baine, L., & Shah, P. S. 2013. Withdrawal of artificial nutrition and hydration in the Neonatal Intensive Care Unit: Parental perspectives. *Archives of Disease in Childhood, Fetal and Neonatal Edition*, 98(1): F21–F25.

Henoch, I., Axelsson, B., & Bergman, B. 2010. The Assessment of Quality of life at the End of Life (AQEL) questionnaire: A brief but comprehensive instrument for use in patients with cancer in palliative care. *Quality of Life Research*, 19(5): 739–750.

Hickson, M. & Frost, G. 2004. An investigation into the relationships between quality of life, nutritional status and physical function. *Clinical Nutrition*, 23(2): 213–221.

Hildebrand, A. J. 2000. Masked intentions: The masquerade of killing thoughts used to justify dehydrating and starving people in a persistent vegetative state and people with other profound neurological impairments. *Issues in Law and Medicine*, 16(2): 143–165.

Hughes, N. & Neal, R. D. 2000. Adults with terminal illness: A literature review of their needs and wishes for food. *Journal of Advanced Nursing*, 32(5): 1101–1107.

Kaasa, S. & Loge, J. H. 2003. Quality of life in palliative care: Principles and practice. *Palliative Medicine*, 17(1): 11–20.

Karnofsky, D. & Burchenal, J. 1949. The clinical evaluation of chemotherapeutic agents in cancer. In C. Macleod (Ed.), *Evaluation of Chemotherapeutic Agents* (pp. 199–205). Columbia University Press, New York.

Kir, S. & Spiegelman, B. M. 2016. Cachexia and brown fat: A burning issue in cancer. *Trends in Cancer*, 2(9): 461–463.

Kutner, J. 2005. Terminal care: The last weeks of life. *Journal of Palliative Medicine*, 8(5): 1040–1041.

Larcher, V. 2013. Ethical considerations in neonatal end-of-life care. *Seminars in Fetal and Neonatal Medicine*, 18(2): 105–110.

LCP. 2008. Liverpool Care Pathway for the Dying Patient. Marie Curie Palliative Care Institute. www.mcpcil.org.uk

Locker, L. S., & Lübbe, A. S. 2015. Quality of life in palliative care: An analysis of quality-of-life assessment. *Progress in Palliative Care*, 23(4): 208–219.

Mailhot Vega, R., Zullig, L., Wassung, A., Walters, D., Berland, N., Du, K. L., ... Schiff, P. B. 2016. Food as medicine: A randomized controlled trial (RCT) of home delivered, medically tailored meals (HDMTM) on quality of life (QoL) in metastatic lung and non-colorectal GI cancer patients. *Journal of Clinical Oncology*, 34(29): 155.

Marin Caro, M. M., Laviano, A., & Pichard, C. 2007. Nutritional intervention and quality of life in adult oncology patients. *Clinical Nutrition*, 26(3): 289–301.

Mehanna, H., Nankivell, P. C., Moledina, J., & Travis, J. 2009. Refeeding syndrome—Awareness, prevention and management. *Head and Neck Oncology*, 1(1): 4.

Morita, T., Miyashita, M., Shibagaki, M., Hirai, K., Ashiya, T., Ishihara, T., ... Nakashima, N. 2006. Knowledge and beliefs about end-of-life care and the effects of specialized palliative care: A population-based survey in Japan. *Journal of Pain and Symptom Management*, 31(4): 306–316.

Mystakidou, K., Tsilika, E., Kouloulias, V., Parpa, E., Katsouda, E., Kouvaris, J., & Vlahos, L. 2004. The "Palliative Care Quality of Life Instrument (PQLI)" in terminal cancer patients. *Health and Quality of Life Outcomes*, 2(1): 8.

National Institute for Health and Care Excellence (NICE). 2006, updated 2017. Clinical guideline 32: Nutrition support for adults: oral nutrition support, enteral tube feeding and parenteral nutrition. https://www.nice.org.uk/CG032NICEguideline

Neuberger, J., Guthrie, C., & Aaronovitch, D. 2013. *More Care, Less Pathway: A Review of the Liverpool Care Pathway*. London: Department of Health.

Nursing Midwifery Council. 2010. *Standards for Pre-Registration Nursing Education*. London: NMC.

Oliver, J., Huxley, P., & Bridges, K. 1996. *Quality of Life and Mental Health Services*. London: Routledge.

Orrevall, Y. 2015. Nutritional support at the end of life. *Nutrition*, 31(4): 615–616.

Pais-Ribeiro, J. 2004. Quality of life is a primary end-point in clinical settings. *Clinical Nutrition*, 23(1): 121–130.

Pazart, L., Cretin, E., Grodard, G., Cornet, C., Mathieu-Nicot, F., Bonnetain, F., ... Aubry, R. 2014. Parenteral nutrition at the palliative phase of advanced cancer: The ALIM-K study protocol for a randomized controlled trial. *Trials*, 15(1): 370.

Pittiruti, M., Hamilton, H., Biffi, R., MacFie, J., & Pertkiewicz, M. 2009. ESPEN Guidelines on Parenteral Nutrition: Central venous catheters (access, care, diagnosis and therapy of complications). *Clinical Nutrition*, 28(4): 365–377.

Pols, J. & Limburg, S. 2016. A matter of taste? Quality of life in day-to-day living with ALS and a feeding tube. *Culture, Medicine, and Psychiatry*, 40(3): 361–382.

Ravasco, P., Monteiro-Grillo, I., Vidal, P. M., & Camilo, M. E. 2005. Dietary counseling improves patient outcomes: A prospective, randomized, controlled trial in colorectal cancer patients undergoing radiotherapy. *Journal of Clinical Oncology*, 23(7): 1431–1438.

Ruggeri, M., Bisoffi, G., Fontecedro, L., & Warner, R. 2001. Subjective and objective dimensions of quality of life in psychiatric patients: A factor analytical approach. *British Journal of Psychiatry*, 178(3): 268–275.

Saiki, C., Zorzi, J., Stearns, V., & Wolff, A. C. 2016. Piloting survivorship care planning with the metastatic breast cancer patient. *Journal of Clinical Oncology*, 34(29): 146.

Schildmann, J., Doyal, L., Cushing, A., & Vollmann, J. 2006. Decisions at the end of life: An empirical study on the involvement, legal understanding and ethical views of preregistration house officers. *Journal of Medical Ethics*, 32(10): 567–570.

Schneider, S., Pouget, I., Staccini, P., Rampal, P., & Hebuterne, X. 2000. Quality of life in long-term home enteral nutrition patients. *Clinical Nutrition*, 19(1): 23–28.

Scott, N., Fayers, P., Aaronson, N., Bottomley, A., de Graeff, A., Groenvold, M., ... Sprangers, M. 2008. *EORTC QLQ-C30. Reference Values*. Brussels: EORTC.

Sobotka, L., Schneider, S., Berner, Y., Cederholm, T., Krznaric, Z., Shenkin, A., ... Volkert, D. 2009. ESPEN guidelines on parenteral nutrition: Geriatrics. *Clinical Nutrition*, 28(4): 461–466.

Somogyi-Zalud, E., Zhong, Z., Hamel, M. B., & Lynn, J. 2002. The use of life-sustaining treatments in hospitalized persons aged 80 and older. *Journal of the American Geriatrics Society*, 50(5): 930–934.

Spitzer, W. O., Dobson, A. J., Hall, J., Chesterman, E., Levi, J., Shepherd, R., ... Catchlove, B. R. 1981. Measuring the quality of life of cancer patients: A concise QL-index for use by physicians. *Journal of Chronic Diseases*, 34(12): 585–597.

Tian, J. & Chen, J.-S. 2005. Nutritional status and quality of life of the gastric cancer patients in Changle County of China. *World Journal of Gastroenterology*, 11(11): 1582.

Todorovic, V., Russell, C., Stratton, R., Ward, J., & Elia, M. 2003. *The "MUST" Explanatory Booklet: A Guide to the "Malnutrition Universal Screening Tool" ("MUST") for Adults*. British Association for Parenteral and Enteral Nutrition (BAPEN), Redditch.

Vigano, A., Kasvis, P., Di Tomasso, J., Gillis, C., Kilgour, R., & Carli, F. 2017. Pearls of optimizing nutrition and physical performance of older adults undergoing cancer therapy. *Journal of Geriatric Oncology*, 8(6): 428–436.

Ware, J., Snow, K., Kosinski, M., & Gandek, B. 1993. *SF-36 Health Survey Manual and Interpretation Guide*. Boston, MA: The Health Institute, New England Medical Center Hospitals.

Wenhold, F. A. 2017. Nutrition screening: Science behind simplicity. *South African Journal of Clinical Nutrition*, 30(3): 5–6.

World Health Organization (WHO). 2004. *Palliative Care: The Solid Facts*. Geneva, Switzerland: WHO.

6 Refractory Cancer Cachexia

David Blum and Florian Strasser

CONTENTS

INTRODUCTION

Involuntary weight loss is a common consequence of advanced cancer. Cachexia is a paraneoplastic syndrome and a major cause of involuntary weight loss. Cancer cachexia is a metabolic disorder that leads to an ongoing loss of skeletal muscle mass with or without fat mass and a negative protein and energy balance often associated with reduced food intake. In cancer cachexia, not only weight, but also physical functions declines. Cancer cachexia affects patients and their loved ones.

PREVALENCE AND SIGNIFICANCE OF CANCER CACHEXIA

Cancer cachexia and its consequences are among the most common problems of advanced cancer patients (Blum et al. 2014). Depending on the source, the prevalence of cancer cachexia in cancer patients ranges from 24% to 80%. Survival is often limited to a few weeks to months. The difficulty in clinical practice is not only recognizing cancer cachexia and its underlying problems of reduced nutritional intake, but managing cancer cachexia and its consequences like fatigue and decreased physical functioning (Evans et al. 2008). Accompanying symptoms like early satiety, nausea, and dysgeusia are major challenges for the treating healthcare professionals. The emotional and existential burden of the patients and their carers is often underestimated and can be overwhelming.

PHASES

Different phases of cancer cachexia have been proposed (Fearon et al. 2011). Early or pre-cachexia is defined as presenting early clinical and metabolic signs without the presence of significant involuntary weight loss. Cachexia syndrome is reached when weight loss reaches more than 5% or is ongoing. In patients with refractory cachexia, the prognosis of survival is too short to reverse depletion (Figure 6.1).

Multimodal Management of Cachexia

Current management of cancer cachexia includes basic cachexia management, which includes general symptom management that depends on the presence or absence of secondary nutritional impact symptoms and the phase. Pre-cachexia and cachexia demand standard cachexia management including pharmacologic, nutritional, psychological, and physical interventions (Table 6.1). This approach is conceptualized as multimodal therapy, and it is generally accepted that a single intervention cannot reverse cachexia (Fearon 2008).

Refractory Cachexia

The decline of physical function and the decrease of nutritional intake are part of the natural dying process. Therefore, it is paramount in clinical practice in palliative care to identify the point of no return in this decline. If this point of the disease has been diagnosed, cachexia is called *refractory*. There are completely different priorities in treatment of cachexia syndrome and refractory cachexia. The aim of this chapter is to help in the diagnosis of refractory cachexia.

Diagnosing Cachexia

In a Delphi consensus a new definition of cancer cachexia was proposed based on the generic wasting disease definition for chronic illnesses (Evans et al. 2008). The consensus defines cancer cachexia as a multifactorial syndrome defined by an ongoing loss of skeletal muscle mass and a characteristic

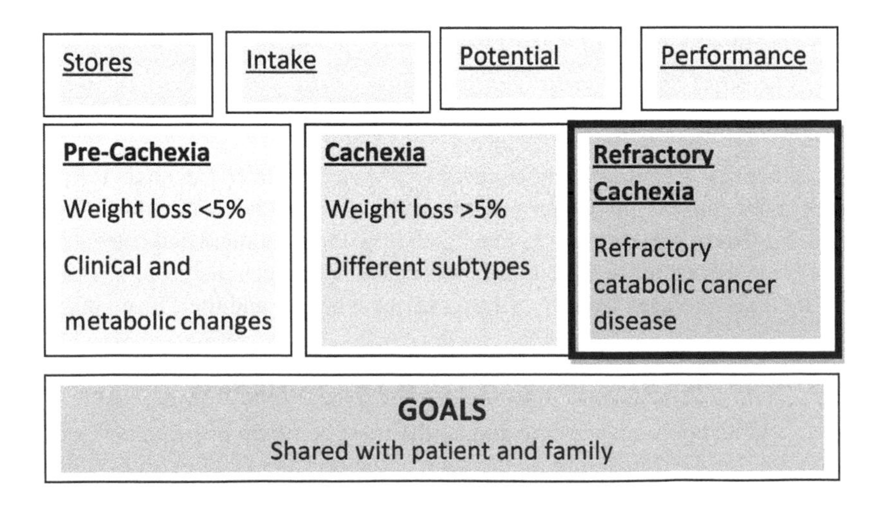

FIGURE 6.1 Stages of cachexia and refractory cachexia.

TABLE 6.1
Multimodal Management According to Cachexia Stage

Pre-Cachexia	Cachexia	Refractory Cachexia
Monitor weight	Multimodal therapy	Symptom control
Prevention	Anticancer therapy	Symptom prevention
	Anti-cachexia therapy	Psychosocial/spiritual care
	Physical therapy	Physical therapy active/passive
	Psychosocial therapy	

Note: Pre-cachexia and cachexia demand standard cachexia management including pharmacological, nutritional, psychological, and physical interventions.

pathophysiology including a negative protein and energy balance, driven by a variable combination of reduced food intake and abnormal metabolism. Cancer cachexia cannot be fully reversed by conventional nutritional support and leads to progressive functional impairment.

Four domains are used to assess cancer cachexia:

- Stores
- Intake
- Potential
- Performance

TABLE 6.2
Assessment According to Cachexia Domain

	Basic	Specialists
	Storage	
Weight loss	PG-SGA Module—Weight loss	Weight loss history
Muscle mass loss	Change of mid-arm circumference	Native CT L4
	Intake	
Eating-related symptoms	PG-SGA presence of symptoms	Symptom quantitative scale
Nutritional intake	PG-SGA Module – Intake	1–2 day record (kcal, protein)
Secondary causes for decreased intake	PG-SGA Module – Presence NIS	Secondary-NIS quantitative scale
	Potential	
Tumor catabolic activity	Presence of anticancer treatment	Tumor type, activity, response
Inflammation	Clinical signs	C-reactive protein
	Performance	
Muscle strength	KPS	Chair raise time, get up and go
Physical functioning	KPS	Subjective, mobility checklist
Psychosocial adaptation	Single-item question	Cachexia-related suffering

Note: A set of key variables used to describe different phases of cancer cachexia, as a minimal data set and helps in terms of a clinical decision-guiding instrument to introduce or improve cancer cachexia treatment accordingly.

Abbreviations: CT, computed tomography; KPS, Karnofsky Performance Status; PG-SGA, patient-generated subjective global assessment; S-NISs, secondary nutritional intake symptoms.

The assessment of these four domains is designed for use as a screening tool to detect patients with cancer cachexia. It defines a set of key variables used to describe different phases of cancer cachexia, as a minimal data set, and helps in terms of a clinical decision-guiding instrument to introduce or improve cancer cachexia treatment accordingly (Table 6.2).

Pre-cachexia, as a condition with no or very little weight loss (less than 5% of body weight loss in six months), is associated with anorexia, inflammation, and/or metabolic changes. These patients are at risk for progression to the cachexia syndrome. Therefore, pre-cachectic patients are the target group for cachexia prevention and intervention trials. Patients with greater than 5% weight loss in the last six months or with body mass index (BMI) less than 20 kg/m^2 and ongoing weight loss greater than 2% are considered to be cachectic. Furthermore, in obese patients, muscle loss can be masked by fat or fluid mass loss (Tan et al. 2009).

DIAGNOSING REFRACTORY CACHEXIA

Refractory cachexia is diagnosed clinically. Cachexia becomes refractory if the underlying disease is far advanced, rapidly progressive, and unresponsive to treatment, and the catabolism increased so that weight loss management is not possible or indicated. Refractory cachexia can often only be diagnosed after a defined treatment attempt. Diagnosing refractory cachexia is close to diagnosing dying. However, the symptoms associated with cachexia (i.e., anorexia, weight loss) are often used to diagnose approaching death even when cachexia is potentially still treatable. In general, the dying patient becomes bedbound, does not swallow food or drugs, and is comatose or semi-comatose. But all of these symptoms are ambiguous and can occur in non-dying patients as well. Many different prognostication tools have been developed and validated (Simmons et al. 2017). However, the clinical judgement is still the most important factor (Fairchild et al. 2014).

Several classification systems have been investigated. In an early system, the final classification into stages was left to clinical judgement (Vigano et al. 2012), but then it was further developed (Vigano et al. 2017). Another classification used a cluster analysis and proved the relevance of a classification system (Wallengren et al. 2013). In clinical practice, the use of the proposed domains of cachexia has proven to be helpful.

STORES

Weight loss is a key feature of cachexia. With weight loss above 5% the definition is reached (Martin et al. 2010). Due to an increase of adiposity in our population, weight loss can be substantial even when a normal BMI is still present. Weight loss measured by a scale is an easy-to-measure surrogate marker for the cachexia-defining muscle loss, because there is no clear consensus on how to assess muscle loss in clinical practice. However, a variety of methods are applicable: muscle loss can be assessed by clinical judgment, mid-arm circumference measurement, computed tomography (CT) scan of the lumbar spine, magnetic resonance imaging (MRI) or dual X-ray absorptiometry (DEXA), and bioimpedance analysis. If muscle loss exceeds 10% of muscle mass, the likelihood of refractory cachexia is strong.

INTAKE

Social retreat and refusal of food are further common signs of approaching death. Living without food is possible up to three months and death occurs due to protein homeostasis. Anorexia per se does not define refractory cachexia, because it can often be surmounted by conscious control of eating. Intake can be impaired by a variety of symptoms other than anorexia. Epidemiology studies support correlations between symptoms and weight loss (Teunissen et al. 2007). Symptoms like mucositis and constipation occur frequently in advanced cancer. Other factors can impair the integrity from mouth to anus and act as secondary causes of impaired nutritional intake (secondary nutritional intake symptoms [S-NISs]). Further, S-NISs involve shortness of breath, pain, fatigue, or depression and may also contribute to cachexia (Omlin et al. 2013). The predominance of secondary nutrition intake symptoms is inversely related with refractory cachexia. Such S-NISs are treatable and potentially reversible. If there is severe structural or functional damage to the gastrointestinal tract, parenteral nutrition can be introduced if the treatment is monitored closely and a goal is defined.

Potential

The tumor per se is the main influence on survival, because high tumor activity and unresponsiveness to antitumor treatment are key features of a poor prognosis. Even though estimation of prognosis in a specific case is very difficult, stage and tumor types are predictive. C-reactive protein (CRP) as a marker for the inflammatory response in cancer has been proved to be prognostic for survival (Pantano et al. 2016). In the absence of infections, CRP can be a useful prognostication marker. Although a specific threshold for refractory cachexia is not defined, measurements above 150 mg/L are associated with high catabolic drive. Because of the potential influence of other underlying conditions (i.e., ongoing infection), it should never be used on its own. However, repetitive measurements can strengthen its prognostic value.

Performance

To estimate the impact of cachexia on patients' physical functioning, routine assessment of physical activity is recommended. The method of choice is patient-reported physical functioning (e.g., EORTCQLQ-C30, patient- completed Eastern Cooperative Oncology Group [ECOG]). Other methods may be physician reported (e.g., Karnofsky Score) or objective methodologies (e.g., activity meter, checklists of specific activities). Low performance status is strongly associated with refractory cachexia, but possible reversible causes (like delirium, depression, etc.) must be excluded first. Decrease of hand grip strength has been proven to be prognostic (Kilgour et al. 2013). For the assessment of psychosocial impact of cancer cachexia, a single screening question such as, 'How much do you feel distressed about your inability to eat?' is proposed. The Functional Assessment of Anorexia/Cachexia Therapy (FAACT) scale involves questions about psychosocial impact also (Ribaudo et al. 2000). Cachexia-related distress can arise as long as cachexia persists and resolve close to death due to other priorities. Not only weight loss, appetite loss and loss of function are distressing, likewise the change of body image adds to suffering (Rhondali et al. 2015). The assessment and treatment of cachexia-related suffering (CRS) are described in a separate chapter in this book.

TREATMENT

Palliative Cancer Care

For careful decision-making in palliative care, the patient with cancer cachexia must be assessed. Decision-making leads to the definition of a common intervention goal in general, and it is paramount to ensure that the patient and the family understand and share these goals. Decision-making is based on adequate communication. Antineoplastic therapy can reduce the catabolic stimulus of the tumor and ameliorate cachexia (Giordano and Jatoi 2005). However, side effects from antineoplastic therapy can also aggravate symptoms. High catabolism can be reduced by antineoplastic therapies. Slow tumor progression due to tumor characteristics or chemotherapy with palliative intention does not necessarily lead to catabolism and can be overcome by nutritional interventions. An attempt to increase nutritional intake is warranted if refractory cachexia is not proven. Secondary nutritional impact symptoms are actively searched and treated. Conscious control of eating habits is fundamental to any nutritional intervention. Enriched nutrition like protein drinks is commonly used. Taste preferences may vary between patients and in a patient over time. If there is a severe structural barrier in the upper gastrointestinal tract, a percutaneous endoscopic gastrostomy (PEG) tube may be the device of choice in this situation. In severe structural or functional barriers in the intestines, as seen in chronic subileus due to peritoneal metastasis, parenteral nutrition may be preferable. Patients should be monitored for signs of refeeding syndrome. An evaluation after 10–14 days with measurement of pre-/albumin is indicated. If there is an increase in these parameters in the absence of complications, total parenteral nutrition (TPN) is continued and evaluated over time. However, with such interventions, weight gain is not the target outcome, due to interference with fluid retention. Muscle mass, physical function, and well-being should improve if an attempt to improve nutritional intake is undertaken. If anticancer treatment and nutritional interventions do not reach their predefined goals, refractory cachexia is evident. In refractory cachexia, therapeutic interventions have to focus on alleviating symptoms and avoiding complications and side effects (Figure 6.2).

Treatment of Refractory Cachexia

Nutritional Interventions

In refractory cachexia, TPN should be stopped because the additional supply of calories in this situation is no longer effective and causes only side effects. All efforts by the nutritionist to increase nutritional intake including behavioral interventions (conscious control of eating) should be reduced. Patients and their families are comprehensively informed that loss of appetite at this stage is often observed and attempts to force-feed the patient are futile. Possibilities of sharing other than sharing meals should be explained, for instance massages, reading, or listening to music.

Pharmacologic Interventions

In refractory cachexia, it is important that pharmacologic treatment does not replace other modes of care, that is, psychological, social, or spiritual. A few drugs can play a role in alleviation of symptoms.

Corticosteroids

Corticosteroids improve appetite, oral food intake, and well-being in patients with advanced cancer. They are widely used to alleviate symptoms in refractory cachexia. Their exact mechanism of action

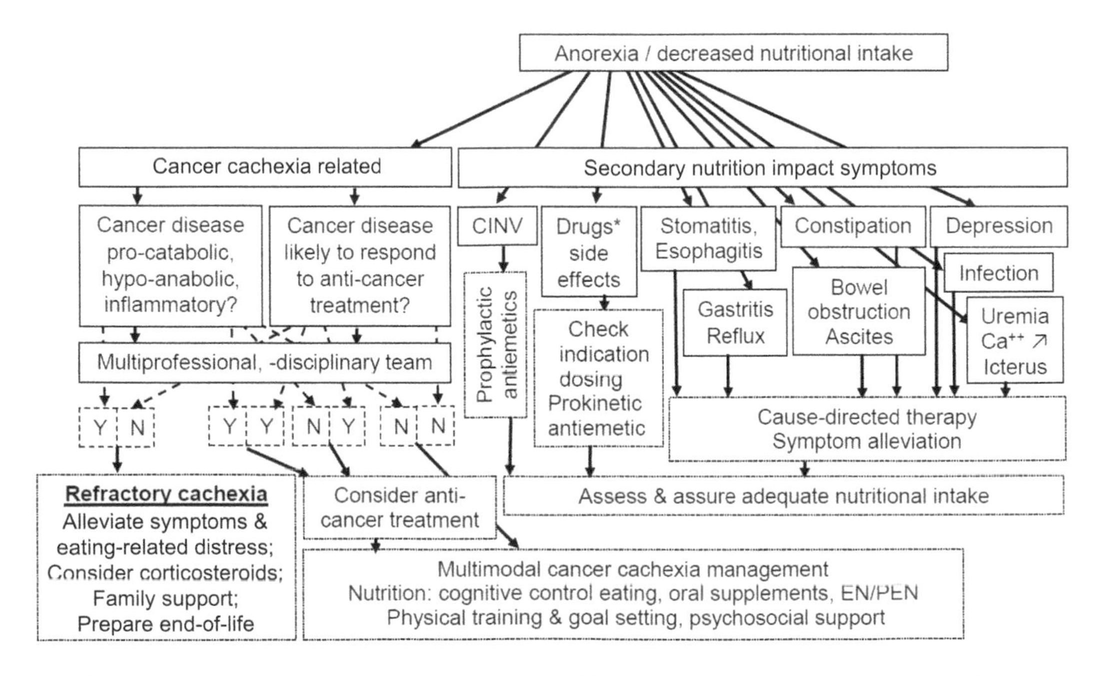

FIGURE 6.2 Cachexia treatment tree. (*Abbreviations:* CINV, Echemotherapy-induced nausea and vomiting; EN, enteral nutrition; N, no; PEN, parenteral nutrition; Y, yes.)

is unclear, but their effects on mood are well known. An interaction with orexigenic hormones in the hypothalamus is discussed. Several studies have shown improvements in appetite, food intake, and quality of life in advanced cancer patients taking corticosteroids. A meta-analysis summarizes six double-blind randomized controlled trials (Yavuzsen 2005). Study duration ranges from 6 to 12 weeks and doses from 300 to 1200 mg methylprednisolone. However, in five of six studies, benefits were dismissed over time (Metz et al. 1989). Due to their broad effect, corticosteroids have a wide range of negative side effects like muscle myopathy, insulin resistance, and immune suppression. Adrenal insufficiency due to withdrawal can occur. Corticosteroids are recommended to alleviate symptoms in refractory cachexia for a short time.

Antidepressant 5-HT-Antagonists

Antidepressants are widely used in advanced cancer. Appetite gain is a common side effect of antidepressants. A study with mirtazapine in patients with advanced cancer showed appetite stimulation (Riechelmann et al. 2009). The atypical neuroleptic drug olanzapine, used in anorexia nervosa, stimulated cachectic patients' appetite and raised ghrelin levels in a phase I study (Braiteh et al. 2008).

Progestins

Synthetic progestagens have been used in the treatment of hormone-sensitive tumors. Due to their side effects, like appetite increase, they were investigated in cancer cachexia. Several prospective controlled randomized trials have been published in a Cochrane meta-analysis (Berenstein and Ortiz 2003). Several randomized controlled trials have shown that progestins improve appetite, caloric intake, and loss of fat tissue in patients with advanced cancer. However, improvements of physical function, fatigue, and lean body mass have not been demonstrated, but there are limited data for the use of progestins in refractory cachexia. Progestins are mainly recommended in cachexia when anorexia is the main cause for suffering after careful patient education. In refractory cachexia, progestins have limited benefit due to the relative overweight of other symptoms. Clinically relevant side effects such as thromboembolic events and edema, and the costs of the therapy have to be taken into account.

Cannabinoids

Throughout history mankind has used extracts from the plant *Cannabis sativa* as a recreational and therapeutical drug. Endocannabinoids are involved in the natural regulation of appetite. The synthetic cannabinoid dronabinol (Delta-9THC) is approved as an antiemetic drug and as an appetite stimulant in HIV wasting. In cancer cachexia, after promising phase II trial results, two large placebo-controlled trials showed no clear improvement in appetite or quality of life (Strasser et al. 2006). Psychological symptoms like confusion and somnolence, and physiological symptoms like tachycardia or hypotension occur in terms of adverse effects. In selected patients with predominantly chronic nausea or anxiety, the use of cannabinoids can be an option.

Prokinetics

Long-acting prokinetics show an effect in patients suffering from chronic nausea, but they do not help in all patients. Still, based on good overall tolerability, prokinetics can be used in refractory cachexia if nausea is a predominant symptom.

Other Agents

Eicosapentaenoic acid (EPA) and cyclo-oxygenase inhibitors play a role in the treatment of cachexia but not in refractory cachexia.

Recent trials showed an increase in appetite and food intake with ghrelin analogues, but the substances did not get approval by European Medicines Agency (EMEA) and the U.S. Food and Drug Administration (FDA) for the treatment of cachexia (Pietra et al. 2014). Careful discussion is needed about which agents should be researched in this vulnerable patient population.

Physical Interventions

Physical activity can influence quality of life and is safe and without negative side effects, even in far advanced cancer (Stene et al. 2013). Two-thirds of patients are interested in physical activity and half of the patients participate in physical training (Lowe et al. 2016). In refractory cachectic patients, especially when they are pre-terminal or dying, activation attempts have to be well-considered; well-being is essential, and more passive interventions like care and massage are more important.

PSYCHOSOCIAL INTERVENTIONS AND EMOTIONAL SUPPORT

In refractory cachexia, patients and families should be carefully educated about the irreversible nature of their disease and be given time for acceptance. Meanwhile, patients and families are supported in finding ways other than sharing a meal to show their love and their care for each other.

APPLICATIONS TO OTHER AREAS OF TERMINAL OR PALLIATIVE CARE

Wasting disease was a major problem in HIV/AIDS patients in the first world and still is in the third world. Since the introduction of triple antiretroviral agents, loss of weight has become reversible in most AIDS patients. Patients who seemed to have refractory cachexia started to gain weight and physical function after having received antiretroviral therapy. Translated into cancer research, this may indicate that along with successful anticancer therapy, cancer cachexia might be resolved. However, there are anticancer therapies that can worsen cachexia per se or increase secondary nutritional impact symptoms and outweigh any benefit. There were anticachectic trials that were positive in AIDS and negative in cancer, challenging the straightforward comparability of these diseases. Wasting and cachexia in other end-stage diseases like advanced chronic obstructive pulmonary disease (COPD), cardiopathy or renal insufficiency have different dynamics than in advanced cancer patients. The point of no return where cachexia becomes refractory might be more difficult to define, because the decline might be slower or the phases of the disease more variable.

PRACTICAL METHODS AND TECHNIQUES

The first step is an active comprehensive multidimensional physical, psychological, social, and spiritual assessment of the patient and his family. This includes a good prognostication process with an estimation of survival and a discussion with the patient and his or her family. Cachexia assessment covers the following four domains.

Stores: A normal calibrated scale is sufficient to measure body weight. Patients should wear usual clothing without shoes. For repeated measurements the same scale should be used. Repeated measurements over time may increase accuracy. In patients with significant fluid retention, large tumor mass or obesity (BMI >30 kg/m^2), significant muscle wasting may occur in the absence of weight loss. In such patients a direct measure of muscularity is recommended. Muscle loss can be measured by an L4/5 native CT scan or DEXA, but the same method should be applied each time.

Intake: Anorexia is usually measured on a visual analogue scale (VAS) (0 no problem, 10 maximal problem). A score greater than 3/10 or impaired oral nutritional intake (less than 75% of normal or less than 20 kcal/kg body weight) is part of the historic definition. Patients' estimation of overall food intake in relation to their normal intake may better reflect the actual amount of food intake, although this can be affected by recollection bias. The capacity to improve food intake by checking causes for simple starvation/secondary nutritional impact symptoms should be an integral part of the assessment. There are several nutritional assessment tools in use. The patient-generated subjective global assessment (PG-SGA) is a frequently used validated method of nutritional assessment. Full nutritional assessment in clinical practice is commonly done using a food diary analyzed by a nutritionist. Other methods such as a digital balance or photographs may also be used. In refractory cachexia patients or proxies, estimation may be sufficient.

Potential: Patients suffering from certain cancer types are more prone to develop cancer cachexia, such as carcinomas from the gastrointestinal tract. Gastrointestinal and head and neck cancers are often associated with secondary nutritional impact symptoms due to disease or therapy. Different tumor dynamics or tumor burden (stable or progressive disease, stage, tumor kinetics, metastasis) have an impact on cachexia. During progressive disease the tumor burden is a driver of increased metabolism and catabolism. A key component of cancer cachexia is this (hyper-) catabolic drive caused by systemic inflammation. CRP proved to be a robust marker to measure systemic inflammation. Sweating and night sweats or fever are a clinical sign.

Performance: A systematic review identified 135 different assessment tools (Helbostad et al. 2009). Simple and frequently used tools are the Karnofsky Performance Status (KPS) scale and ECOG, which are based on a physician's estimation. Patient-reported physical functioning is part of the EORTC-OLQ-C30. Psychosocial impact should be assessed (e.g., items such as 'how much do you feel distressed about your inability to eat?', 'have you experienced feelings of pressure, guilt, or relational distress related to cachexia and weight loss?'). A single question asking about concerns regarding eating or the FAACT may be helpful for screening purposes. A validated tool, however, is lacking to date. Refractory cachexia is suggested by significant weight loss, low intake, and low performance status, and proven by unresponsiveness to anti-cachexia treatment.

Interventions

In refractory cachexia, therapeutic interventions focus on alleviating symptoms and avoiding complications. This often includes discontinuation of anticancer and nutritional treatment. Steroids and antidepressants are commonly used drugs. Pharmacologic treatment becomes less important. Psychosocial counselling at this stage becomes essential. Patients and their families are educated in possibilities of sharing other than taking meals together and supported in finding other ways to care.

ETHICAL ISSUES

Diagnosing refractory cachexia is often a matter of debate. Cultural, religious, or legal issues arise. To admit that therapeutic attempts are no longer beneficial can be difficult for a treating team. Starting a therapeutic attempt is easier than stopping therapeutic attempts like chemotherapy or TPN, because it can be overestimated as a symbol of hope, especially by relatives. Careful education about the nature of the disease and its trajectory prevents conflicts and reduces distress in teams or families.

KEY FACTS: REFRACTORY CACHEXIA

- Cancer cachexia has a big impact on patients and families.
- Assessment of patients involves psychological, social, and spiritual issues.
- Monitor weight and muscle mass.
- Monitor and treat for secondary nutritional impact symptoms.
- Assess tumor dynamics and catabolism, and prognosticate carefully.
- Refractory cachexia is defined by unresponsiveness to anti-cachexia treatment.
- In refractory cachexia interventions alleviate symptoms and suffering.
- Complications are avoided by cessation of futile therapeutic attempts.
- Cachexia-related suffering is assessed and treated.

SUMMARY POINTS

- Cachexia is a paraneoplastic syndrome and is a common cause of involuntary weight loss in advanced cancer.
- Associated symptoms like early satiety, nausea, and dysgeusia can impair nutritional intake. Other symptoms like pain or depression can impair nutritional intake. They are called secondary nutritional impact symptoms and require standardized assessment and management due to their reversibility.
- Manifest cachexia requires both standard management and pharmacologic and nutritional interventions.
- Cachexia becomes refractory if the underlying disease is far advanced, rapidly progressive and unresponsive to treatment, and catabolism so increased that weight loss management is not possible or indicated.
- Refractory cachexia can often only be diagnosed after a defined treatment attempt.
- The emotional and existential burden of the patients and their carers is often underestimated and can be overwhelming.
- In refractory cachexia therapeutic interventions focus on alleviating symptoms and avoiding complications. This often includes discontinuation of nutritional treatment attempts.
- Psychosocial counseling at this stage becomes essential.

ACKNOWLEDGEMENTS

We thank the international cancer cachexia experts, and last but not least we thank our patients.

LIST OF ABBREVIATIONS

BMI	Body Mass Index
COPD	Chronic Obstructive Pulmonary Disease
CPS	Clinical Prediction of Survival
CRP	C-Reactive Protein
DEXA	Dual-Energy X-ray Absorptiometry
ECOG	Eastern Cooperative Oncology Group
FAACT	Functional Assessment of Anorexia/Cachexia Therapy
GI	Gastrointestinal
KPS	Karnofsky Perfomance Status
PG-SGA	Patient-Generated Subjective Global Assessment
PPI	Prognostic Index
S-NIS	Secondary Nutritional Intake Symptoms
TPN	Total Parenteral Nutrition

REFERENCES

Berenstein EG and Z Ortiz. 2003. Megestrol Acetate for the Treatment of Anorexia-Cachexia Syndrome. In: *Cochrane Database of Systematic Reviews*. Wiley-Blackwell, doi:10.1002/14651858.cd004310.

Blum D, GB Stene, TS Solheim, P Fayers, MJ Hjermstad, VE Baracos, K Fearon, F Strasser, S Kaasa, and Euro- Impact. 2014. Validation of the Consensus-Definition for Cancer Cachexia and Evaluation of a Classification Model—A Study Based on Data from an International Multicentre Project (EPCRC-CSA). *Annals of Oncology*, 25(8): 1635–1642.

Braiteh F, S Dalal, A Khuwaja, H David, E Bruera, and R Kurzrock. 2008. Phase I Pilot Study of the Safety and Tolerability of Olanzapine (OZA) for the Treatment of Cachexia in Patients with Advanced Cancer. *Journal of Clinical Oncology*, 26(15_suppl): 20529.

Evans WJ, JE Morley, J Argilés, C Bales, V Baracos, D Guttridge, A Jatoi et al. 2008. Cachexia: A new definition. *Clinical Nutrition*, 27(6): 793–799.

Fairchild A, B Debenham, B Danielson, F Huang, and S Ghosh. 2014. Comparative Multidisciplinary Prediction of Survival in Patients with Advanced Cancer. *Supportive Care in Cancer*, 22(3): 611–617.

Fearon K, F Strasser, SD Anker, I Bosaeus, E Bruera, RL Fainsinger, A Jatoi et al. 2011. Definition and Classification of Cancer Cachexia: An International Consensus. *Lancet Oncology*, 12(5): 489–495.

Fearon KCH. 2008. Cancer Cachexia: Developing Multimodal Therapy for a Multidimensional Problem. *European Journal of Cancer*, 44(8): 1124–1132.

Giordano KF and A Jatoi. 2005. The Cancer Anorexia/Weight Loss Syndrome: Therapeutic Challenges. *Current Oncology Reports*, 7(4): 271–276.

Helbostad JL, JC Hølen, MS Jordhøy, GI Ringdal, L Oldervoll, and S Kaasa. 2009. A First Step in the Development of an International Self-Report Instrument for Physical Functioning in Palliative Cancer Care: A Systematic Literature Review and an Expert Opinion Evaluation Study. *Journal of Pain and Symptom Management*, 37(2): 196–205.

Kilgour RD, A Vigano, B Trutschnigg, E Lucar, M Borod, and JA Morais. 2013. Handgrip Strength Predicts Survival and Is Associated with Markers of Clinical and Functional Outcomes in Advanced Cancer Patients. *Supportive Care in Cancer*, 21(12): 3261–3270.

Lowe SS, B Danielson, C Beaumont, SM Watanabe, and KS Courneya. 2016. Physical Activity Interests and Preferences of Cancer Patients with Brain Metastases: A Cross-Sectional Survey. *BMC Palliative Care*, 15(1): 7.

Martin L, S Watanabe, R Fainsinger, F Lau, S Ghosh, H Quan, M Atkins, K Fassbender, GM Downing, and V Baracos. 2010. Prognostic Factors in Patients with Advanced Cancer: Use of the Patient-Generated Subjective Global Assessment in Survival Prediction. *Journal of Clinical Oncology*, 28(28): 4376–4383.

Metz CA, T Popiela, R Lucchi, and F Giongo. 1989. Methylprednisolone as Palliative Therapy for Female Terminal Cancer Patients. *European Journal of Cancer and Clinical Oncology*, 25(12): 1823–1829.

Omlin A, D Blum, J Wierecky, SR Haile, FD Ottery, and F Strasser. 2013. Nutrition Impact Symptoms in Advanced Cancer Patients: Frequency and Specific Interventions, a Case-Control Study. *Journal of Cachexia, Sarcopenia and Muscle*, 4(1): 55–61.

Pantano NdP, BSR Paiva, D Hui, and CE Paiva. 2016. Validation of the Modified Glasgow Prognostic Score in Advanced Cancer Patients Receiving Palliative Care. *Journal of Pain and Symptom Management*, 51(2): 270–277.

Pietra C, Y Takeda, N Tazawa-Ogata, M Minami, X Yuanfeng, EM Duus, and R Northrup. 2014. Anamorelin HCl (ONO-7643), a Novel Ghrelin Receptor Agonist, for the Treatment of Cancer Anorexia-Cachexia Syndrome: Preclinical Profile. *Journal of Cachexia, Sarcopenia and Muscle*, 5(4): 329–337.

Rhondali W, GB Chisholm, M Filbet, D-H Kang, D Hui, MC Fingeret, and E Bruera. 2015. Screening for Body Image Dissatisfaction in Patients with Advanced Cancer: A Pilot Study. *Journal of Palliative Medicine*, 18(2): 151–156.

Ribaudo JM, D Cella, EA Hahn, SR Lloyd, NS Tchekmedyian, J Von Roenn, and WT Leslie. 2000. Re-Validation and Shortening of the Functional Assessment of Anorexia/Cachexia Therapy (FAACT) Questionnaire. *Quality of Life Research*, 9(10): 1137–1146.

Riechelmann RP, D Burman, IF Tannock, G Rodin, and C Zimmermann. 2009. Phase II Trial of Mirtazapine for Cancer-Related Cachexia and Anorexia. *American Journal of Hospice and Palliative Medicine*, 27(2): 106–110.

Simmons CPL, DC McMillan, K McWilliams, TA Sande, KC Fearon, S Tuck, MT Fallon, and BJ Laird. 2017. Prognostic Tools in Patients with Advanced Cancer: A Systematic Review. *Journal of Pain and Symptom Management*, 53(5): 962–970.e10.

Stene GB, JL Helbostad, TR Balstad, II Riphagen, S Kaasa, and LM Oldervoll. 2013. Effect of Physical Exercise on Muscle Mass and Strength in Cancer Patients During Treatment—A Systematic Review. *Critical Reviews in Oncology/Hematology*, 88(3): 573–593.

Strasser F, D Luftner, K Possinger, G Ernst, T Ruhstaller, W Meissner, Y-D Ko, M Schnelle, M Reif, and T Cerny. 2006. Comparison of Orally Administered Cannabis Extract and Delta-9-Tetrahydrocannabinol in Treating Patients with Cancer-Related Anorexia-Cachexia Syndrome: A Multicenter, Phase III, Randomized, Double-Blind, Placebo-Controlled Clinical Trial from the Cannabi. *Journal of Clinical Oncology*, 24(21): 3394–3400.

Tan BHL, LA Birdsell, L Martin, VE Baracos, and KCH Fearon. 2009. Sarcopenia in an Overweight or Obese Patient Is an Adverse Prognostic Factor in Pancreatic Cancer. *Clinical Cancer Research*, 15(22): 6973–6979.

Teunissen SCCM, W Wesker, C Kruitwagen, HCJM de Haes, EE Voest, and A de Graeff. 2007. Symptom Prevalence in Patients with Incurable Cancer: A Systematic Review. *Journal of Pain and Symptom Management*, 34(1): 94–104.

Vigano A, E Del Fabbro, E Bruera, and M Borod. 2012. The Cachexia Clinic: From Staging to Managing Nutritional and Functional Problems in Advanced Cancer Patients. *Critical Reviews in Oncogenesis*, 17(3): 293–304.

Vigano AAL, JA Morais, L Ciutto, L Rosenthall, J di Tomasso, S Khan, H Olders, M Borod, and RD Kilgour. 2017. Use of routinely available clinical, nutritional, and functional criteria to classify cachexia in advanced cancer patients. *Clinical Nutrition*, 36(5): 1378–1390.

Wallengren O, K Lundholm, and I Bosaeus. 2013. Diagnostic Criteria of Cancer Cachexia: Relation to Quality of Life, Exercise Capacity and Survival in Unselected Palliative Care Patients. *Supportive Care in Cancer*, 21(6): 1569–1577.

Yavuzsen T. 2005. Systematic Review of the Treatment of Cancer-Associated Anorexia and Weight Loss. *Journal of Clinical Oncology*, 23(33): 8500–8511.

7 Sedation in Palliative Care and Its Impact on Nutrition and Fluid Intake

Carel M. M. Veldhoven, Kris C. P. Vissers, Jeroen H. Hasselaar, and Constans A. V. H. H. M. Verhagen

CONTENTS

INTRODUCTION

According to the definition of the World Health Organization, palliative care's objective is to improve the quality of life of patients suffering incurable diseases and their relatives. The focus is on symptom control and, where possible, symptom prevention.

When symptoms such as pain, delirium, agitation, dyspnoea, nausea/vomiting or psychological distress prove to be refractory to other treatment options, sedation may be considered.

When sedation is considered to be started, questions regarding the utility of nutrition and hydration in sedated patients arise. It should be stressed that several patients in palliative care already need specific feeding arrangements, because the disease itself may be responsible for changes in digestion, absorption and the possibility of food intake.

WHAT IS PALLIATIVE SEDATION?

The definition of palliative sedation is, "deliberately reducing consciousness so that the patient no longer experiences discomfort" (Levy and Cohen 2005). This describes the fact that patients are sedated to palliate unacceptable refractory symptoms. Symptoms are considered refractory when all conventional symptom treatment has failed to alleviate suffering within the available time frame and at an acceptable risk-benefit ratio (de Graeff and Dean 2007). Somewhere in the palliative phase, palliative care is no longer directed towards quality of life but towards quality of dying and treatment of discomfort. This mainly occurs in the last few weeks of life. Only when a symptom or a combination of symptoms becomes overwhelming and untreatable, suffering could interfere with different domains of quality of dying: communication or expressing availabilities, feeding possibilities and experiencing proximity of next of kin. In these cases, palliative sedation may be an option of last resort to provide relief.

Sedation can be continuous and intermittent. Furthermore, sedation can be light or deep. In proportional sedation, the patient's consciousness is deliberately lowered to an extent that the refractory symptoms are no longer felt to be intolerable. If possible, sedation will not be complete, and communication may be preserved as long as experiencing discomfort is balanced against complete loss of consciousness. Continuous deep sedation (CDS) is an extreme form of palliative sedation used in those patients who continue to suffer from refractory symptoms, despite efforts to optimize the patient's comfort. This type of sedation is only acceptable in a patient with a short life expectancy of maximally two weeks. Intermittent sedation can be discontinued to permit reflection and discussion about the benefits and burdens of the sedation intervention by the healthcare team and the family and, if feasible, the patient. Theoretically, intermittent sedation may break an escalating cycle of refractory symptoms and permit the resumption of non-sedating palliation (Vissers et al. 2007). Table 7.1 gives a summary of the characteristics of deep continuous and intermittent sedation.

Palliative sedation is an extraordinary sedation, because most physicians do not use this technique frequently. Although the incidence of palliative sedation is increasing, it is estimated that an individual physician performs this technique only a few times (zero to five) a year (Hasselaar J. G. et al. 2008). This results in a relatively low level of expertise, making the choice between the different types of palliative sedation difficult. The choice of the type of sedation will depend on the severity of symptoms in all dimensions, the patient's general condition and life expectancy. Special attention should be given to personal care for the patient and the patient's relatives. Lodging facilities should consist of a nice, domestic room, with possibility for privacy for the relatives, and a place to rest. Finally, a dedicated team should be permanently available with attention for the multidimensional aspects of the palliative care trajectory. This team will be composed of a treating physician with expertise in palliative care and palliative sedation, nurses trained in palliative care, and as needed psychologists and/or a consultant in spiritual care. Relatives remain involved and attend the patient. The staff involved in the patient's care should be informed and engaged (Vissers et al. 2007).

The criteria for selecting patients for sedation are outlined in Table 7.2.

CURRENT PRACTICE IN PALLIATIVE SEDATION

In 2005, the Royal Dutch Medical Association (RDMA) published a national guideline for palliative sedation that was revised in 2009. In this guideline, palliative sedation is considered a common medical practice as laid down in the Dutch Medical Treatment Act, making it mandatory for all physicians within the country.

A review of the role of sedation in palliative care (Hasselaar J. G. et al. 2009b; van der Heide et al. 2017) clearly showed the increasing interest in this technique during the past two decades.

Three consecutive surveys conducted in the Flemish part of Belgium regarding the practices of end of life show that in 1998 deep sedation was not reported, whereas in 2001 and 2008 it was reported in, respectively, 8.2% and 14.5% of cases (Bilsen et al. 2009). Surveys conducted

TABLE 7.1
Characteristics of Light Sedation, Intermittent Sedation, and Deep Continuous Sedation

Domain	Characteristics	Light Sedation	Intermittent	Deep Continuous
Medical	Imminent death	Often near future	Often near future	Prerequisite
	Refractory symptoms[a]	Often or difficult	Often difficult	Prerequisite
	Titration of sedatives	Proportionally[b]	Proportionally	Until deep sleep
	Other medication (as indicated)	Full spectrum often orally	Full spectrum often orally	Limited for comfort only parenterally (subcutaneous or intravenous)
	Eating and/or drinking	Possible: often independently	Possible: often independently	Impossible
	Artificial feeding and/or hydration	If indicated	If indicated	Often counterproductive
Care	Monitoring symptom relief	Yes, input patient	Yes, input patient	Yes, observational
	Adequate feeding and/or hydration	Requires attention	Mainly intact	No issue (anymore)
	Special interventions (bladder catheter, bedsore prevention, mouth care, etc.)	Attention required	Seldom necessary	Always necessary
Social	Communication with patient	Slightly restricted	Normal at awakening	Impossible
	End-of-life rituals	Not yet necessary	Not yet necessary	Just before sedation
	Relatives are prepared for dying process	In principle but not inevitably imminent	In principle but not inevitably imminent	Yes
Ethical	Autonomy of patient	Still expressible	Still expressible	Must be cared for
	Life shortening	Not in effect of meant	Not in effect of meant	Not in effect of meant
	Less harmful/rigid alternatives are not available	Prerequisite	Prerequisite	Prerequisite
	Sedation is proportional to level of patient discomfort	Yes	Yes	Yes[c]
Legal	Objectives	No legal restrictions	No legal restrictions	No legal restrictions
	Regulations	According to medical guidelines and good clinical praxis	According to medical guidelines and good clinical praxis	According to medical guidelines and good clinical praxis
Other	Recommendations	Consultation if experience is limited	Consultation if experience is limited	Consultation if experience is limited

[a] No sedation for psycho-existential problems exclusively.

[b] Proportional sedation demands a careful titration of sedatives at the lowest dose possible aimed at symptom relief balanced with preservation of communication possibilities.

[c] Even deep and continuous sedation must be proportional. A less rigid sedation protocol is not effective or sound and ample reasoning suggests it is not effective.

in the Netherlands in 2003–2005, 2007 and 2015 provide information regarding the increasing frequency of use and the practice of palliative sedation (Onwuteaka-Philipsen et al. 2012). Current figures for the Netherlands estimate continuous deep sedation to be applied in 18% of all dying persons (van der Heide et al. 2017). These surveys also indicate that the implementation of national guidelines changes the practice of palliative sedation. Besides the increasing frequency of sedation, it is seen that more physicians discussed sedation with patients in advance. Patient request for euthanasia before sedation occurred significantly less often after the introduction of the guideline (Hasselaar J. et al. 2009a).

TABLE 7.2
Criteria for Selecting Patients for Sedation

1. The illness is irreversible, and death is expected imminently.
2. The symptoms for which relief is sought are clearly defined and understood.
3. These defined symptoms are unbearable for the patient and are truly refractory.
4. Informed consent must be obtained from the patient or the patient's proxy.
5. The patient and proxies have received extensive information relative to complete or deep sedation and the potential alternatives such as light sedative measures.
6. Contraindications for sedation are absent.
7. If not already in place, an order to withhold cardiopulmonary resuscitation must be instituted before sedation is initiated.
8. Consultation should be sought from palliative care experts who are skilled in the use of sedation.
9. Family members remain involved at the behest of the patient.
10. The staff involved in the patient's care should be informed and engaged.
11. Basic healthcare actions are maintained (such as prevention of bedsores, mouth care, continuation of essential drugs to prevent exaggeration of preventable symptoms under sedation, bladder catheter, and timely evacuation of stools).
12. Attention should be paid to personal care for the patient and proxies, with the availability of psychological support.
13. Specifics of sedation medications and patient response will be documented in the medical record on a regular basis.
14. After the patient has passed away, mourners and attending nurses must be offered an opportunity to discuss their feelings, remaining questions and experiences with the deceased.

GUIDELINES FOR PALLIATIVE SEDATION

There are very few guidelines on (the application of) palliative sedation, mainly because of the absence of randomized controlled trials, which are impossible to perform in this frail population. Moreover, there is no reference treatment for the management of refractory symptoms at the end of life. Besides the already mentioned guidelines issued by the RDMA, other guidelines are worth mentioning (Abarshi et al. 2017; Cherny and Group 2014; Cherny et al. 2009; Dean et al. 2012; de Graeff and Dean 2007; Kirk et al. 2010; Morita et al. 2005; RDMA 2009). These guidelines provide comparable recommendations regarding the different steps before, during and after palliative sedation, considering the care for the patient, relatives and caregivers. However, the subject of nutrition and hydration of sedated patients remains complicated and controversial.

The Dutch guidelines indicate that medically assisted nutrition in patients with continuous deep sedation for palliative symptom control should not be used, because of the patient's condition and the commonly observed fact that terminally ill patients hardly have food intake prior to sedation. For hydration, however, the issue is much more difficult. The above-mentioned guidelines differentiate between patients who already had an insufficient fluid intake prior to sedation and those who still have sufficient oral or parenteral fluid intake. Depending on the condition and consciousness of the patient, the issue of continuing or stopping will be discussed with the patient and/or his legal representatives. Food and fluid administration should only be considered when it does not harm the patient, does not cause unnecessary suffering and does not represent a useless medical act (RDMA 2009).

The Japanese guidelines take a comparable but more moderate point of view, whereby artificial food and fluid administration must be made possible when the patient or the relatives request it. As in the Dutch guidelines, it is made clear that the patient and his relatives can only form an informed decision when all aspects of the sedation and consequences of nutrition and hydration are clearly and realistically explained (Morita et al. 2005).

NUTRITIONAL PATTERNS OF TERMINALLY ILL PATIENTS

Many terminally ill patients have a reduced oral intake that may be attributed to anorexia/cachexia syndrome, generalized weakness/sickness, bowel obstruction or loss of appetite (Good et al. 2008).

The most important obstruction for nutritional intake is the fact that the patient usually becomes lethargic when death is imminent by a natural loss of physiological processes in the dying phase and therefore is less able to take or receive nutrition orally.

Management of this condition may include medically assisted nutrition, which can be given via a tube inserted into any part of the gastrointestinal tract or intravenously. Benefit from medical interventions and artificial feeding has not been proven (Bally et al. 2016; Guo et al. 2005). Moreover, in a Cochrane review this technique was judged to involve ethical controversies (Brody et al. 2011; Fatati 2015; Geppert et al. 2010; Good et al. 2008). First, there is no unanimity regarding the perception of medically assisted hydration and nutrition as a medical intervention or a basic provision of comfort. Second, the problem arises as to who should decide on artificial feeding and hydration in patients who are no longer competent to make their own decisions. The Cochrane review focused on the value of medically assisted nutrition in palliative care patients in general. The main findings are that there are no randomized or prospectively controlled trials on the subject and the prospective non-controlled trials are judged to be of poor quality. Hence, no recommendations regarding medically assisted hydration and nutrition can be made for palliative care patients according to the methods accepted by Cochrane reviews.

FEEDING AND HYDRATION IN TERMINALLY ILL PATIENTS

Beneficial Effects of Nutrition and Hydration

Hydration and feeding are considered essential for survival. Indeed, laymen consider nutrition and hydration a necessary part of basic human treatment of any patient at any stage of any disease. Nutrition and hydration are judged important to allow organs to function normally and to prevent hunger and thirst. Feeding and hydration are also considered signs of love and caring. This explains the perception of people that withdrawing nutrition and, even more so, hydration will hasten death, which is considered not to be true.

Detrimental Effects of Nutrition and Hydration

The elemental knowledge in medicine that hydration and feeding are considered essential for survival may not hold true for patients in an end stage of their disease or dying patients. In terminally ill patients the objective of the treatment is treating discomfort and symptom control (van Adrichem et al. 2017). Moreover, these patients often have renal and other organ failure. Liquid administration may cause fluid retention resulting in nausea, vomiting, aspiration, oedema and increased secretions. These conditions may in turn cause intolerable symptoms and even iatrogenic cardiac or lung failure.

There is no compelling evidence that withholding nutrition or hydration either increases or diminishes suffering in the dying patient. Table 7.3 summarizes the points to consider when making the decision on hydration.

Ethical Concerns Regarding Nutrition and Hydration

In the second edition of the International Association for Hospice and Palliative Care (IAHPC) Manual of Palliative Care (Doyle and Woodruff 2009), the ethical dimension of hydration and nutrition is brought back to a medical question: ‘Will this particular intervention restore or enhance the quality of life of the particular patient?’ If the answer is yes, and it can be justified on the basis of clinical grounds, then it is ethically right to do it. When, on the contrary, the answer is no, it should not be done.

There are other arguments to consider in the discussion of artificial hydration in patients in an end stage of their lives. Withholding fluids from a terminally ill patient may result in a dry mouth, but this can be well palliated topically by adjusted mouth care. Normally, withholding hydration should result in thirst, but most dying patients do not complain of thirst.

TABLE 7.3
Points to Consider When Making the Decision on Artificial Feeding and Hydration

Question

1. Is the patient capable of autonomous feeding/drinking?
2. Is the patient dehydrated?
3. Is the patient cachectic?
4. Is the life expectancy longer than two weeks?
5. What are the symptoms caused or aggravated by dehydration?
6. Do the expected advantages of feeding outweigh the expected disadvantages?
7. Do the expected advantages of hydration outweigh the expected disadvantages?
8. Do the patient and family agree to artificial feeding/hydration?

TABLE 7.4
Possible Administration Routes of Nutrition and Fluids

Route	Nutrition	Fluid	Comments
Subcutaneous		√	24-hour continuous infusion or intermittent administration
Intravenous	√	√	Peripheral or central line (may be present for other purposes)
Enteral	√	√	Nasogastric tube or gastrostomy
Proctoclysis		√	When other routes of hydration are not possible

A second concern in withholding fluids could be the fact that dehydration may also provoke a diminished conscious state. Several reports and one randomized controlled trial, however, showed no correlation between hydration and cognition in terminally ill patients (Dalal and Bruera 2004).

Dehydration may be responsible for reduced urine output, which means less need for movement and less incontinence. Also, pulmonary secretions are diminished, thus possibly reducing dyspnoea, terminal congestion and death rattle. The reduced gastrointestinal secretions may lessen nausea, vomiting and diarrhoea. Finally, the risk of oedema and effusions is possibly reduced, and existing ascites may be absorbed. When the patient is not capable of independent oral intake, artificial feeding and hydration may be considered on specific well-thought-out indications. The modalities for artificial feeding and hydration are outlined in Table 7.4.

Another aspect of artificial feeding and hydration (by means of a drip) might be that it creates a 'false hope of a reversible situation', and the drip forms a barrier between the patient and the relatives. Because the effects of artificial hydration in a terminal patient seem limited from a medical perspective, in general there is no reason to recommend continuing or starting it during palliative sedation and the issue seems best decided on within the individual physician-patient relationship, as one guideline recommends (Morita et al. 2005). In discussing this issue with the patient and the patient's relatives, the potential benefits and disadvantages of artificial feeding and hydration in terminally ill patients as summarized in Table 7.5 can be helpful.

NUTRITION IN SEDATED PATIENTS

There are no guidelines on nutrition in patients under palliative sedation. Therefore, the following recommendations are only expert opinion.

TABLE 7.5
Advantages and Disadvantages of Nutrition and Hydration

Advantages	Disadvantages
	Medical
Provides basic needs	Fluid increases urine output, pulmonary secretions, risk of edema and ascites
Nutrition relieves hunger	
Fluid relieves thirst	
Fluid prevents/alleviates symptoms such as: confusion, agitation and neuromuscular irritability	Sedated patient does not present such symptoms
	Emotional
Response to family's emotional concerns	Instrumentation may give the impression of a curative intervention – generates false hope for reversibility of the patient's situation
	Instrumentation creates barrier between patient and relatives

Important Points to Consider

A distinction should be made between continuous sedation (CS) and intermittent sedation. Only CS will make autonomous feeding by the patient him- or herself impossible and could, therefore, theoretically harm the patient.

Continuous Sedation

Patients eligible for (deep) continuous palliative sedation have a life expectancy that normally will not exceed two weeks. It has been estimated that seven or eight out of 10 patients who are indicated for continuous palliative sedation have already stopped oral intake before the start of sedation (Hasselaar J. et al. 2009b). Therefore, most controversy surrounds patients with artificial hydration or with considerable oral intake at the time of starting continuous sedation. Many patients, even early on in their disease, express disgust and aversion for food as it makes them nauseated and oppressed and induces vomiting and/or causes cramps and diarrhoea. In these cases, parenteral or intravenous feeding is not indicated. Artificial feeding is expected to be a futile medical intervention in a dying patient and may even harm the patient with potential side effects.

In patients who already receive artificial oral or parenteral nutrition, the administration of food supplements will be halted for the same reasons as have been discussed for initiating artificial feeding.

The controversy lies in the need for hydration (Dalal and Bruera 2004; Dalal et al. 2009). In contrast to inadequate feeding for a restricted episode, withholding fluids from patients may be considered as an act that may shorten life, particularly when these patients have considerable oral intake at the start of continuous sedation and a longer prognosis, that is, an expected life of more than two weeks. As long as the dying process induces the patient to stop the intake of fluids and death has been accepted, no ethical controversy will arise. But in cases where sedation prevents adequate intake, uneasiness considering artificial hydration may arise. If death is expected within due time, artificial hydration may not change the outcome. Moreover, a nasal gastric drip or intravenous hydration may have numerous adverse effects including lung aspiration, worsening oedema, increasing secretions and unnecessarily prolonging the naturally evolving dying process (Plonk and Arnold 2005). All these acts may have an important negative impact on the quality of life and the quality of dying. If death is not expected within a short time frame, continuous sedation that interrupts adequate intake of fluids should not be undertaken as long as the patient him- or herself is willing to continue intake. In that case, respite sedation (e.g., during night) could be an alternative.

On pure medical indications, it seems logical to stop food and fluid administration in patients whose death is imminent. When, however, death cannot be predicted to be imminent, intermittent sedation should be preferred.

Intermittent Sedation

For patients with refractory symptoms where intermittent sedation proves to be adequate, oral food and liquid intake will be possible and acceptable between periods of sleep. During intermittent sedation, the patient has some respite and the general condition may improve to such a point that sedation is no longer needed or evolve to a natural dying phase. Intermittent sedation preserves the possibility of food and fluid intake as far as the function of the body to digest and absorb remains intact to a certain degree. This mainly will be restricted to a form of comfort diet (van Adrichem et al. 2017). This form of sedation does not influence the natural course of dying and the patient him- or herself will be able to express to what extent he or she may experience benefit and/or harm from any intake. Nevertheless, during intermittent sedation, signs and symptoms of inadequate intake should be monitored carefully (Dalal et al. 2009). When feeding, the patient should be fully awake, reactive and able to swallow normally. Thus, there have to be adequate periods of awake time. This is especially true when signs of imminent dying are absent. On the contrary, as the condition of the patient deteriorates following the natural evolution of the underlying disease to a dying phase, feeding and fluid intake should not be forced, in order to prevent medically induced harm to the patient (Dalal and Bruera 2004).

Light Sedation

For those patients who have light or superficial sedation, oral feeding and drinking may be considered. However, it is absolutely necessary that the patient be able to swallow normally, and that he or she remains in a phase in which feeding and drinking may be beneficial, and this will not often be the case. All remarks under intermittent sedation hold true for this condition also. The main difference will be that the depth of superficial sedation may be changed according to the needs of the patient in order to sedate in proportion to the suffering experienced. Such a step-wise approach may evolve to a stage at which the patient is no longer able to maintain adequate food and fluid intake. Attending nurses and the responsible physicians should monitor intake cautiously.

ETHICAL CONSIDERATIONS OF NUTRITION

From an ethical point of view, the patient has the right to decide if fluid and food intake should be continued or stopped. The majority of patients under proportional, superficial, or intermittent sedation are capable of continuing or stopping drinking and eating according to their wishes and biological needs. In case of a need for artificial feeding and hydration, the decision to start or withhold such an intervention should be an act of shared decision-making. Even potentially beneficial interventions should always be weighed against potential disadvantages. But as soon as a medical intervention has been judged advantageous, the patient or next of kin may insist on the proper execution of such treatment. The patient always can refuse any intervention on personal grounds, even if a potential benefit can be expected. No patient or family, however, has the right to force a medical intervention to be executed if the indication is missing or if it is clearly harmful. Of course, any decision by the patient or next of kin can only be made based on accurate information provided by healthcare professionals. In cognitively impaired patients, who may no longer be able to express their own wishes, the next of kin have the obligation to reconstruct the most likely choice of their beloved one. In cases where the evidence for and against an intervention is less clear, or in cases where important patient values are at stake, shared decision-making between professionals and the patient/family seems the best way to attain a good medical policy. Any conscious and decisive patient has the right to exert his or her autonomous will to forego life-prolonging interventions.

When a patient, suffering incurable disease, has deliberately stopped eating and drinking in an attempt to hasten his or her death, the patient's decision should be respected. This may not limit access to palliative sedation, provided that there is a clear medical indication for it.

In some cases, ethical and moral problems arise in those situations where culture or religion dictate that life should be respected and maintained with medical interventions regardless of the terminal condition of the patient or his or her own wishes for withdrawal of medical treatment. Indeed, life should be respected, but medically this does not by definition include the provision of artificial hydration. In dying patients, caregivers should never abandon the patient, but medicalization of dying needs to be avoided. In several cultures, feeding and providing drink is synonymous with love and caring. The idea that a beloved, terminally ill patient suffers from hunger and thirst is considered unacceptable, even if it is not true from a medical point of view. However, dying patients under sedation usually do not experience thirst as long as proper mouth care is provided.

Cultural and religious differences should of course be respected, but efforts should be made by the caregiver to explain the potential benefits and risks of medically assisted nutrition and hydration in continuously sedated patients. In addition, worries should be addressed carefully; for example, mouth care may be a very important treatment for both patient and relatives to show that the patient is still a valued person during his or her final days or hours. This shared decision making is reflected in the EAPC framework definition of palliative sedation that states that the sedation should be ethically acceptable to the patient, family, and the healthcare providers (Cherny and Radbruch 2009).

APPLICATIONS TO OTHER AREAS OF TERMINAL OR PALLIATIVE CARE

Palliative sedation is mainly an intervention aimed at controlling symptoms of the dying patient. In this stage of life, considerations of maintaining organ functioning are no longer applicable. In earlier stages of palliative care (or curative care), the decisions will be made based on the patient's general condition, the life expectancy, and the patient's own will.

PRACTICAL METHODS AND TECHNIQUES

Intermittent and light sedation as a technique can be considered as a sedation in the operation room. The medications and the doses will be adapted according to the patient's needs. Care should be taken to switch essential oral medications to a parenteral route when the patient becomes unable to take them orally.

When the indication for continuous deep palliative sedation is clearly established and the patient and/or his or her proxies have provided informed consent, care should be taken to make sure that the patient and family clearly understand that once the sedation is started there is no possibility for communication left. When necessary, the essential medication should be administered parenterally, mainly by the subcutaneous route.

In principle, sedation will be started with benzodiazepines, preferably midazolam. When this induces insufficient symptom control, additional hypnotics and antipsychotic drugs may be considered. It is advised to follow a national or local protocol. For hospitalized or institutionalized patients where the treatment can be supervised by an anaesthesiologist, the use of a narcoleptic drug such as propofol can be considered. In some cases, sedation can be achieved by increasing the dose of the sedatives already used by the patient.

The use of morphine to reduce the patient's consciousness, for example, by increasing the dose of already used morphine, is judged to be a medical error because the patient may become confused and agitated but not (enough) sedated. Moreover, increasing the dose of morphine may induce neurotoxicity, also indicated as 'morphine-induced hyperalgesia', which is characterized by hyperalgesia, delirium, and myoclonus.

All caregivers, especially the nurses, should follow a care program dedicated to patients under sedation. This includes observation of the primary symptoms that were the reason for applying sedation, and potential new problems. They should monitor the general sense of comfort and peace of the patient and next of kin. In patients with intermittent or superficial sedation they will monitor the duration of sedation, depth of sedation, and balance between preserving communication and palliation of existing complaints more intensively. Especially in these cases, they should also monitor adequate intake and the level of consciousness during intake to prevent complications.

KEY FACTS

- Palliative sedation may be considered for patients with a short life expectancy (two weeks) who suffer from refractory symptoms.
- Intermittent sedation allows patients to be awake and have food and liquid intake if needed. In some cases, intermittent sedation can provide symptom relief, whereafter the patient can be kept awake.
- Before starting continuous sedation, informed consent from the patient and/or relatives is required.
- Patients and family must realize that, once continuous deep sedation is started, contact is not possible.
- All caregivers, especially nurses, should follow a care program dedicated to patients under sedation. This includes observation of the primary symptoms that were the reason for applying sedation, and potential new problems. They should monitor the general sense of comfort and peace of the patient and next of kin.
- Due to the natural evolution of a terminal disease, patients at the end of life experience less thirst and hunger and have, in most cases, compromised food and liquid intake.
- The elemental knowledge in medicine that hydration and feeding are considered essential for survival may not hold true for patients in an end stage of their disease or dying patients.

SUMMARY POINTS

- Palliative sedation consists of deliberately reducing the patient's level of consciousness to control refractory symptoms in order to assure comfort.
- Palliative sedation in the strict sense of continuous deep sedation is only indicated in patients whose death is imminent and who suffer symptoms that cannot be controlled otherwise.
- There are three levels of palliative sedation that cover the whole spectrum of proportionally applied sedation in the palliative phase:
  - Intermittent sedation with restricted periods of induced sleep and consequently symptom control.
  - Light sedation, whereby the degree of sedation is adapted to the patient's need, but communication and intake remain (partially) intact.
  - Deep continuous sedation.
- The role of nutrition and hydration depends on the patient's general condition, ability, and willingness to accept food and beverages.
- Deeply sedated patients cannot take oral food and drinks. In CDS in the palliative phase, artificial feeding and hydration have no documented added medical value, and they may even induce complications.
- For intermittent and lightly sedated patients, nutrition and hydration will be administered according to the patient's will and when no risk of aspiration is present.

LIST OF ABBREVIATIONS

CDC Continuous Deep Sedation
IAHPC International Association for Hospice & Palliative Care
RDMA Royal Dutch Medical Association

REFERENCES

Abarshi, E., J. Rietjens, L. Robijn, A. Caraceni, S. Payne, L. Deliens, L. Van den Block and I. Euro. 2017. International Variations in Clinical Practice Guidelines for Palliative Sedation: A Systematic Review. *BMJ Support Palliat Care* 7(3): 223–229.

Bally, M. R., P. Z. Blaser Yildirim, L. Bounoure, V. L. Gloy, B. Mueller, M. Briel and P. Schuetz. 2016. Nutritional Support and Outcomes in Malnourished Medical Inpatients: A Systematic Review and Meta-analysis. *JAMA Intern Med* 176(1): 43–53.

Bilsen, J., J. Cohen, K. Chambaere, G. Pousset, B. D. Onwuteaka-Philipsen, F. Mortier and L. Deliens. 2009. Medical End-of-Life Practices Under the Euthanasia Law in Belgium. *N Engl J Med* 361(11): 1119–1121.

Brody, H., L. D. Hermer, L. D. Scott, L. L. Grumbles, J. E. Kutac and S. D. McCammon. 2011. Artificial Nutrition and Hydration: The Evolution of Ethics, Evidence, and Policy. *J Gen Intern Med* 26(9): 1053–1058.

Cherny, N. I. and E. G. W. Group. 2014. ESMO Clinical Practice Guidelines for the Management of Refractory Symptoms at the End of Life and the Use of Palliative Sedation. *Ann Oncol* 25(Suppl 3): iii143–iii152.

Cherny, N. I., L. Radbruch and C. Board of the European Association for Palliative. 2009. European Association for Palliative Care (EAPC) Recommended Framework for the Use of Sedation in Palliative Care. *Palliat Med* 23(7): 581–593.

Dalal, S. and E. Bruera. 2004. Dehydration in Cancer Patients: To Treat or Not to Treat. *J Support Oncol* 2(6): 467–479, 483.

Dalal, S., E. Del Fabbro and E. Bruera. 2009. Is There a Role for Hydration at the End of Life? *Curr Opin Support Palliat Care* 3(1): 72–78.

Dean, M. M., V. Cellarius, B. Henry, D. Oneschuk and S. L. Librach Canadian Society of Palliative Care Physicians Taskforce. 2012. Framework for Continuous Palliative Sedation Therapy in Canada. *J Palliat Med* 15(8): 870–879.

de Graeff, A. and M. Dean. 2007. Palliative Sedation Therapy in the Last Weeks of Life: A Literature Review and Recommendations for Standards. *J Palliat Med* 10(1): 67–85.

Doyle, D. and R. Woodruff. 2009. *The IAHPC Manual of Palliative Care*, 3rd edition. Doyle, D. and Woodruff, R. IAHPC Press. https://hospicecare.com/uploads/2013/9/The%20IAHPC%20Manual%20of%20 Palliative%20Care%203e.pdf

Fatati, G. 2015. [Artificial Nutrition: Technical, Scientific and Ethical Considerations]. *Recenti Prog Med* 106(2): 81–84.

Geppert, C. M., M. R. Andrews and M. E. Druyan. 2010. Ethical Issues in Artificial Nutrition and Hydration: A Review. *J Parenter Enteral Nutr* 34(1): 79–88.

Good, P., J. Cavenagh, M. Mather and P. Ravenscroft. 2008. Medically Assisted Nutrition for Palliative Care in Adult Patients. *Cochrane Database Syst Rev* 8(4): CD006274.

Guo, Y., J. L. Palmer, G. Kaur, S. Hainley, B. Young and E. Bruera. 2005. Nutritional Status of Cancer Patients and Its Relationship to Function in an Inpatient Rehabilitation Setting. *Support Care Cancer* 13(3): 169–175.

Hasselaar, J., S. Verhagen, R. Reuzel, E. van Leeuwen and K. Vissers. 2009a. Palliative Sedation Is Not Controversial. *Lancet Oncol* 10(8): 747–748.

Hasselaar, J. G., R. P. Reuzel, M. E. van den Muijsenbergh, R. T. Koopmans, C. J. Leget, B. J. Crul and K. C. Vissers. 2008. Dealing with Delicate Issues in Continuous Deep Sedation. Varying Practices among Dutch Medical Specialists, General Practitioners, and Nursing Home Physicians. *Arch Intern Med* 168(5): 537–543.

Hasselaar, J. G., S. C. Verhagen, A. P. Wolff, Y. Engels, B. J. Crul and K. C. Vissers. 2009b. Changed Patterns in Dutch Palliative Sedation Practices After the Introduction of a National Guideline. *Arch Intern Med* 169(5): 430–437.

Kirk, T. W., M. M. Mahon, H. Palliative Sedation Task Force of the National and C. Palliative Care Organization Ethics. 2010. National Hospice and Palliative Care Organization (NHPCO) Position Statement and Commentary on the Use of Palliative Sedation in Imminently Dying Terminally Ill Patients. *J Pain Symptom Manage* 39(5): 914–923.

Levy, M. H. and S. D. Cohen. 2005. Sedation for the Relief of Refractory Symptoms in the Imminently Dying: A Fine Intentional Line. *Semin Oncol* 32(2): 237–246.

Morita, T., S. Bito, Y. Kurihara and Y. Uchitomi. 2005. Development of a Clinical Guideline for Palliative Sedation Therapy Using the Delphi Method. *J Palliat Med* 8(4): 716–729.

Onwuteaka-Philipsen, B. D., A. Brinkman-Stoppelenburg, C. Penning, G. J. de Jong-Krul, J. J. van Delden and A. van der Heide. 2012. Trends in End-of-Life Practices Before and After the Enactment of the Euthanasia Law in the Netherlands from 1990 to 2010: A Repeated Cross-Sectional Survey. *Lancet* 380(9845): 908–915.

Plonk, W. M., Jr. and R. M. Arnold. 2005. Terminal Care: The Last Weeks of Life. *J Palliat Med* 8(5): 1042–1054.
Royal Dutch Medical Association (RDMA). 2009. *Guideline for Palliative Sedation*. KNMG guideline.
van Adrichem, V., M. Ariëns, S. Beijer, P. Delsink, N. Doornink A. Droop, et al. 2017. Guideline nutrition and cancer (Richtlijn voeding bij kanker). Oncoline.
van der Heide, A., J. J. M. van Delden and B. D. Onwuteaka-Philipsen. 2017. End-of-Life Decisions in the Netherlands over 25 Years. *N Engl J Med* 377(5): 492–494.
Vissers, K. C., J. Hasselaar and S. A. Verhagen. 2007. Sedation in Palliative Care. *Curr Opin Anaesthesiol* 20(2): 137–142.

8 Pain Control in Palliative Care

Marcin Chwistek

CONTENTS

INTRODUCTION

Pain and palliative care are interlinked in many nuanced ways. Pain is a complex, multidimensional experience that is common in patients with an advanced disease, including cancer, advanced heart failure, chronic obstructive pulmonary disease (COPD), AIDS and neurologic diseases. It is estimated that around 50% of patients with advanced illness suffer from pain (Bostwick et al. 2017). Pain is rarely an isolated symptom and often presents as part of a cluster of symptoms, all negatively affecting patients' quality of life. In fact, pain, breathlessness and fatigue occur in more than half of patients with cancer, COPD, chronic renal disease, heart disease and AIDS (Solano, Gomes, and Higginson 2006). Pain that is persistent and severe enough may be a source of substantial suffering for patients with advanced illness who already struggle with a high level of distress. The experience of pain is isolating and can threaten a person's sense of "wholeness," of being an authentic human being (Cassel 1982). The key tenet of palliative care is the relief of suffering; relief of pain, therefore, becomes one of the most important tasks for palliative care practitioners. Naturally, not all pain leads to suffering, but there is evidence for a strong association between pain reports and suffering in advanced illness, especially cancer. Only a framework that addresses the physical, psychological, social and spiritual dimensions of pain and suffering, the "total pain" as expressed eloquently by Cicely Saunders, can bring real relief to patients with advanced illness (Figure 8.1) (Twycross 1997; Goebel et al. 2009).

PATHOPHYSIOLOGY OF PAIN

The experience of pain resists language. In fact, as Elaine Scarry writes in *The Body in Pain*, "physical pain does not simply resist language but actively destroys it, bringing about an immediate reversion to a state anterior to language, to the sounds and cries a human being makes before language is learned"

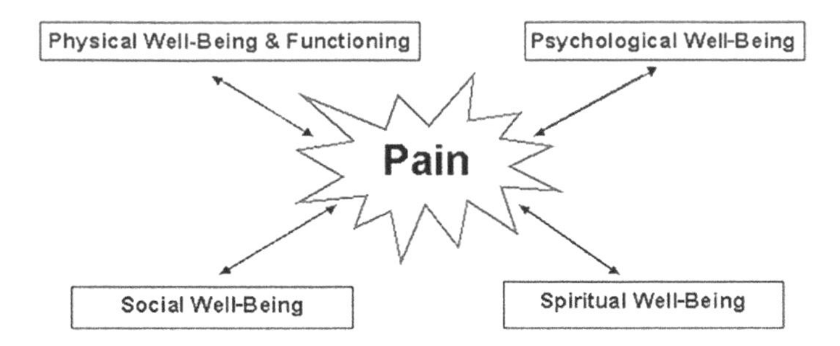

FIGURE 8.1 Pain impacts quality of life. The concept of "total pain," first articulated by Cicely Saunders, to describe the suffering experienced by patients faced with terminal disease. (Adapted with permission from John Wiley and Sons. Goebel, Joy R et al. 2009. *Nursing Forum* 44[3]: 175–85. Blackwell.)

(1985). In the clinical world, a description of a complex phenomenon such as pain is nevertheless necessary for proper diagnosis and treatment. The most broadly accepted definition of pain is the one provided by the International Association for the Study of Pain (IASP), which defines pain as "unpleasant sensory and emotional experience associated with actual or potential tissue damage, or described in terms of such damage" (Merskey and Bogduk 1994). Pain in patients with advanced disease can be classified based on the underlying disease (e.g., cancer versus noncancer pain), temporal characteristics (acute versus chronic), intensity (mild, moderate, severe), location (e.g., abdominal, lower extremity, etc.) and putative pathophysiology (nociceptive or neuropathic) (Boland, Mulvey, and Bennett 2015; Bonica 1990; Portenoy 2011).

Acute pain occurs as a result of nociceptive activity generated by typically clearly identifiable peripheral tissue damage, such as injury to muscles or bones or growth of a tumor. In chronic pain, the relationship between the noxious phenomena and the level of pain experienced is complicated and transformed by neuroplastic processes (known as *sensitization*) that can happen at various levels of the peripheral and central nervous systems. In other words, chronic pain is not just a temporal extension of acute pain (although arbitrarily, chronic pain is often defined as pain that lasts longer than three months) but, some argue, a separate disease entity that can exist even without any apparent tissue damage (Davis and Mehta 2016; Kent et al. 2017). Nociceptive pain is defined as pain that arises from the activation of the peripheral nociceptors and can be further subdivided into somatic and visceral (Table 8.1). Somatic pain comes from activation of cutaneous or deep musculoskeletal nociceptors. Examples may include pain from surgery or bone metastases. Visceral pain results from infiltration, compression, distention of thoracic or abdominal viscera (e.g., pain arising from liver metastasis and capsular distention or pain related to bowel obstruction). This type of pain is poorly localized and usually described as "deep, squeezing or pressure." Neuropathic pain (NP) is defined as pain "from the disease or lesion of the somatosensory system" (IASP). NP is associated with poor outcomes, has a worse prognosis than nociceptive pain and typically does not raespond as well to opioids and non-steroidal anti-inflammatory drugs (NSAIDs) when compared to somatic pain (Levy, Chwistek, and Mehta 2008). NP is commonly seen in cancer patients or diseases of the peripheral or central nervous systems, (e.g., nerve injury, amyotrophic lateral sclerosis [ALS] or multiple sclerosis [MS]) (Cohen and Mao 2014; Mulvey et al. 2017).

PAIN ASSESSMENT

Pain is a dynamic experience that requires an ongoing comprehensive assessment to help characterize it, identify the underlying pathophysiology and examine the effects of pain on the patient's life

TABLE 8.1
Classification of Neuropathic and Nociceptive Pain

Clinical Characteristic	Neuropathic Pain	Nociceptive Pain
Cause	Injury to the nervous system, often accompanied by maladaptive changes in the nervous system	Damage or potential damage to tissues
Descriptors	Lancinating, shooting, electric-like, stabbing pain	Throbbing, aching, pressure-like pain
Sensory deficits	Common—for example, numbness, tingling, prickling	Uncommon; if present they have a non-dermatomal or non-nerve distribution
Motor deficits	Neurological weakness may be present if a motor nerve is affected; dystonia or spasticity may be associated with central nervous system lesions and sometimes peripheral lesions (such as complex regional pain syndrome)	May have pain-induced weakness
Hypersensitivity	Pain often evoked by non-painful (allodynia) or painful (exaggerated response) stimuli	Uncommon except for hypersensitivity in the immediate area of an acute injury
Character	Distal radiation common	Distal radiation less common; proximal radiation more common
Paroxysms	Exacerbations common and unpredictable	Exacerbations less common and often associated with activity
Autonomic signs	Color changes, temperature changes, swelling, or sudomotor (sweating) activity occur in a third to half of patients	Uncommon

Source: Adapted with permission from BMJ Publishing Group Ltd. Cohen S P and J Mao. 2014. *BMJ* (Clinical Research Ed.) 348(February): f7656: 1–12.

and function. When assessing pain, a clinician should focus on sensory, affective and cognitive dimensions of pain. The sensory dimension includes aspects of pain such as intensity, location, radiation, temporal, and aggravating and relieving factors. The affective dimension addresses the psychosocial aspects of pain. The cognitive dimension focuses on patients' perceived meaning of pain and its impact on quality of life (QOL) (Portenoy 2011). A functional assessment focusing on the impact of pain on abilities and sleep can provide a helpful therapeutic target. Exploration of the meanings of pain has particular importance in palliative care. For example, to this day many cancer patients believe that pain is an inseparable and unavoidable consequence of having cancer (and such strong-held beliefs may affect the patient's reports of pain and even the response to therapy) (Lemay et al. 2011). This multidimensional approach ensures the comprehensive assessment of pain and helps palliative care clinicians determine the appropriate treatment (Breivik et al. 2008).

PAIN MEASUREMENT

Pain is a subjective experience, and as such, its measurement relies almost solely on self-reports through either clinical questionnaires or visual, numerical or verbal scales that measure the intensity of pain from "no pain" to the "most excruciating pain" ever (Caraceni et al. 2002). It is important to remember that measurement of pain intensity is most useful in acute pain or pain at the end of life, and it becomes less helpful in chronic pain (Ballantyne and Sullivan 2015; Sullivan and Ballantyne 2016). Many validated pain questionnaires can help clinicians assess patients' pain (Caraceni et al. 2002). The most commonly used are the McGill Pain Questionnaire or the Brief Pain Inventory (Cleeland and Ryan 1994; Melzack and Katz 2001). Also, there are various screening tools for NP. Although they are not diagnostic, they can help clinicians detect NP in patients with advanced illness (Boland, Mulvey, and Bennett 2015; Freynhagen et al. 2016; Nandi 2012).

ETIOLOGY OF PAIN IN ADVANCED DISEASE

CANCER PAIN

Despite tremendous progress in early detection and treatment of oncologic diseases, the effectiveness of treatment of cancer pain (CP) has changed little in the last 30 years. CP still is the most feared aspect of the disease (Lemay et al. 2011). More than half of cancer patients receiving anti-cancer treatment and two-thirds of patients with advanced and metastatic cancer report pain (van den Beuken-van Everdingen et al. 2016). Pain in cancer patients is not a homogenous pathologic process. It is an umbrella term for a diverse group of pain states that typically are classified as pain caused by the tumor itself (60%–75%), its treatment, e.g., chemotherapy, surgery or radiation therapy (10%–20%) or unrelated to the cancer diagnosis (10% caused by comorbid conditions) (Bennett 2017; Nandi 2012). For example, a cancer patient with metastatic colon cancer may have visceral pain related to metastatic liver disease, neuropathic pain from compression of the lumbosacral plexus caused by a primary pelvic tumor, chemotherapy-induced painful peripheral neuropathy caused by the use of neurotoxic chemotherapy and chronic mechanical low back pain unrelated to his or her cancer. Another classic example of cancer pain is cancer-induced bone pain, which is now understood as a complex pain state that has nociceptive, inflammatory and neuropathic characteristics (Falk and Dickenson 2014; Heo et al. 2017; Kane, Hoskin, and Bennett 2015).

PAIN IN ADVANCED NON-CANCER DISEASES

Recent epidemiologic studies have shown that patients with advanced disease also often report chronic pain across various non-cancer conditions. For example, 63%–80% of patients with AIDS report pain and 10%–15% of these patients have painful distal neuropathy. Patients with COPD also report pain in 34%–77% of cases (Solano, Gomes, and Higginson 2006). One group of researchers showed that patients with chronic lung diseases have similar degrees of pain and dyspnea as those with lung cancer (Bostwick et al. 2017; Moens et al. 2014). Almost half of patients with chronic renal disease report pain that is often associated with high degrees of fatigue, anorexia, dyspnea and depression (Davison 2007). Patients with advanced heart failure experience various types of pain. Pain can be related to cardiovascular health, such as chest pain associated with angina, or peripheral vascular disease. One study found 89% of end-stage heart failure patients have pain (Lowey 2017). Pain in neurologic disorders is quite common and diverse in its underlying pathophysiology and clinical presentation. In some conditions, such as painful peripheral neuropathies, pain is neuropathic, although even within this category there are considerable phenotypic variations. The neurologic conditions most associated with pain are painful peripheral neuropathy including diabetic neuropathy, HIV-associated neuropathy and postherpetic neuralgia; complex regional pain syndrome; MS; Parkinson disease and central poststroke pain (Nandi 2012). However, not all pain in neurologic disease is neuropathic. For example, nociceptive pain is common in conditions affecting the motor system. Patients with advanced illness may also suffer from chronic and common musculoskeletal pain (e.g., low back pain and degenerative joint disease), which may be compounded by frailty and limitations in mobility.

MANAGEMENT OF PAIN IN ADVANCED ILLNESS

Pain is a dynamic and complex phenomenon, and its practical management requires an individualized, multimodal plan of treatment based on comprehensive and ongoing assessment coupled with close monitoring of the outcomes of therapy and management of its adverse effects. In recent years, the landscape of chronic, incurable disease has been transformed by the development of new non-curative options for treatment. In cancer, HIV and cardiology treatments have considerably prolonged survival, in some instances by years. Unfortunately, for some patients, prolonged survival means that patients may need to live and cope with pain and other symptoms for extended periods of time. Therefore, it is essential to evaluate the effectiveness of pain control and modify its treatment in the context of patients' prognosis and functional status, with the primary goal of improving overall well-being (Figure 8.2).

Opioid Therapy

Opioids remain the mainstay of pharmacologic pain management in patients with advanced illness (Figure 8.3). Yet, their role in treatment has been evolving, principally due to a growing understanding of their adverse effects associated with chronic use. This is especially important in the context of more prolonged survival in patients with incurable diseases. Chronic opioid therapy (defined as greater than three months) has been associated with increased risk of endocrinopathies, depression, sleep-disordered breathing, impaired wound healing, substance use disorders and cognitive impairment (Davis 2010; Paice et al. 2016). Finding the proper balance between appropriate analgesia and the risks associated with opioid therapy may be particularly challenging due to a number of factors. Patients with incurable diseases live longer, are older in general, suffer from often multiple comorbid illnesses and are taking multiple medications. Additionally, palliative care practitioners increasingly find themselves taking care of patients with substance use and mental health disorders, which in turn requires specialized knowledge, skills and resources that are often not readily available (Reisfield, Paulian, and Wilson 2009; Sacco et al. 2017).

Treatment of Neuropathic Pain

NP is more difficult to treat than nociceptive pain. There is consistent evidence that shows that NP is associated with worse quality of life of patients and its management is typically challenging. NP is present on average in 40% of cancer patients, but may also affect patients with other advanced conditions (Cruccu and Truini 2017; Mulvey et al. 2014). For example, patients with end-stage heart failure may suffer from neuropathic pain caused by thoracotomy. Similarly, patients with ALS may

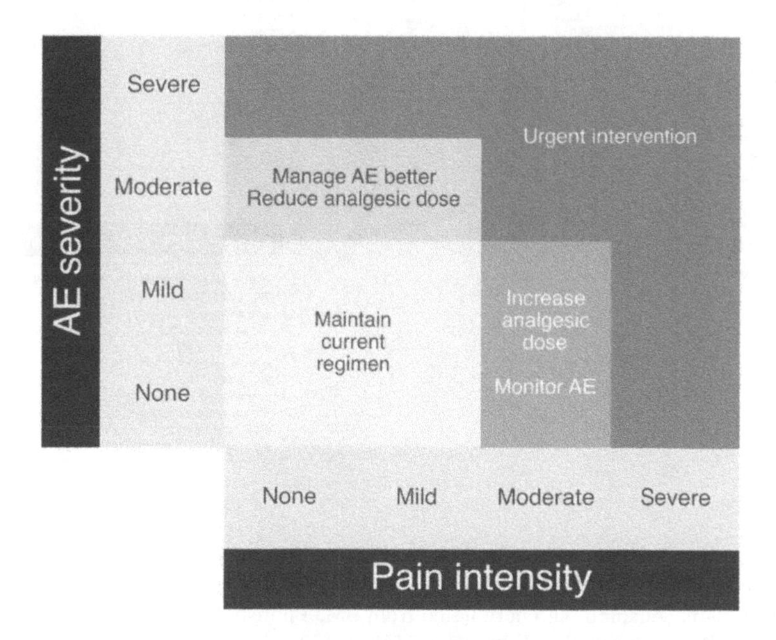

FIGURE 8.2 Opioids for cancer pain – an overview of Cochrane reviews. The goal of treatment of cancer pain is to maximize pain relief while minimizing adverse event severity. The concept and the need for measurement of pain and assessment of the severity of adverse events. (Wiffen P J et al. Opioids for cancer pain - an overview of cochrane reviews. *Cochrane Database of Systematic Reviews. 2017. 7,* CD012592. Copyright Wiley-VCH Verlag GmbH & Co. KGaA. Reproduced with permission.)

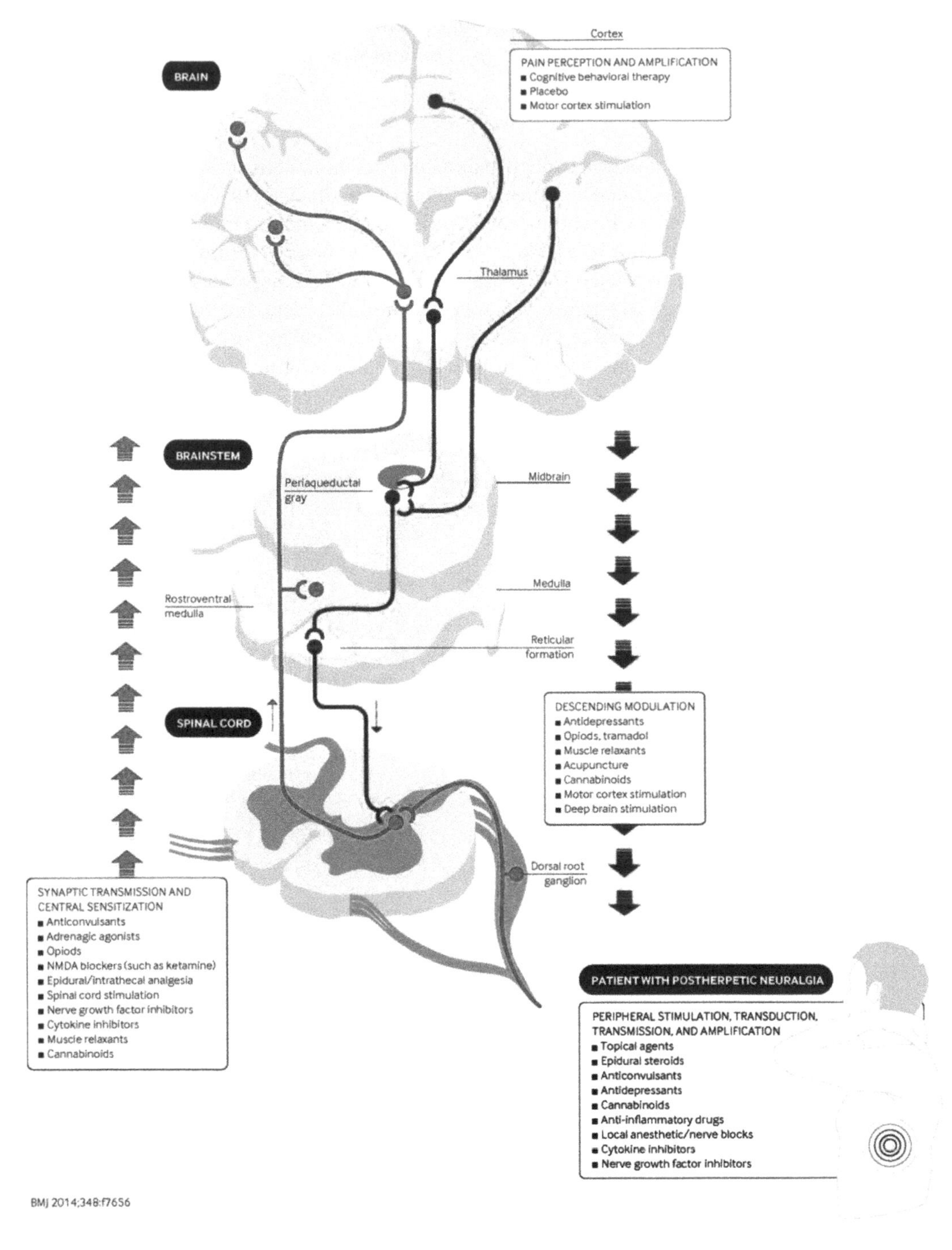

FIGURE 8.3 The site of action of various classes of analgesics. Schematic representation of the ascending (arrow ↑) and descending (arrow ↓) pain pathways and the site(s) of action of various classes of analgesics used in the treatment of pain. (Adapted with permission from BMJ Publishing Group Ltd. Cohen S P and J Mao. 2014. *BMJ* [Clinical Research Ed.] 348[February]: f7656: 1–12.)

TABLE 8.2
Currently Recommended Neuropathic Pain Drugs[a]

Drug	Total Daily Dose and Dose Regimen	Recommendations
	Strong Recommendations for Use	
Gapabentin	1200–3600 mg, in three divided doses	First line
Gabapentin extended release or enacarbil	1200–3600 mg, in two divided doses	First line
Pregabalin	300–600 mg, in two divided doses	First line
Serotonin-norepinephrine reuptake inhibitors duloxetine or venlafaxine[b]	60–120 mg, once a day (duloxetine); 150–225 mg, once a day (venlafaxine extended release)	First line
Tricyclic antidepressants	25–150 mg, once a day or in two divided doses	First line[c]
	Weak Recommendations for Use	
Capsaicin 8% patches	One to four patches to the painful area for 30–60 minutes every three months	Second line (peripheral neuropathic pain)[d]
Lidocaine patches	One to three patches to the region of pain once a day for up to 12 hours	Second line (peripheral neuropath pain)
Tramadol	200–400 mg, in two (tramadol extended release) or three divided doses	Second line
Botulinum toxin A (subcutaneously)	50–200 units to the painful area every three months	Third line; specialist use (peripheral neuropathic pain)
Strong opioids	Individual titration	Third line[e]

Source: Reprinted from *Mayo Clinic Proceedings*, 90(4), Gilron I et al., Neuropathic pain: principles of diagnosis and treatment, Copyright 2015, with permission from Elsevier.

[a] GRADE = Grading of Recommendations Assessment, Development, and Evaluation.

[b] Duloxetine is the most studied, and therefore recommended, of the serotonin-norepinephrine reuptake inhibitors.

[c] Tricyclic antidepressants generally have similar efficacy; tertiary amine tricyclic antidepressants (amitriptyline, imipramine, and clomipramine) are not recommended at doses >75 mg/d in adults aged 65 y and older because of major anticholinergic and sedative adverse effects and potential risk of falls (Backonja and Galer 1998); an increased risk of sudden cardiac death has been reported with tricyclic antidepressants at doses >100 mg/d (Hanson and Haanpää 2007).

[d] The long-term safety of repeated applications of high-concentration capsaicin patches in patients has not been clearly established, particularly with respect to the degeneration of epidermal nerve fibers, which might be a cause for concern in progressive neuropathy.

Sustained-release oxycodone and morphine have been the most-studied opioids (maximum doses of 120 and 240 mg/d, respectively, in clinical trials); long-term opioid use might be associated with abuse, particularly at high doses, cognitive impairment, and endocrine and immunological changes (Baron and Tölle 2008; Feldman et al. 1994).

have neuropathic pain related to the development of a central nervous system lesion. Pharmacologic treatment of neuropathic pain consists of the use "adjuvant analgesics"—a group of medications that were approved for treatment of other conditions (e.g., seizures) but were found to have analgesic properties (Table 8.2) (Boland, Mulvey, and Bennett 2015; Cohen and Mao 2014; Mulvey et al. 2017).

Non-Pharmacologic Options

Pharmacologic options for treatment of pain in advanced illness are not always sufficient for adequate pain control (Table 8.3). When designing a treatment plan, palliative care clinicians need to take into account a range of potential treatment options, including non-pharmacologic treatments that may include behavioral approaches (e.g., cognitive behavioural therapy), mindfulness techniques, neuromodulation techniques, interventional approaches, medical marijuana and cannabinoids and

TABLE 8.3
Categories of Treatments for Pain in Patients with Advanced Illness

Pharmacological
- Opioid analgesics
- Non-opioid analgesics
- Non-traditional analgesics (adjuvant analgesics)

Interventional
- Injection therapies
- Neural blockade
- Implant therapy

Rehabilitative
- Modalities
- Therapeutic exercise
- Occupational therapy
- Hydrotherapy
- Treatment for specific disorders (e.g., lymphoedema)

Psychological
- Psychoeducational interventions
- Cognitive behavioural therapy
- Relaxation therapy, guided imagery, other types of stress management
- Other forms of psychotherapy

Neurostimulation
- Transcutaneous
- Transcranial
- Implanted

Integrative (complementary or alternative)
- Acupuncture
- Massage
- Physical or movement
- Others

Source: Reprinted from *Lancet*, 377(9784), Portenoy R K. Treatment of Cancer Pain, 2236–47, Copyright 2011, with permission from Elsevier.

complementary medicine. Many of these techniques and treatments can be an integral part of an individualized plan of treatment and can be used alongside medications (Bostwick 2012; Chwistek 2017; Deer et al. 2013; Goroszeniuk and Pang 2014; Lamer, Deer, and Hayek 2016).

GLOBAL ISSUES

Unrelieved pain remains a public health concern in many areas of the world. Patients with advanced illness face many barriers to effective pain control including access to pain and palliative care practitioners and availability and accessibility of analgesics. Lack of access to opioids is a global problem. The World Health Organisation (WHO) estimates that 80% of the world's population, including patients with terminal cancer and end-stage AIDS, do not have adequate access to pain treatment. In light of apparent inadequacies in the management of pain in advanced illness around the world, the international pain and palliative care communities began to frame the problem in the context of human rights. Many organizations issued statements that framed the problem of inadequate pain management as a human rights issue, which, in turn, led to its acknowledgment and affirmation by bodies within the United Nations (Brennan, Carr, and Cousins 2007, 2016; Cousins and Lynch 2011; Hall and Boswell 2009).

OPIOID MISUSE AND ABUSE

As worldwide advocacy efforts promoting pain management as a human right continued, the United States increasingly faced a significant crisis of prescription opioid abuse (Benzon and Anderson 2017). There is omnipresent discourse in medical and lay publications discussing the crisis and its tragic consequences. New guidelines on pain management and safe opioid prescribing have been issued. Surprisingly, guidelines have focused primarily on patients with chronic non-cancer pain and have provided minimal direction on how best to manage safe opioid prescribing in patients with advanced cancer and terminal illness (Dowell, Haegerich, and Chou 2016). In fact, these populations of patients have been excluded from most of the publications, despite new data showing that rates of opioid abuse, misuse and addiction are basically the same as those seen in the general public (Copenhaver, Karvelas, and Fishman 2017). The WHO analgesic ladder was written in 1986 to address the largely inadequate treatment of cancer pain and later revised in 1996, well before the groundswell of the epidemic of opioid overdoses. The most recent edition of the National Comprehensive Cancer Network guidelines for the management of cancer pain to an extent addresses safety issues regarding opioid prescribing. But it but does not provide specific recommendations, for example, how and when to taper opioids, or how to switch patients to treatment with buprenorphine (Swarm 2013). Despite the progress made in our understanding of pain, pain management is still not considered a priority, and research, guidelines and resources are limited. Advancing pain care as a basic human right and understanding how to balance this with an epidemic of opioid overdoses will require widespread and concerted efforts of key stakeholders, including medical communities, legislators, patient advocacy groups and professional medical organizations.

KEY FACTS: PAIN CONTROL IN PALLIATIVE CARE

- Pain is a complex multidimensional experience common in patients with advanced disease, especially cancer, but also in patients with advanced heart failure, COPD, AIDS and neurologic diseases.
- Opioid-based pharmacotherapy remains the mainstay of pain treatment in patients with advanced illness, although the use of other agents such as NSAIDs, glucocorticoids, antidepressants and anticonvulsants may be necessary and helpful.
- Many non-pharmacologic treatments such as interventional approaches, neurostimulation techniques and complementary approaches should be considered and may be implemented into the treatment regimen if necessary.
- There is a paucity of data addressing the issues of opioid misuse, abuse and addiction in patients with advanced and terminal diseases.

SUMMARY POINTS

- Pain is one of the most common symptoms in patients with advanced illness, and yet despite significant progress in the understanding of its pathophysiology, many patients worldwide still do not receive adequate analgesia.
- Pain is a complex phenomenon that is best understood in the biopsychosocial context and addressed through comprehensive multidimensional assessment and treatment.
- The relief of suffering is the cardinal goal of palliative medicine in patients with incurable and progressive disease; numerous effective therapies (pharmacologic, interventional, behavioral, complementary) exist for the treatment of pain in patients with advanced illness.
- Opioids remain the most effective and commonly used medication for the treatment of pain associated with advanced illness, and their widespread use needs to be balanced with safe prescribing.

LIST OF ABBREVIATIONS

ALS	Amyotrophic Lateral Sclerosis
CAM	Complementary and Alternative Therapies
CIBP	Cancer-Induced Bone Pain
CIPN	Chemotherapy-Induced Painful Neuropathy
COT	Chronic Opioid Therapy
CP	Cancer Pain
fMRI	Functional MRI
IAHPC	International Association of Hospice and Palliative Care
IASP	International Association for the Study of Pain
MS	Multiple Sclerosis
NCCN	National Comprehensive Cancer Network
NP	Neuropathic Pain
NSAIDs	Non-Steroidal Antiinflammatory Drugs
PC	Palliative Care
QOL	Quality of Life
SNRIs	Serotonin-Norepinephrine Reuptake Inhibitors
TCAs	Tricyclic Antidepressants
UN	United Nations
WHO	World Health Organization
WPCA	Worldwide Palliative Care Alliance

REFERENCES

Backonja M M and B S Galer. 1998. Pain Assessment and Evaluation of Patients Who Have Neuropathic Pain. *Neurologic Clinics* 16(4): 775–90.

Ballantyne J C and M D Sullivan. 2015. Intensity of Chronic Pain—The Wrong Metric? *New England Journal of Medicine* 373(22): 2098–99.

Baron R and T R Tölle. 2008. Assessment and Diagnosis of Neuropathic Pain. *Current Opinion in Supportive and Palliative Care* 2(1): 1–8.

Bennett, M I. 2017. Mechanism-Based Cancer-Pain Therapy. *Pain* 158 Suppl 1(April): S74–78.

Benzon, H T and T A Anderson. 2017. Themed Issue on the Opioid Epidemic: What Have We Learned? Where Do We Go from Here? *Anesthesia and Analgesia* 125(5): 1435–37.

Boland E G, M R Mulvey, and M I Bennett. 2015. Classification of Neuropathic Pain in Cancer Patients. *Current Opinion in Supportive and Palliative Care* 9(2): 112–15.

Bonica J J. 1990. Definition and Taxonomy Pain. In: Bonica J (ed.) *The Management of Pain* 2: 18–27.

Bostwick D, S Wolf, G Samsa, J Bull, D H Taylor, K S Johnson, and A H Kamal. 2017. Comparing the Palliative Care Needs of Those with Cancer to Those with Common Non-Cancer Serious Illness. *Journal of Pain and Symptom Management* 53(6): 1079–1084.e1.

Bostwick J M. 2012. Blurred Boundaries: The Therapeutics and Politics of Medical Marijuana. *Mayo Clinic Proceedings* 87(2): 172–86.

Breivik, H, P C Borchgrevink, S M Allen, L A Rosseland, L Romundstad, E K B Hals, G Kvarstein, and A Stubhaug. 2008. Assessment of Pain. *British Journal of Anaesthesia* 101(1): 17–24.

Brennan F, D B Carr, and M Cousins. 2007. Pain Management: A Fundamental Human Right. *Anesthesia and Analgesia* 105(1), 205–21. doi:10.1213/01.ane.0000268145.52345.55

Brennan F, D Carr, and M Cousins. 2016. Access to Pain Management—Still Very Much a Human Right. *Pain Medicine* 17(10): 1785–89.

Caraceni A, N Cherny, R Fainsinger, S Kaasa, P Poulain, L Radbruch, and F De Conno. 2002. Pain Measurement Tools and Methods in Clinical Research in Palliative Care: Recommendations of an Expert Working Group of the European Association of Palliative Care. *Journal of Pain and Symptom Management* 23(3): 239–55.

Cassel E J. 1982. The Nature of Suffering and the Goals of Medicine. *New England Journal of Medicine* 306(11): 639–45.

Chwistek M. 2017. Recent Advances in Understanding and Managing Cancer Pain. [Version 1; Referees: 3 Approved]. *F1000Research* 6(June): 945.

Cleeland C S and K M Ryan. 1994. Pain Assessment: Global Use of the Brief Pain Inventory. *Annals of the Academy of Medicine, Singapore* 23(2): 129–38.
Cohen S P and J Mao. 2014. Neuropathic Pain: Mechanisms and Their Clinical Implications. *BMJ* (Clinical Research Ed.) 348(February): f7656: 1–12.
Copenhaver D J, N B Karvelas, and S M Fishman. 2017. Risk Management for Opioid Prescribing in the Treatment of Patients with Pain from Cancer or Terminal Illness: Inadvertent Oversight or Taboo? *Anesthesia and Analgesia* 125(5): 1610–15.
Cousins M J and M E Lynch. 2011. The Declaration Montreal: Access to Pain Management Is a Fundamental Human Right. *Pain* 152(12): 2673–74.
Cruccu G and A Truini. 2017. A Review of Neuropathic Pain: From Guidelines to Clinical Practice. *Pain and Therapy* 6(Suppl 1): 35–42.
Davis M P. 2010. Recent Advances in the Treatment of Pain. *F1000 Medicine Reports* 2(August): 63.
Davis M P and Z Mehta. 2016. Opioids and Chronic Pain: Where Is the Balance? *Current Oncology Reports* 18(12): 71.
Davison S N. 2007. The Prevalence and Management of Chronic Pain in End-Stage Renal Disease. *Journal of Palliative Medicine* 10(6): 1277–87.
Deer T R, E Grigsby, R L Weiner, B Wilcosky, and J M Kramer. 2013. A Prospective Study of Dorsal Root Ganglion Stimulation for the Relief of Chronic Pain. *Neuromodulation* 16(1): 67–71; discussion 71.
Dowell D, T M Haegerich, and R Chou. 2016. CDC Guideline for Prescribing Opioids for Chronic Pain—United States, 2016. *Journal of the American Medical Association* 315(15): 1624–45.
Falk S and A H Dickenson. 2014. Pain and Nociception: Mechanisms of Cancer-Induced Bone Pain. *Journal of Clinical Oncology* 32(16): 1647–54.
Feldman E L, M J Stevens, P K Thomas, M B Brown, N Canal, and D A Greene. 1994. A Practical Two-step Quantitative Clinical and Electrophysiological Assessment for the Diagnosis and Staging of Diabetic Neuropathy. *Diabetes Care* 17(11): 1281–89.
Freynhagen R, T R Tölle, U Gockel, and R Baron. 2016. The PainDETECT Project – Far More than a Screening Tool on Neuropathic Pain. *Current Medical Research and Opinion* 32(6): 1033–57.
Gilron Ian, Ralf Baron, and Troels Jensen. 2015. Neuropathic pain: principles of diagnosis and treatment. *Mayo Clinic Proceedings* 90(4). Elsevier.
Goebel J R, L V Doering, K A Lorenz, S L Maliski, A M Nyamathi, and L S Evangelista. 2009. Caring for Special Populations: Total Pain Theory in Advanced Heart Failure: Applications to Research and Practice. *Nursing Forum* 44(3): 175–85.
Goroszeniuk T and D Pang. 2014. Peripheral Neuromodulation: A Review. *Current Pain and Headache Reports* 18(5): 412.
Hall J K and M V Boswell. 2009. Ethics, Law, and Pain Management as a Patient Right. *Pain Physician* 12(3): 499–506.
Hansson P and M Haanpää. 2007. Diagnostic Work-up of Neuropathic Pain: Computing, Using Questionnaires or Examining the Patient? *European Journal of Pain* 11(4): 367–69.
Heo M H, J Y Kim, I Hwang, E Ha, and Keon Uk Park. 2017. Analgesic Effect of Quetiapine in a Mouse Model of Cancer-Induced Bone Pain. *Korean Journal of Internal Medicine* 32(6): 1069–74.
Kane C M, P Hoskin, and M I Bennett. 2015. Cancer Induced Bone Pain. *BMJ* (Clinical Research Ed.) 350(January): h315.
Kent M L, P J Tighe, I Belfer, T J Brennan, S Bruehl, C M Brummett, C C Buckenmaier et al. 2017. The ACTTION-APS-AAPM Pain Taxonomy (AAAPT) Multidimensional Approach to Classifying Acute Pain Conditions. *Journal of Pain* 18(5): 479–89.
Lamer T J, T R Deer, and S M Hayek. 2016. Advanced Innovations for Pain. *Mayo Clinic Proceedings* 91(2): 246–58.
Lemay K, K G Wilson, U Buenger, V Jarvis, E Fitzgibbon, K Bhimji, and P L Dobkin. 2011. Fear of Pain in Patients with Advanced Cancer or in Patients with Chronic Noncancer Pain. *Clinical Journal of Pain* 27(2): 116–24.
Levy M H, M Chwistek, and R S Mehta. 2008. Management of Chronic Pain in Cancer Survivors. *Cancer Journal* 14(6): 401–9.
Lowey S E. 2017. Palliative Care in the Management of Patients with Advanced Heart Failure. *Advances in Experimental Medicine and Biology*, doi:10.1007/5584_2017_115.
Melzack R and J Katz. 2001. *The McGill Pain Questionnaire: Appraisal and Current Status*. New York, NY: Guilford Press.
Merskey H and N Bogduk (Eds.). 1994. Classification of Chronic Pain: Descriptions of Chronic Pain Syndromes and Definitions of Pain Terms, 2nd edn. Seattle: IASP Press.

Moens K, I J Higginson, R Harding, and EURO IMPACT. 2014. Are There Differences in the Prevalence of Palliative Care-Related Problems in People Living with Advanced Cancer and Eight Non-Cancer Conditions? A Systematic Review. *Journal of Pain and Symptom Management* 48(4): 660–77.

Mulvey M R, E G Boland, D Bouhassira, R Freynhagen, J Hardy, M J Hjermstad, S Mercadante, C Pérez, and M I Bennett. 2017. Neuropathic Pain in Cancer: Systematic Review, Performance of Screening Tools and Analysis of Symptom Profiles. *British Journal of Anaesthesia* 119(4): 765–74.

Mulvey M R, R Rolke, P Klepstad, A Caraceni, M Fallon, L Colvin, B Laird, M I Bennett, and IASP Cancer Pain SIG and the EAPC Research Network. 2014. Confirming Neuropathic Pain in Cancer Patients: Applying the NeuPSIG Grading System in Clinical Practice and Clinical Research. *Pain* 155(5): 859–63.

Nandi P R. 2012. Pain in Neurological Conditions. *Current Opinion in Supportive and Palliative Care* 6(2): 194–200.

Paice J A, R Portenoy, C Lacchetti, T Campbell, A Cheville, M Citron, L S Constine et al. 2016. Management of Chronic Pain in Survivors of Adult Cancers: American Society of Clinical Oncology Clinical Practice Guideline. *Journal of Clinical Oncology* 34(27): 3325–45.

Portenoy R K. 2011. Treatment of Cancer Pain. *Lancet* 377(9784): 2236–47.

Reisfield G M, G D Paulian, and G R Wilson. 2009. Substance Use Disorders in the Palliative Care Patient #127. *Journal of Palliative Medicine* 12(5): 475–76.

Sacco P, J G Cagle, M L Moreland, and E A S Camlin. 2017. Screening and Assessment of Substance Use in Hospice Care: Examining Content from a National Sample of Psychosocial Assessments. *Journal of Palliative Medicine* 20(8): 850–56.

Scarry E. 1985. *From the Body in Pain: The Making and Unmaking of the World*. New York, NY: Oxford University Press.

Solano J P, B Gomes, and I J Higginson. 2006. A Comparison of Symptom Prevalence in Far Advanced Cancer, AIDS, Heart Disease, Chronic Obstructive Pulmonary Disease and Renal Disease. *Journal of Pain and Symptom Management* 31(1): 58–69.

Sullivan M D and J C Ballantyne. 2016. Must We Reduce Pain Intensity to Treat Chronic Pain? *Pain* 157(1): 65–69.

Swarm R A. 2013. The Management of Pain in Patients with Cancer. *Journal of the National Comprehensive Cancer Network* 11(5 Suppl): 702–4.

Twycross R. 1997. Cancer Pain Classification. *Acta Anaesthesiologica Scandinavica* 41(1 Pt 2): 141–45.

van den Beuken-van Everdingen M H J, L M J Hochstenbach, E A J Joosten, V C G Tjan-Heijnen, and D J A Janssen. 2016. Update on Prevalence of Pain in Patients with Cancer: Systematic Review and Meta-Analysis. *Journal of Pain and Symptom Management* 51(6): 1070–1090.e9.

Wiffen P J, B Wee, S Derry, R F Bell, and R A Moore. 2017. Opioids for cancer pain—an overview of cochrane reviews. *Cochrane Database of Systematic Reviews*, 7, CD012592. doi:10.1002/14651858.CD012592.pub2

9 Communication in Palliative and End-of-Life Care

Blair Henry

CONTENTS

We speak not only to tell other people what we think, but to tell ourselves what we think. Speech is a part of thought.

Oliver Sacks (Sacks 1989)

INTRODUCTION

The modern concept of palliative and hospice care has only been around for the past 60 years. In the 1950s, medicine specifically in the field of oncology focused singularly on the potential for cure, such that a patient who was considered to be dying from their disease would be avoided and subsequently abandoned by their healthcare team (Clark 2007). As patients approached the end stages of their disease, physicians felt they had little to offer in the form of treatment and would frequently tell their patients to go home as there was nothing more that medicine had to offer (Clark 2007).

However, in the 1950s and 1960s new research started to emerge in Europe, identifying important new insights into the components of care for the dying (Clark 2007). In North America it would be the work of a clinical psychiatrist named Elizabeth Kubler Ross who brought to the fore the importance of care of the dying in her seminal book, published in 1969, entitled: *On Death and Dying* (Kubler Ross 1969; Doka et al. 2011). These events ushered in a new field of study known as *thanatology*, the scientific study of death and the practices associated with it, including the recognition of a response to needs of the dying patient and their families (Doka et al. 2011).

In its nascency, palliative care (PC) was only offered to patients in the last weeks to months of life, when all attempts at cure had been exhausted. However, in the intervening years palliative and hospice care has continued to grow and evolve, and has slowly received a modest degree of acceptance within the medical and lay communities. In fact, over the past decade, it has been noted that early palliative care can improve quality of life and reduce unnecessary hospitalizations for patients when they receive appropriate integrative care early in the disease process (Bacon 2012).

The World Health Organization (WHO) first formally defined the term *palliative care* in 1989; however, its most recent articulation in 2017 defined palliative care as "an approach that improves the quality of life of patients and their families facing the problem associated with life-threatening illness, through the prevention and relief of suffering by means of early identification and impeccable assessment and treatment of pain and other problems, physical, psychosocial and spiritual" (WHO 2017).

Communication has come to be recognized as an essential component of delivering palliative care (Dunne and Sullivan 2000; Kennedy-Sheldon, Barrett, and Ellington 2006). If, based on the WHO the goal of PC is to improve quality of life by prevention of or relief of physical, psychological, social and spiritual suffering then effective communication is essential to it achieving its desired ends. To accomplish these goals clinicians need to help their patients and families to openly express their fears and concerns, assess needs effectively, and elicit honest and appropriate plans of care going forward (Perrin 2001). In addition the ability to communicate well is known to effect good patient care in general and reduce patient and family member distress, and has even proven to improve patient satisfaction (Granek et al. 2013).

Additional challenges to engaging communication will also come about from the changing face of palliative care. As the population ages and demands increase, reliance on a specialist palliative care service alone will not be sustainable. To ensure quality and accessible access to services, a palliative care system needs to be integrated into primary healthcare, community and home-based levels of care (Bacon 2012).

This chapter attempts to look into the current academic literature on the status of communication in the field of palliative care. To improve understanding and awareness of the underpinnings of interpersonal communications, a popular communication theory will be used, as an example, to illustrate the complexities inherent in the art of communications. PC/end-of-life (EOL) care involves communication events critical in success or failure of palliative care, regardless of where it is introduced in the illness trajectory. Second a review of known barriers and potential tools to improve communication skills are discussed.

COMMUNICATION THEORY

A reductionist understanding of communication would be to state that it is simply the process whereby information can be exchanged. This oversimplification leaves barren the nature and power of what communication truly entails. Contemporary communication theories, specifically looking at interpersonal communications, represent a focused area of research that attempts to better understand how humans use both verbal and non-verbal symbols to accomplish their personal, professional and relational goals (Berger 2008).

Good or effective communications might best be described as a generic process that involves a two-way process between two or more individuals in which ideas, feelings and information are shared with the aim being to reduce uncertainty and clarify issues (Parker and Coiera 2000).

However, communication only becomes complete when there is feedback to ensure the message has been received and understood. To be truly effective, communication in health serves the following ends (Parker and Coiera 2000):

- Advises on the resources available to address holistic needs and concerns
- Provides patients with a sense of security, consistency and comfort
- Educates family members and care providers on caring aspects
- Aims to improve relationships at all levels
- Ensures a good flow of information within and between organizations involved in service delivery

Any number of communication theories could serve the education purposes of this chapter; however, to illustrate the complexities inherent in the process of communication, the model developed by Berlo in 1960 serves as a good example to consider for this purpose. Unlike his contemporaries, Berlo took a different approach to modeling communication by electively categorizing and studying the individual ingredients involved in the four stages of the communication process: source, message, channel, and receiver (SMCR). This became known as the SMCR communication model (Berlo 1960).

In this model, the source (aka the sender) is the one from whom the thought originates. The source is the one who transfers the information to the receiver after carefully putting thoughts into words. The process of transferring occurs with the aid of the sender's communication skills, attitude, knowledge, social system and culture. Suffice to say that when an individual converts his or her thoughts into words, a message is created. Berlo posits these messages are typically composed of the following elements: content, element, treatment, structure, and code (body movement, expressions, gestures). The channel he describes actually refers to the medium – how the information flows from the sender to the receiver. In this model any of the five senses (sight, sound, touch, smell and taste) can form the channels that help human beings to communicate with each other. Finally, the model considers the receiver of the intended message; not surprisingly the ingredients for the receiver are similar to those of the source. As the theory holds, if the receiver's communication skills, attitudes, knowledge, social and cultural backgrounds differ, and remain unattended, we can expect communications problems to ensue (Berlo 1960).

The complexities and nuances of communication can only be partially illustrated using a theoretical model such as Berlo's. Though informative in its provided structure and component elements, what is truly missing from such a mode is consideration for the context from which communication occurs – medicine, specifically at the EOL. This charged context for communication involves strong emotions, religious and culture heterogeneity, institution settings and policies, an account of the varying power dynamics between the messenger and receiver, and the interplay of underlying psychological factors such as coping skills, grief and maturity.

As suggested, no single text could do justice to the complexities that underpin communications challenges in the context of palliative care. Even the type of communication plays a significant role. Take by example research into verbal and non-verbal messaging. UCLA Psychologist Alan Mehrabian outlined three elements in a message that can account differently to our trusting our degree of liking for the person who puts forward a message concerning their feelings. His work showed that words account for 7%, tone of voice accounts for 38%, and body language accounts for 55% of the liking. Otherwise known as "the 7%–38%–55% Rule," see Figure 9.1, his research goes on to suggest that the receiver will most likely trust the predominant form of communications, the non-verbal impact of tone + gestures (38% + 55%), rather than the literal meaning of the words (7%) (Mehrabian 1971).

In addition to Mehrabian's work, the influence of non-verbal forms of communication in healthcare has been well studied and can attest to helping build rapport and empathic communication between all parties (Bylund and D'Agostino 2014; Ruben and Hall 2016). Providing one's undivided attention through non-verbal channels, such as directly facing the patient, being at eye level, and avoiding distractions sends the message that what the patient is conveying is important. As challenging as it can be in a busy clinical environment, avoiding interruption and giving patients undivided attention can communicate that the healthcare professional is fully present and ready to listen (Moore 2005).

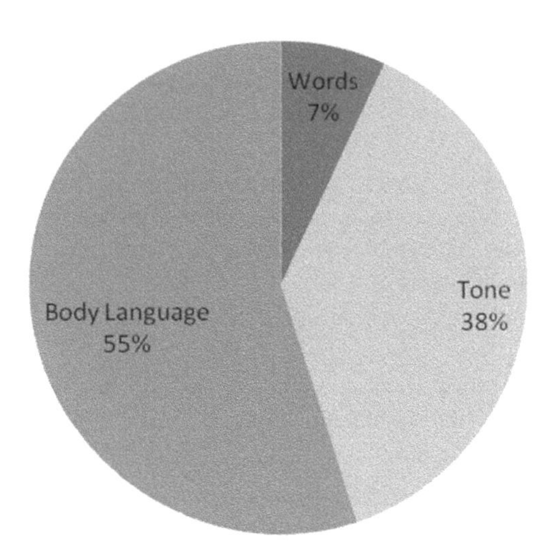

FIGURE 9.1 Impact of elements in interpersonal communications. Illustrating the *7%–38%–55%*. (From Mehrabian, A. 1971. *Rule based on the work of Mehrabian A. Silent Messages*. Belmont, CA: Wadsworth.)

Eye contact is another important component of non-verbal communication. Looking patients in the eyes while talking and listening signals emotional connection and psychological presence and the provider is truly listening to, connected with, and concerned about the patient. However, it is important to note that the importance of direct eye contact is valued in the dominant Western culture, and may not be appropriate when interacting with patients and families from diverse backgrounds (Ruben and Hall 2016).

ILLNESS TRAJECTORY AND KEY CONVERSATION EVENTS

The illness trajectory and experience, from diagnosis to death, will be unique for each patient. However, collective wisdom has shown that most journeys will involve a series of key conversational events that will greatly impact the quality of the relationships and the direction of care. Though not meant to be complete, Table 9.1 identifies nine such key events where reliance on a clinician's interpersonal and communication skills will surely be tested (Hudson et al. 2006).

TABLE 9.1
Major Clinical Events in EOL Communications Based on Stages of Typical Disease Progression

- Breaking bad news
- How long do I have? (Prognostication)
- Introducing palliative care
- Advance care planning
- "Lane changing" (from curative to comfort)
- "Do not resuscitate" conversations
- Goals of care
- Addressing request/desire for hastened death
- Saying goodbye

Note: This listing of major clinical events is based on the author's EOL experience in hospice and palliative care.

In a world where candor is considered an essential component of the clinical encounter it is equally important to remember that the words and gestures we use can have long-lasting impact (Gueguen et al. 2009). In offering to elaborate more on this topic the reader is directed to pay heed to a quote by Carl Buehner: People may forget what you said, they may forget what you did – but people will never forget how you made them feel (Buehner 1971).

Breaking Bad News

Though each of the 10 events present unique challenges, breaking bad news is often considered to be a key moment in the patient-physician relationship. An important aspect of the disclosure process involves evaluating the patient's attitudes, knowledge, wishes and needs before breaking bad news to the patient. Establishing how much they currently know, and how much they want to know is key to undertaking this conversation (Han and Kagan 2012).

A meta-synthesis published in 2015 provides a thorough and structured understanding of oncologists' perspectives and experiences of delivering bad news to patients who have cancer (Bousquet et al. 2015). Though directed to cancer, it is suggested that the findings can be extrapolated to the disclosure of other life-limiting conditions. In their report, the authors identified two broad themes: the essential aspects of the communication between the two parties; and impact of external factors shaping the patient-oncologist encounter (Bousquet et al. 2015).

The report identified and delved into the following themes found persistent in the literature they reviewed:

> Breaking bad news requires a balancing act between informing patients and sustaining their hope. Terminology used and sustaining hope was noted to be particularly challenging for patients who are going to die, and the potential for collusion in maintaining unrealistic expectations during the stages of terminal illness was noted. In addition, breaking bad news means facing strong emotions—both the patient's and the oncologist's. Oncologists mentioned difficulties in dealing with their patients' emotional reactions to their announcement (Bousquet et al. 2015).
>
> Systemic and institutional factors such as lack of time, space, and their perceptions of insufficient training in breaking bad news were noted as influencing the process. The culture, not only of the patient but also of the oncologist, strongly influences how bad news is both given and received. Despite all the programs to improve a clinician's ability to deliver bad news, this emotional experience remains invasive and complex for the physician (Bousquet et al. 2015).

Prognostication

Communicating prognosis, with patients suffering from life-limiting illness, can be a difficult process. While many patients with advanced or life-limiting illness need prognostic information to better accept their disease, and to make decisions regarding treatment, this information is often not conveyed to the patient effectively (Hagerty et al. 2005).

Errors in over-estimation and under-estimation of survival can lead to adverse consequences, in which patients believing they have more time obtain more aggressive treatment than warranted, ultimately leading to increased morbidity. Conversely, when a prognosis has been underestimated in the past and exceeded, patients and families lack confidence in future prognostic estimates.

Failure to communicate patients' prognoses may be related to the healthcare providers' fear of making patients unnecessarily upset or causing patients to lose hope, as well as uncertainty regarding how to present prognostic information, and lack of confidence.

Many providers are inadequately trained in prognostication, or may have had limited experience with a particular disease. When uncertain about these conversations with patients and families, it has been suggested that the clinician should seek support from an appropriate specialist, such as a palliative care specialist (Christakis and Lamont 2000; Chang et al. 2014).

Introducing Palliative Care

In practice, many clinicians are reluctant to bring up the idea of palliative care to their patients – based on past experiences where patients and families became visibly upset when this was mentioned – equating the word palliative with death and dying. Undoubtedly a stigma around palliative care services does exist, but the importance of educating patients on the true scope of palliative care, and its role early in the curative stages of treatment requires a different approach on how this topic can be broached with patients and families. Simply changing the term from *palliative care* to *supportive care* is not the answer – education is (Moore 2005).

Advance Care Planning

The importance of advance care planning (ACP) on assisting family members to act in accordance with a patient's wishes has gained considerable attention (Moore 2005). Many countries have federal-level initiatives promoting ACP and offer educational material to assist individuals in starting the conversations.

It was initially assumed that the primary care setting was the most appropriate venue for this conversation to be discussed – and that when patients appeared in the hospital it would be too late in timing to be of benefit. Though still considered true, the introduction of ACP for patients with a chronic life-limiting disease at the point of hospital discharge can provide an opportunity for these conversations to occur. However, engaging in effective ACP conversations requires skill and training.

It is known that many patients experience the EOL receiving aggressive care they did not want, in locations they wanted to avoid (Hudson et al. 2006). ACP conversations should not address treatments in the form of a checklist for acceptability or not. The ACP should elicit a patient's wishes – a fulsome discussion of what gives their lives meaning and conversely what conditions would they not want to see themselves in. Broader discussion on what brings quality to life will be most informative to care decisions as well as having the person who will be the substitute decision-making (SDM) be a part of this conversation (Moore 2005).

Lane Changing

Moving from a curative approach to care to a level of care that is primarily comfort focused requires sensitive communication – and the assistance of a trained palliative care colleague may be of assistance in navigating this emotionally laden terrain. Too often these lane changes occur in the middle of the night when the concepts of medical futility become the driver for these conversations to occur. Having ACP conversations earlier in the disease trajectory can help (Bousquet et al. 2015).

Do Not Resuscitate (DNR) Conversations

The abbreviation DNR is often considered a composite of the three most troubling letters in medicine – and the need to bring up code status often evokes anxiety and dread in equal measure to clinicians, patients and family. Unfortunately the letters DNR have been symbolically associated with giving up (Henry 2016). New trials are underway to provide better patient information in the form of an objective video educational tool that attempts to provide accurate information on what is involved and potential outcomes and risks involved. DNR conversations are treatment conversations and should only precede a clear goals-of-care talk (Field et al. 2014).

Goals of Care

Clinical attention on the need to conduct effective goals-of-care (GoC) conversations has garnered more attention in both the internal medicine and palliative care literature. GoC conversations when properly conducted focus on identifying the current understanding of illness and providing education and updates if needed such that an alliance between patient, family and healthcare team can focus on the overall goals of a healthcare encounter. The outcome of an effective GoC conversation yields nicely into the development of a treatment plan and consent process that becomes the intended purpose of the hospitalization. In this sense it provides for a trial of therapy to ensue to attempt to reach these goals and if they are unattainable a further set of meetings can potentially navigate new goals (Perrin 2001).

In the setting of palliative care, where disease progression is the norm, conversations aimed at re-adjustment of the GoC become an important step to maintain alliance between the team and the patient and family (Perrin 2001; Granek et al. 2013).

Addressing Request/Desire for Hastened Death

Ultimately, responding to requests for assistance in dying will depend on the jurisdiction (state, country) one lives in. Self-administered and clinically administered forms of medical assistance in dying are legal options in some parts of the world. However, even in these areas, a request for hastened death needs to be responded to in a non-judgmental and compassionate manner. Special communication skills are required to hear the subtle difference between the expression of a desire, centered in despair and grief over the requests that represent a clear and articulate autonomous desire (Abrahm 2008).

In some cases, expressions for hastened death may be motivated by a readiness to die, or fear of a prolonged dying process and require education and appropriate EOL planning. Best practice guidelines to date suggest that responding to statements expressing a desire to die should touch on the following key components: respond professionally and compassionately; assess to identify treatable problems or concerns especially psychological or spiritual issues; assess and explore current feelings and fears; respond appropriately to specific issues identified; summarize the discussion and seek feedback to ensure shared understanding; and document and advise other team members (Pollak et al. 2007).

Saying Goodbye

The act of making closure, within the context of EOL care, brings with it strong and often sad emotions. Outside of the palliative care context, few are trained in this often forgotten or overlooked ritual. As clinicians, we need to help families and patients say their goodbyes, and for us to also acknowledge the end of a relationship as a patient approaches death. Palliative care specialist Byock's work in this area is helpful. He delineated the process of saying goodbye into four simple phrases: "Please forgive me," "I forgive you," "Thank you," and "I love you" (Byock 2016).

PRACTICAL METHODS

The following represents three well-known practical tools used by clinicians to support EOL communication when navigating key conversation events.

Responding to Emotions

There are five types of empathic statements that can be used by clinicians in response to a patient's expression of emotions. Developed at Duke University, the use of a "continuer statement" continues to find favor in training programs (Baile et al. 2000).

The mnemonic "NURSE" effectively gives a label to the following five continuer statements (Baile et al. 2000):

- *Name*: name the emotion you see the patient is struggling with
- *Understand*: empathize with and legitimize the emotion

- *Respect*: praise the patient for his or her strength
- *Support*: show support explicitly
- *Explore*: with open-ended questions

Breaking Bad News

A moment most frequently dreaded by healthcare professionals is the moment where bad or unwanted news needs to be delivered to a patient. A protocol that continues to be instructive is the SPIKES protocol developed at the M.D. Anderson Cancer Center (Schapira 2008).

The SPIKES acronym used to describe the protocol invites the clinician to consider the following six steps (Schapira 2008):

- *Setting*: Plan ahead for details such as being sure that you are in a private, comfortable setting.
- *Perception*: Assess the patient's perception about their illness, such that you can correct any misunderstanding the patient has and tailor the news to the patient's understanding and expectations.
- *Invitation*: Obtain the patient's invitation to provide more information.
- *Knowledge*: Give knowledge and information to the patient: communicate in ways that help the patient process the information.
- *Empathy*: Address the patient's emotions with empathic responses.
- *Strategize and summarize*: Providing a clear strategy will lessen the patient's anxiety and uncertainty. Let the patient know that he or she can come back if he or she has further questions or concerns.

Conducting a Family Meeting

A well-conducted family/team meeting can provide an important opportunity to bring the inter-professional team, family and patient together to re-assess plans of care, address new issues, and alert everyone to concerns that may be arising before they become an issue (Gueguen et al. 2009).

Running an effective family meeting requires good planning and communication skills. A blueprint of potential strategies to consider in the development of an agenda for the conduct of a family meeting in the setting of palliative care should consider the following (Gueguen et al. 2009):

- Plan and set up prior to the meeting (decide what needs to be addressed and who should attend, conduct pre-meeting with staff)
- Welcome and outline the agenda for the meeting
- Check each family member's understanding of the illness and current prognosis, see if they have other issues they want to discuss
- Review and check in for consensus on the current goals of care
- Identify family and team outstanding concerns on care needs
- Clarify the family's view of what the future holds
- Check in to see how the family is coping and feeling emotionally
- Confirm and identify family strengths and offer supports
- Close the family meeting (summary and review next steps)

APPLICATIONS TO OTHER AREAS OF TERMINAL OR PALLIATIVE CARE

The need for effective and skilled communication extends beyond the realm of terminal or palliative care. In fact, this chapter's basic premise has been that palliative care needs to move beyond the role of only responding to a specific phase of the disease and that it needs to grow as an approach that is used across all sectors or primary and acute care. At any point that patients and families encounter the healthcare team, the need to build shared understanding underpins every aspect of the therapeutic relationship. A plan of care needs to be based on more than a response to disease (from diagnosis to treatment options); it needs to consider the patient's culture, beliefs and experience of suffering, as well as the family who will often shoulder the main responsibility and burden of the care. To succeed in the development of a plan of care that respects the needs to all requires good communication skills (Collins, McLachlin, and Philip 2017).

ETHICAL ISSUES

In navigating the moral terrain pertaining to EOL care, stakeholders will frequently be asked to face a myriad of potential ethical issues, such as truth telling, self-disclosure, withholding or withdrawing treatments, the use of artificial hydration and nutrition, informed consent and challenging a substitute decision-maker (SDM) who may not be acting in the patient's best interest.

In its operationalization, palliative care can simply be reframed as value care. Larger questions enter the moral space surrounding the team, patient and family: Should we value the quantity over the quality of life? What constituents of futility should be prioritized: physiological or psychological? What constitutes a good death?

CONCLUSION

Undoubtedly, EOL is one of the more emotionally fraught and sensitive areas in healthcare. It requires equal measures of exceptional acumen, skill and compassion to maneuver successfully. To date, the process of what I call the natural self-selection of professionals into the field of palliative care has helped to ensure those with the "right heart" find themselves most involved in the final stages of life. However, as previously noted, the demand for palliative care will increase; this along with the movement towards the introduction of a palliative approach integrated earlier into the treatment process will require that primary care physicians as well as hospitalists be more adept and comfortable in the provision of palliative care and communications related to palliative care that will fall outside the domain of specialist purposes. These skills can be learnt, but concerted effort needs to be put into adding these into the curricula of not just physicians but of nurses and all other members of the interprofessional team.

KEY FACTS

- Communication is an activity that incorporates both verbal and non-verbal signals.
- The choice of words accounts for only 7% of the impact our communication receives.
- Embracing the holistic philosophy of palliative care requires the ability to entrust activities and communication roles to all members of the inter-professional team.
- Communication processes involve four distinct stages: source, message, channel, and receiver.
- Knowledge and experience in running a family meeting are a core competency for all healthcare providers working in palliative care.
- The journey from diagnosis to the EOL entails movement through a series of emotionally powerful events that require empathy and good communication skills.

SUMMARY POINTS

- Effective communication is the bedrock for the delivery of EOL care that meets the needs of the patient and family.
- Patients and families reported the need to maintain hope during advanced illness, and the importance of physicians not removing all hope during the communication of bad news.

- Understanding the theory underpinning effective communications can enhance the appreciation for the nuances imbedded in all interpersonal communications.
- Palliative and EOL communications involve navigating known challenging situations (breaking bad news, ACP, etc.). These should form the basis of entrustable professional competencies that should be evaluated in education programs.
- Earlier engagement of PC into the patient's healthcare journey provides an opportunity for conversations to focus on quality over quantity of life.
- Effective PC requires the support of a larger inter-professional team. Clear and cohesive communications by all team members are needed.

LIST OF ABBREVIATIONS

ACP	Advance Care Planning
DNR	Do Not Resuscitate
EOL	End of Life
GoC	Goals of Care
PC	Palliative Care
SDM	Substitute Decision-Maker
WHO	World Health Organization

REFERENCES

Abrahm, J. L. 2008. Patient and Family Requests for Hastened Death. *Hematology American Society of Hematology. Education Program* 2008 (1): 475–480.

Bacon, J. 2012. *The Palliative Approach: Improving Care for Canadians with Life-Limiting Illnesses*. Ottawa, ON: Canadian Hospice Palliative Care Association.

Baile, W. F., R. Buckman, R. Lenzi, G. Glober, E. A. Beale, and A. P. Kudelka. 2000. SPIKES – A Six-Step Protocol for Delivering Bad News: Application to the Patient with Cancer. *The Oncologist* 5 (4): 302–311.

Berger C. 2008. Interpersonal Communications. In *The International Encyclopedia of Communications*, edited by W. Donsbach, 3671–3682. New York: Wiley-Blackwell.

Berlo, D. 1960. *The Process of Communication: An Introduction to Theory and Practice*. New York: Holt, Rinehart and Winston.

Bousquet, G., M. Orri, S. Winterman, C. Brugière, L. Verneuil, and A. Revah-Levy. 2015. Breaking Bad News in Oncology: A Metasynthesis. *JCO* 33 (22): 2437–2443.

Buehner, C. 1971. *Quote Book*, edited by R. Evans. Lebanon Junction, KY: Publishers Press.

Bylund, C. L. and T. A. D'Agostino. 2014. Nonverbal Accommodation in Health Care Communication. *Health Communication* 29 (6): 563–573.

Byock, I. R. 2016. *The Four Things that Matter Most: A Book about Living*. 10th ed. New York: Simon & Schuster.

Chang, A., I. Datta-Barua, B. McLaughlin, and B. Daly. 2014. A Survey of Prognosis Discussions Held by Health-Care Providers Who Request Palliative Care Consultation. *Palliative Medicine* 28 (4): 312–317.

Christakis, N. A. and E. B. Lamont. 2000. Extent and Determinants of Error in Physicians' Prognoses in Terminally Ill Patients: Prospective Cohort Study. *The Western Journal of Medicine* 172 (5): 310–313.

Clark, D. 2007. From Margins to Centre: A Review of the History of Palliative Care in Cancer. *The Lancet Oncology* 8 (5): 430–438.

Collins, A., S. McLachlin, and J. Philip. 2017. Communication about Palliative Care: A Phenomological Study Exploring Patient Views and Responses to Its Discussion. *Palliative Medicine* 32 (1): 133–142.

Doka, K. J., E. N. Heflin-Wells, T. L. Martin, L. M. Redmond, and S. R. Schachter. 2011. The Organization of Thanatology. *Omega* 63 (2): 113–124.

Dunne, K. and K. Sullivan. 2000. Family Experiences of Palliative Care in the Acute Hospital Setting. *International Journal of Palliative Nursing* 6 (4): 170–178.

Field, R. A., Z. Fritz, A. Baker, A. Grove, and G. D. Perkins. 2014. Systematic Review of Interventions to Improve Appropriate Use and Outcomes Associated with Do-Not-Attempt-Cardiopulmonary-Resuscitation Decisions. *Resuscitation* 85 (11): 1418–1431.

Granek, L., M. K. Krzyzanowska, R. Tozer, and P. Mazzotta. 2013. Oncologists' Strategies and Barriers to Effective Communication about the End of Life. *Journal of Oncology Practice* 9 (4): e129–e135.

Gueguen, J. A., C. L. Bylund, R. F. Brown, T. T. Levin, and D. W. Kissane. 2009. Conducting Family Meetings in Palliative Care: Themes, Techniques, and Preliminary Evaluation of a Communication Skills Module. *Palliative and Supportive Care* 7 (2): 171–179.

Hagerty, R. G., P. N. Butow, P. M. Ellis, S. Dimitry, and M. H. N. Tattersall. 2005. Communicating Prognosis in Cancer Care: A Systematic Review of the Literature. *Annals of Oncology* 16 (7): 1005–1053.

Han, J. and A. R. Kagan. 2012. Breaking Bad News. *American Journal of Clinical Oncology* 35 (4): 309.

Henry, B. 2016. A Reasoned Argument for the Demise of the "Do Not Resuscitate" Order. *Annals of Palliative Medicine* 5 (4): 303–307.

Hudson, P. L., P. Schofield, B. Kelly, R. Hudson, M. O'Connor, L. J. Kristjanson, M. Ashby, and S. Aranda. 2006. Responding to Desire to Die Statements from Patients with Advanced Disease: Recommendations for Health Professionals. *Palliative Medicine* 20 (7): 703–710.

Kennedy-Sheldon, L., R. Barrett, and L. Ellington. 2006. Difficult Communications in Nursing. *Journal of Nursing Scholarship* 38 (2): 170–179.

Kubler Ross, E. 1969. *On Death and Dying.* London: Tavistock.

Mehrabian, A. 1971. *Silent Messages.* Belmont, CA: Wadsworth.

Moore, C. D. 2005. Communication Issues and Advance Care Planning. *Semin Oncol Nursing* 21 (1): 11–19.

Parker, J. and E. Coiera. 2000. Improving Clinical Communications: A View from Psychology. *Journal of the American Medical Informatics Association. American Medical Informatics Association* 7 (5): 453–461.

Perrin, K. O. 2001. Communication with Seriously Ill and Dying Patients, Their Families and Their Providers. In *Palliative Care Nursing. Quality to the End of Life*, edited by M. L. Matzon and D. W. Sherman, 219–244. New York: Springer.

Pollak, K. I., R. M. Arnold, A. S. Jeffreys, S. C. Alexander, M. K. Olsen, A. P. Abernethy, C. Sugg Skinner, K. L. Rodriguez, and J. A. Tulsky. 2007. Oncologist Communication about Emotion during Visits with Patients with Advanced Cancer. *Journal of Clinical Oncology* 25 (36): 5748–5752.

Ruben, M. A. and J. A. Hall. 2016. Healthcare Providers' Nonverbal Behavior Can Lead Patients to Show Their Pain More Accurately: An Analogue Study. *Journal of Nonverbal Behavior* 40 (3): 221–234.

Sacks, O. 1989. *Seeing Voices: A Journey into the World of the Deaf.* Toronto: Stoddart.

Schapira, L. 2008. Communication: What Do Patients Want and Need? *Journal of Oncology Practice* 4 (5): 249–253.

World Health Organization. 2017. Definition of Palliative Care. http://www.who.int/cancer/palliative/definition/en/.

Section II

Cultural Aspects

10 Enteral Feeding in Palliative Care: Cultural Aspects and Beyond

Helen Yue-Lai Chan and Kitty Ka Yee Wong

CONTENTS

INTRODUCTION

Enteral feeding is a type of artificial nutrition and hydration (ANH) treatment for delivering nutrition directly to the gut via a tube. The tube may be introduced through the nostril (nasogastric tube) or percutaneously into the stomach (percutaneous endoscopic gastrostomy). Enteral feeding is considered when individuals cannot meet their nutritional needs through oral intake. However, clinical evidence suggests that the risks and harms brought by enteral feeding may outweigh its benefits, particularly in terminally ill conditions (Brody et al. 2011; Krishna 2011; Stiles 2013).

In recent years, increasing attention has been geared towards the need to provide information support to patients or their family members for making decisions related to enteral feeding. A number of decision aids, with the use of multimedia, were developed to explain the nature and purpose of enteral feeding and its potential complications (Hanson et al. 2011; Snyder et al. 2013). Despite these efforts, the feeding decision remains difficult as it intertwines with the socio-cultural context. This chapter describes how the cultural values of feeding in a Chinese community affect organisational policies and the perceived roles and responsibilities of family members and health professionals.

TO TUBE FEED OR NOT TO TUBE FEED?

In recent years, making feeding decisions for people with advanced diseases often emerges as an ethical quandary in the healthcare services. Although enteral feeding has been defined as a treatment for life sustenance, it is also widely understood as a kind of basic care for offering food and fluid and hence cannot be withheld or withdrawn (Stiles 2013). The two following cases were brought up for discussion in a clinical ethics seminar and a geriatric care symposium for health professionals, respectively. Both discussions on each case eventually resulted in fierce debate rather than formulation of a solution.

> An old lady was diagnosed with terminal cancer, with grave prognosis. She understood the illness trajectory, and thus, she told her children and her medical team that she preferred comfort care in the last phase of her life. Weeks later, she became comatose, and her health condition worsened progressively. Despite knowing her condition and care wishes, her son pleaded with the doctor to insert a nasogastric tube so that the son could feed his mother with her favourite homemade sweet soup. The son believed that feeding her favourite food was the last thing he can do for his mother. The medical team was hesitant and implored the son to discuss the matter with his elder sister again. The old lady died before her children reached a consensus.

> An old man diagnosed with dementia cannot tolerate oral feeding for months. He often choked during mealtime although the food texture is adjusted. The old man had been admitted to the hospital several times due to aspiration pneumonia. The speech therapist noted that oral feeding was no longer a safe practice for him. Thus, the medical doctor proposed tube feeding to the old man's family members. The old man's wife thought that inserting a feeding tube was cruel as it induces discomfort and deprives his enjoyment for eating. However, his children thought otherwise: continual oral feeding is cruel as the old man will be susceptible to starvation, malnutrition and aspiration pneumonia. The nurses and care assistants were hesitant to feed him for fear of liability.

In the first case, the medical team was relieved because they managed to protect the patient's care wishes from being overridden. However, this resolution was not ideal because the son felt guilt for failing to feed his mother with her favourite food in the last days of her life. Given the increased prevalence of dementia, the second case became more common in geriatric care, but the medical community still explores means of resolving this kind of situation.

CULTURAL MEANING OF FEEDING

The complexities of feeding decisions are rooted in the cultural meaning associated with eating. The Chinese tradition values eating as the most important part of living, as illustrated by the metaphor, "eating is the sky of man." A television documentary titled, "A Bite of China," ran viral in the Chinese communities in recent years because the documentary illustrates the stories and spirit behind Chinese dishes. Foods, for example, fruit, soup, dried seafood or boxes of biscuits or chocolates, owing to the influence of Western culture, are constantly given as gifts to show love and concern for others. Food is given during festivals or on other special occasions, such as visiting the sick or after a woman giving birth. Treating people with a meal and hosting banquets imply hospitality, gratitude or simply sharing of joy. Therefore, food carries the important symbolic meaning of "doing something special for a person" in the culture (Stiles 2013).

Filial piety is a key concept in Confucianism (Krishna 2011). Under this concept, preparing food for senior family members is the cultural way of expressing filial piety as traditional tales, including *The Twenty-four Paragons of Filial Devotion* (Wang 1992), illustrate this concept. For example, Luji, a six-year-old child, who hid two oranges from a banquet, explained to the host that he wanted to bring the fruits for his mother. Tanzi was nearly killed in the forest by a hunter because he was dressed in deerskin while milking a deer to provide food for his elderly parents. Wangxiang lay naked on ice during winter to catch fish for his stepmother. Yu fed his sick father with flesh from his son and his own body. Such treatment was ineffective, and his father died. Soon after, Yu and his son also died from exhaustion. Despite this tragedy, their act was highly commended by the emperor and by their neighbours. A monument was eventually built to commemorate Yu's unconditional love and devotion.

One key theme in these stories is that the children tried every means they could to satiate their parents. Until now, the symbolic meaning of caregiving through offering food remains prevalent in the Chinese culture. Hence, in the aforementioned cases, failing to fulfil the filial obligation of "doing something for the sick or senile parents" may contribute to thoughts of abandonment and guilt in the adult children (Ho, Krishna and Yee 2010).

WHEN PROFESSIONAL JUDGEMENT MEETS PERSONAL VALUE

The previous sections mainly illustrate the challenges in making feeding decisions from the perspective of a layperson. However, one should not misinterpret that such challenges are related to inadequate knowledge of enteral feeding. The discordance between clinical practice and personal preference over the use of enteral feeding revealed that the decisional conflict is more prominent among health professionals. Wong and Chan (2012) conducted a survey to examine the attitudes of medical doctors and nurses towards ANH for the terminally ill in a Chinese community. The 115 respondents included medical doctors and nurses from acute wards of various hospitals. Findings showed that ANH was generally administered to patients with terminal illness as a standard procedure in the current practice although most of the respondents are aware that ANH cannot improve survival rates and may increase the risk of chest infection. When considering the factors for feeding decision-making listed in Table 10.1, family views and preferences on ANH were ranked higher by more respondents than patients' preferences.

The paradox is that wide application of ANH does not necessarily mean that health professionals absolutely support its use. As shown in Table 10.2, when comparing the proportion of usage of ANH in the current practice, a significantly smaller portion of respondents was willing to receive it in case they were the patients. One plausible explanation is that health professionals tended to err on the side of life preservation in conventional care. Health professionals also feel ethically obliged

TABLE 10.1
Considering Factors in Artificial Nutrition and Hydration (ANH) Decision-Making

Factors[a]	*n* (%)
Benefits of ANH	106 (92.2)
Quality of life of patient	87 (75.7)
Family view/preference on ANH	80 (69.6)
Patient's preferences on ANH	79 (68.7)
Life expectancy	64 (55.7)
Professional guidelines	63 (54.8)
Ethical concerns	61 (53.0)
Likelihood of disease complications	60 (52.2)
Legal concerns	59 (51.3)
Burdens of ANH	58 (50.4)
Age	53 (46.1)
Underlying co-morbidities	47 (40.9)
Healthcare resources	28 (24.3)
Personal experiences	27 (23.5)

[a] Respondents can select more than one option.

Note: This table summarizes the number and proportion of participants who selected the factors to be considered in ANH decision-making. (Unpublished)

TABLE 10.2
Attitudes Towards Providing or Receiving Artificial Nutrition and Hydration

Clinical Scenario	In the Role of Health Professional n (%)	In the Role of Patient n (%)	p-Value
Terminal cancer	96 (83.5)	75 (65.2)	<0.001*
Persistent vegetative state	93 (80.9)	62 (53.9)	<0.001*
Advanced dementia	86 (74.8)	55 (47.8)	<0.001*

Note: Presented are the number and proportion of participants who were willing to provide and receive artificial nutrition and hydration in three different clinical scenarios if they were in the capacity of care providers and care recipients, respectively. There were significant differences between their responses, with a significantly lower acceptance rate if they were the patients.

* $p \leq 0.05$.

to provide ANH though they realise that the potential benefits of this method may not outweigh its risks and harms.

IS ENTERAL FEEDING IN THE PATIENT'S BEST INTERESTS?

According to guidelines on the use of life-sustaining treatments in life-limiting conditions, decisions should be made while considering the best interests of the patients, if they have not clarified their preference before they lost decisional capacity. However, defining the concept of best interests will unavoidably involve the subjective quality-of-life considerations. For example, in the second case mentioned previously, although dementia is a terminal condition, median survival after diagnosis varies between four and nine years, whereas that of the advanced stage is 1.3 years, depending on age, type of dementia and co-morbidities. In this condition, enteral feeding may be generally considered an appropriate option to improve the old man's nutritional status while preventing him from choking rather than letting him suffer from hunger and thirst (Palecek et al. 2010). The issue is more controversial when medication has to be administered through the feeding tube. Withholding or withdrawing enteral feeding in this case may deprive the patient from receiving the medication as needed, thus resulting in poor disease or symptom control. A nurse shared another case on one occasion:

> A patient suffered from metastatic brain cancer. He refused all life-sustaining treatments, including enteral feeding, in the end-of-life care. He lost his consciousness afterwards, and all invasive treatments were withheld. However, the patient experienced repeated seizures several times a day because the anticonvulsant medication cannot be given to him orally. His wife felt perplexed because she hoped to free her husband from physical suffering in the last days of his life. Eventually, in balancing between the distress from tube insertion and physical problems, the wife and the healthcare team agreed that inserting a nasogastric tube to deliver drugs will be a more acceptable means of achieving the patient's goal of end-of-life care.

The accountability of performing comfort feeding has seldom been discussed openly. Comfort feeding refers to continuous oral feeding of a person for as long as he or she can, depending on tolerance (Palecek et al. 2010). In this case, the question is whether oral feeding with specific careful hand-feeding techniques is appropriate if the speech therapist has advised against the procedure due to poor swallowing ability of the patient. The nurses and nursing assistants owed a duty of care to the old man and were held responsible for taking care of the old man. In this therapeutic relationship, the nurses and nursing assistants were bound to follow the standard of care expected for a reasonable level of competence in their positions. In the traditional manner of determining malpractice using the *Bolam* test, individuals should act in accordance with practices accepted as proper in the field. Remoteness of damage can be easily established because the old man was susceptible to aspiration due to poor swallowing ability, and it was foreseeable that oral feeding would cause choking easily. Liability for malpractice will be determined based on whether comfort feeding is supported as a proper practice by a body of medical opinion. In the previous case, the nurses and nursing assistants were hesitant to hand-feed the old man. Notwithstanding, this practice is supported by some care settings, and literature. However, guidelines about comfort feeding are unavailable at the organisational level. Decisions are further complicated when medical staff knowingly administered medication through ineffective means. Hence, feeding decisions should be made on a case-by-case basis as no one-size-fits-all solution is available.

The new legal approach for medical decision shed light on this kind of situation, which involves a benefit-risk balance. The *Montgomery* case highlights that the healthcare team has the responsibility of informing patients of significant risks that will affect the judgement of a reasonable patient. In other words, it is not a professional medical judgement to determine the need to discuss the risk of treatments or an alternative treatment with a patient. Patients are entitled to information relating to the risks involved in the medical decision. This new approach emphasises the importance of person-centred care through information giving and thorough communication with the patient in the decision-making process (Lee 2017).

APPLICATIONS TO OTHER AREAS OF TERMINAL OR PALLIATIVE CARE

Discussions about enteral feeding in palliative care should not be limited to its applicability in patients with terminal cancer. The feeding decision becomes more challenging in patients with chronic progressive diseases due to the difficulty in prognostication.

GUIDELINES

- Policies and guidelines for supporting decision-making of enteral feeding should be developed. These guidelines will provide guidance to health professionals on supporting patients or family members in the decision-making process.
- The concept of advance care planning should be promoted to allow individuals to participate in planning their own future care, including the use of enteral feeding.
- Both patients and family members should engage in open discussion about their personal values and beliefs towards the goal of care in the advance care planning. The deliberation process facilitates shared decision-making.
- Public education about the nature, purposes and harms of enteral feeding options bears importance in clarifying myths and misunderstandings.

ETHICAL ISSUES

Enteral feeding is often confused as part of basic care for offering food and fluid to people who cannot meet nutritional needs through oral intake. Enteral feeding seems unethical as it may only provide marginal benefits to the patients. Family members often consider it is a filial obligation to prevent their loved ones from experiencing hunger or thirst, whereas health professionals felt obliged to err on the side of life preservation through every means they can. There is a lack of consensus defining benefits and harms of enteral feeding to patients.

KEY FACTS: DECISION-MAKING IN ENTERAL FEEDING

- Evidence suggests that the risks and harms brought by enteral feeding may outweigh its benefits in life-limiting conditions.
- Offering food and drinks features symbolic cultural meanings of caregiving and love.
- Enteral feeding is widely understood as a kind of basic care for offering food and fluid.
- Family members often experience conflicts and frustration in the feeding decision-making process.
- The liability of careful hand-feeding for patients with swallowing difficulties has been seldom discussed.
- Professional judgement is important but not the only consideration in the determination of a patient's best interests.

SUMMARY POINTS

- Enteral feeding is commonly used in the current clinical practice for people with dysphagia or cognitive impairment to meet their nutritional needs.
- Enteral feeding is a life-sustaining treatment with marginal benefits and risks for complications in individuals with life-limiting conditions.
- Decisions about the use of enteral feeding often emerged as ethical dilemmas in the recent decade.
- Withholding and withdrawing enteral feeding is misunderstood as not providing care to patients.
- A discordance exists between clinical practice and personal preference over the use of enteral feeding among health professionals.
- There should not be a one-size-fits-all solution for tube-feeding decisions.
- Defining the concept of best interests involves quality-of-life considerations and may occasionally reach beyond cultural issues.
- There are insufficient discussions on the risks of malpractice when healthcare providers maintain oral feeding against professional advice.
- The healthcare team holds the responsibility of informing patients of the significant risks of enteral feeding during the decision-making process.
- Patients are entitled to information related to the potential benefits and risks involved in medical decisions.
- Patients and family members must be engaged in advance for a thorough discussion about personal values on the use of enteral feeding.

LIST OF ABBREVIATION

ANH Artificial Nutrition and Hydration

REFERENCES

Brody H, Hemer LD, Scott LD, Grumbles LL, Kutoc JE, McCommon SD. 2011. Artificial nutrition and hydration: The evolution of ethics, evidence, and policy. *Journal of General Internal Medicine*, 26(9): 1063–8.

Hanson, LC, Carey, TS, Caprio, AJ, Lee, TJ, Ersek, M, Garrett, J, Mitchell, SL. 2011. Improving decision-making for feeding options in advanced dementia: A randomized, controlled trial. *Journal of the American Geriatrics Society*, 59(11): 2009–16.

Ho ZJM, Krishna LKR, Yee CPA. 2010. Chinese familial tradition and Western influence: A case study in Singapore on decision making at the end of life. *Journal of Pain and Symptom Management*, 40(6): 932–7.

Krishna L. 2011. Nasogastric feeding at the end of life: A virtue ethics approach. *Nursing Ethics*, 18(4): 485–94.

Lee A. 2017. Bolam to Montgomery is result of evolutionary change of medical practice towards "patient-centred care." *Postgraduate Medical Journal*, 93(1095): 46–50.

Palecek, EJ, Teno, JM, Casarett, DJ, Hanson, LC, Rhodes, RL, Mitchell, SL. 2010. Comfort feeding only: A proposal to bring clarity to decision-making regarding difficulty with eating for persons with advanced dementia. *Journal of the American Geriatrics Society*, 58(3): 580–4.

Snyder, EA, Caprio, AJ, Wessell, K, Lin, FC, Hanson, LC. 2013. Impact of a decision aid on surrogate decision-makers' perceptions of feeding options for patients with dementia. *Journal of the American Medical Directors Association*, 14(2): 116–8.

Stiles E. 2013. Providing artificial nutrition and hydration in palliative care. *Nursing Standard*, 27(20): 35–42.

Wang, Z. (ed.). 1992. *Er shi si xiao (The Twenty-four Paragons of Filial Devotion)*. Hong Kong: Xing Hui Tu Shu. [in Chinese].

Wong KKY, Chan HYL. 2012. Attitudes of Hong Kong physicians and nurses towards artificial nutrition and hydration for patients with terminal cancer. *Newsletter of the International Society of Nurses in Cancer Care*, 24(3): 7.

11 An Overview of the Indian Perspective on Palliative Care with Particular Reference to Nutrition and Diet

Nanda Kishore Maroju, Vikram Kate, and N. Ananthakrishnan

CONTENTS

INTRODUCTION

Provision of care as a palliative measure implies catering not only to the physical requirements of patients but also their spiritual, religious and personal beliefs. This definition seeks to affirm life and regard dying as a normal process while offering a support system to the patient and the patient's family to allow the patient to live as actively as possible until death (World Health Organization [WHO] 2010).

Feeding the terminally ill has strong emotional elements for patients, relatives and doctors. For patients, it is symbolic of their ability to survive their illness or gain more time. For their families, it is the most basic act of caring, and for doctors it is about providing succour and improving the quality of life (Jackson 2000). While the emotional elements of nutrition are very important, it is also important to realise that in the early stages of disease, the requirements of these patients are no less than a patient of any other reversible illness and a proper assessment and support have definite impact on their quality of life. There is also increasing evidence that diet and nutrition impact not only the quality of life but the overall patient health, and possibly, cancer progression and recurrence (Bazzan et al. 2013).

In putting together an Indian perspective on diet and nutrition in palliative care, it is essential to consider whether an Indian perspective is different from the global view and standards of care as established in the West. The vast differences, in terms of availability of resources, infrastructural and financial, may have contributed to the Indian healthcare system attempting to provide quality curative services rather than develop reliable palliative care support. However, it is encouraging to note that the unique model of community-driven, and predominantly home-based palliative care model that emerged in small pockets of the country, especially in the state of Kerala, is increasingly being adopted across the country, in addition to gaining traction with international agencies.

RELEVANCE OF PALLIATIVE CARE IN INDIA

India is among the most populous nations of the world, accounting for close to one-fifth of the world's population. The WHO estimates an annual incidence of 1 million new cancer patients in India. About three-quarters of these patients present at an advanced stage of malignancy where cure is almost impossible. That would tentatively put a figure of 750,000 new patients requiring palliative care yearly. The Government of India spends a mere 1.15% of its gross domestic product (GDP) on health, only a fraction of which is spent on cancer care (Chidambaram 2008). Ninety percent of resources allocated for cancer are spent on curative services. Of the noncancer patients requiring palliative care, such as HIV/AIDS patients, end-stage renal disease patients and patients with chronic medical diseases, only 10% receive reasonable care.

Palliative care is an emerging area of interest on India's healthcare map. There is improved awareness among the medical fraternity as well as laypeople regarding palliative care (Koshy 2009). Further, among the South Asian countries, the largest body of published literature regarding palliative care is from India. Available literature identifies the greater attention towards palliative services, and attempts to establish regionally relevant models of care. The existing evidence predominantly includes service descriptions, with very little outcome data being available (Singh and Harding 2015). However, against the backdrop of the sheer number of patients requiring palliative care, there are huge gaps in services, which need to be filled.

DIFFICULTY OF PALLIATIVE CARE IN INDIA

Resource Deficit

The most important obstacle in improving the reach and quality of palliative care in India is the mismatch between the demand and resources available. Of the 5% of GDP spent on healthcare, close to 4% is through private providers (WHO Statistical Information System 2010). This care is essentially profit oriented, cure centric and inaccessible to the poor of the country. A very large segment of the population is dependent on government-provided services, which are simply insufficient.

Government Policy

The only policy framed by the government for palliative care is as a component of the National Cancer Control Program. As a result, palliative care is invariably linked to advanced cancers alone. HIV/AIDS has received considerable attention but the stress here too is on awareness, prevention and antiretroviral therapy (Rajagopal and Venkateswaran 2003).

Attitudes of the Medical Fraternity

There is no dearth of advanced medical technology or know-how in the country and several centres have technology and expertise that match some of the best in the world. Most hospitals aspire towards a technology-intensive healthcare model. In several instances, rather than focusing on a symptom-based approach to these patients, doctors often prescribe anticancer medications or treatments which are costly, painful and ineffective. Ironically, while most chemotherapeutic drugs used in the West are easily available in the Indian market, it is near impossible to procure morphine owing to a very strict drug control policy (Mazza and Lipman 2003).

Lack of Open Communication

More than half of patients in India seeking cancer treatment are unaware of their diagnosis or treatment (Chandra et al. 1998). A major reason for this is explained by the phenomenon of collusion. In healthcare, collusion implies any information being withheld or not shared among individuals involved (Chaturvedi, Loiselle, and Chandra 2009). The family is a close-knit unit and can provide sustained and committed support. At the same time, it can hamper effective open communication between the patient, physician and relatives, making it difficult and time consuming. In centres that are busy, communication is therefore half-hearted or absent (Rajagopal and Venkateswaran 2003).

Attitudes Towards Hospices

The hospices movement never really took off in India, in contrast to the developed countries where most of the care for dying is provided in hospices. Most patients who are terminally ill die either at their homes or in hospitals. The main reason for this is the perception of hospices as places where people without families die. Looking after the old and infirm is the norm in Indian families and the inability to do so is counted as failure on the part of the family.

FACTORS CONDUCIVE TO A GOOD PALLIATIVE CARE MODEL IN THE COUNTRY

Family

Families live as close-knit units in India and extended family members provide assistance where required. This is a very useful asset as there is a universal trend towards shifting end-of-life care from hospital settings where healthcare professionals are in charge to the home-care setting where the family members are in charge of the care (Yates 1999).

Support Structures

Families can provide effective care only when backed by strong and sustained support from a palliative care unit. In the absence of such support, there may be a negative impact on the patients as well as their families. The experiment in the Indian state of Kerala called the Neighbourhood Network in Palliative Care (NNPC) is an initiative of the Pain and Palliative Care Society. This experiment involves a symbiosis between the existing government facilities, nongovernmental organisations, volunteers and patients' families (Figure 11.1). The huge success of this programme has set this as the benchmark of care in developing countries with limited resources. Kerala is now a WHO demonstration site for palliative care, and serves to educate the international community in affordable palliative care (Laurence 2017).

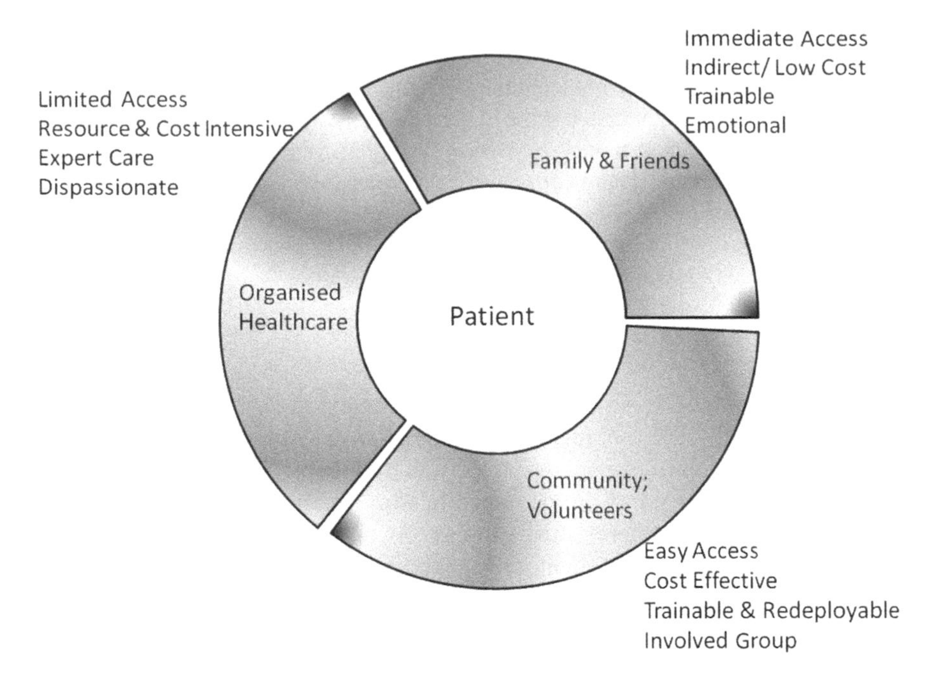

FIGURE 11.1 Integrated unit of care for palliation. The different providers of palliative care with the advantages and drawbacks of each group of providers. Complete and effective care is achieved by proportional inputs from the different groups. This proportional input depends on cultural, social and economic factors.

Cancer Epidemiology

Among Indians residing all over the world, the lowest overall cancer incidence is among those residing in India. This is attributed to lifestyle and environmental factors. There are unique aspects of diet with a relative preponderance of vegetarianism and a high consumption of spices such as turmeric, which have anticarcinogenic properties (Rastogi et al. 2008).

Complementary and Alternate Forms of Medicine

Alternative Indian systems of medicine like Ayurveda and Siddha have popular appeal and are also supported by government initiatives. Some principles of these forms of medicine are deeply ingrained in the culture of most Indians and are reflected in good food and lifestyle choices. Another area with positive impact is the practice of yoga. While there is no definite evidence regarding these forms of medicine or lifestyle on cancers or progressive diseases, their value in enriching the quality of life, physically and spiritually, is well established (Table 11.1).

TABLE 11.1
Key Features of Ayurvedic Medicine

1. Ayurveda literally means the "science of life" and is an ancient system of medicine which originated in India.
2. It is a comprehensive system of medicine and attempts to maintain or restore health by achieving harmony between the individual and his environment.
3. Ayurvedic medicine includes natural therapies including herbal medications, yoga, breathing exercises, massage and meditation.
4. "Shaman" refers to a step in Ayurvedic disease management specifically related to palliation where the focus is more on the spiritual aspects of healing.

OVERVIEW OF DIETARY AND NUTRITIONAL PRACTICES IN INDIA

A good description of the Indian diet was provided by Shetty in 2002. An average Indian consumes a diet to provide 2321 kcal/day, 70 g of protein and 31.3 g of fat. Cereals form a large component of the habitual Indian diet. Rice and wheat and their derivatives are the most common cereals consumed. A typical Indian diet consists of 488.1 g of cereals per consumption unit (CU) per day. In terms of weight, milk and milk products come second at 125.9 g/CU/day. Pulses and legumes are a very important source of vegetable proteins in the Indian diet. Animal fat accounts for only 27.5% of total fat consumed. Meat is restricted or avoided in several communities for religious reasons (Shetty 2002).

NUTRITIONAL ISSUES IN PALLIATIVE CARE

The goals of nutritional support as a part of palliative care change with progression of the disease. In the initial stages of the disease, food contributes to maintaining quality of life, and helps to provide for body's defences and healing, as well as meet metabolic requirements. As the disease progresses food has more of a social function than a nutritional one. Caregivers need to be aware of these changes and set realistic nutritional targets (Watson, Lucas, and Hoy 2005).

In forming an approach to designing a nutritional programme for patients, we classify the patients based on their needs and abilities as follows (Figure 11.2):

a. Patients who are eating well
b. Patients who do not want to eat (due to cancer-associated anorexia)
c. Patients who cannot eat. This group can be further classified as:
   i. Troubled by nausea, vomiting and constipation
   ii. Obstructed due to oropharyngeal, laryngeal, oesophageal, gastric growth (common in India)
   iii. Have disease- or treatment-related complications: intestinal obstruction, enterocutaneous fistulae (common in India)

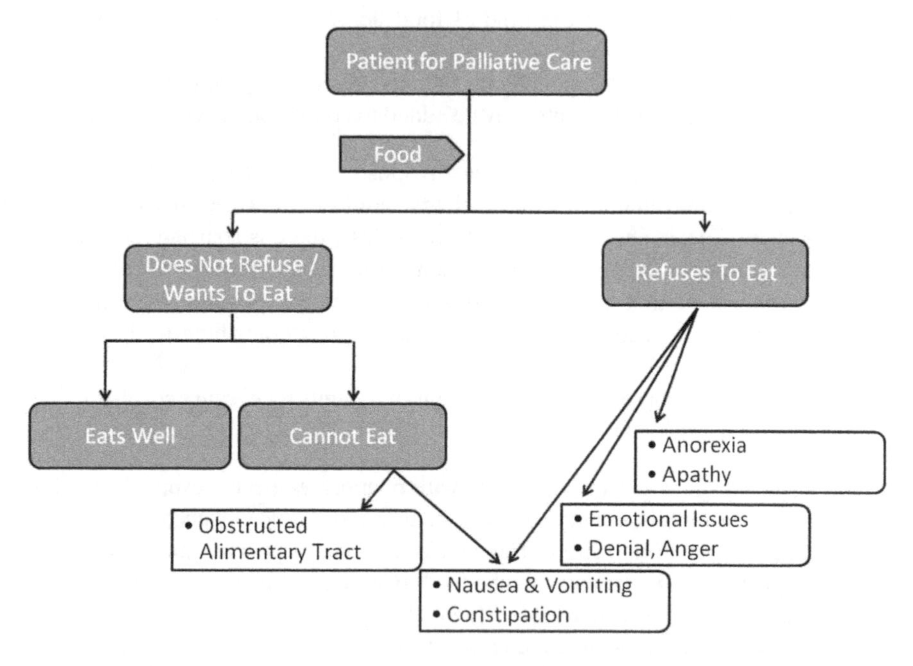

FIGURE 11.2 Classification of patients based on their needs and abilities. The response of different groups of patients to food. This pathway can help providers choose the appropriate line of care.

Patients in the first two groups are usually at either end of the spectrum of patients requiring palliative care and can be managed without specialised care. Specialised care is required for patients who desire to eat but are unable to for various reasons.

a. Patients who are eating well

These patients are reasonably healthy and are receptive to the idea of making a comprehensive plan for their care. The main issues in the management of these patients are as follows:

1. Nutritional assessment to account for daily requirements and additional provision to cater for the illness and the treatment
2. Nutritional supplements like mineral and vitamin supplements
3. A plan for home management
4. Preparing the patient and the family for the natural course of the disease

b. Patients who do not want to eat

This group of patients needs a much more supportive assessment of their condition. A failure to provide food to a patient is often perceived as a failure to provide care. Second, good intake provides some hope of improvement for the caregivers and patients. Reduced intake is seen as a sign of deterioration. These problems are especially common where open communication between patients, doctors and relatives is not encouraged.

There is increased recognition that anorexia may develop as a secondary effect of the heightened breakdown of protein and fat in cancer patients, resulting in the vicious cycle of cachexia and sarcopenia. The role of appetite stimulants like steroids, megestrol acetate and other newer agents needs to be recognized in this group of patients (Shrikant Atreya, personal communication).

Anorexia as a component of advanced cancer has to be accepted and common-sense strategies to address this have to evolve. Some common techniques to encourage intake in patients with anorexia are as follows:

1. Smaller meals may appear more feasible to an anorexic, disinterested patient.
2. Limited exercise may stimulate appetite.
3. Patient's wishes with regard to the kind of food he or she wants to consume should be respected.
4. Metoclopramide and domperidone may be used to control early satiety.
5. Dexamethasone or megestrol acetate may be added to counter anorexia (Gullett et al. 2011).

As the disease progresses the patient may be less responsive to feeding efforts. Evidence suggests that the best course of management in these patients should be to avoid invasive modes of nutritional support (Watson, Lucas, and Hoy 2005). Nevertheless, there is a strong tendency to resort to tube feeding or to intravenous support in these patients. Enteral and parenteral routes of nutritional supplementation are invasive and are associated with definite complications. Restraining agitated patients to enable intravenous access and its maintenance may contribute to the suffering of the family and the patient.

The reasons tube feeding continues to be prevalent in patients receiving end-of-life care are multiple. Some of the arguments are as follows:

1. *For prolonging life*: This is true in patients with nonprogressive or reversible conditions. In patients who are terminally ill with advanced cancer, there is no evidence for prolongation of life with tube feeds (Ackerman 2006). There is also evidence supporting an increased incidence of aspiration pneumonia in patients on tube feeds (Campbell-Taylor and Fisher 1987).
2. *Patients who are fed have a better quality of life*: This may be true for patients who have an appetite and yet are unable to eat due to causes like obstruction to the alimentary tract. In patients who are cachectic, no change in the quality of life is seen. The tube may be an irritant and make life miserable for the patient.

The use of intravenous fluids for hydration in the palliative setting is still a common occurrence in most parts of the country. Many hospitals create a semblance of care by connecting an intravenous drip to the patient. This in most instances satisfies the relatives that "something is being done." However, intravenous hydration has its own complications, does not benefit the patient and may well increase the patient's discomfort and pain. Good, open communication is the key in avoiding unnecessary interventions.

c. Patients who cannot eat

This group of patients benefits from interventions of some kind. Among these patients, a large number are troubled by symptoms of nausea, vomiting, sore mouth and constipation. These complaints need to be addressed sympathetically. While complete relief is difficult, an attempt must be made to alleviate these symptoms.

Nausea and vomiting can be managed by taking small portions of food and eating it slowly. Some patients seem to tolerate cold foods better. The 5-HT3 antagonists are reliable drugs to manage chemotherapy-associated vomiting and generic ondansetron tablets are effective.

There are a number of Ayurvedic preparations that are considered alternatives to allopathic drugs in the management of nausea, vomiting and constipation. A controlled clinical trial using a combination of an Ayurvedic (herbal) preparation (Misrakasneham) with a conventional laxative tablet (Sofsena) found this to be an acceptable alternative in morphine-induced constipation (Ramesh et al. 1998). Fresh ginger is one among several preparations with multiple beneficial properties used in controlling symptoms of nausea and vomiting (Ali et al. 2008).

Patients with an obstructed alimentary tract are the ones for which a considered decision needs to be made in order to provide nutritional support. Cancers of the oral cavity, pharynx, larynx and oesophagus are extremely common in India. The majority of these cancers are advanced and are considered for palliative radiotherapy (Babu 2001).

Patients with oral cavity cancers present with large ulceroproliferative growths and intractable pain. A considered assessment of patients must be taken to quantify the amount of oral intake. Where oral intake is severely impaired, a nasogastric tube may be placed for providing nutritional support during the period of treatment. Patients usually tolerate an oral diet on completion of radiotherapy.

In patients with obstructing lesions of the larynx and pharynx, the options are limited to feeding by a nasogastric tube, a gastrostomy or a jejunostomy, at least until palliative radiotherapy facilitates oral feeding. A 16 or 18 Fr nasogastric tube can be inserted if there is a patent upper alimentary lumen. On successful insertion, the position of the tip of the tube in the stomach must be confirmed by a radiograph before the initiation of feeds. Most patients with appetite and thirst accept the tube easily despite the initial discomfort. Tube blockage is prevented by giving blenderised and strained feeds. The advantage over feeding gastrostomy or feeding jejunostomy is that an operative procedure can be avoided. Complications are tube blockage requiring change of tube, oesophageal ulceration and pain, nasal discomfort, sinusitis and aspiration pneumonia.

Feeding gastrostomy needs to be placed operatively as the proximal obstruction precludes placement of the tube endoscopically. A pharyngeal growth may render intubation difficult and hence a gastrostomy is placed operatively under local anaesthesia and sedation. The procedure is technically simple and inexpensive. The wide-bore Malecots catheter, which is used as the feeding tube, will accept incompletely blenderised food and makes feeding an uncomplicated process. The number of times that a feed has to be administered is also reduced as a relatively larger volume can be given at a time. However, very large volumes carry the risk of regurgitation or reflux and should be avoided. A slipped gastrostomy tube can be easily replaced as a reliable epithelised gastrocutaneous track is formed.

Feeding jejunostomy is superior to a feeding gastrostomy in having a lower incidence of oesophageal regurgitation after feeds. Another indication for a feeding jejunostomy is delayed gastric emptying or an obstructing pyloric growth. The procedure is technically more difficult as compared to gastrostomy. Jejunostomy feeds need to be blenderised completely and administered slowly as a drip

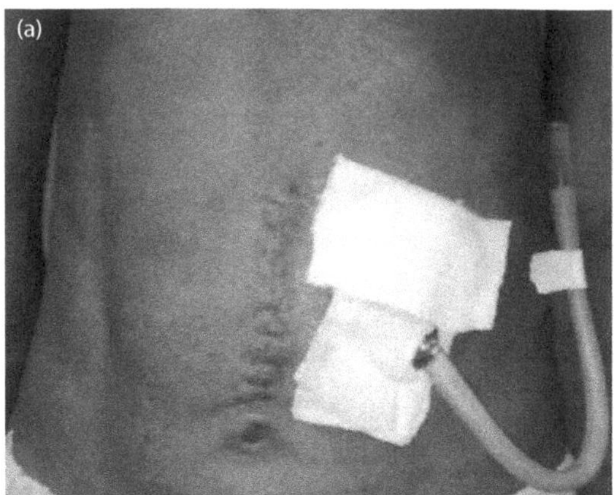

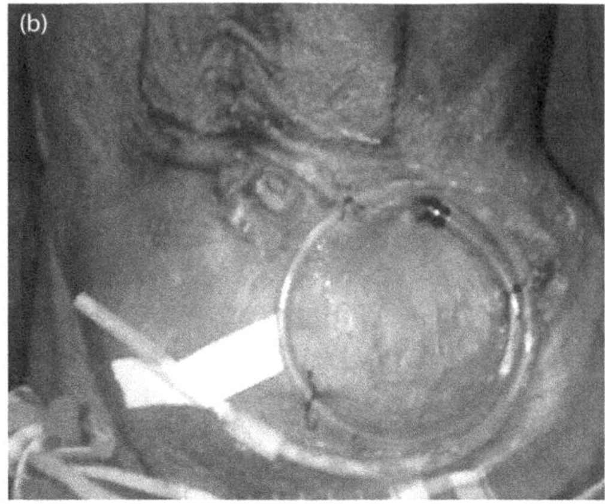

FIGURE 11.3 Enteral access for nutritional support. Enteral access can be achieved by (a) feeding gastrostomy or (b) feeding jejunostomy. Malecot's catheter for gastrostomy and nasogastric tube for jejunostomy are inexpensive options of achieving enteral nutrtion in patients with oesophageal carcinoma. The difference in the calibre of the two tubes can be appreciated in this photograph. (Courtesy Dr Vishnu Kumar)

over 12–18 hours. A slipped jejunostomy tube can only be replaced operatively. The literature does not provide any guidance in choosing one procedure over the other and the choice of a jejunostomy or a gastrostomy depends on an individual assessment of each case. In our experience, when not contraindicated, patients find a gastrostomy easier to manage than a jejunostomy and it meets the nutritional demands of the patient (Figure 11.3).

Patients with obstructing lesions of the oesophagus have a number of procedures for palliation. The oesophagus has a relatively narrow lumen and the tumour usually obstructs the lumen relatively early in the course of the disease. These patients retain true hunger and thirst but are unable to take anything by mouth. An ideal palliative procedure should open up the lumen of the oesophagus rapidly and reliably to allow oral intake and swallowing of saliva.

Endoscopic placement of self-expanding metallic stents with or without dilation of the lumen achieves an immediate and lasting improvement in dysphagia. A study done at our centre recorded dysphagia scores and quality-of-life scores before and after the procedure and found significant improvement on all counts. There was no procedure-related mortality and morbidity was acceptable (Maroju et al. 2006) (Figure 11.4).

Radiotherapy, either external beam alone or combined with intraluminal brachytherapy, is another option that is performed regularly in patients with advanced inoperable carcinoma oesophagus. However, this mode of palliation requires the patient to undergo therapy over 30–35 days and may require intermittent endoscopic dilatation. A study performed at our centre found good relief of symptoms with radiotherapy (Vivekanandam et al. 2001).

Endoscopic laser therapy using neodymium:yttrium-aluminium-garnet (Nd:YAG) laser photocoagulation of tumour tissue is yet another technique available to relieve distressing dysphagia. A large study from Chennai, India, found that, on average, 2.7 sessions of laser photocoagulation were required to relieve dysphagia in these patients (Rau, Harikrishnan, and Krishna 1994).

Another inexpensive alternative attempted by our centre is endoscopic injection of ethanol into the tumour. The drawback with this technique is the shorter period of relief from dysphagia.

NUTRITIONAL ISSUES IN NON-CANCER PATIENTS

There is evidence to indicate that the severity of nutritional deficiency is proportional to the severity of disabilities. In a study of patients with cerebral palsy and anaemia, vitamin B, A, and D deficiencies were significantly common. This is compounded by lower socioeconomic status, suboptimal care,

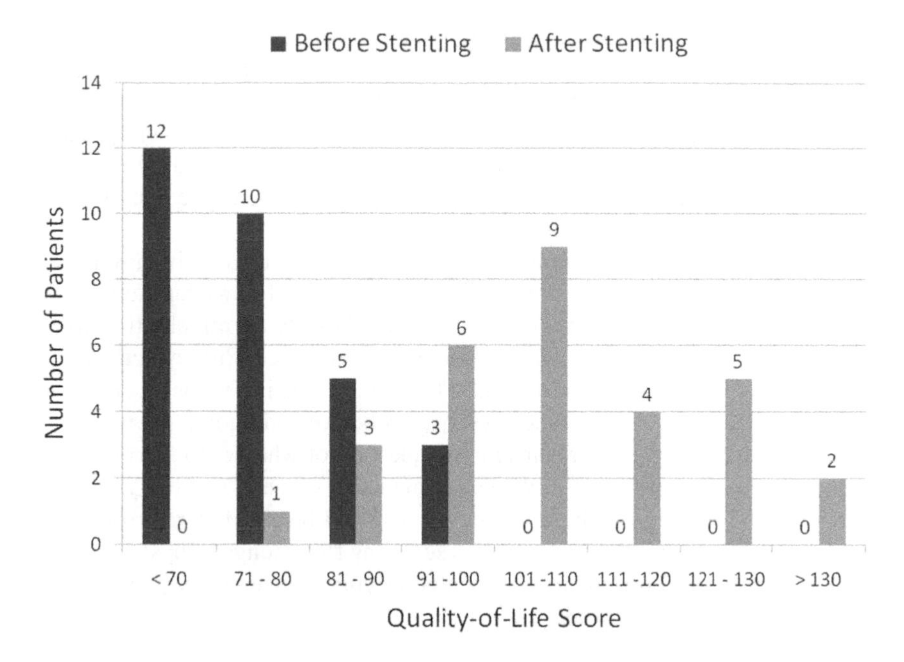

FIGURE 11.4 Quality of Life after placement of self-expanding metallic stent in patients with oesophageal carcinoma. The Quality of Life was assessed by a self prepared questionnaire (modified European Organisation for Research and Treatment of Cancer, QLQ C30), and higher scores indicate a better quality of life. The figure shows a marked improvement in quality of life after placement of the stent.

and gross motor and functional disabilities. These findings emphasize the need for a focused nutritional programme that aims to provide a complete package of nutritional supplementation, and physical and financial rehabilitation (Hariprasad et al. 2017).

FOCUSED NUTRITIONAL INTERVENTION

Kapoor et al. studied the role of IAtta (improved atta), a nutritious flour mix using locally available and acceptable ingredients, in improving the quality of life among adult female cancer patients with symptoms of cachexia. They observed that over a six-month period, patients who received IAtta had significantly better body weight, upper arm circumference and body fat compared to the control group. Further, patients reported a significant improvement in fatigue and appetite scores at the end of the intervention. The success of this intervention was attributed to the use of flour for flatbread, which is commonly consumed in the region. The authors improved this flour by using a mix of grains that included Bengal gram, barley, soy and flax seeds along with amaranth leaves, and was designed to provide the minimum requirements of calories, protein, fat, and fibre in addition to anti-inflammatory, and immunomodulatory activity (Kapoor et al. 2017).

ETHICAL ISSUES

Informed consent is the cornerstone of all medical treatments. It requires the capacity to retain and weigh information as well as the ability to communicate a decision. In patients with severe neurological impairment like stroke disease or dementia these requirements are often not met. Depending on local law, a legal guardian or the treating physician might have to make a decision for the patient based on the patient's best interest. In palliative care situations, it can be especially difficult to ascertain what constitutes this best interest.

Second, the amount of information required for the consent to be informed may worsen the already anxious or depressed patient's mood. It therefore requires careful consideration how much and which information is provided to the patient to not increase anxiety levels and mood problems. Ethical issues might also arise surrounding the availability of palliative care treatments. The best treatment might not be locally available or might not be funded.

Stents have superior results in the short term compared to radiotherapy (oesophageal obstruction) and surgery (gastric outlet obstruction), while long-term results favour radiotherapy and surgery, respectively. To advise on treatment, the physician needs to judge life expectancy well. This can be extremely difficult.

Whether to advise prophylactic treatment to prevent dysphagia (radiotherapy for oesophageal cancer for example) or an expectant strategy also needs ethical consideration. A prophylactic approach might take up valuable, high-quality time in a relatively asymptomatic patient, while an expectant approach only takes up time when a problem has occurred. Prophylactic treatment might also have negative psychological effects (increased feeling of being ill), while an expectant approach might lead to the patient experiencing a lot of symptoms before undergoing the intervention.

Difficult ethical issues often arise regarding the question of whether to start enteral feeding in patients with advanced or severe disease. While the evidence suggests that early tube feeding after severe strokes and tube feeding in advanced dementia should be avoided, relatives might push for such an intervention in the belief that the patient is suffering from hunger. Physicians face an ethical dilemma while trying not to upset relatives when conveying the treatment plan and acting in the patient's best interests at the same time.

KEY FACTS

- Nutrition is one of the central elements in palliative care.
- Cost and availability of care is an important issue in a resource deficit setup in the Indian context.
- Community-driven initiatives have been tested and proven to be effective in ensuring adequate nutritional and supportive care in India; these are applicable to countries that are similarly placed.
- Interventional procedures for nutritional support are used only as a last resort.

SUMMARY POINTS

- Feeding the terminally ill has strong emotional elements for patients, relatives and doctors.
- Regional economic, social and cultural factors render the availability and provision of palliative care in India different from the Western models of care.
- The unique family structure in India, availability of support structures and acceptance of alternate forms of medicine are conducive to the development of a good palliative care model in the country.
- The main components of an Indian diet are cereals, pulses, fresh vegetables, fruits and milk.
- Patients can be classified as those who do not want to eat, those who cannot eat and those patients who consume a normal diet.
- Focused nutritional interventions, which provide a combination of locally available and acceptable nutritional supplements, may be a reliable and cost-effective option.
- Overall, invasive procedures in the terminally ill should be avoided as they increase patient suffering without much nutritional benefit.

ACKNOWLEDGEMENTS

We acknowledge the contribution of Dr. Shrikant Atreya, Consultant, Pain and Palliative Medicine, Tata Medical Centre, Kolkata, India, for his insights into the nutritional issues in palliative care in the Indian context.

LIST OF ABBREVIATIONS

GDP Gross Domestic Product
NNPC Neighbourhood Network in Palliative Care
WHO World Health Organization

REFERENCES

Ackerman, R. J. 2006. Withholding and withdrawing potentially life-sustaining treatment. In *Principles and practice of palliative care and supportive oncology*, eds. A. M. Berger, J. L. Schister, and J. H. von Roenn, 697–706. Philadelphia: Lippincott, Williams, and Wilkins.

Ali, B. H., G. Blunden, M. O. Tanira, and A. Nemmar, 2008. Some phytochemical, pharmacological and toxicological properties of ginger (*Zingiber officinale* Roscoe): A review of recent research. *Food Chem Toxicol* 46:409–20.

Babu, K. G. 2001. Oral cancers in India. *Semin Oncol* 28:169–73.

Bazzan, A. J., Newberg, A. B., Cho, W. C., and D. A. Monti, 2013. Diet and nutrition in cancer survivorship and palliative care. *Evid Based Complement Alternat Med* 2013:917647.

Campbell-Taylor, I., and R. H. Fisher. 1987. The clinical case against tube feeding in palliative care of the elderly. *J Am Geriatr Soc* 35:1100–4.

Chandra, P. S., S. K. Chaturvedi, A. Kumar, S. Kumar, D. K. Subbakrishna, S. M. Channabasavanna, and N. Anantha. 1998. Awareness of diagnosis and psychiatric morbidity among cancer patients: A study from South India. *J Psychosom Res* 45:257–61.

Chaturvedi, S. K., C. G. Loiselle, and P. S. Chandra. 2009. Communication with relatives and collusion in palliative care: A cross-cultural perspective. *Indian J Palliat Care* 15:2–9.

Chidambaram, P. Budget 2008–09. *Government of India: Union budget and economic survey*. National Informatics Centre, Web. 16 January 2010. http://indiabudget.nic.in/ub2008-09/bs/speecha.htm.

Gullett, N. P., Mazurak, V., Hebbar, G., and T. R. Ziegler. 2011. Nutritional interventions for cancer-induced cachexia. *Curr Probl Cancer* 35:58–90.

Hariprasad, P. G., Elizabeth, K. E., Valamparampil, M. J., Kalpana, D., and T. S. Anish. 2017. Multiple nutritional deficiencies in cerebral palsy compounding physical and functional impairments. *Indian J Palliat Care* 23:387–92.

Jackson, K. C., II. 2000. Nutrition and hydration problems in palliative care patients. *J Pharm Care Pain Symptom Control* 8:183–97.

Kapoor, N., Naufahu, J., Tewfik, S., Bhatnagar, S., Garg R., and I. Tewfik. 2017. A prospective randomized controlled trial to study the impact of a nutrition-sensitive intervention on adult women with cancer cachexia undergoing palliative care in India. *Integr Cancer Ther* 16:74–84.

Koshy, C. 2009. The palliative care movement in India: Another freedom struggle or a silent revolution? *Indian J Palliat Care* 15:10–13.

Laurence, J. 2017. India's movement to help people die better. *The Atlantic*. 28 February. https://www.theatlantic.com/health/archive/2017/02/india-palliative-care/517995/.

Maroju, N. K., P. Anbalagan, V. Kate, and N. Ananthakrishnan. 2006. Improvement in dysphagia and quality of life with self-expanding metallic stents in malignant esophageal strictures. *Indian J Gastroenterol* 25:62–65.

Mazza, D. and A. C. Lipman. 2003. Commentary: Palliative care in India, more than a matter of resources. In *Pain and palliative care in the developing world and marginalized populations: A global challenge*, eds. M. R. Rajagopal, D. Mazza, and A. C. Lipman, 129. New York: Haworth Medical Press.

Rajagopal, M. R. and C. Venkateswaran. 2003. Palliative care in India, more than a matter of resources. In *Pain and palliative care in the developing world and marginalized populations: A global challenge*, eds. M. R. Rajagopal, D. Mazza, and A. C. Lipman, 121–128. New York: Haworth Medical Press.

Ramesh, P. R., K. S. Kumar, M. R. Rajagopal, P. Balachandran, and P. K. Warrier. 1998. Managing morphine-induced constipation: A controlled comparison of an Ayurvedic formulation and senna. *J Pain Symptom Manage* 16:240–44.

Rastogi, T., S. Devesa, P. Mangtani, A. Mathew, N. Cooper, R. Kao, and R. Sinha. 2008. Cancer incidence rates among South Asians in four geographic regions: India, Singapore, UK and US. *Int J Epidemiol* 37:147–60.

Rau, B. K., K. M. Harikrishnan, and S. Krishna. 1994. Oesophageal carcinoma: Laser palliation in 231 cases. *Ann Acad Med Singapore* 23:32–34.

Shetty, P. S. 2002. Nutrition transition in India. *Public Health Nutrition* 5:175–82.
Singh T. and R. Harding, 2015. Palliative care in South Asia: A systematic review of the evidence for care models, interventions, and outcomes. *BMC Res Notes* 8:172.
Vivekanandam, S., K. S. Reddy, K. Velavan, V. Balasundaram, S. Rangarao, K. S. V. K. Subbarao, and M. Nachiappan. 2001. External beam radiotherapy and intraluminal brachytherapy in advanced inoperable esophageal cancer: JIPMER experience. *Am J Clin Oncol* 24:128–30.
Watson, M., C. Lucas, and A. Hoy. 2005. *Oxford handbook of palliative care.* New York: Oxford University Press.
WHO definition of palliative care. *World Health Organization.* WHO, Web. 16 January 2010. http://www.who.int/cancer/palliative/definition/en/.
WHOSIS WHO statistical Information system. *World Health Organization.* WHO, Web. 16 January 2010. http://apps.who.int/whosis/data/search.jsp.
Yates, P. 1999. Family coping: Issues and challenges for cancer nursing. *Cancer Nursing* 22:63–71.

12 Italian Aspects of Linking Nutritional Support in Cancer

Riccardo Caccialanza, Emanuele Cereda, and Paolo Pedrazzoli

CONTENTS

INTRODUCTION

Malnutrition is a frequent problem in oncology, particularly within the growing population of elderly cancer patients, and its prevalence and severity primarily depend on tumor stage and site (Hébuterne et al. 2014). Its negative consequences are prolonged hospitalization, a greater degree of treatment-related toxicity, reduced response to cancer treatment, lower activity level, impaired quality of life and a worse overall prognosis (Van Cutsem and Arends 2005; Prado et al. 2011; Aoyama et al. 2015; Jung et al. 2015; Suzuki et al. 2016; Strulov Shachar et al. 2017).

Despite robust evidence that nutritional status deterioration negatively affects survival and tolerance of anti-cancer treatments, and the availability of updated international guidelines for nutritional care in cancer patients (Arends et al. 2017), cancer patients still do not receive adequate nutritional support (Hébuterne et al. 2014). Furthermore, nutritional support has been traditionally considered as part of palliative care for advanced cancer patients, so that its potential in enhancing active treatment efficacy has been almost completely overlooked. This could be related to insufficient awareness of nutritional issues among healthcare professionals, a lack of structured collaboration between oncologists and clinical nutrition specialists and the almost complete lack of evidence supporting the notion that nutritional support improves clinically relevant outcome measures beyond nutritional parameters, in malnourished or at-risk cancer patients. This last issue is critical since, as very few intervention trials are currently underway (Qiu et al. 2015; Gavazzi et al. 2016; Cereda et al. 2018), the efficacy of nutritional support in different care settings for cancer patients, especially during the early phases of disease, still needs to be properly elucidated.

In view of these considerations, the Italian Association of Medical Oncology (AIOM), the Italian Society of Artificial Nutrition and Metabolism (SINPE) and the Italian Federation of Volunteer-based Cancer Organizations (FAVO) initiated a structured collaborative project named "Integrating Nutritional Therapy in Oncology (INTO)," with the aim of increasing awareness of nutritional issues among oncologists and, consequently, improving the nutritional care of cancer patients (Caccialanza et al. 2017).

ITALIAN INITIATIVES TO IMPROVE NUTRITIONAL CARE IN CANCER PATIENTS

A working group, composed of a panel of experts and representatives from AIOM, SINPE and FAVO, was established with the aim of elaborating and recommending a series of initiatives.

First, a national web-based exploratory survey was conducted to investigate the attitude of oncologists towards malnutrition and the management of nutritional support (Caccialanza et al. 2016a).

A survey conducted in the United Kingdom in 2006 showed that while oncologists recognize that nutritional status and intervention are important to outcome in patients receiving active anti-cancer therapy, they fail to identify patients at nutritional risk or to refer to clinical nutrition specialists, those who may benefit from early nutritional intervention. This was reported to be mainly due to a lack of knowledge and clear guidelines, and time constraints (Spiro et al. 2006). Another study tried to identify barriers to, and ways of improving, the implementation of nutrition care in head and neck and esophageal cancer patients (Martin et al. 2016). The main barriers were identified as a perceived lack of evidence for the benefit of nutrition interventions, a lack of standardized protocols for nutrition care, attitudinal differences, inadequate knowledge and poor training of healthcare providers.

The results of the recent Italian survey were consistent with those previously reported, and confirmed that poor nutrition care in cancer patients is still an alarming problem. In particular, only 135 (5.7%) out of 2,375 AIOM members participated in the survey. This very low response rate confirmed the lack of awareness and consideration of nutritional issues among Italian oncologists.

Moreover, the survey showed that oncologists may be convinced that nutritional status is important and often crucial in deciding if oncologic treatment is going to be practicable or tolerated, but they find it difficult to identify patients at nutritional risk. The evidence that nutritional assessment was carried out only upon patient request in about half of the cases, was of concern. The use of nutritional screening tools was reported only by 16% of responders, despite early detection of nutritional problems being essential for appropriate nutritional management of cancer patients (Arends et al. 2017).

The criteria for the identification of candidates needing nutritional support and artificial nutrition, appeared to be adequate since almost 80% of oncologists reported the availability of all the possible types of nutritional support in their institutions. Nutritional counseling and nutritional supplements appeared to be the most common nutritional treatments in all the clinical settings, and this was consistent with their proven efficacy in increasing protein-calorie intake, body weight and improving body composition in malnourished cancer patients (Baldwin et al. 2012; Caccialanza et al. 2015). Nevertheless, although clinical nutrition specialists were reported to be available by most oncologists, nutritional support varied considerably and whether all the reported nutritional treatments were appropriate, remains unclear. Hence, the lack of collaboration between specialists may be one of the first obstacles to overcome. In the next scheduled survey, the questions will be addressed to single oncology center referees to allow a more accurate and reliable picture to emerge.

GUIDELINES IN ITALY

An inter-society consensus document was published in order to provide suitable, concise and practical recommendations for the appropriate nutritional approach in cancer patients (Caccialanza et al. 2016b).

The document emphasized that malnutrition is an important issue in cancer patients, which should be appropriately managed by structured collaboration between oncologists and clinical nutrition specialists. It recommended validated nutritional screening upon diagnosis and at regular time points, and emphasized that cancer type, stage or treatment all potentially affect nutritional status. The document also recommended prompt referral to clinical nutrition services or medical personnel with documented skills in clinical nutrition, for comprehensive nutritional assessment and artificial nutrition prescription. In addition, it stated that well-designed clinical trials are needed to

TABLE 12.1
Summary of the Italian Association of Medical Oncology/Italian Society of Artificial Nutrition and Metabolism Practical Recommendations for Nutritional Support in Cancer Patients

- Nutritional screening should be performed using validated tools (NRS 2002, MUST, MST, MNA) upon diagnosis and systematically repeated at regular time points in patients with cancer type, stage or treatment potentially affecting nutritional status.
- Patients at nutritional risk should be promptly referred for comprehensive nutritional assessment and support to clinical nutrition services or medical personnel with documented skills in clinical nutrition, specifically for cancer patients.
- Nutritional support should be actively managed and targeted for each patient according to nutritional conditions, clinical status, planned treatment and expected outcome. It should comprise nutritional counseling with the possible use of oral nutritional supplements and/or artificial nutrition (enteral nutrition, total or supplemental parenteral nutrition) according to spontaneous food intake, tolerance and effectiveness.
- Nutritional support and dietary modifications should aim to assist the maintenance or recovery of nutritional status by increasing or preserving protein and calorie intake. "Alternative hypocaloric anti-cancer diets" (e.g., macrobiotic or vegan diets) are not recommended.
- Nutritional support may be integrated into palliative care programs, according to individual-based evaluations, quality-of-life implications, life expectancy and patients' awareness.
- Home artificial nutrition should be prescribed and regularly monitored using defined protocols shared between oncologists and clinical nutrition specialists.
- Nutritional parameters should be considered as relevant outcomes or potential confounders in outcome assessment in clinical oncology research.
- Well-designed clinical trials are needed to improve the evidence in favour of nutritional support in different care settings for cancer patients.

Abbreviations: MNA, mini nutrition assessment; MST, malnutrition screening tool; MUST, malnutrition universal screening tool; NRS, nutritional risk screening.

improve the evidence in favour of nutritional support in different care settings for cancer patients and that nutritional parameters should be considered as relevant outcomes or potential confounders in outcome assessment in clinical oncology research. A summary of the AIOM-SINPE practical recommendations is reported in Table 12.1.

INFORMATION AND EDUCATION

Disinformation is a critical point with regards to nutrition for cancer patients. A worrying issue, which may hamper objective nutritional care, is the expanding market of "alternative" hypocaloric anti-cancer diets with putative anti-cancer effects, which are promoted in hundreds of books and websites despite the lack of any supporting scientific evidence. This is a serious and potentially harmful problem, which may negatively interfere with cancer patients' care, as these dietary regimens could decrease protein-calorie intake and have no proven benefits on cancer recurrence rates (Sierpina et al. 2015). Moreover, the uncontrolled use of such unproven remedies could negatively interfere with active treatments. In view of these considerations, the working group decided to plan a press campaign and a web-based communication strategy, in order to provide patients with appropriate and verifiable information, and to initiate a further survey to investigate the modification of nutrition habits among cancer patients during treatment.

Education is key to improving awareness and in implementing appropriate clinical practice, so a series of courses on the nutritional management in oncology was implemented around the country and a specific session on nutritional support was permanently introduced in the national AIOM congress.

THE CANCER PATIENTS' BILL OF RIGHTS FOR APPROPRIATE AND PROMPT NUTRITIONAL SUPPORT

A key initiative of the INTO project has been the elaboration of the "Cancer Patients' Bill of Rights for appropriate and prompt Nutritional Support," which consists of the following statements:

1. *Right to correct information and nutritional counseling*: every cancer patient has the right to comprehensive evidence-based clinical information on her/his nutritional status, any possible associated consequences, the available nutritional therapeutic options, together with nutritional counseling to adapt her/his diet to suit ensuing medical, surgical or radiotherapeutic treatment.
2. *Right to nutritional screening and assessment*: every cancer patient has the right to nutritional screening to reduce the risk of malnutrition, using validated tools, both at diagnosis and at regular time points, while ensuring that the cancer type and stage are taken into account along with any treatment likely to affect nutritional status. Every cancer patient at nutritional risk, has the right to prompt referral for comprehensive nutritional assessment and support to Clinical Nutrition Services or to medical personnel with documented skills in clinical nutrition. Nutritional assessment must be an integral part of any diagnostic-therapeutic regimes developed by oncology units.
3. *Right to dietary prescriptions*: every cancer patient at nutritional risk or malnutrition has the right to receive personalized dietary prescriptions by medical personnel with documented skills in clinical nutrition.
4. *Right to oral nutritional supplements*: every cancer patient at nutritional risk has the right, according to clinical conditions and specific nutrient deficiencies, to receive oral nutritional supplements, including vitamins and minerals.
5. *Right to appropriate and prompt artificial nutrition*: artificial nutrition is a complex therapeutic procedure that requires specific medical skills, as it may be associated with severe complications if not carried out according to evidence-based standard operating protocols. Every cancer patient at nutritional risk, who is unable maintain an adequate nutritional status despite nutritional counseling and oral nutritional support, has the right to receive appropriate and swift artificial nutrition in every health care setting, as part of continuing care.
6. *Right to appropriate and safe home artificial nutrition*: every cancer patient, who needs to continue artificial nutrition after hospital discharge, has the right to receive appropriate and safe home artificial nutrition, prescribed by Clinical Nutrition Services or medical personnel with documented skills in clinical nutrition.
7. *Right to nutritional support monitoring*: every cancer patient requiring nutritional support has the right to periodic reassessment of treatment adequacy and efficacy using established integrated healthcare regimes supervised by collaborating Oncologists and Clinical Nutritionists.
8. *Right to treatment for overweight-related health problems during or after cancer treatment*: every cancer patient has the right to be referred to Clinical Nutrition Services, during or after oncologic rehabilitation programs, so that ideal body weight can be recovered or maintained, to avoid the negative impact of increased weight on prognosis and the clinical course of many cancer types.
9. *Right to psychological support*: malnutrition and overweight considerably affect body image and can cause problems within families. Any patient likely to experience such problems has the right to receive appropriate and swift psychological support.
10. *Right to participate in clinical nutrition trials*: every cancer patient has the right to be enrolled in clinical studies on nutritional support, at different stages of the disease.

Pain management has significantly improved in the last few years (Bhaskar 2012), and general awareness on this issue has significantly increased, even if it may still be suboptimal (Fisch et al. 2012). The Cancer Patients' Bill of Rights implies that nutritional support should be considered in the same manner as pain management and integrated into the framework of simultaneous care (Zagonel et al. 2016). This evidence-based approach to pain relief has been demonstrated to give improved survival and quality of life of cancer patients and their families (Temel et al. 2017), whereas the current situation of inadequate nutritional care in oncology may have negative consequences not only on clinical outcomes, but also on the distress suffered by patients, their families and their caregivers (Amano et al. 2016).

Hence, the document aims first at making cancer patients aware of their rights with regards to nutritional care, as well as sensitizing public opinion and institutions to the problem of malnutrition in oncology. It has been submitted to the Italian Ministry of Health and to the European Cancer Patient Coalition for subsequent international promotion.

FUTURE PERSPECTIVES

Finally, the INTO project called for the development of multicentre observational studies and clinical trials investigating the role of nutritional support in different oncologic settings, new cost-effective and non-invasive methods of assessing body composition in cancer patients, and for standardized diagnostic-therapeutic protocols for appropriate nutritional management in different cancer types.

Improving awareness and clinical practice is not an easy process. It takes time, and considerable effort is required, particularly at the institutional level. Inadequate nutritional management for cancer patients should be considered ethically unacceptable and appropriate nutritional support in the context of simultaneous care should become a guaranteed right for all cancer patients, as it can bring many clinical and economic advantages, while improving the quality of life of patients and caregivers.

KEY FACTS

- Malnutrition is a frequent and overlooked problem in cancer patients.
- Consequences include a greater degree of treatment-related toxicity, reduced response to cancer treatment, impaired quality of life and a worse overall prognosis.
- Nutritional screening and assessment are not systematically performed in cancer patients.
- Prompt and appropriate nutritional support may not, currently, be guaranteed to all cancer patients.
- Nutritional support may bring many clinical and economic advantages, while improving the quality of life of patients and caregivers.

SUMMARY POINTS

- This chapter focuses on malnutrition and nutritional care in cancer patients in Italy, which are often overlooked.
- Italian oncologists, clinical nutritionists and cancer patient organizations initiated a structured collaborative project aimed at increasing awareness of nutritional issues among oncologists and, consequently, improving the nutritional care of cancer patients.
- A national web-based exploratory survey, which investigated the attitude of Italian oncologists towards malnutrition and the management of nutritional support, showed that poor nutrition care in cancer patients is an alarming problem in Italy.
- An inter-society consensus document provided suitable, concise and practical recommendations for the appropriate nutritional approach in cancer patients.

- A key initiative of the project has been the elaboration of the "Cancer Patients' Bill of Rights for appropriate and prompt Nutritional Support," which aims at making cancer patients aware of their rights with regards to nutritional care, as well as sensitizing Italian public opinion and institutions to the problem of malnutrition in oncology.
- The design of multicentre studies could be a useful strategy to increase the awareness of oncologists, to increase referral to nutrition specialists, to integrate nutritional care in the clinical workup of cancer patients, and to identify cost-effective nutritional interventions.

LIST OF ABBREVIATIONS

AIOM Italian Association of Medical Oncology
INTO Integrating Nutritional Therapy in Oncology
FAVO Italian Federation of Volunteer-Based Cancer Organizations
SINPE Italian Society of Artificial Nutrition and Metabolism

REFERENCES

Amano K, Maeda I, Morita T, Okajima Y, Hama T, Aoyama M, Kizawa Y, Tsuneto S, Shima Y, Miyashita M. Eating-related distress and need for nutritional support of families of advanced cancer patients: A nationwide survey of bereaved family members. *J Cachexia Sarcopenia Muscle*. 2016; 7: 527–34.

Aoyama T, Kawabe T, Fujikawa H, Hayashi T, Yamada T, Tsuchida K, Yukawa N et al. Loss of lean body mass as an independent risk factor for continuation of S-1 adjuvant chemotherapy for gastric cancer. *Ann Surg Oncol*. 2015; 22: 2560–6.

Arends J, Bachmann P, Baracos V et al. ESPEN guidelines on nutrition in cancer patients. *Clin Nutr*. 2017; 36: 11–48.

Baldwin C, Spiro A, Ahern R, Emery PW. Oral nutritional interventions in malnourished patients with cancer: A systematic review and meta-analysis. *J Natl Cancer Inst*. 2012; 104: 371–85.

Bhaskar AK. Interventional management of cancer pain. *Curr Opin Support Palliat Care*. 2012; 6: 1–9.

Caccialanza R, Cereda E, Pinto C, Cotogni P, Farina G, Gavazzi C, Gandini C, Nardi M, Zagonel V, Pedrazzoli P. Awareness and consideration of malnutrition among oncologists: Insights from an exploratory survey. *Nutrition*. 2016a; 32:1028–32.

Caccialanza R, De Lorenzo F, Pedrazzoli P. The integrating nutritional therapy in oncology (INTO) project: Rationale, structure and preliminary results. *ESMO Open*. 2017 July 19; 2(3): e000221.

Caccialanza R, Palladini G, Cereda E et al. Nutritional counseling improves quality of life and preserves body weight in systemic immunoglobulin light-chain (AL) amyloidosis. *Nutrition*. 2015; 31: 1228–34.

Caccialanza R, Pedrazzoli P, Cereda E et al. Nutritional support in cancer patients: A position paper from the Italian Society of Medical Oncology (AIOM) and the Italian Society of Artificial Nutrition and Metabolism (SINPE). *J Cancer*. 2016b; 7: 131–5.

Cereda E, Cappello S, Colombo S et al. Nutritional counseling with or without systematic use of oral nutritional supplements in head and neck cancer patients undergoing radiotherapy. *Radiother Oncol*. 2018; 126(1): 81–8.

Fisch MJ, Lee JW, Weiss M et al. Prospective, observational study of pain and analgesic prescribing in medical oncology outpatients with breast, colorectal, lung, or prostate cancer. *J Clin Oncol*. 2012; 30: 1980–8.

Gavazzi C, Colatruglio S, Valoriani F, Mazzaferro V, Sabbatini A, Biffi R, Mariani L, Miceli R. Impact of home enteral nutrition in malnourished patients with upper gastrointestinal cancer: A multicentre randomised clinical trial. *Eur J Cancer*. 2016; 64: 107–12.

Hébuterne X, Lemarié E, Michallet M, de Montreuil CB, Schneider SM, Goldwasser F. Prevalence of malnutrition and current use of nutrition support in patients with cancer. *JPEN*. 2014; 38: 196–204.

Jung HW, Kim JW, Kim JY et al. Effect of muscle mass on toxicity and survival in patients with colon cancer undergoing adjuvant chemotherapy. *Support Care Cancer*. 2015; 23: 687–94.

Martin L, de van der Schueren MA, Blauwhoff-Buskermolen S, Baracos V, Gramlich L. Identifying the barriers and enablers to nutrition care in head and neck and esophageal cancers: An international qualitative study. *JPEN* 2016; 40: 355–66.

Prado CM, Antoun S, Sawyer MB, Baracos VE. Two faces of drug therapy in cancer: Drug-related lean tissue loss and its adverse consequences to survival and toxicity. *Curr Opin Clin Nutr Metab Care*. 2011; 14: 250–4.

Qiu M, Zhou YX, Jin Y et al. Nutrition support can bring survival benefit to high nutrition risk gastric cancer patients who received chemotherapy. *Support Care Cancer.* 2015; 23(7): 1933–9.
Sierpina V, Levine L, McKee J et al. Nutrition, metabolism, and integrative approaches in cancer survivors. *Semin Oncol Nurs.* 2015; 31: 42–52.
Spiro A, Baldwin C, Patterson A et al. The views and practice of oncologists towards nutritional support in patients receiving chemotherapy. *Br J Cancer.* 2006; 95: 431–4.
Strulov Shachar S, Deal AM, Weinberg M, Nyrop KA, Williams GR, Nishijima TF, Benbow JM, Muss HB. Skeletal muscle measures as predictors of toxicity, hospitalization, and survival in patients with metastatic breast cancer receiving taxane based chemotherapy. *Clin Cancer Res.* 2017; 23: 658–65.
Suzuki Y, Okamoto T, Fujishita T, Katsura M, Akamine T, Takamori S, Morodomi Y, Tagawa T, Shoji F, Maehara Y. Clinical implications of sarcopenia in patients undergoing complete resection for early non-small cell lung cancer. *Lung Cancer.* 2016; 101: 92–97.
Temel JS, Greer JA, El-Jawahri A et al. Effects of early integrated palliative care in patients with lung and GI cancer: A randomized clinical trial. *J Clin Oncol.* 2017; 35: 834–841.
Van Cutsem E, Arends J. The causes and consequences of cancer-associated malnutrition. *Eur J Oncol Nurs.* 2005; 9: S51–63.
Zagonel V, Torta R, Franciosi V et al. Early integration of palliative care in oncology practice: Results of the Italian Association of Medical Oncology (AIOM) Survey. *J Cancer.* 2016; 7: 1968–78.

Section III

General Aspects

13 Stents in the Gastrointestinal Tract in Palliative Care

Iruru Maetani

CONTENTS

INTRODUCTION

Many gastrointestinal malignancies are significantly advanced and incurable at presentation. Unresectable malignancies frequently lead to luminal obstruction, and reobstruction after surgical resection caused by local recurrence or lymph node metastasis may occur.

The consequences of gastrointestinal obstruction can be serious, including intolerance of oral intake and deterioration of quality of life. Stents now play a significant role in relieving obstructive symptoms in these patients. With regard to the esophagus, plastic prostheses have been used for a long time. Self-expandable metallic stents (SEMSs) introduced in the early 1990s have enabled stenting procedures in the gastroduodenum and colorectum. Although conventional treatment for obstruction of the gastrointestinal tract has been palliative surgery, such as gastroenterostomy or colostomy, the fact that unresectable gastrointestinal obstruction is often a preterminal event may make less invasive stent placement preferable. Therefore, the use of SEMSs is significantly increasing in the area.

ESOPHAGUS

Malignant Esophageal Stricture

The main etiology of esophageal obstruction is esophageal cancer, but some cases are caused by cancer extension or metastasis from other malignancies. The rising incidence of esophageal cancer over the past two decades has coincided with a change in histologic type and primary tumor location, owing to the increasing incidence of adenocarcinoma of the esophagus in the United States and Western Europe. However, in Asia and the Middle East, the proportion of squamous cell carcinoma remains high.

Such obstructions often cause dysphagia. Approximately 50%–60% of esophageal cancer patients cannot undergo resection at diagnosis due to distant metastases, extensive invasion, or a poor health condition. Most of these patients have short life expectancy, and the primary goal of palliative care is rapid relief of dysphagia. Although a variety of palliative treatments for relieving malignant dysphagia, including stents, brachytherapy, radiotherapy with or without chemotherapy, and ablative procedures, are available, the use of stents has increased markedly.

Stent Placement

Given the straight anatomy of the esophagus, efforts to place a stent in this organ have a long history. Semirigid plastic prostheses were commonly used in the 1970s and 1980s, but they were associated with a higher rate of critical complications like perforation. Advancements in stent technology have led to the development of SEMSs for the esophagus, with the first experience reported in 1990 (Domschke et al. 1990). Flexible SEMSs mounted in a thinner delivery system have made stenting procedures much easier and safer. A systematic review concluded that SEMSs provided greater dysphasia improvement with lesser risk of adverse events than plastic stents (Dai et al. 2014). Thus, SEMSs now account for most endoprostheses used for esophageal obstruction. Self-expandable plastic stents have also recently become commercially available, but they may be associated with higher risk of migration.

The first generation of uncovered SEMSs (USEMSs) had the drawback of allowing tissue growth through the wire mesh of the stent, leading to recurrent dysphagia in 20%–30% of cases. Therefore, USEMSs have been mostly replaced with covered SEMSs (CSEMSs), but CSEMSs are more likely to migrate. In addition, CSEMSs are generally used as an effective treatment in sealing esophagorespiratory fistula caused by cancer development. When the fistula cannot be sealed off with esophageal stent alone, application of both esophageal and airway stents may be required (Shin et al. 2004).

Practical Methods and Techniques

The procedure can be performed under conscious sedation. SEMSs are usually placed using the over-the-wire (OTW) placement procedure with or without endoscopic assistance. A guidewire is passed through the endoscope across the stricture. Then, a delivery system is introduced along the guidewire to the stenotic lesion. The stent is gradually deployed with position adjustment under fluoroscopic control. Finally, the endoscope is then reinserted to confirm correct stent positioning (Figure 13.1).

Efficacy and Complications

The technical success rate of stent placement in the esophagus is approximately 100%, and an improvement in dysphagia score is obtained in 83%–100% of patients. In terms of esophagorespiratory fistula, successful closure with CSEMSs is achieved in 75%–100% of patients (Spaander et al. 2016). Brachytherapy has a greater quality-of-life improvement and survival benefit than SEMS placement;

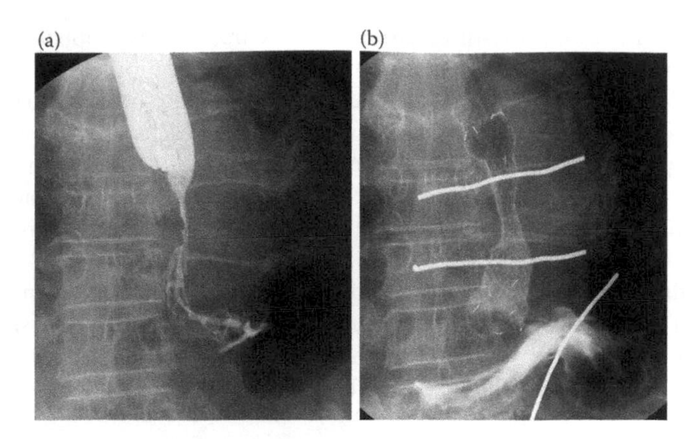

FIGURE 13.1 Stent placement for esophageal cancer. (a) Contrast study showing stricture of the lower esophagus. (b) A metallic stent was placed and deployed at the optimal position. Upper, middle, and lower external radiopaque markers indicate the proximal end of the stricture, distal end of the stricture, and esophagogastric junction, respectively.

thus, it is recommended for patients with longer life expectancy (Spaander et al. 2016). Gastrostomy does not allow patients to resume oral diet, but the patients are expected to continue nutritional support with lower need for reintervention until death. A recent retrospective study has shown that gastrostomy is associated with longer overall survival, more stabilized nutritional status, and less frequent reinterventions compared with SEMS insertion (Min et al. 2017). By contrast, another study assessing only patients with esophagorespiratory fistula showed that compared with gastrostomy/jejunostomy, SEMS insertion significantly improves overall survival, presumably due to better infection control by sealed fistula with SEMS placement (Chen et al. 2012). These two studies are retrospective, so these issues warrant future randomized comparison.

Various early or delayed AEs occur during or after the procedure. Early AEs include pain, migration, gastroesophageal reflux, bleeding, and perforation. Delayed AEs include recurrent dysphagia (e.g., migration, ingrowth, overgrowth, food impaction, and benign tissue hyperplasia), reflux, fistula, and perforation. Among these delayed AEs, recurrent dysphagia occurs most frequently with a rate of 29%–41% (Spaander et al. 2016). Most recurrent dysphasia can be treated with placement of an additional stent.

Cervical Esophagus and Gastroesophageal Junction

Two specific methodological conditions require consideration. SEMS insertion for esophageal stricture close to the upper esophageal sphincter was technically difficult and associated with higher risks of prolonged chest pain and globus sensation, which may require stent removal. Recently, some experts have proposed the use of SEMS with smaller diameter for proximal esophageal stricture to decrease pain and/or globus sensation. The other condition is stenting across the gastroesophageal junction, usually performed for esophageal adenocarcinoma or cardiac cancer. The main problems associated with this procedure are possible migration and gastroesophageal reflux. Placement of USEMS may prevent stent migration, and placement of stent with an anti-reflux valve may prevent reflux. However, a systematic review failed to demonstrate the advantage of an anti-reflux SEMS over a standard open SEMS (Dai et al. 2014).

Concomitant Palliative Radiotherapy/Prior Palliative Chemotherapy and Radiotherapy

As palliative radiotherapy takes four to six weeks to relieve dysphasia, a combination of SEMS and palliative radiotherapy has been suggested to increase survival and immediate symptom relief. However, a higher risk of life-threatening AEs occurs, such as esophagorespiratory fistula and bleeding, in those who receive stenting and concurrent radiotherapy. Thus, the clinical guidelines by the European Society of Gastrointestinal Endoscopy (ESGE) (Spaander et al. 2016), American College of Gastroenterology (Sharma et al. 2010), and Japan Esophageal Society (Japan Esophageal Society 2017) do not recommend the concurrent use of radiotherapy if an esophageal stent is present. In contrast to external radiotherapy, single-dose brachytherapy combined with SEMS placement has been reported to be acceptable, as it does not cause significant AEs (Amdal et al. 2013).

Prior chemoradiotherapy is generally considered to increase life-threatening complications after placement of SEMS. However, a prospective study with 200 patients suggests that prior chemoradiotherapy does not affect the incidence of life-threatening complications and survival after stenting (Homs et al. 2004), indicating the need for further evaluation of this issue.

STOMACH AND DUODENUM

Gastric Outlet Obstruction

Gastric outlet obstruction (GOO) is common in patients with unresectable malignancies, such as gastric and periampullary cancers. GOO often causes a variety of obstructive symptoms, including nausea, vomiting, and bloating, and usually leads to poor or no oral intake in affected patients. In patients with severe GOO through which gastric juice cannot pass, dehydration and electrolyte dehydration are often present.

The conventional therapy in patients with unresectable malignant GOO is palliative surgery, such as gastrojejunostomy (GJJ). However, this surgery is somewhat invasive in patients with limited life expectancy. Most patients unsuitable for surgical palliation do not ingest food orally and often require placement of a decompression tube (i.e., nasogastric or gastrostomy tube). Furthermore, chemotherapy and radiotherapy are often still unsatisfactory despite recent advancements in chemotherapy regimens. In this context, stent placement has recently emerged as a new alternative to surgical palliation.

Stent Placement

Stent placement for GOO is technically difficult due to anatomical reasons (long access route, sharp angulation). Initial reports were for patients with post-operative anatomy (Kozarek et al. 1992). We first reported duodenal stenting in a patient with normal anatomy using a peroral placement technique in 1994 (Maetani et al. 1994).

The initial lack of dedicated systems meant that the OTW method was mostly performed in the early period. However, the placement technique was markedly complicated and difficult. First-generation dedicated enteral stents became available in the late 1990s (Soetikno et al. 1998). This type of stent is mounted in a slim delivery system, which can be inserted through the operating channel of the endoscope. The through-the-scope (TTS) method facilitates SEMS placement in the pyloro-duodenal region. A variety of TTS-type SEMSs are now commercially available.

Most patients with pancreatobiliary cancers have both biliary and gastroduodenal obstruction. Such patients may require combined duodenal and biliary stenting, which is generally a challenging procedure that entails considerable expertise. Among many variations, biliary SEMS insertion via the ampulla is highly difficult due to obscured ampulla in patients with preexisting duodenal stents covering the papilla. A multinational retrospective study revealed that the success rate of endoscopic biliary cannulation for such patients is only 34.2%, but most patients with endoscopic retrograde cholangiopancreatography failure are successfully managed with endoscopic ultrasound (EUS)-guided biliary drainage or percutaneous transhepatic biliary drainage (Khashab et al. 2014).

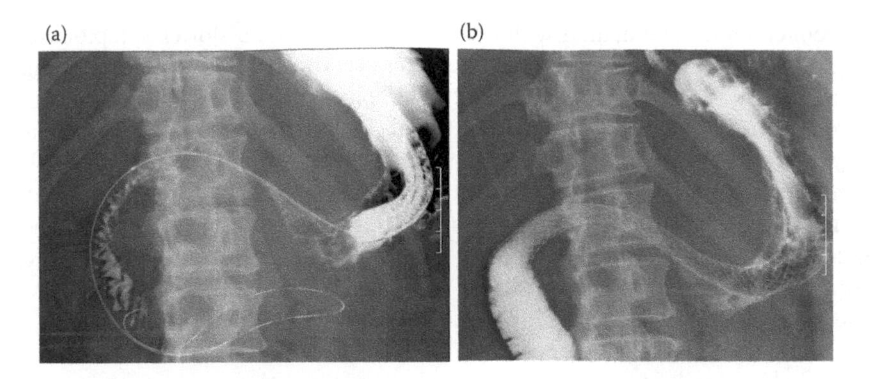

FIGURE 13.2 Stent placement for gastric cancer. (a) Contrast study through the endoscope showing marked antral stenosis. (b) Plain x-ray image showing a successfully placed stent.

Practical Methods and Techniques

TTS procedure is now generally performed because of its significant ease of use. However, it requires a therapeutic endoscope with a large working channel that accommodates a 10-Fr delivery catheter. A guidewire is passed across the stricture under endoscopic and fluoroscopic control. Then, the delivery system is advanced along this guidewire, then positioned and deployed in the stricture. Finally, a contrast dye is injected to confirm correct SEMS placement (Figure 13.2).

Efficacy and Complications

A review of 1,046 published cases reported technical and clinical success rates of 96% and 89%, respectively (Jeurnink et al. 2007). Reasons for clinical failure were the presence of duplicated distal stenosis, dissemination, and deteriorated peristalsis due to neural invasion. Previous studies assessing efficacy of SEMS insertion in patients with carcinomatosis reported divisive results (Mendelsohn et al. 2011; Shin et al. 2016). However, these are retrospective studies; future prospective studies are warranted to verify the findings.

The most frequently used system to score oral intake is the Gastric Outlet Obstruction Scoring System (GOOSS), with 0 = no oral intake, 1 = liquid only, 2 = soft solids, and 3 = low-residue or full diet (Adler and Baron 2002). A systematic review suggested that the GOOSS score is significantly improved following stent placement (Jeurnink et al. 2007).

According to a systematic review (Jeurnink et al. 2007), major early complications occur in 7%, and major late complications in 18%. These late complications are mostly stent migration and obstruction caused by tumor in- or over-growth, hyperplasia, or food impaction. Stent obstruction occurs more frequently than stent migration. Stent obstruction or migration is usually managed by placement of a second stent. Minor complications, such as pain, nausea, and vomiting, are not frequent (9%) (Jeurnink et al. 2007), and life-threatening complications, such as perforation and bleeding, are rare.

CSEMSs may prevent tumor ingrowth and mucosal hyperplasia, but they are more likely to migrate than USEMSs. A systematic review (Pan et al. 2014) failed to show an advantage of stent patency for CSEMSs. An anti-migration feature might be necessary to take advantage of the covering membrane of the CSEMS.

Stent Placement versus Gastrojejunostomy

Only three randomized comparisons of stent placement and GJJ in patients with GOO have been published to date (Fiori et al. 2004b; Mehta et al. 2006; Jeurnink et al. 2010). Among them, the latest and largest study (Jeurnink et al. 2010) showed that GJJ is associated with better long-term outcome from fewer reinterventions compared with SEMS insertion, despite slower symptom relief. SEMS tends to require reinventions for delayed AEs like stent occlusion or migration developing over time. Therefore, the authors of this study proposed that SEMS placement should be selected in patients with less than two months of life expectancy (Jeurnink et al. 2010). The authors also found that the World Health Organization performance score was the only significant predictor for survival in patients with malignant GOO (Jeurnink et al. 2011). Patients with good performance status and longer life expectancy may be considered as good candidates for GJJ, which should be confirmed in future studies.

EUS-guided gastroenterostomy has recently emerged as a new therapeutic alternative to SEMS insertion or surgical GJJ in patients with GOO. This new procedure has yet to be fully established despite several successful reports. In addition to sufficient investigation on its feasibility and safety, comparison with SEMS or GJJ is warranted.

COLORECTUM

Colorectal Obstruction

Acute colorectal obstruction usually requires decompressive procedures and can be life-threatening if left untreated. It is most frequently caused by colorectal cancer and rarely by extrinsic invasive tumors. There are two main indications of stenting using SEMS in the colorectum: palliative treatment in patients with unresectable colorectal obstructions and presurgical decompression for potentially curable patients. The present section focuses only on palliative indication, and SEMS placement as a bridge to elective surgery is not discussed.

Stent Placement

The first application of a SEMS for the colorectum was reported in 1991 (Dohmoto 1991). Since no dedicated stent system was available at that time, the placement procedure was difficult like GOO, and was significantly complicated by the need for various modifications and accessories. However, current dedicated TTS stents facilitate SEMS insertion even for the proximal colon.

Practical Methods and Techniques

The TTS procedure under both endoscopic and fluoroscopic guidance is commonly selected and recommended because of its use of ease. The TTS placement procedure for colorectal obstruction is almost the same as for GOO stenting (Figure 13.3). The OTW procedure without an endoscopy is also feasible, but it is used particularly in cases of left-sided colonic obstruction.

Efficacy and Complications

In a systematic review of 96 previously published series involving 1,198 cases (palliation, 791 patients), the technical and clinical success rates in patients treated palliatively were 93% and 91%, respectively (Sebastian et al. 2004). Compared with primary colorectal cancer, stenting extracolonic obstruction is considered to have lower success rate and higher risk of complications (Keswani ct al. 2009). However, the ESGE guidelines state that "SEMS insertion is generally advisable to attempt palliative stenting of extracolonic malignancies to avoid surgery in these patients who have a relatively short survival" (Van Hooft et al. 2014).

A more recent meta-analysis assessing 4,086 patients on 86 studies has shown a relatively high perforation rate (7.4%) and a significant association with stent design, benign etiology, and bevacizumab use (Van Halsema et al. 2014). Stricture dilation is considered to be a risk factor for perforation, and thus, should be generally avoided (Van Hooft et al. 2014). The majority of patients with perforations require surgical interventions. Migration was the most frequent problem, occurring in 11.8% of the patients (Sebastian et al. 2004); two-thirds of the patients developed this complication

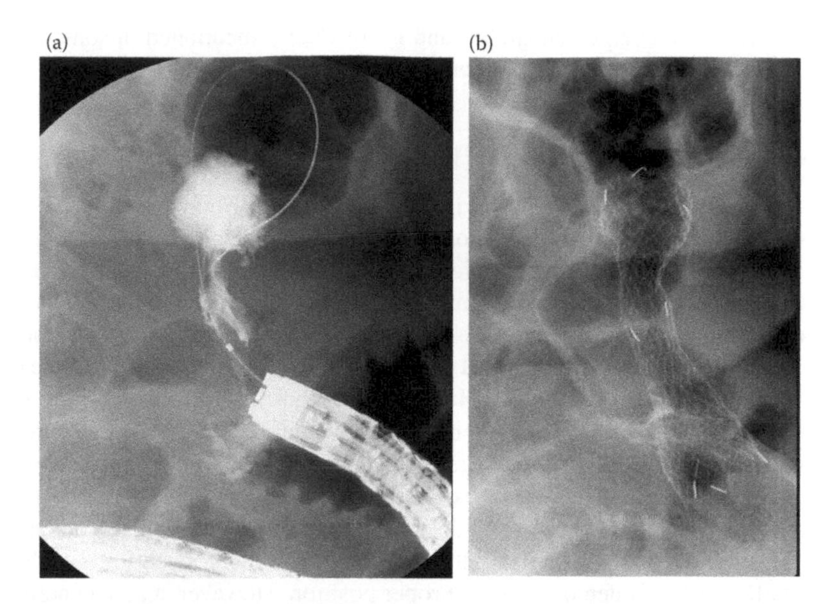

FIGURE 13.3 Colonic stenting for primary incurable colon cancer. (a) Contrast study through the endoscope showing obstructive colon cancer in the descending colon. A guidewire was passed across the stricture. (b) A self-expandable metallic stent was successfully placed and deployed.

within a week after stent placement. Migrated stents are usually excreted from the anus. The review indicated that the rate of reobstruction mostly caused by tumor ingrowth was 7.3% (Sebastian et al. 2004). Stent migration or reobstruction can be generally treated by placement of a second stent.

Aside from sealing off the colorectal fistula, CSEMS is infrequently used for treating malignant colorectal obstruction because of more frequent migration.

Other complications, including pain, diarrhea, and minute bleeding, occur less frequently and are often not serious. No consensus exists on whether stent placement in the lower rectum provides effective and comfortable palliation. These patients should be counseled about possible risk of pain, incontinence, and tenesmus before considering stent placement.

Procedure-related mortality is quite rare. A systematic review reported a mortality rate of 0.6%, and most cases were associated with perforation (Sebastian et al. 2004).

Stent Placement versus Surgical Alternatives

Three randomized controlled trials compared palliative stenting and surgical intervention (Fiori et al. 2004a; Xinopoulos et al. 2004; Van Hooft et al. 2008). Results of two studies showed that stent placement offers better outcomes, such as shorter hospital stay and shorter procedure time, than colostomy (Fiori et al. 2004a; Xinopoulos et al. 2004). However, both studies comprised a limited number of patients; thus, larger randomized studies are warranted. Another randomized clinical trial compared endoscopic stenting and palliative resection or fecal diversion. The trial was prematurely terminated because of the high rate of perforation in the SEMS group (Van Hooft et al. 2008). Recent meta-analyses assessing previously published comparative analyses of patients with incurable colorectal obstruction treated using SEMS or palliative surgery show higher incidence of late complications in the SEMS group (Zhao et al. 2013; Liang et al. 2014), despite shorter hospital stay (Zhao et al. 2013; Liang et al. 2014) and less chance of stoma creation (Zhao et al. 2013). With regard to early complications, one meta-analysis indicated no difference between the two groups (Liang et al. 2014), whereas the other indicated significantly lower rates of early complications in the SEMS group (Zhao et al. 2013). A meta-analysis by Zhao et al. revealed that SEMSs are associated with lower clinical success than palliative surgery (Zhao et al. 2013). However, the definition of clinical success differs among pooled studies and is not clearly mentioned in some articles. Thus, this issue warrants a large randomized comparison.

APPLICATION OF STENTING TO OTHER AREAS OF PALLIATIVE CARE

Small bowel obstruction can occur due to various malignancies: primary, metastasis, or peritoneal carcinomatosis. This is an untapped area for SEMS insertion because complete assessment of stenosis status (e.g., location, severity, and length) is difficult to perform and the lesion is quite difficult to reach from the mouth or the anus, making SEMS insertion extremely challenging or impossible. Currently, three types of device-assisted enteroscopy, namely, double-balloon enteroscopy, single-balloon enteroscopy, and spiral enteroscopy, are available. These enteroscopy systems can reach the deep small bowel. However, they have a 2.8 mm working channel that cannot accommodate a 10-Fr delivery system of the conventional TTS stent. Therefore, SEMS insertion in the small bowel requires a complicated process as follows. First, a guidewire is traversed through the stricture using an enteroscope. Second, the enteroscope is withdrawn while leaving the guidewire in place. Third, a stent delivery system is fluoroscopically advanced through the overtube for enteroscopy (Ross et al. 2006), or through the conventional endoscope (Lee et al. 2012). Finally, SEMS is deployed at the proper position. However, a new-generation double-balloon enteroscopy with a 3.2 mm working channel and a new enteral stent with 9-Fr delivery system have been recently launched. The combination of these devices allows small bowel stenting using the TTS technique to be performed. However, many patients with small bowel obstruction, particularly due to metastasis or peritoneal carcinomatosis, are likely to have multiple sites of obstruction and/or significant decrease in bowel movement, in which SEMS placement may be of little or no help to relieve obstructive symptoms. Thus, careful evaluation using computed tomography and/or small bowel series using water-soluble contrast agent should be carried out before considering small bowel stenting.

ETHICAL ISSUES

As noted, stent placement is a safe and effective procedure in patients with incurable gastrointestinal obstructions. However, 10%–30% of patients may encounter complications over time, including migration and occlusion. These complications usually require reintervention. Thus, this procedure should not be performed as prophylaxis. As some severe AEs like perforation are possibly associated with improper procedures, SEMS insertion should be performed by experienced personnel using gentle manipulation. In addition, 5%–15% of patients may not obtain symptom relief even after stent placement. Provision of appropriate information, including potential complications, ineffectiveness, and the inability to remove a stent, before the procedure is therefore important.

KEY FACTS

- Various malignancies may cause gastrointestinal obstruction, which generally deteriorate quality of life of patients.
- Self-expandable metallic stents are now widely used in treating malignant esophageal, gastroduodenal and colorectal obstructions.
- Stent placement takes generally only a short time under conscious sedation.
- Technical and clinical success rate is high.
- A stent is very effective to relieve obstructive symptoms and resume oral diet soon after the procedure.
- Procedure-related critical adverse events or mortalities are quite rare.

SUMMARY POINTS

- Currently, self-expandable metallic stents play an important role in the palliation of gastrointestinal obstruction.
- The main advantage of this treatment is less invasiveness and faster symptom relief compared with surgical alternatives.
- The success rate of stenting is relatively high even in a tortuous and tight stricture.
- Serious adverse events are rare. However, 10%–30% of patients may encounter recurrent obstruction due to stent migration or occlusion, which may occur more frequently over time than palliative surgery.
- A larger randomized comparison with surgical alternatives is warranted for further verification of this procedure.

LIST OF ABBREVIATIONS

AE	Adverse Event
CSEMS	Covered Self-Expandable Metallic Stent
GJJ	Gastrojejunostomy
GOO	Gastric Outlet Obstruction
GOOSS	Gastric Outlet Obstruction Scoring System
OTW	Over-the-Wire
SEMS	Self-Expandable Metallic Stent
TTS	Through-the-Scope
USEMS	Uncovered Self-Expandable Metallic Stent

REFERENCES

Adler, D. G. and Baron, T. H. 2002. Endoscopic palliation of malignant gastric outlet obstruction using self-expanding metal stents: Experience in 36 patients. *Am J Gastroenterol*, 97, 72–8.

Amdal, C. D., Jacobsen, A. B., Sandstad, B., Warloe, T. and Bjordal, K. 2013. Palliative brachytherapy with or without primary stent placement in patients with oesophageal cancer, a randomised phase III trial. *Radiother Oncol*, 107, 428–33.

Chen, Y. H., Li, S. H., Chiu, Y. C., Lu, H. I., Huang, C. H., Rau, K. M. and Liu, C. T. 2012. Comparative study of esophageal stent and feeding gastrostomy/jejunostomy for tracheoesophageal fistula caused by esophageal squamous cell carcinoma. *PLOS ONE*, 7, e42766.

Dai, Y., Li, C., Xie, Y., Liu, X., Zhang, J., Zhou, J., Pan, X. and Yang, S. 2014. Interventions for dysphagia in oesophageal cancer. *Cochrane Database Syst Rev*, 10, CD005048.

Dohmoto, M. 1991. New method—Endoscopic implantation of rectal stent in palliative treatment of malignant stenosis. *Endoscopia Digestiva*, 3, 1507–1512.

Domschke, W., Foerster, E. C., Matek, W. and Rodl, W. 1990. Self-expanding mesh stent for esophageal cancer stenosis. *Endoscopy*, 22, 134–6.

Fiori, E., Lamazza, A., De Cesare, A., Bononi, M., Volpino, P., Schillaci, A., Cavallaro, A. and Cangemi, V. 2004a. Palliative management of malignant rectosigmoidal obstruction. Colostomy vs. endoscopic stenting. A randomized prospective trial. *Anticancer Res*, 24, 265–8.

Fiori, E., Lamazza, A., Volpino, P., Burza, A., Paparelli, C., Cavallaro, G., Schillaci, A. and Cangemi, V. 2004b. Palliative management of malignant antro-pyloric strictures. Gastroenterostomy vs. endoscopic stenting. A randomized prospective trial. *Anticancer Res*, 24, 269–71.

Homs, M. Y., Hansen, B. E., Van Blankenstein, M., Haringsma, J., Kuipers, E. J. and Siersema, P. D. 2004. Prior radiation and/or chemotherapy has no effect on the outcome of metal stent placement for oesophagogastric carcinoma. *Eur J Gastroenterol Hepatol*, 16, 163–70.

Jeurnink, S. M., Steyerberg, E. W., Van Hooft, J. E., Van Eijck, C. H., Schwartz, M. P., Vleggaar, F. P., Kuipers, E. J., Siersema, P. D. and Dutch, S. S. G. 2010. Surgical gastrojejunostomy or endoscopic stent placement for the palliation of malignant gastric outlet obstruction (SUSTENT study): A multicenter randomized trial. *Gastrointest Endosc*, 71, 490–9.

Jeurnink, S. M., Steyerberg, E. W., Vleggaar, F. P., Van Eijck, C. H., Van Hooft, J. E., Schwartz, M. P., Kuipers, E. J., Siersema, P. D. and Dutch, S. S. G. 2011. Predictors of survival in patients with malignant gastric outlet obstruction: A patient-oriented decision approach for palliative treatment. *Dig Liver Dis*, 43, 548–52.

Jeurnink, S. M., Van Eijck, C. H., Steyerberg, E. W., Kuipers, E. J. and Siersema, P. D. 2007. Stent versus gastrojejunostomy for the palliation of gastric outlet obstruction: A systematic review. *BMC Gastroenterol*, 7, 18.

Keswani, R. N., Azar, R. R., Edmundowicz, S. A., Zhang, Q., Ammar, T., Banerjee, B., Early, D. S. and Jonnalagadda, S. S. 2009. Stenting for malignant colonic obstruction: A comparison of efficacy and complications in colonic versus extracolonic malignancy. *Gastrointest Endosc*, 69, 675–80.

Khashab, M. A., Valeshabad, A. K., Leung, W., Camilo, J., Fukami, N., Shieh, F., Diehl et al. 2014. Multicenter experience with performance of ERCP in patients with an indwelling duodenal stent. *Endoscopy*, 46, 252–5.

Kozarek, R. A., Ball, T. J. and Patterson, D. J. 1992. Metallic self-expanding stent application in the upper gastrointestinal tract: Caveats and concerns. *Gastrointest Endosc*, 38, 1–6.

Lee, H., Park, J. C., Shin, S. K., Lee, S. K. and Lee, Y. C. 2012. Preliminary study of enteroscopy-guided, self-expandable metal stent placement for malignant small bowel obstruction. *J Gastroenterol Hepatol*, 27, 1181–6.

Liang, T. W., Sun, Y., Wei, Y. C. and Yang, D. X. 2014. Palliative treatment of malignant colorectal obstruction caused by advanced malignancy: A self-expanding metallic stent or surgery? A system review and meta-analysis. *Surg Today*, 44, 22–33.

Maetani, I., Ogawa, S., Hoshi, H., Sato, M., Yoshioka, H., Igarashi, Y. and Sakai, Y. 1994. Self-expanding metal stents for palliative treatment of malignant biliary and duodenal stenoses. *Endoscopy*, 26, 701–4.

Mehta, S., Hindmarsh, A., Cheong, E., Cockburn, J., Saada, J., Tighe, R., Lewis, M. P. and Rhodes, M. 2006. Prospective randomized trial of laparoscopic gastrojejunostomy versus duodenal stenting for malignant gastric outflow obstruction. *Surg Endosc*, 20, 239–42.

Mendelsohn, R. B., Gerdes, H., Markowitz, A. J., Dimaio, C. J. and Schattner, M. A. 2011. Carcinomatosis is not a contraindication to enteral stenting in selected patients with malignant gastric outlet obstruction. *Gastrointest Endosc*, 73, 1135–40.

Min, Y. W., Jang, E. Y., Jung, J. H., Lee, H., Min, B. H., Lee, J. H., Rhee, P. L. and Kim, J. J. 2017 Comparison between gastrostomy feeding and self-expandable metal stent insertion for patients with esophageal cancer and dysphagia. *PLOS ONE*, 12, e0179522.

Pan, Y. M., Pan, J., Guo, L. K., Qiu, M. and Zhang, J. J. 2014. Covered versus uncovered self-expandable metallic stents for palliation of malignant gastric outlet obstruction: A systematic review and meta-analysis. *BMC Gastroenterol*, 14, 170.

Ross, A. S., Semrad, C., Waxman, I. and Dye, C. 2006. Enteral stent placement by double balloon enteroscopy for palliation of malignant small bowel obstruction. *Gastrointest Endosc*, 64, 835–7.

Sebastian, S., Johnston, S., Geoghegan, T., Torreggiani, W. and Buckley, M. 2004. Pooled analysis of the efficacy and safety of self-expanding metal stenting in malignant colorectal obstruction. *Am J Gastroenterol*, 99, 2051–7.

Sharma, P., Kozarek, R. and Practice Parameters Committee of American College of Gastroenterology. 2010. Role of esophageal stents in benign and malignant diseases. *Am J Gastroenterol*, 105, 258–73; quiz 274.

Shin, J. H., Song, H. Y., Ko, G. Y., Lim, J. O., Yoon, H. K. and Sung, K. B. 2004. Esophagorespiratory fistula: Long-term results of palliative treatment with covered expandable metallic stents in 61 patients. *Radiology*, 232, 252–9.

Shin, Y. S., Choi, C. W., Kang, D. H., Kim, H. W., Kim, S. J., Cho, M., Hwang, S. H. and Lee, S. H. 2016. Factors associated with clinical failure of self-expandable metal stent for malignant gastroduodenal obstruction. *Scand J Gastroenterol*, 51, 103–10.

Soetikno, R. M., Lichtenstein, D. R., Vandervoort, J., Wong, R. C., Roston, A. D., Slivka, A., Montes, H. and Carr-Locke, D. L. 1998. Palliation of malignant gastric outlet obstruction using an endoscopically placed Wallstent. *Gastrointest Endosc*, 47, 267–70.

Spaander, M. C., Baron, T. H., Siersema, P. D., Fuccio, L., Schumacher, B., Escorsell, A., Garcia-Pagan, J. C. et al. 2016. Esophageal stenting for benign and malignant disease: European Society of Gastrointestinal Endoscopy (ESGE) Clinical Guideline. *Endoscopy*, 48, 939–48.

The Japan Esophageal Society. 2017 XI. Palliative treatment. In Society, T. J. E. (Ed.) *Guidelines for Diagnosis and Treatment of Carcinoma of the Esophagus: 2017 edition* Tokyo, Kanehara & Co., Ltd.

Van Halsema, E. E., Van Hooft, J. E., Small, A. J., Baron, T. H., Garcia-Cano, J., Cheon, J. H., Lee, M. S. et al. 2014. Perforation in colorectal stenting: A meta-analysis and a search for risk factors. *Gastrointest Endosc*, 79, 970–82 e7; quiz 983 e2, 983 e5.

Van Hooft, J. E., Fockens, P., Marinelli, A. W., Timmer, R., Van Berkel, A. M., Bossuyt, P. M., Bemelman, W. A. and Dutch Colorectal Stent, G. 2008. Early closure of a multicenter randomized clinical trial of endoscopic stenting versus surgery for stage IV left-sided colorectal cancer. *Endoscopy*, 40, 184–91.

Van Hooft, J. E., Van Halsema, E. E., Vanbiervliet, G., Beets-Tan, R. G., Dewitt, J. M., Donnellan, F., Dumonceau, J. M. et al. and European Society of Gastrointestinal, E. 2014. Self-expandable metal stents for obstructing colonic and extracolonic cancer: European Society of Gastrointestinal Endoscopy (ESGE) Clinical Guideline. *Endoscopy*, 46, 990–1053.

Xinopoulos, D., Dimitroulopoulos, D., Theodosopoulos, T., Tsamakidis, K., Bitsakou, G., Plataniotis, G., Gontikakis et al. 2004. Stenting or stoma creation for patients with inoperable malignant colonic obstructions? Results of a study and cost-effectiveness analysis. *Surg Endosc*, 18, 421–6.

Zhao, X. D., Cai, B. B., Cao, R. S. and Shi, R. H. 2013 Palliative treatment for incurable malignant colorectal obstructions: A meta-analysis. *World J Gastroenterol*, 19, 5565–74.

14 Artificial Nutrition, Advance Directives and End of Life in Long-Term Care

Cheryl Ann Monturo

CONTENTS

INTRODUCTION

Up to one-third of older adults will suffer and die from or with dementia (Weuve et al. 2014). Of those, half will die in long-term care (LTC) settings (Houttekier et al. 2010), highlighting the need for a focus on palliative care services. A significant part of this care requires consideration of the resident's preferences for life-sustaining treatment. One manner in which these preferences are communicated is through advance directives (ADs) executed by the residents. Although a variety of treatments may be addressed, artificial nutrition (AN) has attracted significant attention through numerous legal cases highlighting society's ambivalence with the underlying issues related to this medical treatment. This chapter addresses LTC, ADs and AN for those at the end of life.

LONG-TERM CARE FACILITIES

Personnel to Meet the Demands

As individuals live longer with serious illness, many require skilled care that can be found in LTC facilities also known as nursing homes or care homes (The Care Commission 2009). Increasingly, these facilities are becoming the place for approximately 25% of Americans to die (Gruneir et al. 2007; National Center for Health Statistics 2008). With these numbers comes an increased demand for staff to care for more residents. The Centers for Medicare and Medicaid Services (CMS) in the United States presented minimum guidelines on appropriate staffing for nursing homes, concluding that 90% of the homes were already deficient in meeting these standards (Abt Associates 2001). Poorer staffing translates into more residents per staff member, causing the potential for significant workplace stress and higher rates of staff turnover. This lack of stability further erodes the quality of care in general, and palliative care in particular.

In some instances residents who are capable of eating may receive AN due to poor staffing. These residents require hand feeding and in the absence of family or volunteers to assist, may not receive adequate nutrition because of the time it takes to feed them. Although some may feel that AN is more expedient and will provide all the necessary nutrients, residents are deprived of the innate social nature of mealtime.

Palliative Care Services

More residents not only demand higher staffing ratios, but staff capable of providing overall as well as palliative care. The needs of older adults requiring palliative care often remain unmet (Graham et al. 2010) and care is often inconsistent with high (Marie Curie Cancer Care 2009) or suboptimal (Brennan 2007) quality standards. In addition, staff may lack awareness that palliative care should be delivered to specific residents (The Care Commission 2009). Statistics are available on multiple aspects of palliative care; however, for the purposes of this chapter, the focus remains on life-sustaining treatments, specifically AN.

Palliative Care Education

The deficiency of palliative care in LTC may be attributed to inadequate attention by staff development departments within homes (International Council of Nurses 2002), the absence of proper education within basic nursing curricula (McDonnell et al. 2009; The Care Commission 2009) and the lack of formal end-of-life or palliative care programs and protocols (Oliver, Porock and Zweig 2004; Temkin-Greener et al. 2009). Further, with higher staff turnover rates, the effectiveness of educational programs is limited, requiring continual re-education. Consideration of these needs is important to fostering appropriate educational programs (Table 14.1).

Although there is a significant body of literature on the palliative care educational needs of LTC staff, there are few studies on the effect of systematic organized education. In one study, the presence of a palliative care program in a group of nursing homes positively impacted the knowledge level and attitudes of staff (Stillman et al. 2005). It is clear that education is a positive force in improving palliative care; however, historical events in the regulation of LTC facilities may add to the difficulty in realizing appropriate palliative care.

Regulations

LTC regulations exist for the protection and welfare of residents. In Ireland, both publicly and privately owned facilities are subject to regulations (Health Information and Quality Authority 2008) recognizing the need for palliative care knowledge and basic skills (An Bord Altranais 2009). Scotland's Commission for the Regulation of Care recently reported mixed results on the provision of palliative care in care homes (The Care Commission 2009).

Abuse and neglect in mid-twentieth century U.S. LTC facilities necessitated the institution of regulations to insure adequate nutrition and hydration. These regulations utilized resident weight as an indicator of nutritional adequacy unless further documentation identified a reason that this goal could not be achieved (Omnibus Budget Reconciliation Act [OBRA] 1987). A resident's refusal to

TABLE 14.1
Palliative Care Education in Long-Term Care Facilities

- Examine the underlying culture of the institution
  - Survey staff and administrators
  - Capture beliefs and values
  - Include a values clarification exercise
- Develop a plan for palliative care education
  - Use multiple strategies
  - Provide the basics first
  - Include plans for remediation
  - Provide support for staff to attend
  - Plan ahead for continuing education
- Include all parts of the organization in educational sessions
  - Administration, clinical and support staff
  - "Buy in" is essential for success
- Develop an advance care planning protocol
  - Identify key staff who will approach residents and families
  - Identify a timeline for completion of the process from admission
  - Reinforce need for consistency of message to residents and families
- Develop a standard advance directive
  - Begin with a standardized document to avoid omissions
  - Allow for additions by residents and families
- Reinforce necessary documentation
  - Document advance care planning process
  - Document resident's preferences on an advance directive
  - Standardize the location for all documentation
- Reinforce the ongoing process
  - Preferences may change so continuous communication is key
  - Support of resident and family

Note: Presented here are key steps in the process of initiating a palliative care education program in a LTC facility. The process includes the mechanics as well as the need to incorporate psychosocial and cultural aspects of program development. In addition, ongoing support, evaluation, and readjustment of the program are necessary to maintain a healthy and viable palliative care education program.

eat or drink was not considered in applying this regulation, thereby increasing the possibility that AN would be instituted to maintain compliance. In addition to OBRA (1987), U.S. nursing homes receiving funds from Medicare (a federally funded program) or Medicaid (a state-funded program) must collect specific nutritionally related data on each resident as part of the Minimum Data Set (MDS) (Table 14.2).

Although weight may be one indicator of poor nutrition, it is one of many that must be assessed in the palliative care population. Difficulty in standardization of procedures and equipment leads to inaccuracies in the reporting of actual weights. Disease processes and aging also affect the weight in terms of measuring lean body mass, fat and extracellular fluid changes (Monturo and Strumpf 2007). Fear of litigation and/or loss of institutional accreditation may increase the use of AN without considering the residents' preferences, quality of life, or that weight loss is a common indicator of impending death (Center for Gerontology and Health Care Research Brown Medical School 2004).

Recent updates to the interpretive guidelines for LTC facility surveyors focus on AN and ADs in new Survey and Certification Letters (S&C 13-17-NH, S&C 13-16-NH) which may ameliorate the previous fears of litigation and loss of accreditation. The guideline directs that "any feeding tube

TABLE 14.2
Minimum Data Set (MDS) Nutritional Parameters

- Oral problems
- Height and weight
- Weight change
- Altered taste
- Hunger
- Uneaten meals
- Food intake
- Use of nutrition support
- Use of mechanically altered food
- Use of therapeutic diets

Note: The MDS is a data repository for information collected on all residents in U.S. nursing homes receiving state or federal funding. The data are used to assess residents, and are also extensively used for research purposes as the data are easily accessible through Internet sites.

used to provide enteral nutrition to a resident by bypassing oral intake" (S&C12-46-NH) should be limited to situations in which a benefit outweighs the potential risks through documented evidence (S&C 13-17-NH). In addition, the updated guidelines focused on ADs and clarifying the importance of assisting in and respecting resident's end-of-life decisions (S&C 13-16-NH).

Cognitive Impairment

Dementia results in many neurodegenerative impairments including difficulties in decision-making and eating, particularly in its final stages. In the United Kingdom, approximately 400,000 people with dementia reside in care homes providing long-term care (Laing and Buisson 2013). Statistics show that 70% of those with dementia are expected to receive end-of-life care in nursing homes (Mitchell et al. 2005). The use of AN in residents with dementia is variable, with older reports showing a higher likelihood of the treatment (Mitchell et al. 2003) as compared to more recent reports noting a lower chance of receiving AN in LTC residents with Alzheimer's disease and an AD (Tschirhart et al. 2014). In addition to dementia, those with other forms of cognitive impairment such as individuals in a persistent vegetative state, a minimally conscious state, or a coma, are unable to eat normally and therefore AN may be provided.

ADVANCE DIRECTIVES

ADs are considered the written result of advance care planning and must not exist in isolation as simple documents (Figure 14.1, Table 14.3). ADs may be standardized to include certain language, such as those in individual U.S. states, or may be available to the general public. Routinely, ADs contain directions to allow or refuse specific medical treatments. In this manner they may also be called "living wills." Another form of AD is the power of attorney for healthcare decisions. This AD identifies an individual who will make decisions for the resident should the resident no longer be able to communicate his or her own wishes. These two ADs may also be combined into one document, such as Five Wishes offered by the organization *Aging with Dignity.* Alternately, 22 U.S. states use some form of the Physician Orders for Life-Sustaining Treatment (POLST), a portable set of medical orders identifying patient preferences (National POLST Paradigm 2016). In some Asian cultures, ADs are viewed as a liberal model for decision-making, one that is not central to normal familiar

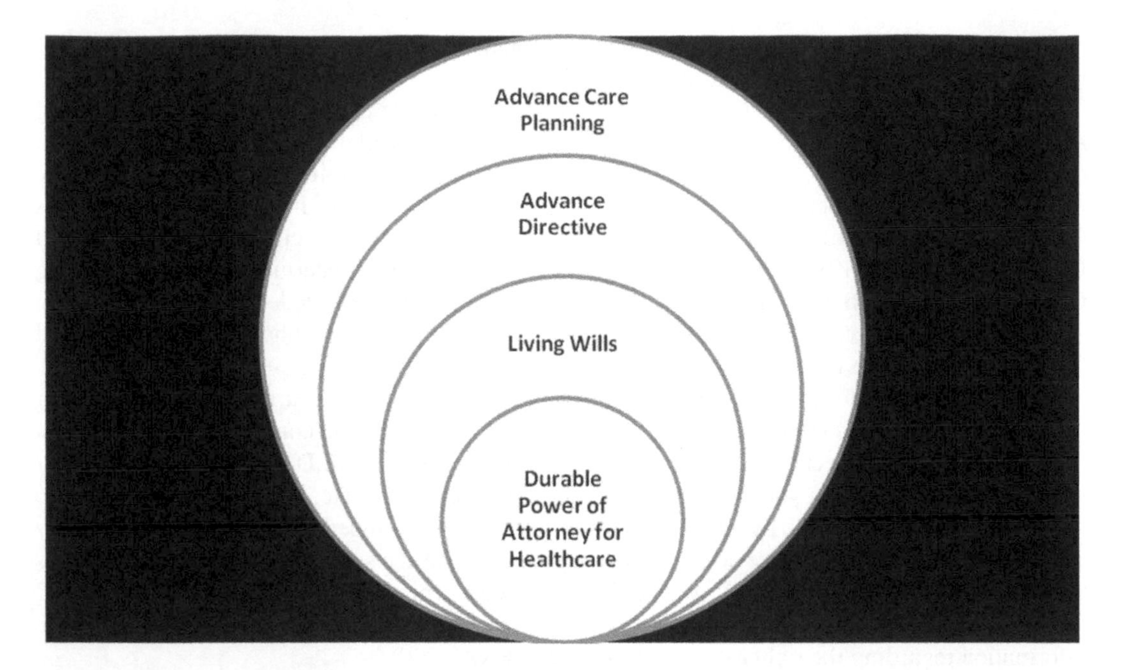

FIGURE 14.1 Advance directives. Advance care planning is the overarching and inclusive approach to advance directive development.

relationships (Chan 2004), and therefore not utilized as widely (Tsai, Tsai and Liu 2017). For these reasons, much of this section is dedicated to information derived from the United States.

Historical Evolution

Literature focused on advance care planning and specifically ADs in the United States originated from legal mandates and the right-to-die movement in the latter part of the twentieth century, unlike the previous focus on do-not-resuscitate orders and a less autonomous environment. The first right-to-die case was that of Karen Ann Quinlan, a young nursing home resident in a persistent vegetative state supported on a respirator. Although the case involved discontinuation of a respirator, removal

TABLE 14.3
Key Facts of an Advance Directive (AD)

- It is a document but should be supported by a plan of care.
- An AD provides directions for care when an individual is unable to communicate.
- ADs may be modified over time.
- Actual templates or documents vary with country/state.
- ADs may be developed using two basic forms: a living will and a durable power of attorney for healthcare.
- ADs are considered legally valid in some areas.
- ADs may also be seen as an "individual's voice."
- Enforceability of advance directives also varies with locale.
- There is no expiration date on an AD.
- ADs require preparation prior to execution of the document.

Note: ADs vary according to locale; however, they contain basic information necessary to communicate the preferences of residents no longer able to describe their wishes.

of AN was also an option, but one that was not acceptable to her family at that time. Quinlan died nine years later of pneumonia while still receiving AN.

Numerous cases arose after Quinlan focused on withdrawal of treatment, sometimes including AN. At this time, some believed there was a difference between withdrawal of AN and withdrawal of antibiotics, respirators, or other medical treatments. Seven years after the Quinlan decision, medical and ethical experts found no difference between AN and other life-sustaining treatments (The President's Commission for the Study of Ethical Problems in Medicine and Biomedical and Behavioral Research 1983). Despite this ruling, societal struggles concerning this life-sustaining treatment continued in the United States. As a result of a newborn case, federal regulations known as the "Baby Doe Directives" were imposed preventing withdrawal or withholding of nutrition and fluids from a newborn based solely on a disability.

In 1990, as a result of the Nancy Cruzan case, the U.S. Supreme Court provided support for individual states' rights in upholding a requirement to provide clear and convincing evidence of an individual's wishes concerning treatment (*In re Cruzan v. Director*, M. D. H. et al. 1990). Similar to Quinlan, Cruzan was a young woman in a persistent vegetative state; however, in this case, the issue was withdrawal of AN. Eventually, Cruzan's AN was discontinued at the request of her family after they provided additional evidence of her wishes. Also at the same time, a U.S. act known as the Patient Self Determination Act was put into place concerning ADs. Upon admission to a LTC facility, staff members were required to ask residents if they possessed an AD, and to provide information regarding the right to complete an AD (OBRA 1990).

Despite court rulings, ethics panel results, and federal acts, other cases involving AN such as that of Terri Schiavo continued to question beliefs versus facts and the supremacy of next-of-kin rights. Schiavo suffered a cardiac arrest in 1990 and fell into a persistent vegetative state where she remained, receiving AN until her husband's wishes were granted to discontinue the treatment, resulting in her death in 2005. In all of these cases, individuals did not have previous documented treatment wishes or ADs; therefore, discussions led to surrogate decision-making, court-appointed guardians and/or a best interest standard.

Usefulness of Advance Directives

The presence and successful use of ADs is variable (Center for Gerontology and Health Care Research Brown Medical School 2004; Monturo and Strumpf 2007; Teno et al. 1997). Some report that given the number of years that ADs have been available, there continues to be poor utilization, and that this venture has essentially failed (Fagerlin and Schneider 2004). Others would argue that the combination of palliative care education, planning and AD can work; however, more focus must be placed on the plan and education than merely on a document (Monturo and Strumpf 2007; Stillman et al. 2005). Recent statistics note a higher level of AD completion by American adults over the age of 60 years from 42% in 2000 to 72% in 2010 (Silveira et al. 2014) as compared to the rare occurrence in Belgium (8.4%) (De Gendt et al. 2013) and the Netherlands (4.9%) (Henriks et al. 2016). The higher rate of AD use in older American adults, however, does not appear to be indicative of the overall acceptance of forgoing some life-sustaining treatments such as AN. In a systematic review of the U.S. literature from 2011 to 2016, statistics reveal that only 36.7% of adults completed an AD (Yadav et al. 2017).

Limited data exist on the incidence or frequency with which preferences for AN appear in ADs. One study reported a high rate of AN preferences (94%) in ADs, although this was likely attributed to the existence of a previously conducted palliative care study in these LTC facilities (Monturo and Strumpf 2007).

ARTIFICIAL NUTRITION

Artificial nutrition (AN) is known by many different names including enteral nutrition, parenteral nutrition and tube feedings. Hydration is frequently included when discussing AN; however, these two treatments are distinct. Although both are delivered as a fluid, hydration is simply intravenous fluids with minimal sodium or dextrose depending on the formulation, whereas enteral (tube feeding) and parenteral nutrition contain micro- and macronutrients necessary to sustain life. AN originated as a means to nourish those unable to ingest food and fluids due to temporary or chronic illness. Although the success of AN is widespread in the literature, its overuse in palliative care and in severe cognitive impairments, such as advanced progressive dementia or persistent vegetative states, may create ethical dilemmas for residents, families and healthcare providers (Monturo 2009).

Enteral Nutrition History

Enteral nutrition or "tube feeding" is more common in LTC and thus will be the focus of this discussion. This treatment dates to ancient times, and throughout the centuries it has taken on a variety of different forms (Randall 1990). Technological advances in surgical procedures led to the development of the percutaneous endoscopic gastrostomy (PEG) tube. Placement of this tube afforded patients a decreased risk of complications. The last available statistics on placement of gastrostomy tubes noted a threefold increase in older adults over a 20-year period (DeFrances et al. 2007), which may be due in part to the relative ease of PEG tube placement.

Enteral Nutrition Use

According to CMS, approximately 5.8% of LTC residents received AN in August 2010 (U.S. Department of Health and Human Services [HHS] 2010). In comparison, the national and individual state rates of AN in those with cognitive impairment range from 18% to 34% and 7.5% to 40%, respectively (Ahronheim et al. 2001; Gessert et al. 2000; Mitchell et al. 2003; Teno et al. 2002). There is little evidence that AN is prescribed for those with dementia in other parts of the world. The rate of AN in the United States may also vary by individual nursing home, community (rural versus urban), and nursing home culture (Gessert et al. 2006; Palan Lopez et al. 2010). Additional research also reported that being older and a resident in a LTC facility were identified as risk factors for not respecting life-sustaining treatment decisions (Biola et al. 2010). Despite the significant number of U.S. nursing home residents receiving AN, there is no evidence to support that this treatment is beneficial to those with dementia (Candy et al. 2009) and in fact is not recommended (Cegelka 2014). In comparison, AN is not started in residents with dementia in LTC settings in the Netherlands (Mehr et al. 2003; Pasman et al. 2004). Conversely, culture appears to play a role in a higher prevalence of AN in Chinese nursing homes, especially at the end of life, to ensure that they have sufficient food near death (Nordin et al. 2015).

Unlike orally ingested food, delivery of AN is not free of complications (Figure 14.2). As a result, efforts should be made to avoid AN in end-of-life care and instead consider viable alternatives.

PRACTICAL GUIDELINES FOR ALTERNATIVES TO ARTIFICIAL NUTRITION

Without the potential for alternatives to AN, practitioners would be forced into a black-and-white decision to initiate, maintain, withhold or withdraw AN in end-of-life situations. In response to this dilemma, some suggest a parallel between the evolution of PEG tubes and cardiopulmonary resuscitation (CPR) (Brauner 2010). As the "do not resuscitate" order limits the use of CPR, Brauner suggests that institution of "comfort feeding only" orders may limit the use of AN (Brauner 2010).

To further avoid this dilemma and to assist the resident and family through the grieving process, guidelines have been developed to address both those residents with an intact gag/swallowing reflex and those with some level of swallowing deficit (Table 14.4).

These guidelines contain ways to provide oral nutrition or fluids for those with intact swallowing function, but more importantly provide other means to comfort residents without the need for food. Historically, eating and feeding are viewed as nurturing or caring functions. For many, food is an

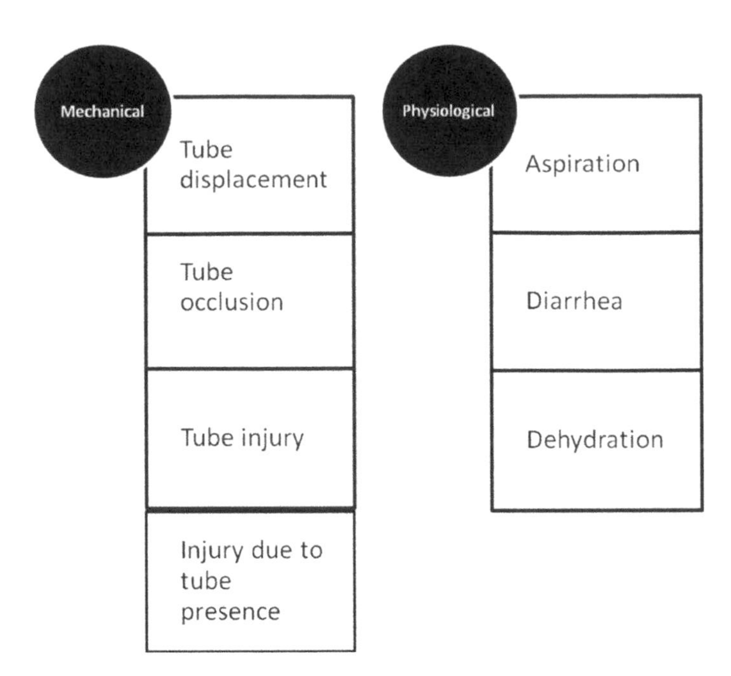

FIGURE 14.2 Enteral nutrition complications. Complications with enteral nutrition are divided into two categories: mechanical and physiological. Mechanical complications are associated with the actual device—the tube, whereas physiological complications encompass the body's reaction to enteral nutrition.

TABLE 14.4
Guidelines for Alternatives to Artificial Nutrition

Intact Swallowing Function	Swallowing Deficit
• Adjust food consistency for ease of ingestion	• Determine limitations for oral intake[a]
• Determine likes/dislikes and tailor menu	• Provide frequent mouth care
• Encourage family/friends to bring appropriate foods	• Provide frequent skin care
• Arrange food attractively on small plates	• Instill lubricant eye drops for dry eyes
• Provide small frequent meals	• Encourage family to assist with physical care
• Medicate as necessary to control pain and/or nausea	• Medicate as necessary to control pain and/or nausea
• Be aware of resident's wishes	• Encourage other nurturing activities in place of food (singing, massage, reading, music, photographs)
• Goal is not nutritional repletion, but comfort or pleasure	• Goal is comfort and helping to replace the "food connection" between resident and family
• Make food and fluid available and accessible to the resident on a regular basis	• If the resident is not being provided with any food or fluids, encourage staff and family to maintain some physical contact (holding hand, gentle touch on shoulder/arm) when present
• When no longer able to feed self, use hand feeding to maintain the social connection	• Encourage family to be "present" when spending time with resident and avoid isolating the resident

Note: For those individuals who choose not to accept artificial nutrition at the end of life, there are alternatives. Suggestions are offered here for those with intact swallowing function as well as those with a swallowing deficit.

[a] For those with a swallowing deficit, families must consult with healthcare providers concerning the limitations for oral intake since the risk of aspiration must be discussed and a decision made to either accept or reject the idea of providing tastes or sips of food/fluids at the request of the resident at end of life.

integral part of secular as well as religious holidays. Food is also central to gatherings for mourning or grieving a loss, assuring that all will be fed and nurtured.

In this respect, practitioners must develop different methods to reconnect or maintain the relationship between residents and families at the end of life. These methods must be based on knowledge of the family and resident, information that may be discovered during the advance care planning process (Monturo and Strumpf 2014).

ETHICAL ISSUES

No research supports the use of AN in end-of-life care, nor does it prove beneficial to those with dementia according to recent results from the Cochrane Collaboration (Candy et al. 2009). Despite this, some may argue that we lack hard evidence in the form of randomized controlled trials examining the benefits and burdens of tube feeding vs hand feeding in those with dementia. This study design would likely be unethical to conduct (Cegelka 2014). Despite this, some nursing home residents with dementia or other terminal illnesses continue to receive AN. Perhaps high profile cases involving AN highlighted an ethical dilemma: is AN a medical treatment or basic life support? Notwithstanding the ethics' panel findings from more than 20 years ago, individuals continue to struggle with the notion of "not feeding" or starving a loved one. Starvation is a highly emotive word and one filled with individual images of pain and suffering. Similarly the emotions connected with the meaning of food are based on individual values and beliefs and comprise one's life story (Monturo 2009; Monturo and Strumpf 2014). Examination of the meaning of food and individual nursing home cultures may provide insight as to the necessary changes and ongoing intensive palliative care education required for compassionate and clinically appropriate end-of-life care for nursing home residents.

APPLICATION TO OTHER AREAS OF TERMINAL OR PALLIATIVE CARE

Although not focused on a LTC population, the issue of voluntarily stopping eating and drinking (VSED) has been considered since 1993 in the Netherlands (Ivanović et al. 2014). In the United States, some suggested this as a plan for those who may suffer from dementia in the future (Span 2015) to avoid the potential challenges of future AN.

KEY FACTS: NURSING HOMES

- Regardless of country, nursing homes, care homes, or long-term care facilities provide care for those unable to care for themselves.
- Some may provide only custodial care, while others may have sub-acute and rehabilitation units.
- Nursing homes are not limited to the care of older adults. Younger adults with life-limiting or severely debilitating and chronic conditions are also treated.
- Nursing homes are regulated so as to provide safe and effective care to all residents. These regulations differ based on country/state.
- Some nursing homes may be modeled after a hospital-type ward with individual rooms off a corridor and no access to a kitchen.
- Other nursing homes offer a more home-like and inviting milieu such as the innovative "Green Houses" featuring central kitchens and great rooms with resident rooms off of this space.
- The cost of long-term care is variable across countries and may be the responsibility of the resident, the family, the insurance company, the health service, the state and federal governments, or a combination of these entities.

SUMMARY POINTS

- Long-term care facilities will increasingly provide a substantial portion of end-of-life care.
- The lack of appropriate palliative care education in nursing homes is well documented.
- Advance directives are one part of the advance care planning process.
- The right-to-die movement began the discussions of withdrawal and withholding of life-sustaining treatments such as artificial nutrition.
- Artificial nutrition is a viable option for treatment of temporary illnesses.
- Artificial nutrition is not beneficial in those with advanced dementia.
- Long-term care facility culture and geographic community may affect the rate of artificial nutrition delivered in that particular home.
- An ethical dilemma exists for some who believe that artificial nutrition is synonymous with food and that withdrawal or withholding this treatment is tantamount to starvation.
- Examination of the meaning of food for residents and families is necessary to plan appropriate end-of-life care.

LIST OF ABBREVIATIONS

AD	Advance Directive
AN	Artificial Nutrition
CMS	Centers for Medicare and Medicaid Services
HHS	U.S. Department of Health and Human Services
LTC	Long-Term Care (also known as Nursing Homes, Skilled Nursing Facilities, Care Homes)
MDS	Minimum Data Set
OBRA	Omnibus Budget Reconciliation Act
PEG	Percutaneous Endoscopic Gastrostomy

REFERENCES

Abt Associates. 2001. *Report to Congress: Appropriateness of minimum nurse staffing ratios in nursing homes.* Phase II Final Report (Center for Medicare and Medicaid Services ed.), Baltimore, MD. https://theconsumervoice.org/uploads/files/issues/CMS-Staffing-Study-Phase-II.pdf). (accessed 4/7/19).

Ahronheim, J. C. et al. 2001. State practice variations in the use of tube feeding for nursing home residents with severe cognitive impairment. *Journal of the American Geriatric Society* 49: 148–152.

An Bord Altranais. 2009. Professional guidance for nurses working with older people (Altranais AB ed.), Dublin. http://www.nursingboard.ie/en/publications_current.aspx (accessed February 14, 2010).

Biola, H. et al. 2010. Preferences versus practice: Life-sustaining treatments in last months of life in long-term care. *Journal of the American Medical Directors Association* 11: 42–51.

Brauner, D.J. 2010. Reconsidering default medicine. *Journal of the American Geriatric Society* 58: 599–601.

Brennan, F. 2007. Palliative care as an international human right. *Journal of Pain and Symptom Management* 33: 494–499.

Candy, B., Sampson, E. L., and Jones, L. 2009. Enteral tube feeding in older people with advanced dementia: Findings from a Cochrane systematic review. *International Journal of Palliative Nursing* 15: 396–404.

Cegelka, A. 2014. American Geriatrics Society feeding tubes in advanced dementia position statement. *Journal of the American Geriatric Society* 62: 1590–1593.

Center for Gerontology and Health Care Research Brown Medical School. 2004. Facts on dying: Policy relevant data on care at end of life. CHCR Brown University. http://www.chcr.brown.edu/dying/usastatistics.htm (accessed December 17, 2004).

Chan, H. M. 2004. Sharing death and dying: Advance directives, autonomy and the family. *Bioethics* 18: 87–103.

DeFrances, C. J., Cullen, K. A., and Kozak, L. J. 2007. National hospital discharge survey: 2005 annual summary with detailed diagnoses and procedure data. *Vital Health Statistics* Series 13: No. 165, 1–209.

De Gendt, C., Bilsen J., Stichele R. V., and Deliens L. 2013. Advance care planning and dying in nursing homes in Flanders, Belgium: A nationwide survey. *Journal of Pain and Symptom Management* 45: 223–234. doi: 10.1016/j.jpainsymman.2012.02.011

Fagerlin, A. and Schneider, C. E. 2004. *Enough: The failure of the living will.* Hasting Center Report 30–42.

Gessert, C. E., Elliott, B. A., and Peden-McAlpine, C. 2006. Family decision-making for nursing home residents with dementia: Rural-urban differences. *Journal of Rural Health* 22: 1–8.

Gessert, C. E. et al. 2000. Tube feeding in nursing home residents with severe and irreversible cognitive impairment. *Journal of the American Geriatric Society* 48: 1593–1600.

Graham, F., Kumar, S., and Clark, D. 2010. Barriers to the delivery of palliative care. In *Oxford Textbook of Palliative Medicine.* 4th ed. Hanks, G., Cherny, N.I., Christakis, N.A. et al. (Eds) Oxford University Press, Oxford.

Gruneir, A., Mor, V., Weitzen, S., Truchil, R., Teno, J., and Roy, J. 2007. Where people die: A multilevel approach to understanding influences on site of death in America. *Medical Care Research and Review: MCRR* 64: 351–378.

Health Information and Quality Authority. 2008. National quality standards for residential care setting for older people in Ireland (HIQUA ed.), Dublin. www.hiqua.ie (accessed February 14, 2010).

Hendriks, S. A., Smalbrugge, M., Deliens, L., Koopmans, R. T. C. M., Onwuteaka-Philipsen, B. D., Hertogh, C. M. P. M., and Steen, J. T. 2017. End-of-life treatment decisions in nursing home residents dying with dementia in the Netherlands. *International Journal of Geriatric Psychiatry* 32: e43–e49. doi: 10.1002/gps.4650

Houttekier, D. et al. 2010. Place of death of older persons with dementia: A study in five European countries. *Journal of the American Geriatric Society* 58: 751–756.

In re Cruzan v. Director, M. D. H. et al. 1990. In the Supreme Court of the United States. No. 88-1503. Nancy Beth Cruzan, by her parents and co-guardians, Lester L. Cruzan, et ux., petitioners, v. Director, Missouri Department Health et al. In *Issues in Law & Medicine.* 453–478.

International Council of Nurses. 2002. Peaceful death: Recommended competencies and curricular guidelines for end-of-life care. http://www.aacn.nche.edu/publications/deathfin.htm (accessed February 14, 2010).

Ivanović, N., Büche, D., Fringer, A. 2014. Voluntary stopping of eating and drinking at the end of life—A "systematic search and review" giving insight into an option of hastening death in capacitated adults at the end of life. *BMC Palliative Care* 13: 421–428.

Laing and Buisson. 2013. *Care of Elderly People. UK Market Survey 2012/2013.* Laing and Buisson, London.

Marie Curie Cancer Care. 2009. End of Life Care for People with Dementia. www.mariecurie.org.uk/documents/healthcare-professionals/innovation/project-report-0210.pdf.

McDonnell, M. M., McGuigan, E., McElhinney, J., McTeggart, M., and McClure, D. 2009. An analysis of the palliative care education needs of RGNs and HCAs in nursing homes in Ireland. *International Journal of Palliative Nursing* 15: 446–455.

Mehr, D. R. et al. 2003. Lower respiratory infections in nursing home residents with dementia: A tale of two countries. *Gerontologist* 43: 85–93.

Mitchell, S. L., Teno, J. M., Miller, S. C., and Mor, V. 2005. A national study of the location of death for older persons with dementia. *Journal of the American Geriatrics Society* 53: 299–305.

Mitchell, S. L., Teno, J. M., Roy, J., Kabumoto, G., and Mor, V. 2003. Clinical and organizational factors associated with feeding tube use among nursing home residents with advanced cognitive impairment. *Journal of the American Medical Association* 290: 73–80.

Monturo, C. 2009. The AN debate: Still an issue…after all these years. *Nutrition in Clinical Practice* 24: 206–213.

Monturo, C. A. and Strumpf, N. E. 2007. Advance directives at end-of-life: Nursing home resident preferences for AN. *Journal of the American Medical Directors Association* 8: 224–228.

Monturo, C. A. and Strumpf, N. E. 2014. Food, meaning and identity among aging veterans at end of life. *Journal of Hospice and Palliative Nursing* 16: 143–149.

National Center for Health Statistics. 2008. *Mortality data, multiple cause-of-death public-use data files. Worktable 309.* Deaths by place of death, age, race and sex/United States, 1999–2005 (Report No. Worktable 309). National Center for Health Statistics. NCHS, CDC, Atlanta, GA.

National POLST Paradigm. 2016. Programs in your state. Retrieved from http://www.polst.org/programs-in-your-state.

Nordin, N. et al. 2015. A descriptive study of nasogastric tube feeding among geriatric inpatients in Malaysia: utilization, complications and caregiver opinions. *Journal of Nutrition in Gerontology and Geriatrics* 34: 34–49.

Oliver, D. P., Porock, D. and Zweig, S. 2004. End-of-life care in U.S. nursing homes: A review of the evidence. *Journal of the American Medical Directors Association* 5: 147–155.

Omnibus Budget Reconciliation Act. 1987. In *Medicare and Medicaid requirements for long-term care facilities*. 42, CFT Part 483.

Omnibus Budget Reconciliation Act. 1990. 42 U.S.C. (1395cc(a) (I)(Q), 1395 mm (c)(8), 1395cc(f), 1396a(a)(57), 1396a(a)(58), and 1396a(w) ed.

Palan Lopez, R., Amella, E. J., Strumpf, N., Teno, J. M., and Mitchell, S. L. 2010. The influence of nursing home culture on the use of feeding tubes. *Archives of Internal Medicine* 170: 83–88.

Pasman, H. R. et al. 2004. Forgoing AN and hydration in nursing home patients with dementia: Patients, decision making and participants. *Alzheimer Disease Association Disorders* 18: 154–162.

Randall, H. T. 1990. The history of enteral nutrition. In *Clinical Nutrition: Enteral and Tube Feeding*, 2nd ed. J. L. Rombeau and M. T. Caldwell (Eds) 614. Saunders, Philadelphia.

Silveira, M. J., Wiitala, W. Piette, J. 2014. Advance directive completion by elderly Americans; A decade of change. *Journal of the American Geriatric Society* 62: 706–710.

Span, P. 2015. Complexities of Choosing an End Game for Dementia. *The New York Times*. https://www.nytimes.com/2015/01/20/health/complexities-of-choosing-an-end-game-for-dementia.html (accessed December 15, 2017).

Stillman, D., Strumpf, N., Capezuti, E., and Tuch, H. 2005. Staff perceptions concerning barriers and facilitators to end-of-life care in the nursing home. *Geriatric Nursing* 26: 259–264.

Temkin-Greener, H., Zheng, N.T., Norton, S.A., Quill, T., Ladwig, S., and Veazie, P. 2009. Measuring end-of-life care processes in nursing homes. *The Gerontologist* 49: 803–815.

Teno, J. M., Branco, K. J., Mor, V., Phillips, C. D., Hawes, C., Morris, J., and Fries, B. E. 1997. Changes in advance care planning in nursing homes before and after the patient Self-Determination Act: Report of a 10-state survey. *Journal of the American Geriatrics Society* 45: 939–944.

Teno, J. M., Mor, V., DeSilva, D., Kabumoto, G., Roy, J., and Wetle, T. 2002. Use of feeding tubes in nursing home residents with severe cognitive impairment. *Journal of the American Medical Association* 287: 3211–3212.

The Care Commission. 2009. Better care every step of the way. Scottish Commission for the Regulation of Care.

The President's Commission for the Study of Ethical Problems in Medicine and Biomedical and Behavioral Research. 1983. *Deciding to Forego Life-Sustaining Treatment*. U.S. Government Printing Office, Washington, DC.

Tsai, H. H., Tsai, Y. F., and Liu, C. Y. 2017. Advance directives and mortality rates among nursing home residents in Taiwan: A retrospective, longitudinal study. *International Journal of Nursing Studies* 68: 9–15.

Tschirhart, E.C., Qingling, D., and Kelley, A. 2014. Factors influencing the use of intensive procedures at the end of life. *Journal of the American Geriatric Society* 62(11): 2088–2094.

U.S. Department of Health and Human Services. August 2010. *CMS*. CASPER 4D Report, CASPER Reporting System: CMS-672, Resident Census and Conditions of Residents.

Weuve, J., Hebert, L. E., Scherr, P. A., and Evans, D. A. 2014. Deaths in the United States among persons with Alzheimer's disease (2010–2050). *Alzheimer's Dementia* 10(2): e40–e46.

Yadav, K. N. et al. 2017. Approximately one in three US adults completes any type of advance directive for end-of-life care. *Health Affairs* 36: 1244.

15 Support for Hydration at End of Life

Robin L. Fainsinger

CONTENTS

INTRODUCTION

The controversial topic of dehydration and rehydration of palliative care patients is complicated and has many different aspects to consider. The divergence of opinion is well illustrated by the following quotes: "Research is limited but suggests that artificial hydration in imminently dying patients influences neither survival nor symptom control" (Soden et al. 2002) and "the best available evidence suggests that hydration of advanced cancer patients plays an important role in maintaining cognitive function and is therefore an important factor in the prevention and reversal of delirium in this population" (Lawlor 2002).

Differences in medical opinions are further complicated by other complex issues illustrated by the following statement: "terminal dehydration is a controversial topic, weighted heavily with historic symbolism and strong religious, societal and cultural conflicts" (Huffman and Dunn 2002). Consideration of a case example can be helpful in illustrating aspects of these issues. A 65-year-old man who has been active and in good health notes that he has lost 4–5 kg of weight over the previous few months. He is investigated, and a liver biopsy confirms liver metastases from a probable pancreatic primary cancer. He develops nausea and vomiting and presents to the emergency room of the local hospital where he is found to have clinical evidence of dehydration. He is given intravenous fluids for rehydration, subsequently improves, and is discharged home. As the patient develops increasing abdominal pain over the next few weeks, he requires increasing morphine doses to keep him comfortable. He expresses a desire to remain at home. He and his wife discuss goals of care and advanced directives with their family physician and indicate that their worldview is that everything possible should be done to maintain life. As the patient develops episodic nausea and vomiting, he is changed to subcutaneous morphine, which is increased up to 120 mg subcutaneously per day. As the patient's oral intake is suboptimal, the palliative home care nurse and family physician suggest the option of parenteral hydration with hypodermoclysis. This is subsequently started to ensure that the patient receives at least 1 L of fluid overnight. At this point, their two children return home to

TABLE 15.1
Issues for Healthcare Professionals to Consider

1. Various expressions of opinion
2. Information on pathophysiology and biochemical changes
3. Conflicting research outcomes
4. Conflicting family and cultural expectations
5. Variability in consensus statements
6. Unique circumstances of each patient and family

provide extra support for their mother in caring for their father. The daughter works as a hospice nurse and does not believe in the value of parenteral hydration. The son is a nephrologist who argues that hydration is essential for normal renal function to avoid the accumulation of morphine metabolites and the associated risk of side effects. The parents are aware of their children's different opinions, but they continue to rely on their relationship with their family physician and home care nurse and their advice and direction as to appropriate management.

This case example demonstrates some of the complex issues that are considered when debating this controversial topic. Regardless of the setting and circumstances, the common ground in the discussion is the desire to keep patients as comfortable as possible and avoid futile management and procedures. Differences of opinion start to emerge when considering what may be futile in the provision of hydration at the end of life. Healthcare professionals trying to make these decisions with patients and families need to consider a variety of expressions of opinion, information on pathophysiology and biochemical changes, a variety of research outcomes, family and cultural expectations and variability in consensus statements. The unique trajectory and circumstances of each patient and family have to be considered as we attempt to make an individual decision on whether or not to use parenteral hydration (Dalal et al. 2009) (Table 15.1).

BACKGROUND TO THE HYDRATION CONTROVERSY

It is important to understand at the outset that encouraging palliative care patients to maintain reasonable oral intake to prevent fluid deficit is not a point of controversy. The opposing viewpoints in literature reports revolve around the use of supplemental parenteral hydration, and include clinical and ethical viewpoints (Craig 1994; Fainsinger and Bruera 1994). The traditional arguments for and against the use of parenteral hydration are summarized in Table 15.2.

The standard medical approach to fluid deficits is to initiate or maintain parenteral hydration. As a result, we can expect that in most countries patients dying in hospitals will have an intravenous line with the exceptions being the patients with a sudden deterioration or unexpected death. This has been demonstrated by a study where 73 of 106 cancer patients dying in a Canadian acute-care hospital had intravenous fluids administered (Burge, King, and Wilson 1990). A report a decade later suggested that artificial hydration may no longer be considered routine hospital practice for palliative care patients. In this retrospective study (Soden et al. 2002) in an English hospital, 65% of patients were hydrated during the last week of life, and only 46% were actually being given hydration when they died. In a survey of 238 Latin American palliative care physicians, 60% prescribed parenteral hydration to 40%–100% of their patients. The difference from traditional hospice philosophy is explained by clinical perceptions of benefit based on individualized treatment decisions (Torres-Vigil et al. 2012).

In our setting in Edmonton, Canada, we sought to understand the routine practice of physicians involved in end-of-life care regarding the application of parenteral hydration for patients in a palliative care unit and an acute-care hospital while being followed or not being followed by the palliative care program at the acute-care site (Lanuke et al. 2004). There were 50 consecutive patients for each of the three cohorts included in this retrospective chart review. The majority of patients received

TABLE 15.2
Arguments for and Against the Use of Parenteral Hydration

No Parenteral Hydration

- Comatose patients do not experience symptom distress.
- Parenteral fluids prolong dying.
- Incontinence and need for catheters will be reduced.
- As a result of decreased gastrointestinal fluid there will be less nausea and vomiting.
- Problems with cough and pulmonary edema will be limited by decreased respiratory secretions.
- Decreased problems with edema and ascites.
- Dehydration may be a natural anesthetic in decreasing patient awareness and suffering.
- Parenteral hydration may limit patient mobility and be uncomfortable.

Use Parenteral Hydration

- Terminally ill patients are more comfortable with parenteral hydration.
- Parenteral hydration does not prolong life.
- Restlessness, confusion and neuromuscular irritability can be increased by fluid deficit.
- Parenteral hydration should be an option for terminally ill patients complaining of thirst.
- This is a minimum standard of care.
- This is a reasonable quality-of-life measure.
- Withholding treatment to other compromised patient groups may begin with withholding parenteral hydration for palliative care patients.

hydration with a range of 66%–98% of patients receiving parenteral hydration during the last week of life. However, the volume of hydration was significantly lower, and the use of hypodermoclysis was significantly higher in the palliative care unit site.

It would seem reasonable to argue that a policy of maintaining intravenous hydration with volumes in excess of 3 L per day in advanced palliative care populations is likely to cause significant problems. In this circumstance, we can anticipate complications such as increased respiratory and gastrointestinal symptoms. Conversely, a review of reports arguing against hydration at the end of life suggest that healthcare professionals looking after palliative care populations may be reacting to overuse of intravenous fluids with the conclusion that the complete opposite approach of no parenteral hydration is preferable. This belief has been reinforced by many anecdotal literature reports suggesting that palliative care patients appear to die comfortably without parenteral hydration. However, review of the literature does indicate that these reports are primarily based on unsubstantiated data.

The argument has been made that there are other issues to consider (Fainsinger and Bruera 1994):

1. Confusion and restlessness in the general population are well recognized as a consequence of fluid deficit. Similar problems of agitated delirium have frequently been reported in palliative care populations.
2. Pre-renal failure is known to be caused by decreased intravascular volume and glomerular filtration rate as a consequence of fluid deficit. We know that opioid metabolites accumulate in patients with renal failure, resulting in confusion, myoclonus and seizures.

The problem of agitated delirium and terminal restlessness is frequently reported and discussed in palliative care literature. The focus of management of these problems is frequently on the need for pharmacological management, including sedation, and often omits consideration of the role of parenteral hydration. We have noted that the severity of agitated delirium requiring sedation decreased to as low as 3% in our palliative care unit. We hypothesized that this was a result of changing our practice to include more frequent use of parenteral hydration with hypodermoclysis, opioid sequential trials when toxicity is noted and less sedating treatments for agitated delirium. Our experience is worth comparing with a retrospective chart review of patients dying at St. Luke's

Hospital in Cape Town, South Africa, where 29% of patients required sedation for agitated delirium. In this setting, no patients were treated with parenteral hydration, and patients requiring sedation were being given significantly higher doses of opioids (Fainsinger et al. 1998). Subsequent reports from our integrated regional palliative care service in Edmonton have suggested that agitated delirium appears to be a less prevalent problem in our different settings where parenteral hydration is common practice, compared with requirements for sedation as reported at other international locations (Fainsinger, deMoissac et al. 2000; Fainsinger, Waller et al. 2000; Lanuke et al. 2004).

Our group has continued to argue that dehydration could be a reversible component of agitated delirium, which may be missed if we focus exclusively on sedative pharmacological solutions to this common and distressing symptom (Fainsinger and Bruera 1997). We do not consider that it is logical for a patient to receive medications for agitated delirium, myoclonus and seizures, if these problems could be prevented or improved for some patients by a more liberal use of parenteral hydration.

CLARIFYING TERMINOLOGY

Reviews on this topic have taken issue with the inaccurate use and description of dehydration (Lawlor 2002). Fluid deficit should be understood as water loss with or without electrolytes that includes subtypes of volume depletion and dehydration. Dehydration is total-body water deficit that is mainly intracellular and is associated with hypernatremia. Volume depletion is deficit in the intravascular fluid volume and may be isotonic, hyponatremic or hypernatremic (Figure 15.1).

A number of factors need to be considered, using history, physical examination and laboratory findings to assess for the risk or presence of fluid deficit. The fluid deficit symptoms to consider include behavior and cognitive changes, fatigue, thirst, nausea and dry mouth. Dry mouth, decreased skin turgor, postural hypotension, tachycardia, decreased jugular venous pressure, sunken eyes and decreased sweating are considered classical signs of fluid deficit. Nevertheless, these problems have to be interpreted with caution as they may be associated with other causes, such as aging, cachexia, advanced cancer and side effects seen with frequently used medications. In some situations laboratory tests can provide further helpful information. Elevated levels of urea, creatinine, plasma proteins, hematocrit and sodium are often seen in volume-depleted patients.

HYDRATION RESEARCH

There are three dimensions that need to be considered when reviewing the research on the use of hydration for palliative care patients (Table 15.3).

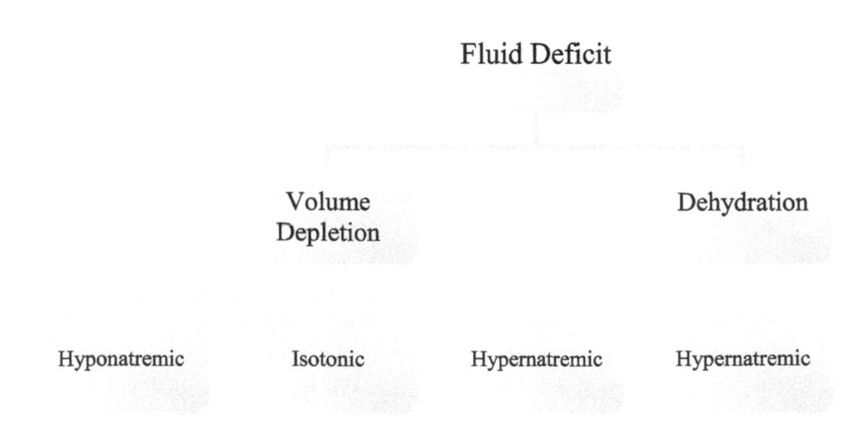

FIGURE 15.1 Fluid deficit subgroups.

TABLE 15.3
Dimensions of Palliative Care Hydration Research

1. Association between biochemical findings and hydration status
2. Association between biochemical findings and clinical symptoms
3. Association between hydration status and clinical symptoms

The acknowledgement of fluid deficit as a cause of renal failure is not considered controversial. Parenteral hydration is accepted as standard management in many settings; however, the impact of fluid deficit and rehydration on renal function and electrolyte balance in palliative care patients, particularly in the last few days of life, is uncertain. There is some evidence that parenteral hydration does have an impact in decreasing abnormal biochemistry, particularly renal function, in the last week of life (Fainsinger 1999; Morita et al. 1998).

While much of the early literature on determining the association between hydration status and clinical symptoms in early literature is based on anecdotal opposing viewpoints in case reports, there have been a number of subsequent reports attempting to look at this issue more carefully. Burge (1993) studied the quantitative assessment of the dehydration experience in advanced cancer patients and concluded that parenteral hydration on the basis of fluid intake and laboratory measures was not helpful if the aim was to reduce thirst. McCann et al. (1994) investigated symptom prevalence and management of hunger and thirst in palliative care patients not receiving parenteral hydration and concluded that the symptoms of hunger, thirst and dry mouth were well managed with oral hydration and mouth care.

Ellershaw et al. (1995) considered the association of symptoms and dehydration in 82 patients where parenteral hydration was not provided. There was no significant association between the level of hydration and the outcome measures of respiratory tract secretions, thirst and dry mouth. However, the association of renal failure and possible consequences of agitated delirium was not assessed.

Our group assessed the impact of our change of practice with regard to parenteral hydration and cognitive impairment in a retrospective chart review of 117 and 162 patients admitted to our palliative care unit in 1988–1989 and 1991–1992. We concluded that our results suggested that routine cognitive assessment, opioid rotation and hydration could reduce the frequency of agitated delirium in our population. Although we believe that parenteral hydration had significant impact, it was not possible to determine relative contributions of our change in practice (Bruera et al. 1995).

Lawlor et al. (2000) reported a prospective delirium study of 113 patients with advanced cancer. Reversibility was associated with psychoactive medications and dehydration. This study concluded that although delirium is multifactorial, the use of hypodermoclysis for parenteral hydration may be a potential useful reversible measure.

An observational study of symptoms and parenteral fluid administered in Swedish hospitals suggested an association with higher volumes and increased documentation of dyspnea in the last week of life (Fritzson et al. 2015).

Bruera et al. (2005) published the first randomized, controlled, double-blind study of parenteral hydration in terminally ill cancer patients. Patients with clinical and biochemical evidence of dehydration, and history of an oral intake of less than 1 L of fluid per day were randomly assigned to receive 1000 mL (treatment group) or 100 mL (placebo group) of normal saline over four hours for two days. Improvement in sedation and myoclonus scores were noted in the hydration treatment group. A more recent similar study by the same group, however, did not demonstrate any improvement in symptoms, quality of life or survival. The authors did acknowledge a number of study limitations and the need for future work to examine subgroups that might still benefit from parenteral hydration (Bruera et al. 2013).

There have been a number of reviews (including three Cochrane Database Systematic reviews) on this topic (Burge 1996; Good et al. 2014; Viola et al. 1997) that have all concluded that it is not possible to draw firm conclusions regarding clinical care based on the research evidence.

SOCIAL, CULTURAL AND ETHICAL ISSUES

Family and patient attitudes, level of comfort with end-of-life issues, education, healthcare professionals' biases and level of education, all have an influence on decisions with regard to parenteral hydration.

It is unfortunate that artificial nutrition and hydration are often considered as the same issue in ethical and clinical discussion papers. This can be confusing as the arguments and rationale for providing nutritional calories via artificial means as opposed to hydration alone deserve to be considered independently.

Morita et al. (1999) considered patient and family perceptions regarding rehydration to identify factors contributing to decision-making. Patient performance status, fluid retention symptoms, denial, physician recommendations, beliefs with regard to hydration effect on patient distress and family anxiety regarding withholding rehydration were all significantly associated with the decision-making process. The most important factors determining rehydration were the patient's performance status, fluid retention symptoms, denial and care receiver's beliefs regarding the effects of rehydration on symptom distress.

Issues of importance to family caregivers regarding parenteral hydration use in advanced cancer patients were considered in a Canadian study (Parkash and Burge 1997). Symptom distress issues, ethical and emotional considerations, information between healthcare professionals and families and culture were all important factors influencing the caregivers. The perceived benefit of parenteral hydration was central to the ethical, emotional and cultural considerations involved in the decisions of caregivers.

An article (Bodell and Weng 2000) on the values of the Jewish faith regarding terminal dehydration provides a good illustration of some of the problems in applying cultural and ethnic research and opinion. This report generated responses varying from descriptions of this as an "excellent article" (Schur 2000) to "extremely offensive in its references to Jewish people" (Rothstein 2000).

A novel study used Q-methodology to identify issues of concern for palliative care patients in regard to decisions about artificial hydration. The need to understand differing patient views and involve them in unbiased, informed decision-making was highlighted (Malia and Bennett 2011). Phenomenological interviews were used to explore how patients and caregivers in home hospice care in the United States viewed parenteral hydration. Contradictory to traditional hospice practice some considered this to enhance comfort, dignity and quality of life (Cohen et al. 2012). A literature review (Gent et al. 2015) on attitudes towards assisted hydration in dying patients identified three core themes: (1) symbolic value; (2) beliefs and misconceptions; and (3) cultural, ethical and legal ideas.

A core ethical principle of healthcare decision-making is the importance of patient autonomy. Using this principle, it has been proposed that voluntary cessation of drinking and the refusal of parenteral hydration is a legal right that could provide an alternative to physician-assisted suicide. Miller and Meier (1998) have suggested that using this option along with standard palliative care treatment, "offers patient's a way to escape agonizing, incurable condition that they consider to be worse than death, without requiring transformation of the law and medical ethics." Quill et al. (1998) argued that voluntary cessation of drinking "may be acceptable to a patient and physician and do not require fundamental changes in the law."

Craig (2008) has argued passionately that a blanket policy of no hydration, as endorsed in a national guideline in the United Kingdom, is ethically indefensible. The primary concern is that the value of hydration is underestimated and could increase deaths associated with palliative sedation. Craig (2004) devoted a book to this issue in which she states, "My personal role in the hydration debate has been to highlight the ethical, legal and medical dangers of a regime of sedation without hydration in the dying and draw attention to the plight of dissenting relatives."

OPTIONS FOR ALTERNATIVE HYDRATION

There is no controversy that the most convenient route for correction of fluid deficits would be improving or increasing oral intake. Where this is not possible or is inadequate, there are some circumstances where the benefits of parenteral hydration need to be considered. We need to

TABLE 15.4
Alternatives to Oral Hydration

1. Intravenous fluids
2. Nasogastric tubes or percutaneous gastrostomy
3. Hypodermoclysis
4. Rectal hydration

understand that we are not necessarily all seeing patients in the same trajectory of illness. Clinical circumstances change over time, and a physically independent and cognitively normal patient at an early stage of a palliative care illness will be viewed differently from the same patient a number of months later who has become physically dependent and cognitively impaired.

If a decision is made to use parenteral hydration (Table 15.4), we need to consider the type of fluid, volume and options for route of administration. In acute-care institutions the traditional route of choice has been intravenous hydration. However, there are many disadvantages such as difficultly finding venous access, pain, infection, mobility limitations and need to replace displaced lines particularly with less cooperative or agitated patients.

Nasogastric Tubes and Gastrostomy

Nasogastric tubes are often uncomfortable for patients, and prolonged use particularly in palliative care populations should be avoided as far as possible. Head and neck or esophageal cancer patients with increasing dysphagia may benefit from nutrition as well as hydration given via a percutaneous gastrostomy. The goals of care with regard to parenteral nutrition need to be reviewed as patients deteriorate. We need to recognize that it can be difficult to discontinue management, and the ease of access with percutaneous gastrostomy can result in ongoing nutrition and hydration in some circumstances where this might otherwise not have been started.

Hypodermoclysis

The use and safety of hypodermoclysis have been well documented and reported, and there have been studies in palliative care populations demonstrating ease of administration with minimal side effects. The application of hypodermoclysis is simple and is associated with minimal discomfort. A subcutaneous needle is inserted and attached to a fluid line that can be run using gravity or an infusion pump. Relatively little training for insertion and surveillance is required, and families can be trained to use this option at home with minimal burden, equipment or technical support (Vidal et al. 2016).

There is evidence that hypodermoclysis is being increasingly used in acute-care settings (Lanuke et al. 2004). The standard recommendation is to use solutions with electrolytes, as nonelectrolyte solutions may draw fluid into the interstitial space. Rates of infusion are usually limited to a maximum of 100–120 mL per hour. However, in some situations, patients can tolerate boluses of up to 500 mL per hour for a maximum of two to three hours per day. These bolus administrations should be administered over one hour at a time every 8–12 hours.

The use of hypodermoclysis has been aided by adding hyaluronidase to promote absorption. The doses used have ranged from 150 to 750 units per liter. However, anecdotal reports suggesting good absorption without hyaluronidase resulted in evidence demonstrating that patients can receive hypodermoclysis without hyaluronidase (Centeno and Bruera 1999). It is now standard practice in our setting to give patients hypodermoclysis without the addition of hyaluronidase with the most common range between 40 and 80 mL per hour. However, recombinant human hyaluronidase has been used in clinical studies and may have a future role in improving the absorption of subcutaneously administered fluids (Pirrello et al. 2007).

Rectal Hydration

Intravenous hydration can be uncomfortable, expensive and difficult to maintain in settings such as the home, while even hypodermoclysis can be too expensive or complicated in some situations. The potential advantage of fluid administered rectally, particularly in resource-limited developing countries prompted reports of rectal hydration use in terminally ill patients (Bruera et al. 1998). Rectal hydration was noted to be well tolerated with minimal side effects in the majority of patients. The mean daily volume, hourly rate and duration of therapy were reported as 1035 ± 150 mL per day, 224 ± 58 mL per hour and 14 ± 8 days, respectively. Rectal hydration appears to be a safe, effective and low-cost technique for rehydration that may have an application in limited poorly resourced terminally ill palliative care populations.

KEY FACTS: SUPPORT FOR HYDRATION AT END OF LIFE

- Fluid deficit, dehydration and rehydration of palliative care patients are complicated and have been a controversial issue in end-of-life care.
- It is important to understand the definitions and use of terminology for fluid deficit, dehydration and volume depletion.
- Artificial nutrition and hydration are not the same issue and should be considered independently in ethical and clinical discussion.
- Individual patient and family social, religious and cultural background can have a major influence in determining clinical management.
- Hypodermoclysis is a safe and convenient alternative when oral hydration is inadequate.
- There is an extensive and growing literature on this topic that includes much opinion and some research and is unlikely to provide any black-and-white answers for the foreseeable future.

SUMMARY POINTS

- The controversial topic of dehydration and rehydration of palliative care patients is complicated and has many different aspects to consider.
- The unique trajectory and circumstances of each patient and family have to be considered as we attempt to make an individual decision on whether or not to use parenteral hydration.
- The opposing viewpoints in literature reports revolve around the use of supplemental parenteral hydration, and include clinical and ethical viewpoints.
- Agitated delirium appears to be a less prevalent problem in settings where parenteral hydration is common practice.
- Terminology regarding fluid deficit, dehydration and volume depletion needs to be understood.
- Hydration research has covered the dimensions of association between biochemical findings and hydration status, association between biochemical findings and clinical symptoms and association between hydration status and clinical symptoms.
- A spectrum of social, cultural and ethical issues needs to be considered.
- The options for supplemental hydration are nasogastric and gastrostomy tubes, intravenous, hypodermoclysis and rectal hydration.

REFERENCES

Bodell, J. and Weng, M.A. 2000. The Jewish patient in terminal dehydration: A hospice ethical dilemma. *Am J Hospice Palliat Care*, 17(3): 185–188.

Bruera, E., Franco, J.J., Maltoni, M., Watanabe, S. et al. 1995. Changing pattern of agitated impaired mental status in patients with advanced cancer: Association with cognitive monitoring, hydration, and opioid rotation. *J Pain Symptom Manage*, 10: 287–291.

Bruera, E., Hui, D., Dalal, S., Torres-Vigil, I. et al. 2013. Parenteral hydration in patients with advanced cancer: A multicenter, double-blind, placebo-controlled randomized trial. *J Clin Oncol*, 31: 111–118.

Bruera, E., Pruvost, M., and Schoeller, T. 1998. Proctoclysis for hydration of terminally ill cancer patients. *J Pain Symptom Manage*, 15: 216–219.

Bruera, E., Sala, R., Rico, M.A., Moyana, J., Centeno, C., Willey, J., and Palmer, J.L. 2005. Effects of parenteral hydration in terminally ill cancer patients: A preliminary study. *J Clin Oncol*, 23(10): 2366–2371.

Burge, F.I. 1993. Dehydration symptoms of palliative care cancer patients. *J Pain Symptom Manage*, 8: 454–464.

Burge, F.I. 1996. Dehydration and provision of fluids in palliative care. What is the evidence? *Can Fam Physician*, 42: 2383–2388.

Burge, F.I., King, D.B., and Wilson, D. 1990. Intravenous fluids and the hospitalized dying: A medical last rite? *Cam Fam Physician*, 86: 883–886.

Centeno, C. and Bruera, E. 1999. Subcutaneous hydration with no hyaluronidase in patients with advanced cancer. *J Pain Symptom Manage*, 17(5): 305–306.

Cohen, M.Z., Torres-Vigil, I., Burbach, B.E., de la Rosa, M., and Bruera, E. 2012. *J Pain Symptom Manage*, 43: 855–865.

Craig, G. 2004. *Challenging Medical Ethics 1: No Water – No Life: Hydration in the Dying*. Fairway Folio (Christian Publishing Services), Cheshire, UK.

Craig, G. 2008. Palliative care in overdrive: Patients in danger. *Am J Hosp Palliat Care*, 25(2): 155–160.

Craig, G.M. 1994. On withholding nutrition and hydration in the terminally ill: Has palliative medicine gone too far? *J Med Ethics*, 20: 139–143.

Dalal, S., Del Fabbro, E., and Bruera, E. 2009. Is there a role for hydration at the end of life? *Curr Opin Support Palliat Care*, 3: 72–78.

Ellershaw, J.E., Sutcliffe, J.M., and Saunders, C.M. 1995. Dehydration and the dying patient. *J Pain Symptom Manage*, 10: 192–197.

Fainsinger, R.L. 1999. Biochemical dehydration in terminally ill cancer patients. *J Palliat Care*, 15(2): 59–61.

Fainsinger, R.L. and Bruera, E. 1994. The management of dehydration in terminally ill patients. *J Palliat Care*, 10: 55–59.

Fainsinger, R.L. and Bruera, E. 1997. When to treat dehydration in a terminally ill patient? *Support Care Cancer*, 5: 205–211.

Fainsinger, R.L., deMoissac, D., Mancini, I., and Oneschuk, D. 2000. Sedation for delirium and other symptoms in terminally ill patients in Edmonton. *J Palliat Care*, 16(2): 5–10.

Fainsinger, R.L., Landman, W., Hoskings, M., and Bruera, E. 1998. Sedation for uncontrolled symptoms in a South African hospice. *J Pain Symptom Manage*, 16(3): 145–152.

Fainsinger, R.L., Waller, A., Bercovici, M., Bengtson, K., Landman, W., Hosking, M., Nunez-Olarte, J.M., and deMoissac, D. 2000. A multi-centre international study of sedation for uncontrolled symptoms in terminally ill patients. *Palliat Med*, 14: 257–265.

Fritzson, A., Tavelin, B., and Axelsson, B. 2015. Association between parenteral fluids and symptoms in hospital end-of-life care: An observational study of 280 patients. *BMJ Support Palliat Care*, 5: 160–168.

Gent, M.J., Fradsham, S., Whyte, G.M., and Mayland, C.R. 2015. What influences attitudes towards clinically assisted dehydration in the care of dying patients? A review of the literature. *BMJ Support Palliat Care* 5: 223–231.

Good, P., Richard, R., Syrmis, W., Jenkins-Marsh, S., and Stephens, J. 2014. Medically assisted hydration for adult palliative care patients. *Cochrane Database Syst Rev*, Issue 4. Art. No.: CD006273.

Huffman, J.L. and Dunn, G.P. 2002. The paradox of hydration in advanced terminal illness. *J Am Col Surg*, 194(6): 835–839.

Lanuke, K., Fainsinger, R.L., and deMoissac, D. 2004. Hydration management at the end of life. *J Palliat Med*, 7(2): 257–263.

Lawlor, P. 2002. Delirium and dehydration: Some fluid for thought? *Support Care Cancer*, 10: 445–454.

Lawlor, P.G., Gagnon, B., Mancini, I.L., Pereira, J.L., Hanson, J., Suarez-Almazor, M.E., and Bruera, E. 2000. Occurrence, causes, and outcome of delirium in patients with advanced cancer. *Arch Int Med*, 160: 786–794.

Malia, C. and Bennett, M. 2011. What influences patient's decisions on artificial hydration at the end of life? A Q-methodological study. *J Pain Symptom Manage*, 42: 192–201.

McCann, R.M., Hall, W.J., and Groth-Juncker, A. 1994. Comfort care for the terminally ill patients. The appropriate use nutrition and hydration. *JAMA*, 272: 1263–1266.

Miller, F.G. and Meier, D.E. 1998. Voluntary death: A comparison of terminal dehydration and physician-assisted suicide. *Ann Intern Med*, 128: 559–562.

Morita, T., Ichika, T., Tsunoda, J., Inoue, S., and Chihara, S. 1998. Biochemical dehydration and fluid retention symptoms in terminally ill cancer patients whose death is impending. *J Palliat Care*, 14(4): 60–62.

Morita, T., Tsunoda, J., Inoue, S., and Chihara, S. 1999. Perceptions and decision-making on rehydration of terminally ill cancer patients and family members. *Am J Hosp Palliat Care*, 16(3): 509–516.

Parkash, R. and Burge, F. 1997. The family's perspective on issues of hydration in terminal care. *J Palliat Care*, 13(4): 23–27.

Pirrello, R.D., Ting Chen, C., and Thomas, S.H. 2007. Initial experiences with subcutaneous recombinant human hyaluronidase. *J Palliat Med*, 10(4):861–864.

Quill, T.E., Meier, D.E., Block, S.D., and Billings, J.A. 1998. The debate over physician-assisted suicide: Empirical data and conversant views. *Ann Intern Med*, 128: 552–558.

Rothstein, J.M. 2000. Out of context? *Am J Hospice and Palliat Care*, 17(5): 297.

Schur, T.G. 2000. Life and afterlife in Jewish tradition. *Am J Hosp Palliat Care*, 17(5): 296–297.

Soden, K., Hoy, A., Hoy, W., and Clelland, S. 2002. Artificial hydration during the last week of life in patients dying in district general hospital. *Palliat Med*, 16: 542–543.

Torres-Vigil, I., Mendoza, T.R., Alonso-Babarro, A., De Lima, L., Cárdenas-Turanzas, M., Hernandez, M., de la Rosa, A., and Bruera, E. 2012. Practice patterns and perceptions about parenteral hydration in the last weeks of life: A survey of palliative care physicians in Latin America. *J Pain Symptom Manage*, 43: 47–58.

Vidal, M., Hui, D., Williams, J., and Bruera, E. 2016. A prospective study of hypodermoclysis performed by caregivers in the home setting. *J Pain Symptom Manage*, 52: 570–574.

Viola, R., Wells, G.A., and Peterson, J. 1997. The effects of fluid status and fluid therapy on the dying: A systematic review. *J Palliat Care*, 13(4): 41–52.

16 Palliative Treatment of Dysphagia

Christian P. Selinger

CONTENTS

INTRODUCTION

The term "dysphagia" means difficulties in swallowing. In a clinical context, "dysphagia" is, however, used to describe a variety of problems that can be encountered while trying to get food and fluid into and through the upper part of the digestive system. Dysphagia can occur because of obstruction in the mouth or head and neck area, through disturbances in the neuro-muscular process that moves fluid or food from the pharynx to the stomach and obstruction of the oesophagus. Gastric outlet obstructions causing regurgitation of stomach contents are also discussed as they are often encountered and the same principles of care apply (Figure 16.1).

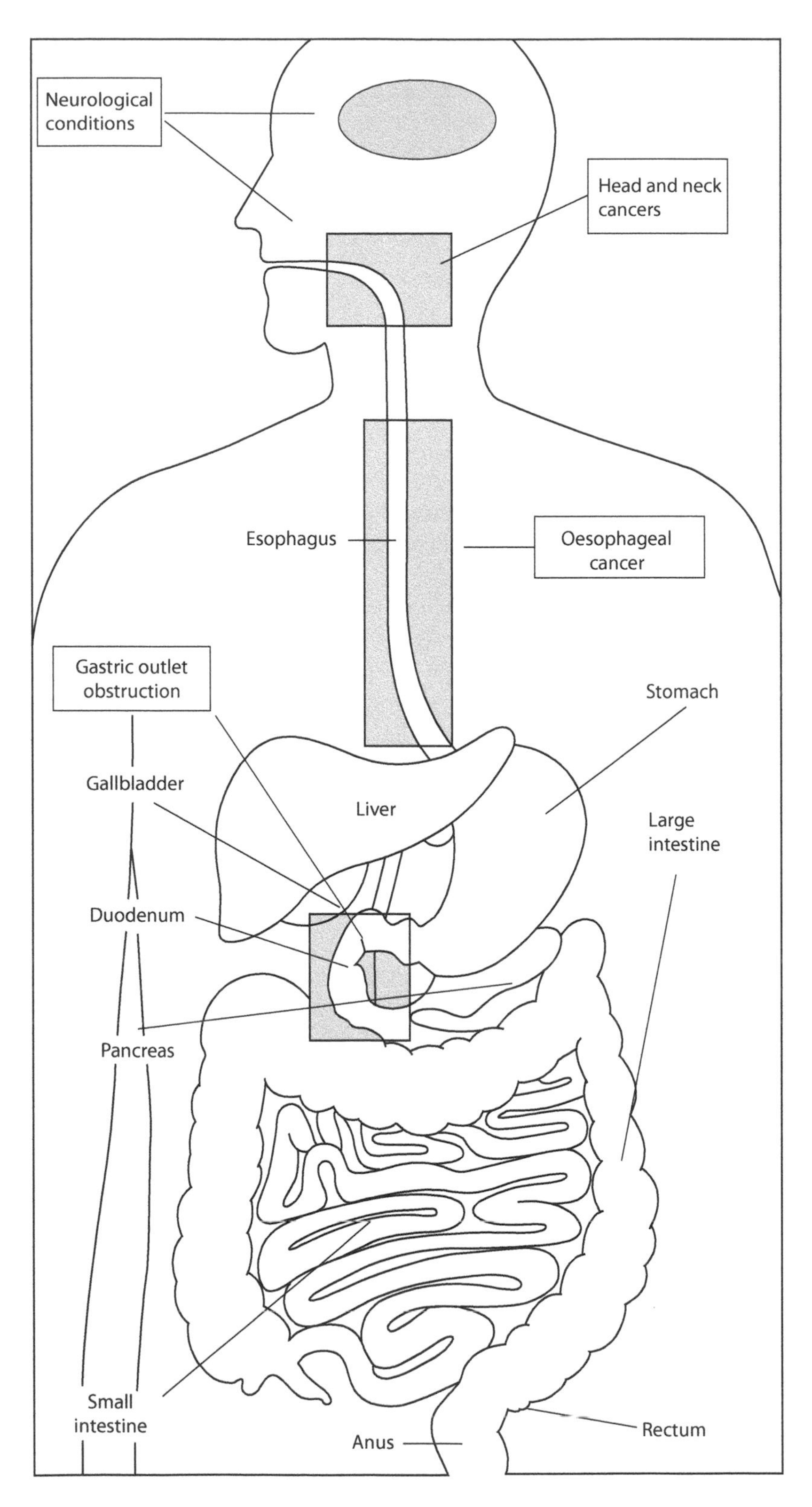

FIGURE 16.1 Pictogram of sites and types of dysphagia. An overview of human anatomy highlighting areas where dysphagia can arise from.

PATHOPHYSIOLOGY AND ANATOMY OF DYSPHAGIA

Neuro-Muscular Dysphagia

To propel food or fluid from the mouth to the stomach, a series of complex neurological and muscular actions is required: Voluntary muscles of the pharynx move the food or fluid to the proximal oesophagus, from where it is moved further by involuntary smooth muscle action to the stomach.

The neurological ability to swallow can be impaired by a variety of conditions encountered in the terminal or palliative care setting. Central or peripheral nervous system illnesses like cerebrovascular disease, intracranial haemorrhages, dementia, primary and secondary cerebral tumours, Parkinson's disease and motor-neuron disease can cause neurological dysphagia at the oropharynx level. Diseases affecting voluntary muscles directly (myotonic dystrophy, for example) can also cause dysphagia. The voluntary swallowing should be assessed clinically by a speech and language therapist and if needed by video-fluoroscopy. Patients might still be able to move the food or fluid to the oesophagus, but they could be at high risk of aspirating the contents into the trachea and lungs, which can lead to aspiration pneumonia. Increasing the viscosity of the food and fluid can increase the safety of swallowing in cases of mild to moderate neuro-muscular dysphagia. Should these measures not lead to a safe swallow, the appropriateness of establishing an alternative enteral feeding route (nasogastric [NG] tube, percutaneous endoscopic gastrostomy [PEG], percutaneous endoscopic jejunostomy [PEJ], radiologically introduced gastrostomy [RIG]) needs to be discussed (Table 16.1). In some circumstances, it might be appropriate to accept a risk of aspiration rather than intervene to establish an alternative feeding route.

A range of diseases can impair the smooth muscle actions of the oesophagus, though they are only infrequently seen in palliative care. In severe cases of systemic sclerosis, for example, an alternative enteral feeding route (NG tube, PEG, PEJ, RIG) can be used.

Dysphagia by Oral, Head and Neck Cancers

Tumours of the mouth, pharynx and larynx can cause direct obstruction prohibiting effective swallowing. Furthermore, surgery or radiotherapy can lead to dysphagia. In most cases, alternative enteral feeding needs to be established via PEG, PEJ, RIG or SPG.

Oesophageal and High Gastric Obstruction

Oesophageal and high gastric tumours can cause direct obstruction of the upper gastrointestinal (GI) tract. However, other intra-thoracic tumours (e.g., lung cancers or lymphadenopathy) can also cause dysphagia by external compression. Palliative efforts will often aim at re-opening the lumen of the oesophagus, which can be achieved by radiotherapy or placing a stent over the tumour (Table 16.2). Alternatively, a different enteral feeding route can be established.

TABLE 16.1
Treatment Options by Cause of Dysphagia

Type of Dysphagia	NG Tube	PEG/RIG Tube	Surgical Jejunostomy	Stent	Surgical Bypass	Radiotherapy
Neuromuscular problems	+	++	(+)	–	–	–
Head and neck cancers	++	+	(+)	–	–	–
Oesophageal cancer	(+)	(+)	(+)	++	–	++
Gastric outlet obstruction	–	–	(+)	++	++	–

Note: An overview of treatments and their feasibility in respect to cause of dysphagia. – not feasible; (+) feasible but rarely advised; + feasible; ++ preferred.

Abbreviations: NG, nasogastric; PEG, percutaneous endoscopic gastrostomy; RIG, radiologically introduced gastrostomy.

TABLE 16.2
Stent versus Radiotherapy for Oesophageal Cancer

	Advantages	Disadvantages
Stent	Quicker improvement of dysphagia Widely available	High rate of late complications Dysphagia improvement not as well sustained
Radiotherapy	Better long-term results Less complications	Slower onset of improvement Need for tertiary referral and travel

TABLE 16.3
Stent versus Gastrojejunostomy for Gastric Outlet Obstruction

	Advantages	Disadvantages
Stent	Quicker improvement of symptoms Relatively minor procedure Short hospital stay	High rate of late complications Improvement not as well sustained
Gastrojejunostomy	Better long-term results Less complications in later phase	Delayed gastric emptying Longer hospital stay Requires fitness for surgery and anaesthesia

Gastric Outlet Obstruction

Obstruction at low gastric or pyloric level is caused by gastric ulceration or malignancy, while duodenal-level obstructions are often caused by pancreatic neoplasms or primary duodenal tumours. Treatment options include re-opening of the narrowed segment by stent placement, surgical gastrojejunostomy or formation of a surgically placed jejunostomy (Table 16.3).

APPLICATIONS TO OTHER AREAS OF TERMINAL OR PALLIATIVE CARE

While maintenance of nutrition is the main aim of dysphagia treatment in a palliative care setting, other aspects also need consideration. If lesions in the upper GI tract cause full or near full obstruction of the lumen, the patient is at high risk of aspiration of saliva and in some cases gastric juices. Treatments that reopen the lumen will allow nutrition but also improve the chest of the patient and greatly reduce the risk of severe aspiration pneumonia. Quality of life (QOL) should also improve. The patient does not need to spit out saliva, which may not be seen as socially acceptable in public spaces. The ability to enjoy at least some oral nutrition should also positively influence QOL.

Furthermore, the ability to take enteral medication can be extremely useful. It avoids the need of an injection when fast-acting pain relief is required and allows the use of medications only available for enteral use.

PRACTICAL PROCEDURES AND TECHNIQUES

Nasogastric Tube Insertion

Nasogastric feeding tubes are fine-bore plastic tubes aimed to produce a safe feeding route for the short to medium term. They can be placed at the bedside, and patients rarely experience any discomfort during placement. Little training is required to learn the technique, making it widely available inside hospitals and hospices. The correct placement of the tube should be established via aspiration and pH-testing of gastric fluid (pH < 5.5) or demonstration of the tube tip below the diaphragm on chest x-rays if pH-testing fails (National Collaborating Centre for Acute Care 2006). NG tubes fall out relatively frequently but can be better secured with a nasal bridle. Occasionally, discomfort is caused by irritation to the throat. In cases of neuro-muscular dysphagia, a risk of regurgitation and aspiration of gastric contents into the lungs remains. Most obstructive upper GI tract pathology is not amenable to NG tube feeding.

Endoscopically Placed Feeding Tubes

Feeding tube placement via a flexible endoscope is normally performed in dedicated endoscopy units (Figures 16.2 and 16.3). In most cases, conscious sedation and antibiotic prophylaxis are used. The endoscope will be passed into the stomach. Via transillumination to the abdominal wall, a suitable site will be identified, and using aseptic technique, a local anaesthetic will be placed. A large-bore cannula gets placed through the abdominal wall into the stomach, and a thread will be fed into the stomach. This thread gets pulled to the mouth, and the feeding tube will be connected to it. By removing the thread back through the abdominal wall, tube placement will be achieved. These tubes can be used long term. The main risks involved in PEG placements are wound infections, perforation and leakage into the peritoneal cavity and bleeding. Complications occur in up to 15.4% of patients (Wollman et al. 1995). Large hiatal hernias, surgical scars in the upper abdomen and previous gastric surgery are relative contraindications. In some cases, an endoscopic placement of a jejunostomy can be feasible.

Radiologically Induced Gastrostomy

Radiological placement requires local anaesthesia but rarely conscious sedation. There is a reduced risk of cardiovascular or respiratory compromise compared to endoscopic placement. An NG tube

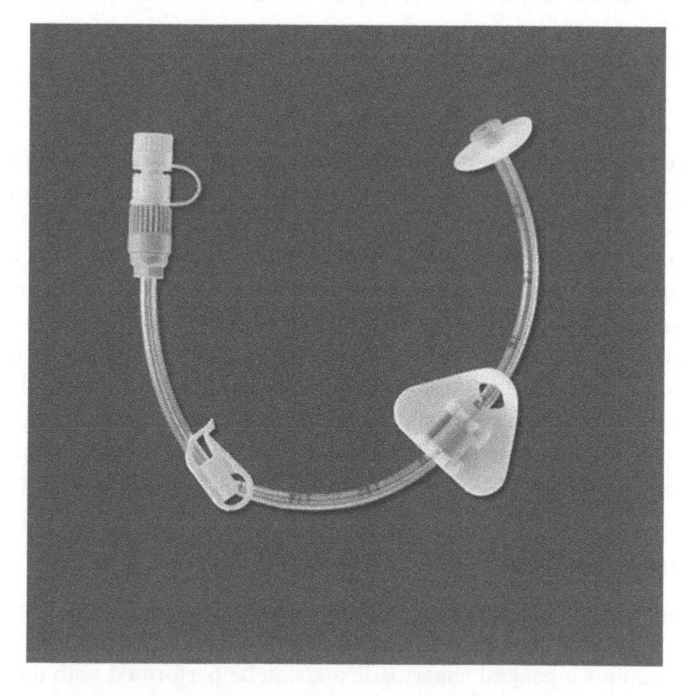

FIGURE 16.2 PEG set. Standard set used for PEG placement. (Reproduced with kind permission from Fresenius Kabi.)

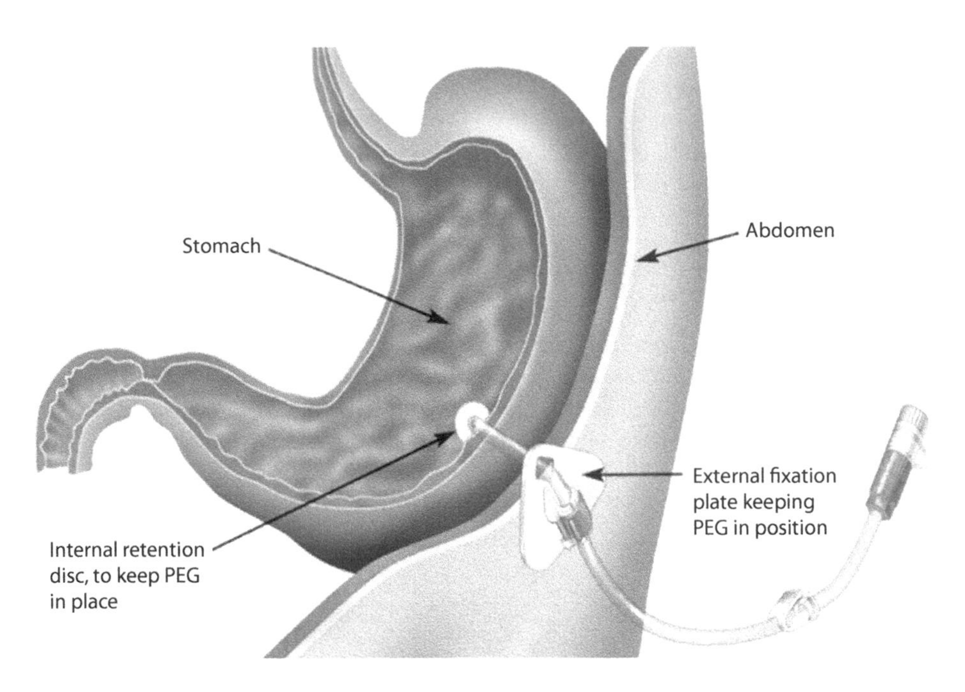

FIGURE 16.3 PEG set and placed in situ. A cut view demonstrating a PEG tube positioned in the stomach. (Reproduced with kind permission from Fresenius Kabi.)

will be used to inflate the stomach to allow radiological detection. Ultrasound can be used to avoid accidental hepatic punctures. The stomach will then be punctured through the abdominal wall, and dilators will be used to open up the puncture site. A tube will then be placed through the stomach wall. Risks involved are the same as for PEG placement, but the complication rate seems lower (Wollman et al. 1995).

Stents

Stents can be placed under radiological or combined endoscopic and radiological guidance. The procedure requires conscious sedation, as pain is experienced frequently during placement. A self-expanding metal stent (SEMS) consists of a tightly knit metal mesh that is rolled onto an introducer measuring 5–7 mm in diameter. Placement of the closed stent over the tumour is guided by x-ray and/or endoscopy. The stent is released, opening up to its full diameter of 16–23 mm, reopening the lumen at the obstruction site and allowing passage of food again. A risk of stent obstruction by food bolus remains, and patients should chew carefully and sometimes stick to a mash-consistency diet. Larger stent diameters seem to reduce the risk of food bolus obstruction (Verschuur et al. 2007). Short-term risks include perforation, heavy bleeding and significant pain, while stent migration and obstruction by tumour overgrowth are longer-term risks (Selinger et al. 2008). Patients experiencing significant acid reflux after oesophageal stent placement should be treated with oral proton pump inhibitors.

Surgically Placed Feeding Tubes

If endoscopic or radiological placement of a feeding tube fails or is impossible due to changes in anatomy, a surgically placed feeding jejunostomy can be used. Though it is a short procedure, placement usually requires a general anaesthetic and can be performed with a mini-laparotomy or using laparoscopy. Wound infection, perforation and leakage into the peritoneal cavity are the main risks.

Surgical Bypass Procedures

In cases of gastric outlet obstruction, a surgical bypass can establish an alternative route allowing food to proceed from the stomach to the proximal intestine. Under general anaesthetic, a proximal small bowel loop will be anastomosed to the stomach. This is a relatively invasive procedure and therefore has a considerable risk (mainly of the anaesthetic, failure of the anastomosis and wound infections) in palliative care patients.

EVIDENCE FOR DYSPHAGIA TREATMENT ACCORDING TO INDICATION

Neurological and Muscular Disorders

Stroke

Strokes caused by either infarction or haemorrhage of the brain can affect swallowing severely. Neurological improvement can often be seen in the first few weeks after a stroke. Alternative feeding routes like NG, PEG or RIG are commonly used to allow nutrition. In a large multi-centre randomized controlled trial (RCT), Dennis et al. (2005) compared early tube feeding versus avoidance of tube feeding for seven days after an acute stroke. A non-significant reduction of death was found in the early feeding group. This reduction, however, came at the expense of an excess of survivors with poor neurological outcome who would have otherwise died. Based on these findings, early tube feeding cannot be recommended. The trial also addressed the issue of NG versus PEG tube insertion in stroke. PEG feeding showed no benefit over NG feeding, and a small non-significant increase in death rate was found in the PEG group (Dennis et al. 2005). The most recent Cochrane review by Gomes et al. (2015) included 11 studies of 735 patients with dysphagia due to a variety of underlying illnesses. They found a significantly lower treatment failure rate of PEG compared with NG tube placement with similar complication rates. PEG tubes offer the advantage of a more secure placement. They do not cause irritation to the patient's throat, and they are the preferred longer-term option. In reality, most patients considered for PEG placement will undergo a period of NG feeding as a bridge to PEG placement.

Motor-Neuron Disease

When motor-neuron disease affects the bulbar region, dysphagia develops. This is of great concern, as dehydration and malnutrition further weaken muscles and thereby hasten the development of respiratory insufficiency and death (Langmore 1996). Poor appetite and the inability to self-feed may also contribute to weight loss. Whether PEG feeding leads to better nutrition, improved QOL and longer survival has not been tested in a RCT. Of seven case-control studies addressing the effect of PEG feeding on survival, four found no difference, while three reported a longer survival. Of the three, two studies with a stronger, prospective desig found a survival benefit (Mazzini et al. 1995; Chio et al. 2002), but this was not evident in the third (Murphy et al. 2008). A Cochrane review by Katzberg and Benatar (2011) confirmed that current data are insufficiently strong to make a routine recommendation. Only three of the seven studies report on nutritional status, but all show positive effects. QOL aspects have not been sufficiently well studied so far. In addition to the opportunity to improve nutrition, PEG placement may also allow for the administration of important enteral medication often required in the palliative care setting. Based on the current level of evidence, PEG feeding should at least be considered in cases of motor-neuron disease.

Dementia

Loss of interest in food and dysphagia occur late in the course of dementia. While over a third of U.S.-based nursing home residents with dementia were tube fed, this practice is not currently used in other parts of the world (Sampson et al. 2009). No RCT has been conducted to assess whether PEG feeding in advanced dementia influences survival, nutritional status or QOL. Based on six case control studies a Cochrane review (Sampson et al. 2009) concluded that there is "insufficient evidence for the effectiveness of enteral feeding for older people with advanced dementia on survival, QOL, nutrition and pressure ulcers, function and behavioural or psychiatric symptoms of dementia." Compared to other indications for PEG placement, dementia sufferers experience higher rates of hospitalisation, and higher 30-day and one-year mortality (Abu et al. 2017). These data also suggest that the risk-benefit profile of PEG insertion in dementia patients is not favourable. The British Society of Gastroenterology advises against the use of PEG in dementia (Westaby et al. 2010).

Other Neuro-Muscular Diseases

Dysphagia caused by other neuro-muscular disorders has not been subject to systematic studies. A case series on PEG placement for neurological indications has included patients suffering from brain tumours, Parkinson's disease and multiple sclerosis (Zalar et al. 2004). A nutritional improvement was seen in all cases, but this heterogenous cohort study without controls does not allow generalisation of this finding. Data remain scarce for these indications, but there is an increasing trend for PEG insertion (with jejunal extension) in Parkinson's disease to allow for direct duodenal delivery of medical treatment with Duodopa rather than for nutrition purposes (Zulli et al. 2016). Owing to the wide variation in prognosis and symptoms in these cases, clinicians should make individual assessments of possible risks and benefits before initiating PEG feeding.

Head and Neck Tumours

Mucositis and dysphagia caused by treatment for head and neck cancers often necessitate temporary or permanent tube feeding (Mekhail et al. 2001). While patients seem to prefer PEG over NG tubes, a retrospective series found that PEG tubes were associated with more dysphagia at three and six months and with a greater need for pharyngoesophageal dilatation of strictures (Mekhail et al. 2001). PEG tubes were required for significantly longer periods than NG tubes. There is a need to confirm these findings in a prospective setting, but a recent trial was terminated prematurely due to patients' reluctance to be randomised (Corry et al. 2008). Early preventative enteral feeding with PEG tubes does not lead to an increased longer-term dependency once cancer treatment is completed (Brown et al. 2017). Metastatic seeding to the PEG site is a major concern in head and neck cancers, which has been reported in up to 0.98% of cases (Ruz et al. 2005). This is generally attributed to the pull technique used in PEG placement, when the tube is pulled through the upper GI tract containing the tumour. The push technique used during RIG placement should avoid this risk, but a case of tumour spread to the RIG site has also been reported (Hawken et al. 2005). Complication rates following RIG placement are higher than those seen after PEG placement (Grant et al. 2009; McAllister et al. 2013). Given the problems associated with PEG use in head and neck cancers, the views of the patient are vital when deciding on the choice of tube feeding method.

Oesophageal and High Gastric Obstruction

In cases of malignant oesophageal and high gastric obstruction, treatment can be focussed on either re-establishing the natural upper GI tract or establishing an alternative feeding route (PEG or RIG). Generally the former is preferred, as this allows the pleasure of eating and eliminates the inability to swallow saliva. The lumen can be re-opened by reducing the tumour bulk (radiotherapy or endoscopic ablative therapy) or by placement of a SEMS. Advances in SEMS have led to a decrease in the use of endoscopic treatment modalities (laser therapy, bipolar cautery, argon plasma coagulation, injection of caustics) (Kozarek 2003). Most patients will be offered palliation by either SEMS or radiotherapy. External palliative radiotherapy is given in one session (Homs et al. 2004b). Endoluminal radiotherapy often requires three sessions (Bergquist et al. 2005). SEMS insertion can be achieved with 48-hour hospital stays in 50% of cases and produces an improvement in dysphagia in 94% of patients (Selinger et al. 2008).

Two RCTs have shown that SEMS leads to a quicker and better improvement in dysphagia at one month when compared to radiotherapy (Homs et al. 2004a,b; Bergquist et al. 2005). Improvement of dysphagia was, however, better sustained at three months in the external radiotherapy group (Homs et al. 2004a,b). The neo-adjuvant use of radiotherapy in addition to SEMS placement leads to a more prolonged improvement in dysphagia and longer survival than SEMS alone, as demonstrated in a RCT of 84 patients (Javed et al. 2012). External and endoluminal brachytherapy were both associated with better overall QOL when compared to SEMS (Homs et al. 2004a,b; Bergquist et al. 2005). Stent insertion is often associated with peri-procedural chest pain (over 10%). Serious acute complications occur in around 5%; longer-term issues including stent migration, food bolus obstruction and tumour overgrowth affect 25% of SEMS patients (Selinger et al. 2008). The main side effects of external radiotherapy are short-lived dysphagia and odynophagia, nausea, a dry mouth and mild skin burns.

A Cochrane review from Dai et al. (2014) concludes that SEMS is safe, effective and provides a quicker method of palliation then other modalities. While thermal and chemical ablation therapies were initially effective, both were associated with a high need for re-intervention (Dai et al. 2014). Given the average life expectancies of these patients, therapies without the need for re-intervention are preferable. Different models of SEMS are available, and anti-reflux stents (potentially less reflux events) or Niti-S stents (potentially longer durability) may have advantages over older models. The authors of the Cochrane review suggest that a combination of SEMS and brachytherapy may provide the best palliation due to a reduced need for re-intervention.

A cost-effectiveness study based on the findings of the endoluminal brachytherapy versus SEMS trial found that due to the higher initial costs of the three sessions of therapy total healthcare-related costs were twice as high as in the SEMS group (Wenger et al. 2005). Cost-effectiveness modelling using U.S. (Medicare)–based healthcare costs suggests that external radiotherapy might be more cost effective than SEMS (Da Silveira and Artifon 2008). The findings of these studies cannot be generalised, as healthcare-related costs and availability of treatments will differ from country to country. In the United Kingdom, SEMS is available in most District General Hospitals, while radiotherapy requires referral to a tertiary centre, leading to a delay in treatment and need for travel. Treatment options should therefore be discussed with the patient, and the patient's preference, local availability of treatment, prognosis, side effects and likelihood of cost effectiveness should be taken into consideration. While patients with a shorter life expectancy will benefit most from SEMS insertion, primary or adjuvant radiotherapy should be considered in individuals with an expected life expectancy of three months or longer.

Gastric Outlet Obstruction

Gastric outlet obstruction (GOO) is most commonly caused by neoplastic processes in the head of the pancreas. Lower gastric and pyloric obstruction due to benign or malignant ulceration and tumour growth as well as hepatobiliary tumours can also cause GOO, which leads to the accumulation of gastric content and subsequent vomiting (Table 16.4). A surgical jejunostomy feeding tube placed distal to the lesion guarantees adequate nutrition. Gastric fluid will, however, continue to cause nausea and vomiting. It is therefore preferable to either re-establish the natural orifice or to construct

TABLE 16.4
Key Facts: Gastric Outlet Obstruction (GOO)

GOO is caused by obstruction of the outflow tract of the stomach.
Common underlying conditions are cancers of the stomach, duodenum and the pancreas and occasionally benign ulceration of the stomach.
GOO leads to accumulation of fluid in the stomach and subsequent vomiting.
Subsequently, dehydration and malnutrition develops.

an alternative route of gastric emptying via a surgical bypass (in most cases a gastrojejunostomy [GOJJ] connecting proximal small bowel to the stomach).

Pancreatic tumours are common, and 15%–20% of patients will experience GOO due to locally advanced tumours (Jeurnink et al. 2007). It is rather controversial whether a prophylactic GOJJ is advisable. Hueser et al. (2009) found in their meta-analysis of two RCTs and one prospective non-randomised study that prophylactic GOJJ at the time of biliary bypass formation leads to significantly lower occurrences of GOO than an expectant strategy (19% versus 1.6%, $p < 0.001$). Morbidity and mortality for the combined procedure including a GOJJ were similar compared to those of a biliary bypass only operation. Given the advances in endoscopic management of biliary obstruction, this seems, however, a comparison with a non-standard treatment: A Cochrane review (Moss et al. 2006) concluded that SEMS insertion should be used as the standard treatment approach for malignant distal biliary tree obstruction. Morbidity and mortality of a GOJJ compare unfavourably to endoscopic biliary SEMS insertion. Given that at least 80% of patients with a pancreatic neoplasm will not experience GOO, major "prophylactic palliative" surgery on the gastric outflow tract should probably not be recommended over a watch-and-wait strategy.

When GOO occurs, treatment choices include SEMS and surgery. SEMS insertion is a relatively minor procedure with a high initial success rate, but around 25% experience late complications like stent occlusion, GI bleeding and intestinal perforation (Kim et al. 2009). Open or laparoscopic GOJJ has a lower risk of late complication and recurrence of obstructive symptoms but is associated with delayed gastric emptying (lasting eight days or longer) in the initial post-operative phase (Jeurnink et al. 2007). Two randomised studies comparing GOJJ and SEMS included only a total of 45 patients and did not allow firm conclusions. A systematic review largely based on non-comparative studies included 1,216 patients and found clinical success rates of 89% for SEMS and 72% for GOJJ ($p = 0.1$) (Jeurnink et al. 2007). Major early and late complications occurred with equal frequency for both interventions, but GOJJ required longer hospital stays (13 versus seven days). Survival was much longer in the GOJJ group. Jang et al. (2017) reached similar findings of shorter hospital stay for SEMS and better survival for GOJJ in a propensity matched, retrospective study of SEMS and GOJJ. This is likely due to selection bias as the majority of patients in this review and the study by Jang et al. (2017) were from non-randomised studies. QOL aspects and cost effectiveness have not been studied well. Patients with shorter life expectancy are likely to benefit more from SEMS, while GOJJ offers preferable longer-term results. An individualised approach taking into account the patient's performance status, co-morbidities and wishes should be applied.

Initial SEMS success rates do not differ for pancreatic or gastric malignancies, but stent collapse occurs significantly more often with gastric carcinomas, while other serious complications (GI bleeding, perforation) are more commonly seen in pancreatic carcinoma patients (Kim et al. 2009). Adjuvant therapy chemotherapy may improve the long-term results of SEMS.

ETHICAL ISSUES

Informed consent is the cornerstone of all medical treatments. It requires the capacity to retain and weigh up information as well as the ability to communicate a decision. In patients with severe neurological impairment like stroke or dementia, these requirements are often not met. Depending on local law, a legal guardian might consent for the patient or the treating physician might have to make a decision for the patient based on what is in the patient's best interest. Especially in palliative care situations, it can be very difficult to ascertain what constitutes this best interest.

In order to make consent informed, a patient needs to be given enough information to understand the procedure, its risks and possible outcomes. Anxiety and low mood occur commonly in palliative patients. Therefore, careful consideration is required when deciding how much and which information should be provided to the patient so as to not increase anxiety levels and mood problems. Furthermore, the patient might be under considerable stress and pressure to make a number of decisions on medical care while also preparing a last will.

Ethical issues might also arise around the availability of palliative care treatments. The best treatment might not be locally available or might not be funded.

Stents provide fast and effective relief from dysphagia caused by upper GI tract obstruction and have superior results in the short term compared to radiotherapy (oesophageal) and surgery (GOO). Results at three months, however, favour radiotherapy and surgery. To advise on treatment, the physician needs to be able to judge life expectancy well. This can be extremely difficult. Judging fitness for and risks of surgery is rather subjective, and ethical issues around this often arise in clinical practice.

Whether to advise prophylactic treatment to prevent dysphagia (radiotherapy for oesophageal cancer, for example) or an expectant strategy also need ethical considerations. A prophylactic approach might take up valuable high-quality time in a relatively asymptomatic patient, while an expectant approach only takes up time when a problem has occurred. Prophylactic treatment might also have negative psychological effects (increased feeling of being ill), while an expectant approach might lead to the patient experiencing a lot of symptoms before undergoing the intervention.

Difficult ethical issues often arise around the question of whether to start enteral feeding in patients with advanced or severe disease. While the evidence suggests that early tube feeding after severe strokes and tube feeding in advanced dementia should be avoided, relatives might push for such an intervention in the belief that the patient is suffering from hunger. Physicians face an ethical dilemma when trying not to upset relatives when conveying the treatment plan and acting in the patient's best interest at the same time.

KEY FACTS

- Dysphagia is a common problem in palliative situations
- Causes of dysphagia vary according to the pathophysiology of the underlying illness
- Treatment needs to be tailored to individual circumstances
- Alternative enteral feeding routes can be established by temporary or permanent approaches
- In some circumstances avoidance of a nutritional intervention is the preferred choice

SUMMARY POINTS

- Dysphagia in the palliative care setting can arise from neuro-muscular problems or obstruction of the upper GI tract.
- Treatment options include the creation of alternative feeding routes (NG, PEG and RIG), therapy to reopen the natural lumen of the GI tract (stents, endoluminal therapy and radiotherapy) and creation of alternative drainage of the stomach with surgery.
- The choice of treatment depends on the patient's overall state of health, fitness to undergo interventions and personal choice.
- PEG, NG and RIG provide a safe feeding route, but the appropriateness of the intervention depends on the underlying condition.
- Stents are a very effective way of treating obstructive dysphagia and have favourable results at one month, but they carry a high risk of long-term complications.
- Surgery or radiotherapy has better long-term results than stents but is not as effective in the short run.

LIST OF ABBREVIATIONS

GI Gastrointestinal
GOJJ Gastrojejunostomy
GOO Gastric Outflow Obstruction
NG Nasogastric Tube

PEG Percutaneous Endoscopic Gastrostomy
PEJ Percutaneous Endoscopic Jejunostomy
RCT Randomised Controlled Clinical Trial
RIG Radiologically Induced Gastrostomy
SEMS Self-Expanding Metal Stent
SPJ Surgically Placed Jejunostomy

REFERENCES

Abu RA, Khoury T, Cohen J, Chen S, Yaari S, Daher S, Benson AA, and Mizrahi M. PEG insertion in patients with dementia does not improve nutritional status and has worse outcomes as compared with PEG insertion for other indications. *Journal of Clinical Gastroenterology* 2017; 51(5): 417–420.

Bergquist H, Wenger U, and Johnsson E. Stent insertion or endoluminal brachytherapy as palliation of patients with advanced cancer of the esophagus and gastroesophageal junction. Results of a randomized, controlled clinical trial. *Disease of the Esophagus* 2005; 18: 131–139.

Brown T, Banks M, Hughes BGM, Lin C, Kenny LM, and Bauer JD. Impact of early prophylactic feeding on long term tube dependency outcomes in patients with head and neck cancer. *Oral Oncology* 2017; 72: 17–25.

Chio A, Mora G, Leone M, Mazzini L, and Cocito DL. Early symptom progression rate is related to ALS outcome: A prospective population based study. *Neurology* 2002; 59: 99–103.

Corry J, Poon W, and McPhee N. Randomized study of percutaneous gastrostomy versus nasogastirc tubes for enteral feeding in head and neck cancer patients treated with (chemo)radiation. *Journal of Medical Imaging Radiation Oncology* 2008; 52: 503–510.

Dai Y, Li C, Xie Y, Liu X, Zhang J, Zhou J, Pan X, and Yang S. Interventions for dysphagia in oesophageal cancer. *Cochrane Database Systematic Reviews* 2014; (10): CD005048.

Da Silveira EB and Artifon EL. Cost-effectiveness of palliation of unresectable esophageal cancer. *Digestive Disease and Science* 2008; 53: 3103–3111.

Dennis MS, Lewis SC, and Warlow C. Effect of timing and method of enteral tube feeding for dysphagic stroke patients (FOOD): A mulitcentre randomised controlled trial. *The Lancet* 2005; 365: 764–772.

Gomes CAR, Andriolo RB, Bennett C, Lustosa SAZ, Matos D, Waisberg DR, and Waisberg J. Percutaneous endoscopic gastrostomy versus nasogastric tube feeding for adults with swallowing disturbances. *Cochrane Database Systematic Reviews* 2015; 22(5): CD008096.

Grant DG, Bradley PT, and Pothier. Complications following gastrostomy tube insertion inpatients with head and neck cancer: A prospective multi-institution study, systematic review and meta-analysis. *Clinical Otolaryngology* 2009; 34: 103–112.

Hawken RM, Williams RW, and Bridger MW. Puncture site metastasis in a radiologically inserted gastrostomy tube: Case report and literature review. *Cardiovascular Interventional Radiology* 2005; 28: 377–380.

Homs MY, Essink-Bot ML and Borsboom GJ. Quality of life after palliative treatment for oesophageal carcinoma – A prospective comparison between stent placement and single dose brachytherapy. *European Journal of Cancer* 2004a; 40: 1862–1871.

Homs MY, Steyerberg EW, and Eijkenboom WM. Single dose brachytherapy versus metal stent placement for the palliation of dysphagia from oesophageal cancer: Multicentre randomised trial. *The Lancet* 2004b; 364: 1497–1504.

Hueser N, Michalski CW, and Schuster T. Systematic review and meta-analysis of prophylactic gastroenterostomy for unresectable pancreatic cancer. *British Journal of Surgery* 2009; 96: 711–719.

Jang SH, Lee H, Min BH, Kim SM, Kim HS, Carriere KC, Min YW, Lee JH, and Kim JJ. Palliative gastrojejunostomy versus endoscopic stent placement for gastric outlet obstruction in patients with unresectable gastric cancer: A propensity score-matched analysis. *Surgical Endoscopy* 2017; 31(10): 4217–4223.

Javed A, Pal S, Dash NR, Ahuja V, Mohanti BK, Vishnubhatla S, Sahni P, and Chattopadhyay TK. Palliative stenting with or without radiotherapy for inoperable esophageal carcinoma: A randomized trial. *Journal of Gastrointestinal Cancer* 2012; 43(1): 63–69.

Jeurnink SM, Van Eijck CHJ, and Steyerberg EW. Stent versus gastrojejunostomy for the palliation of gastric outlet obstruction: A systematic review. *BMC Gastroenterology* 2007; 7: 18.

Katzberg HD and Benatar M. Enteral tube feeding for amyotrophic lateral sclerosis/motor neuron disease. *Cochrane Database Systematic Reviews* 2011; 19(1): CD004030.

Kim JH, Song HY, and Shin JH. Metallic stent placement in the palliative treatment of malignant gastric outlet obstructions: Primary gastric carcinoma versus pancreatic carcinoma. *American Journal of Roentgenology* 2009; 193: 241–247.
Kozarek RA. Endoscopic palliation of esophageal malignancy. *Endoscopy* 2003; 35: S9–S13.
Langmore SE, Kasarskis, EJ, and Manca ML. Enteral tube feeding for amyotrophic lateral sclerosis/ motor neuron disease. *Cochrane Database of Systematic Reviews* 1996; 18(4): CD004030.
Mazzini L, Corra T, and Zaccala M. Percutaneous endoscopic gastrostomy and enteral nutrition in amyotrophic lateral sclerosis. *Journal of Neurology* 1995; 242: 695–698.
McAllister P, MacIver C, Wales C, McMahon J, Devine JC, McHattie G, and Makubate B. Gastrostomy insertion in head and neck cancer patients: A 3 year review of insertion method and complication rates. *British Journal of Oral and Maxillofacial Surgery* 2013; 51(8): 714–718.
Mekhail TM, Adelstein DJ, Rybicki LA, Larto MA, Saxton JP, and Lavertu P. Enteral nutrition during the treatment of head and neck carcinoma: Is a percutaneous endoscopic gastrostomy tube preferable to a nasogastric tube? *Cancer* 2001; 91(9): 1785–1790.
Moss AC, Morris E, and Mac Mathuna P. Palliative biliary stents for obstructing pancreatic carcinoma. *Cochrane Database of Systematic Reviews* 2006; 2: CD004200.
Murphy M, Quinn S, Young J, Parkin P, and Taylor B. Increasing incidence of ALS in Canterbury, New Zealand: A 22-year study. *Neurology* 2008; 71(23): 1889–1895.
National Collaborating Centre for Acute Care. February 2006. Nutrition support in adults. Oral nutrition support, enteral tube feeding and parenteral nutrition. National Collaborating Centre for Acute Care, London. Available from www.rcseng.ac.uk.
Ruz I, Mamel JJ, and Brady PG. Incidence of abdominal wall metastasis complicating PEG tube placement in untreated head and neck cancer. *Gastrointestinal Endoscopy* 2005; 62: 708–711.
Sampson EL, Candy B, and Jones L. Enteral tube feeding for older people with advanced dementia. *Cochrane Database of Systematic Reviews* 2009; 15(2): CD007209.
Selinger CP, Ellul P, and Smith PA. Oesophageal stent insertion for palliation of dysphagia in a UK District General Hospital: Experience from a case series of 137 patients. *QJM* 2008; 101: 545–548.
Verschuur EM, Steyerberg EW, and Kuipers EJ. Effect of stent size on complications and recurrent dysphagia in patients with esophageal or gastric cardia cancer. *Gastrointestinal Endoscopy* 2007; 65: 592–601.
Wenger U, Johnsson E, and Bergquist H. Health economic evaluation of stent or endoluminal brachytherapy as a palliative strategy in patients with incurable cancer of the oesophagus or gastro-oesophageal junction: Results of a randomized trial. *European Journal of Gastroenterology Hepatology* 2005; 17: 1369–1377.
Westaby D, Young A, O'Toole P, Smith G, and Sanders DS. The provision of a percutaneously placed enteral tube feeding service. *Gut* 2010; 59: 1592–1605.
Wollman B, D'Agostino HB, and Walus-Wigle JR. Radiologic, endoscopic, and surgical gastrostomy: An institutional evaluation and meta-analysis of the literature. *Radiology* 1995; 197: 699–704.
Zalar AE, Guedon C, and Piskorz EL. Percutaneous endoscopic gastrostomy in patients with neurological diseases. Results of a prospective multicenter and international study. *Acta Gastroenteroligica Latinoamericana* 2004; 34: 127–132.
Zulli C, Sica M, De Micco R, Del Prete A, Amato MR, Tessitore A, Ferraro F, and Esposito P. Continuous intra jejunal infusion of levodopa-carbidopa intestinal gel by jejunal extension tube placement through percutaneous endoscopic gastrostomy for patients with advanced Parkinson's disease: A preliminary study. *European Review for Medical and Pharmacological Sciences* 2016; 20(11): 2413–2417.

17 Olfaction in Palliative Care Patients

Sagit Shushan and Arkadi Yakirevitch

CONTENTS

INTRODUCTION

Although we are quick to relegate olfaction as an unimportant human sense, it is noteworthy that in our most important decisions we rely on our nose more than on our ears and eyes. For example, we decide what we will and will not eat using smell (Boesveldt et al. 2010), and our mate selection is similarly significantly influenced by smell (Havlicek and Roberts 2009). Adults with impaired sense of smell are profoundly aware of their loss, and helpless in dealing with it (Bojanowski et al. 2012).

Olfactory impairment increases a patient's perception of disability and negatively impacts quality of life. Moreover, self-reported "satisfaction with life" was inversely related to degree of subjective olfactory loss (Miwa et al. 2001). Similar association between chemosensory distortion and decreased quality of life was found among HIV-infected patients (Heald et al. 1998).

Though the majority of research on chemosensory perception in cancer patients has examined the direct effects of anticancer therapies such as radiation and chemotherapy, this symptom is frequently cited among patients with advanced cancer for whom curative therapies have been discontinued in favor of palliative care (Yakirevitch et al. 2006). Evaluation of self-perceived smell and taste functions using a questionnaire among patients receiving palliative care due to advanced cancer revealed that only 14% of them had no chemosensory complaints. The majority of patients reported some degree of chemosensory impairments, and even more specifically 8% of the patients rated their abnormal sense of smell as "severe" or "incapacitating" (Hutton et al. 2007).

Aside of a well-identifiable deteriorating impact on quality of life, one should not ignore the important role that smell and taste play in appetite, food choices, and nutrient intake. While the exact relation between smell and taste variations and malnutrition is still unclear, there are several factors that lead us to assume that those impairments may cause low caloric intake (Hutton et al. 2007) and in turn weight loss, wasting, cachexia and even mortality. Malnutrition frequently contributes to the cause of death in patients with cancer; as many as 20% of patients succumb to progressive nutritional deterioration rather than to the malignancy per se (Ottery 1997).

In this chapter we aim to describe the olfactory alterations that may occur along with palliative care, to overview diagnosis and assessment tools and to outline several treatment strategies.

PHYSIOLOGY OF OLFACTION

Olfaction is organized within a hierarchical network starting from peripheral transduction at the olfactory epithelium (OE) in the nose, onto early processing in the olfactory bulb, then continued processing in the olfactory cortex at the ventral junction of the temporal and frontal lobes, and finally projections to an extensive cortical network (Sela and Sobel 2010) (Figure 17.1).

The OE is spread along the olfactory cleft, and various portions of the nasal cavity, mainly the middle turbinate and septum. This epithelium is composed of several cell types, among them at the base is a thin layer of basal cells that divide and differentiate throughout life, regenerating the other cell types. Throughout the epithelium are supporting cells that are believed to play a maintenance role, although their exact function remains unclear. Scattered within the olfactory epithelium are

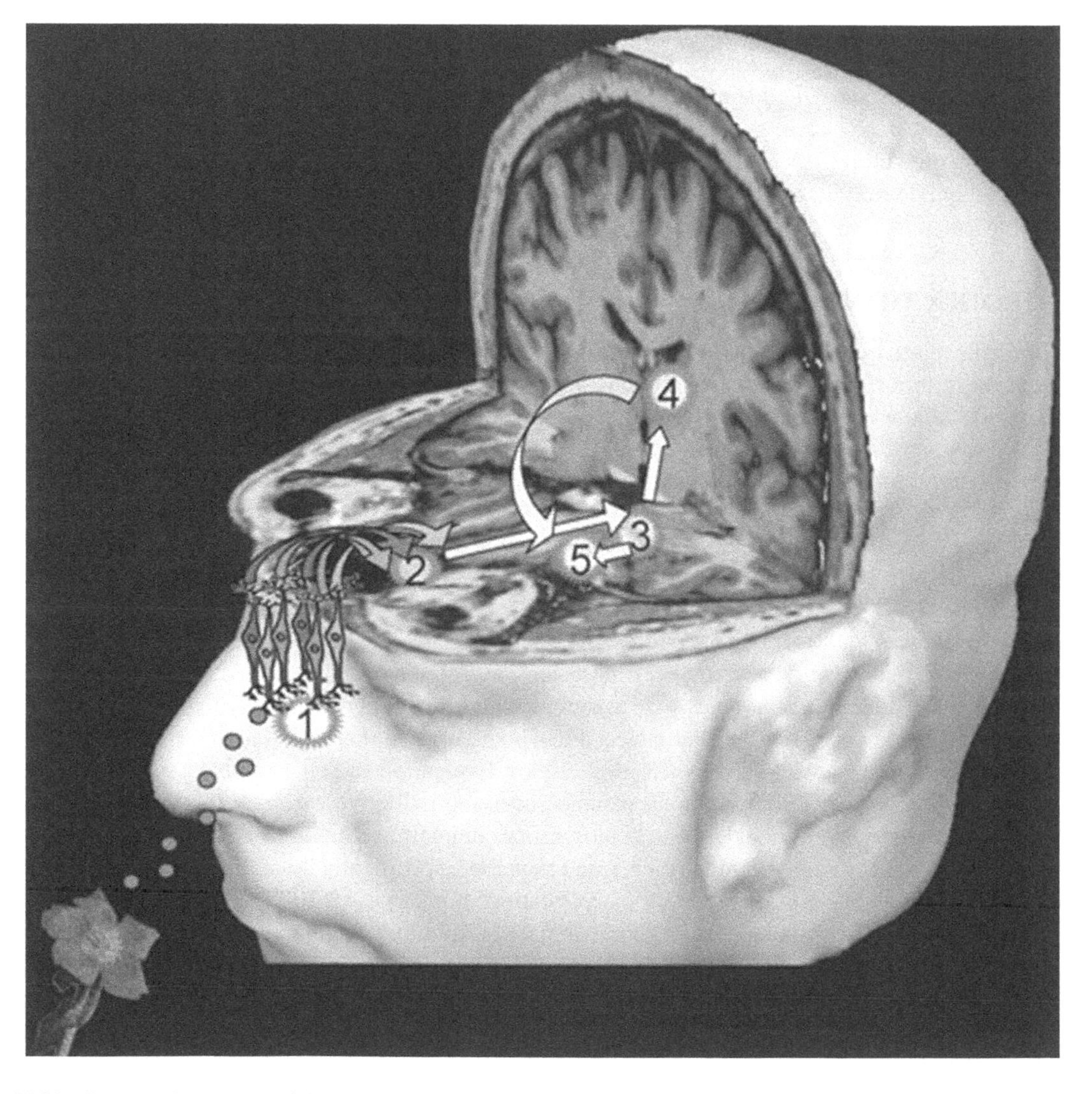

FIGURE 17.1 Schematic of the human olfactory system. Odorants are transduced at the olfactory epithelium (1). Different receptor types (three are illustrated, ~400 in humans) converge via the olfactory nerve onto common glomeruli at the olfactory bulb (2). From here information is conveyed via the lateral olfactory tract to primary olfactory cortex (3). From here, information is further relayed throughout the brain, most notably to insular (not shown) and orbitofrontal cortex (5) via a direct and indirect route through the thalamus (4). (Data from Sela, L. and N. Sobel. 2010. *Experimental Brain Research* 205 (1): 13–29.)

specialized glands known as Bowman's glands that secrete thin, watery mucus that protects the epithelial surface while providing a medium for odorant molecules to act. The majority of cells in this epithelium, however, are the olfactory receptor neurons (ORNs), with an average life span of 30 days and regeneration ability; however, the degree of regeneration depends on the severity of damage. Those neurons are the only neurons that transverse out of the skull to direct contact with the environment.

From each of these bipolar cells, a dendrite extends apically to the surface of the epithelium, giving rise to an olfactory knob. Long, non-motile cilia project from these knobs into the nasal cavity, creating a large surface area for odorant molecules to bind to and interact. Within the membranes of these cilia are the olfactory receptor proteins, a diverse family of G-protein-coupled receptors encoded by the largest gene family in the human genome. Odorant molecules dissolve within the nasal mucus, and then bind to one of these G-protein-coupled receptors. Activation of the G-protein leads to depolarization of the ciliary membrane.

Following transduction in the OE, neural signals progress along the bi-polar neurons, through the cribriform plate, to synapse with dendrites of mitral and tufted cells within the olfactory bulb. Axonal projections from those cells convey into the lateral olfactory tract, to terminate at primary olfactory cortex. Primary cortex is defined as the regions that receive direct projections from the olfactory bulb and includes the anterior olfactory nucleus, ventral tenia tecta, anterior hippocampus, olfactory tubercle, piriform cortex, amygdala, periamygdaloid cortex and entorhinal cortex. The secondary olfactory cortex is defined as regions that receive projections from primary olfactory cortex, either through direct projection or indirect via the thalamic nucleus. This higher-order cortex includes the orbito-frontal cortex, anterior insula, hypothalamus, mediodorsal thalamus and hippocampus. Finally, many of the regions of primary olfactory cortex send dense feedback projections to the olfactory bulb (Uchida et al. 2014). All of these act together to create the perception of smell. The anatomical projection to the hypothalamus emphasizes the importance of olfaction in eating and nutrition.

Olfaction is generally thought to be a "synthetic" sense: its individual components blend creating a holistic sensation different from any of the distinct, individual components.

Any interference with olfaction can also have an impact on taste, because up to 80% of the taste of a meal is related to how it smells (Wrobel and Leopold 2004); thus most experts suggest that olfactory and gustatory disorder should be assessed together.

These neural substrates of olfaction are likewise the neural substrates of olfactory loss. Damage to any one of these neural processing stations could in principle alter or prevent the sense of smell.

OLFACTORY DISORDERS

About 13.3 million adults in the United States suffer from olfactory dysfunction (Hoffman et al. 2016) that includes the following: (1) *anosmia*: inability to detect any odor stimuli; (2) *hyposmia*: decreased sensitivity to odor stimuli; (3) *dysosmia*: distorted odor perception that may be further subdivided to *parosmia* (distorted smell perception, e.g., when lemon smells like rotten fish) and *phantosmia* (perception of smell without odor stimuli as in smell hallucination) (Table 17.1).

TABLE 17.1
Odor-Related Abnormalities

Anosmia	Absence of odor perception
Hyposmia	Decreased sensitivity of odor perception
Dysosmia	Distorted odors perception
Parosmia	Altered odor perception in the presence of odor stimuli
Phantosmia	Odor perception without the presence of any odor

Smell loss was found to be correlated with age; above the age of 50 the prevalence of olfactory loss may be as high as 25% of the population, indicating that age is a major factor in olfactory disorder (Murphy et al. 2002).

As mentioned previously, olfactory disorders can stem from damage to any station along the olfactory path, for example, sinonasal polyposis that obstructs the nasal cavity, thus preventing odor molecules from reaching ORNs (Jafek et al. 1987). Post-viral infection may damage ORNs as well, occasionally and unfortunately in an irreversible manner. Histologic specimens taken from post-viral patients revealed an absence of ORNs or replacement by respiratory epithelium (Jafek et al. 2002). Any head or facial trauma, even minor, may cause acquired anosmia. It remains unclear whether the pathogenesis involves tearing of ORN axons alone, or includes olfactory bulb and cortex injury (Jafek et al. 2002). Finally, toxic chemical inhalation or various pharmacological treatments may also trigger altered olfactory ability (Gobba 2006).

Several medical conditions are associated with altered smell and taste, especially cancer, Alzheimer's and Parkinson's diseases (Table 17.2).

TABLE 17.2
Representative Medical Conditions That Affect the Senses of Taste or Smell

Nervous	Alzheimer's disease
	Bell's palsy
	Damage to chorda tympani
	Epilepsy
	Head trauma
	Korsakoff's syndrome
	Multiple sclerosis
	Parkinson's disease
	Tumors and lesions
Nutritional	Cancer
	Chronic renal failure
	Liver disease including cirrhosis
	Niacin (vitamin B3) deficiency
	Vitamin B12 deficiency
	Zinc deficiency
Endocrine	Adrenal cortical insufficiency
	Congenital adrenal hyperplasia
	Panhypopituitarism
	Cushing's syndrome
	Diabetes mellitus
	Hypothyroidism
	Kallman's syndrome
	Pseudohypoparathyroidism
	Turner's syndrome
Local	Allergic rhinitis, atopy, bronchial asthma
	Sinusitis and polyposis
	Xerostomic conditions including Sjögren's syndrome
Viral infections	Acute viral hepatitis
	Influenza-like infections

Source: Data from Schiffman, S.S. and B.G. Graham. 2000. *European Journal of Clinical Nutrition* 54 (Suppl 3): S54–63.

The exact prevalence of smell and taste disorders among palliative care patients is difficult to establish due to the heterogeneity of studies' participants, treatment modalities and vast variation in the subjective and objective assessment tools that had been used. Nevertheless, reviewing the literature revealed that smell and taste disorder prevalence among cancer patients receiving chemotherapy or radiation ranged between 16%–70% and 50%–70%, respectively (Spotten et al. 2017).

Taste and smell changes are found in untreated patients (Ovesen et al. 1991), as well as in patients treated with chemotherapy (Bernhardson et al. 2009), radiation (Hölscher et al. 2005; Álvarez-Camacho et al. 2017) and immunotherapy. It has been suggested that cancer and its treatment impair the ability to detect the presence of basic tastes, reduce the perceived intensity of suprathreshold concentrations of tastants and interfere with the ability to discriminate and identify tastes and smells. Furthermore, 50% or more of cancer patients may have impaired taste and smell functioning at some point during the course of their disease and treatment (Dewys and Walters 1975). There appears to be individual variability in the time course of recovery (if any) with the duration of losses ranging from several weeks to six months or longer (Ophir et al. 1988).

Possible mechanisms of altered smell in cancer include direct neurotoxic effects involving the OE, demyelination of nerve fibers, immunologic inflammatory reactions or even microvascular injuries. Altered neurotransmitters' levels could constitute an additional mechanism leading to chemosensory disorders.

Along with the direct effects of cancer therapies on the olfactory pathway, any obstruction of airflow by tumor in the nasal cavity or following surgical intervention can have an impact on smell. Surgery can profoundly alter this sense via a variety of mechanisms, such as resection of portions of the oral or nasal cavity (Biazevic et al. 2008) or craniotomy involving the frontal lobe. Laryngectomee patients have a severely reduced sense of smell mostly due to the inability to initiate the olfactory process by sniffing, which is a central component of the olfactory process (Mainland and Sobel 2006). Since laryngectomee patients breathe through their tracheostomy, nasal breathing and sniffing are impossible. The same applies for every tracheotomee individual. When weaning a patient from tube feeding, the obstructive effect of the nasogastric tube should not be overlooked, especially because it is usually placed through a wide side of the nose dominant also in smell perception. Oral complications of cancer such as infections (fungal, viral and bacterial), ulcers, drug-induced stomatitis and dry mouth may also play a role. Contrarily, one should avoid blaming automatically any antineoplastic therapy for chemosensory disorders (as, e.g., cisplatinum was not found to cause olfactory deterioration) (Yakirevitch et al. 2005) and should rule out other possible causes.

Cirrhosis of the liver may be accompanied by olfactory loss. According to the study of Temmel et al. olfactory function was compromised in 76% of cirrhosis patients (Temmel et al. 2005). A significant rate of olfactory loss (56%) was also found among patients with chronic renal failure (Frasnelli et al. 2002).

As the majority of palliative care patients are elderly individuals, aging has a greater role in chemosensory deterioration in this cohort. Most research suggests that the sense of smell is even more impaired by aging than the sense of taste. Olfactory losses occur at both threshold and suprathreshold levels (Lafreniere and Mann 2009).

Drugs in many major pharmacological categories (dopaminergic antagonists, gamma-aminobutyric acid [GABA]-ergic agonists, calcium channel blockers and some orally active local anaesthetic, antiarrhythmic drugs) can impair olfactory function (Henkin 1994) and do so more commonly than presently appreciated. Table 17.3 shows some medications that were reported to alter smell and/or taste. Impairment usually affects sensory function at a molecular level by drug inactivation of receptor function through inhibition of tastant/odorant receptor, causing two major perceptual modifications: decreased perception (i.e., hyposmia or anosmia) and/or perception distortion (i.e., dysosmia) (Table 17.1). Those modifications can impair appetite and food intake, trigger significant lifestyle changes and may even require discontinuation of drug administration. Some sleep-inducing agents are associated with taste and, in rare instances, smell disturbances as potential adverse effects. Zolpidem is listed in the *Physicians' Desk Reference* as producing "taste

TABLE 17.3
Medications That Reportedly Alter Smell and/or Taste[a]

Drug Class	Agent
Antianxiety agents	Alprazolam, buspirone, flurazepam
Antibacterials	Ampicillin, azithromycin, ciprofloxacin, clarithromycin, enoxacin, ethambutol, metronidazole, ofloxacin, sulfamethoxazole, ticarcillin, tetracycline
Antidepressants	Amitriptyline, clomipramine, desipramine, doxepin, imipramine, nortriptyline
Antiepileptic drugs	Carbamazepine, phenytoin, topiramate
Antifungals	Griseofulvin, terbinafine
Antihistamines and decongestants	Chlorphenamine, loratadine, pseudoephedrine
Antihypertensives and cardiac medications	Acetazolamide, amiodarone, amiloride, amiodarone, bepridil, betaxolol, captopril, diltiazem, enalapril, hydrochlorothiazide, losartan, nifedipine, nisoldipine, nitroglycerin, propafenone, propranolol, spironolactone, tocainide
Anti-inflammatory agents	Auranofin, beclomethasone, budesonide, colchicine, dexamethasone, flunisolide, fluticasone propionate, gold, penicillamine
Antimanic drugs	Lithium
Antimigraine agents	Dihydroergotamine mesylate, naratriptan, rizatriptan, sumatriptan
Antineoplastics	Carboplatin, cyclophosphamide, doxorubicin, fluorouracil, levamisole, methotrexate, tegafur, vincristine
Antiparkinsonian agents	Anticholinergics, levodopa
Antipsychotics	Clozapine, trifluoperazine
Antiviral agents	Acyclovir, amantadine, gancyclovir, interferon, pirodavir, oseltamivir, zaicitabine
Bronchodilators	Bitolterol, pirbuterol
Central nervous system stimulants	Amphetamine, dexamfetamine, methylphenidate
Hypnotics	Eszopiclone, zolpidem
Lipid-lowering agents	Atorvastatin, fluvastatin, lovastatin, pravastatin
Muscle relaxants	Baclofen, dantrolene
Pancreatic enzyme preparations	Pancrelipase
Smoking cessation aids	Nicotine
Thyroid drugs	Carbimazole, levothyroxine sodium and related compounds, propylthiouracil, thiamazole

Source: Data from Doty, R.L. et al. 2008. *Drug Safety* 31 (3): 199–215.
[a] Evidence for the involvement of many of these drugs in chemosensory disturbance comes from the *Physicians' Desk Reference*.

perversion" and, more infrequently, "parosmia" (*Physicians' Desk Reference* 2005). Eszopiclone, a nonbenzodiazepine pyrrolopyrazine derivative of the cyclopyrrolone class, is associated with complaints of "unpleasant taste" (Krystal et al. 2003).

Among hospice patients who were previous or current smokers the rate of olfactory impairment was found to be higher than among non-smokers (Yakirevitch et al. 2006).

Dysosmia is a distorted odor perception. It may or may not be accompanied by decreased olfactory thresholds, and is typically unpleasant and very bothering. It may be associated with odor stimuli (*parosmia*) or with no odor stimuli (*phantosmia*). Although the molecular mechanisms leading to phantosmia and the phenomenon localization (olfactory epithelium, olfactory bulb or higher cortical structures) are still unidentified, it may be hypothesized that a decreased number of olfactory bulb neurons is associated with generation of phantosmia (Leopold 2002). A possible mechanism could be the decreased number of olfactory bulb interneurons resulting in a decrease of lateral inhibition (Mori et al. 1999). In turn, this may allow olfactory activation to produce an irregular pattern that may result in a "phantosmic" sensation.

Specialists in endocrinology, nutrition support services, surgery and oncology are well aware that severe chemosensory dysfunction is a primary factor in the development of anorexia, malnutrition and wasting (Hutton et al. 2007).

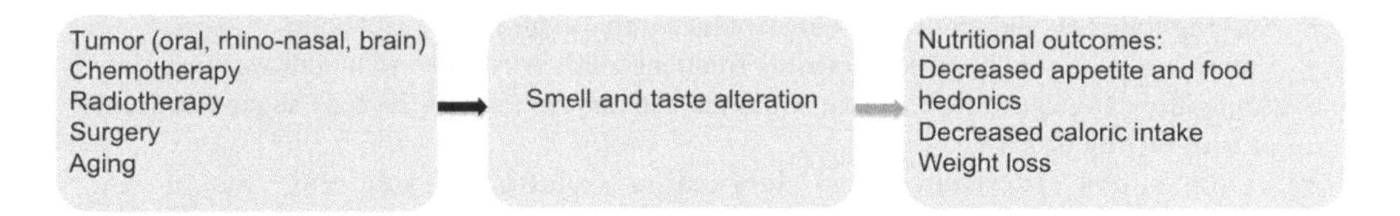

FIGURE 17.2 Cancer-related chemosensory disorder and nutritional outcomes. Smell and taste alterations may be linked to cancer itself, tumor involvement at the oral cavity, olfactory cleft or olfactory cortex, as well as cancer-related treatment modalities. The impact of smell and taste alterations on nutritional outcomes is yet to be established.

First, impaired taste and smell alter the sensations derived from food. Second, food aversions can be learned during the course of cancer when sensory properties of foods are associated with gastrointestinal distress (e.g., nausea) of therapy (Andrykowski and Otis 1990). Learned aversions and decreased food preferences can persist long after all symptoms of discomfort have subsided. The association between olfactory disorder and nutritional outcomes is illustrated in Figure 17.2.

PRACTICAL METHODS AND TREATMENT

The goals of intervention in palliative care are to support nutritional status, immune function, body composition, functional status and quality of life. Understanding and addressing the relationship between abnormal chemosensory function and dietary intake have the potential to improve food enjoyment and nutritional status in palliative care patients. This has been demonstrated in the elderly, for whom the sensory enhancement of foods resulted in increased dietary intake and improved functional status. Recognizing that taste and smell abnormalities are also related to food preference, dietary interventions catering to the unique preferences and chemosensory capacities of palliative care patients may result in improved dietary intake (Hutton et al. 2007).

The first step in improving nutritional state in patients who suffers from abnormal chemosensory function is comprehensive diagnosis of olfactory or gustatory disorder and treatment, if possible, of any underlying cause responsible for it.

Physical examination including nasal endoscopy may reveal any olfactory cleft obstruction that could be reversible. Oral or rhinosinonasal infection should be treated based on the pathogen involved.

Imaging studies may be helpful to rule out brain metastatic spreading, tumors involving the olfactory pathway or sinuses infections. In case no underlying cause was found following the above, any patient who suffers from smell disorder should undergo olfactory tests in order to evaluate olfactory perception.

Olfactory perception is typically measured using three cognitive tasks that vary by their cognitive demands. The first is the basic *detection* of odor, followed by *discrimination* which involves both detection and short-term memory. And finally, *identification* of odors which requires not only detection and discrimination of the stimuli, but also verbal semantic labeling that necessitates long-term memory and depends on previous associations. The majority of olfactory testing relies on this functional hierarchy. The most common commercial tests are the "sniffing sticks" (Hummel et al. 1997), and the University of Pennsylvania Smell Identification Test (UPSIT) (Doty et al. 1984). Olfactory tests may uncover whether anosmia, hyposmia or dysosmia are encountered.

Based on these findings, the following treatment strategies may be undertaken:

- Keeping on a balanced and nutritious diet with adequate calories
- Avoiding use of metallic silverware to reduce the risk of metallic taste
- Reducing the consumption of foods that taste metallic or bitter, such as red meat, coffee or tea, while increasing the consumption of high-protein, mildly flavored foods, such as chicken, fish, dairy products and eggs

- Serving foods at cold temperature may reduce unpleasant flavors and odors
- Practicing good oral hygiene, including frequent tooth brushing and mouth washing
- Applying sialogogues (agents that stimulate salivary secretion), such as sugar-free gums or sour-tasting drops
- Using saliva substitutes and lubricating solutions containing mucin and carboxymethylcellulose
- Adding seasonings and spices
- Utilizing flavors

Flavors are mixtures of odorous molecules that can be extracted or blended from natural products, or they can be synthesized based on chromatographic and mass spectrographic analysis of natural products. Flavors in some cases also contain nonvolatile compounds such as amino acid salts (e.g., monosodium glutamate) that induce taste stimulation. Flavors can be added to food prior to, during or after cooking. For example, simulated beef flavor can be added to beef or beef stock to provide a more intense "beef" sensation. Flavors are analogous to concentrated orange juice or extract of vanilla. Flavor enhancement differs from more traditional methods of increasing odor and taste sensations using spices, herbs and salt. Spices and herbs contribute different flavors to the food rather than intensify actual food flavors. Moreover, flavor-enhanced foods are preferred by frail and sick elderly and can improve immunity, quality of life and functional status (Schiffman and Warwick 1993).

Enteral artificial highly caloric nutritional supplements have an increasing role in palliative care. It has to be kept in mind that, like parenteral products, they may also suffer from inadequate formulation and chemosensory problems. They often have unpleasant tastes and can cause esophageal reflux, especially in bedridden patients.

When drug therapy is responsible for chemosensory disorders, its termination is commonly associated with termination of taste/smell dysfunction, but occasionally effects persist and require specific therapy to alleviate symptoms.

Hyposmia may be treated successfully with olfactory training that involves frequent short-term exposure to different odorants over a period of time (Sorokowska et al. 2017). The origin of the plasticity that governs this acquired ability may be attributed to increased ORNs' regenerative capacity (Youngentob and Kent 1995) or to encouraged neuroplasticity in central components of the olfactory system (Mainland et al. 2002).

As noted previously, tracheotomee patients are unable to smell naturally because they cannot produce adequate sniff. To overcome this problem, a laryngeal bypass with the use of plastic tubing was proposed (Göktas et al. 2008). Another method of olfactory rehabilitation described in the literature is "polite yawning." This maneuver involves inhaling through the nose with the teeth apart but the lips closed. Olfactory rehabilitation was reported as successful in up to 83% of laryngectomees with this maneuver (Risberg-Berlin et al. 2007).

Based on the observation that parosmia is a distorted sense of smell, it can be neutralized with voluntary decrease of olfaction. For example, Muller et al. opted for a simple nasal clip interrupting ortho- and retronasal olfaction, and thus, reducing parosmia, which promptly increased food intake (Müller et al. 2006).

KEY FACTS

- Human can smell 4,000–10,000 odors.
- Each odorant activates a unique set of olfactory receptors called "signature."
- One thousand genes participate in coding of the odor receptors.
- Olfactory receptor cells are true, bipolar neurons. These are the only neurons capable of regeneration, with an average life span of 30 days.
- The anatomical projection of the olfactory pathway to the hypothalamus emphasizes the importance of olfaction in eating and nutrition.

- Olfaction is thought to be a "synthetic" sense: its individual components blend creating a holistic sensation different from any of the distinct, individual components.
- Any interference with olfaction can have an impact on taste, because up to 80% of the taste of a meal is related to how it smells.

SUMMARY POINTS

- The brain mechanism that underlies olfaction exhibits unique features.
- Olfactory dysfunction is an important cause of nutrition problems in palliative care patients.
- Smell and taste disorder should be evaluated and assessed together.
- Smell disorder may result from normal aging, cancer, organic diseases of central neural system, medications, viral insult, obstruction or bypass of nasal airflow and environmental exposure.
- Subjective and objective olfactory tests should be employed for clinical purposes as well as for future studies.
- Apart from addressing its causes, olfactory dysfunction may be compensated with sensory enhancement of food and avoiding unpleasant odors.
- Olfactory training may be considered in hyposmic individuals.

LIST OF ABBREVIATIONS

OE Olfactory Epithelium
ORNs Olfactory Receptor Neurons

REFERENCES

Álvarez-Camacho, M., S. Gonella, S. Campbell, R. A. Scrimger, and W. V. Wismer. 2017. A Systematic Review of Smell Alterations after Radiotherapy for Head and Neck Cancer. *Cancer Treatment Reviews* 54: 110–21.

Andrykowski, M. A. and M. L. Otis. 1990. Development of Learned Food Aversions in Humans: Investigation in a "Natural Laboratory" of Cancer Chemotherapy. *Appetite* 14 (2): 145–58.

Bernhardson, B. M., C. Tishelman, and L. E. Rutqvist. 2009. Olfactory Changes among Patients Receiving Chemotherapy. *European Journal of Oncology Nursing* 13 (1): 9–15.

Biazevic, M. G., J. L. Antunes, J. Togni, F. P. De Andrade, M. B. De Carvalho, and V. Wünsch-Filho. 2008. Immediate Impact of Primary Surgery on Health-Related Quality of Life of Hospitalized Patients with Oral and Oropharyngeal Cancer. *Journal of Oral and Maxillofacial Surgery* 66 (7): 1345–50.

Boesveldt, S., J. Frasnelli, A. R. Gordon, and J. N. Lundström. 2010. The Fish Is Bad: Negative Food Odors Elicit Faster and More Accurate Reactions than Other Odors. *Biological Psychology* 84 (2): 313–17.

Bojanowski, V., T. Hummel, and I. Croy. 2012. Isolierte Congenitale Anosmie – Klinische Und Alltägliche Aspekte Eines Lebens Ohne Geruchssinn. *Laryngo-Rhino-Otologie* 92 (1): 30–33.

Dewys, W. D. and K. Walters. 1975. Abnormalities of Taste Sensation in Cancer Patients. *Cancer* 36 (5): 1888–96.

Doty, R. L., P. Shaman, C. P. Kimmelman, and M. S. Dann. 1984. University of Pennsylvania Smell Identification Test: A Rapid Quantitative Olfactory Function Test for the Clinic. *The Laryngoscope* 94 (2): 176–78.

Doty, R. L., M. Shah, and S. M. Bromley. 2008. Drug-induced taste disorders. *Drug Safety* 31 (3): 199–215.

Frasnelli, J. A., A. F. Temmel, C. Quint, R. Oberbauer, and T. Hummel. 2002. Olfactory Function in Chronic Renal Failure. *American Journal of Rhinology and Allergy* 16 (5): 275–79.

Gobba, F. 2006. Olfactory toxicity: long-term effects of occupational exposures. *International Archives of Occupational and Environmental Health* 79 (4): 322–31.

Göktas, Ö., F. Fleiner, C. Paschen, I. Lammert, and T. Schrom. 2008. Rehabilitation of the Olfactory Sense after Laryngectomy: Long-Term Use of the Larynx Bypass. *Ear, Nose and Throat Journal* 87 (9): 528–36.

Havlicek, J. and S. C. Roberts. 2009. MHC-Correlated Mate Choice in Humans: A Review. *Psychoneuroendocrinology* 34 (4): 497–512.

Heald, A. E., C. F. Pieper, and S. S. Schiffman. 1998 Taste and Smell Complaints in HIV infected Patients. *AIDS* 12: 1667–74.
Henkin, R. I. 1994. Drug-Induced Taste and Smell Disorders. *Drug Safety* 11 (5): 318–77.
Hoffman, H. J., S. Rawal, C. M. Li, and V. B. Duffy. 2016. New Chemosensory Component in the U.S. National Health and Nutrition Examination Survey (NHANES): First-Year Results for Measured Olfactory Dysfunction. *Reviews in Endocrine and Metabolic Disorders* 17 (2): 221–40.
Hölscher, T., A. Seibt, S. Appold, W. Dörr, T. Herrmann, K. B. Hüttenbrink, and T. Hummel. 2005. Effects of Radiotherapy on Olfactory Function. *Radiotherapy and Oncology* 77 (2): 157–63.
Hummel, T., B. Sekinger, S. R. Wolf, E. Pauli, and G. Kobal. 1997. Sniffin' Sticks': Olfactory Performance Assessed by the Combined Testing of Odor Identification, Odor Discrimination and Olfactory Threshold. *Chemical Senses* 22(1): 39–52.
Hutton, J. L., V. E. Baracos, and W. V. Wismer. 2007. Chemosensory Dysfunction Is a Primary Factor in the Evolution of Declining Nutritional Status and Quality of Life in Patients with Advanced Cancer. *Journal of Pain and Symptom Management* 33 (2): 156–65.
Jafek, B. W., D. T. Moran, P. M. Eller, J. C. Rowley, and T. B. Jafek. 1987. Steroid-Dependent Anosmia. *Archives of Otolaryngology–Head and Neck Surgery* 113 (5): 547–49.
Jafek, B. W., B. Murrow, R. Michaels, D. Restrepo, and M. Linschoten. 2002. Biopsies of Human Olfactory Epithelium. *Chemical Senses* 27 (7): 623–28.
Krystal, A. D., J. K. Walsh, E. Laska, J. Caron, D. A. Amato, T. C. Wessel, and T. Roth. 2003. Sustained Efficacy of Eszopiclone over 6 Months of Nightly Treatment: Results of a Randomized, Double-Blind, Placebo-Study in Adults with Chronic Insomnia. *Sleep* 26: 793–99.
Lafreniere, D. and N. Mann. 2009. Anosmia: Loss of Smell in the Elderly. *Otolaryngologic Clinics of North America* 42 (1): 123–31.
Leopold, D. 2002. Distortion of Olfactory Perception: Diagnosis and Treatment. *Chemical Senses* 27 (7): 611–15.
Mainland, J. D., E. A. Bremner, N. Young, and B. N. Johnson. 2002. Olfactory Plasticity: One Nostril Knows What the Other Learns. *Nature* 419: 802.
Mainland, J. D. and N. Sobel. 2006. The Sniff Is Part of the Olfactory Percept. *Chemical Senses* 31 (2): 181–96.
Miwa, T., M. Furukawa, T. Tsukatani, R. M. Costanzo, L. J. DiNardo, and E. R. Reiter. 2001. Impact of Olfactory Impairment on Quality of Life and Disability. *Archives of Otolaryngology–Head and Neck Surgery* 127 (5): 497–503.
Mori, K., H. Nagao, and Y. Yoshihara. 1999. The Olfactory Bulb: Coding and Processing of Odor Molecule Information. *Science* 286: 711–715.
Murphy, C., C. R. Schubert, K. J. Cruickshanks, B. E. K. Klein, R. Klein, and D. M. Nondahl. 2002. Prevalence of Olfactory Impairment in Older Adults. *JAMA* 288 (18): 2307.
Müller, A., B. N. Landis, U. Platzbecker, V. Holthoff, J. Frasnelli, and T. Hummel. 2006. Severe Chemotherapy-Induced Parosmia. *American Journal of Rhinology* 20 (4): 485–86.
Ophir, D., A. Guterman, and R. Gross-Isseroff. 1988. Changes in Smell Acuity Induced by Radiation Exposure of the Olfactory Mucosa. *Archives of Otolaryngology – Head and Neck Surgery* 114 (8): 853–55.
Ottery, F. D. 1997. Nutritional Oncology: A Proactive, Integrated Approach to the Cancer Patient. In *Nutrition Support: Theory and Therapeutic*. Edited by and G.L. Blackburn and S.A. Shikora. New York, NY: Chapman & Hall.
Ovesen, L., M. Smensen, J. Hannibal, and L. Allingstrup. 1991. Electrical Taste Detection Thresholds and Chemical Smell Detection Thresholds in Patients with Cancer. *Cancer* 68 (10): 2260–65.
Physicians' Desk Reference. 2005. 59th edition. PDR publishing, New Jersey.
Risberg-Berlin, B., R. Y. Möller, and C. Finizia. 2007. Effectiveness of Olfactory Rehabilitation with the Nasal Airflow-Inducing Maneuver after Total Laryngectomy: One-Year Follow-up Study. *Archives of Otolaryngology – Head and Neck Surgery* 133 (7): 650–54.
Schiffman, S.S. and B.G. Graham. 2000. Taste and smell perception affect appetite and immunity in the elderly. *European Journal of Clinical Nutrition* 54 (Suppl 3): S54–S63.
Schiffman, S. S. and Z. S. Warwick. 1993. Effect of Flavor Enhancement of Foods for the Elderly on Nutritional Status: Food Intake, Biochemical Indices, and Anthropometric Measures. *Physiology and Behavior* 53 (2): 395–402.
Sela L. and N. Sobel. 2010. Human Olfaction: A Constant State of Change-Blindness. *Experimental Brain Research* 205 (1): 13–29.
Sorokowska, A., E. Drechsler, M. Karwowski, and T. Hummel. 2017. Effects of Olfactory Training: A Meta-Analysis. *Rhinology* 55 (1): 17–26.

Spotten, L. E., C. A. Corish, C. M. Lorton, P. M. Ui Dhuibhir, N. C. O'Donoghue, B. O'Connor, and T. D. Walsh. 2017. Subjective and Objective Taste and Smell Changes in Cancer. *Annals of Oncology* 28 (5): 969–84.

Temmel, A. F., S. Pabinger, C. Quint, P. Munda, P. Ferenci, and T. Hummel. 2005. Dysfunction of the Liver Affects the Sense of Smell. *Wien Klin Wochenschr* 117: 1–2.

Uchida, N., C. Poo, and R. Haddad. 2014. Coding and Transformations in the Olfactory System. *Annual Review of Neuroscience* 37 (1): 363–85.

Wrobel, B. B. and D. Leopold. 2004. Clinical Assessment of Patients with Smell and Taste Disorders. *Otolaryngologic Clinics of North America* 37 (6): 1127–42.

Yakirevitch, A., M. Bercovici, L. Migirov, A. Adunsky, M. R. Pfeffer, J. Kronenberg, and Y. P. Talmi. 2006. Olfactory Function in Oncologic Hospice Patients. *Journal of Palliative Medicine* 9 (1): 57–60.

Yakirevitch, A., Y. P. Talmi, Y. Baram, R. Weitzen, and M. R. Pfeffer. 2005. Effects of Cisplatin on Olfactory Function in Cancer Patients. *British Journal of Cancer* 92 (9): 1611–13.

Youngentob, S. L. and P. F. Kent. 1995. Enhancement of Odorant-Induced Mucosal Activity Patterns in Rats Trained on an Odorant Identification Task. *Brain Research* 670 (1): 82–8.

18 Anorexia in Cancer
Appetite, Physiology and Beyond

Alessio Molfino, Maria Ida Amabile, and Alessandro Laviano

CONTENTS

APPETITE

Appetite is the physiological desire to eat. Anorexia is defined as the reduction or loss of the desire to eat and represents a complex syndrome with a lethal potentiality in several acute and chronic clinical conditions (Laviano et al. 2017b). While in experimental and clinical studies anorexia presents a protective behavior, which confers survival advantage following an acute stress and/or a trauma (Laviano et al. 2017a), the loss of appetite represents a negative prognostic factor when it develops in patients affected by chronic diseases, including cancer (Molfino et al. 2010). Anorexia impacts on a patient's outcome by contributing to weight loss, lean body mass catabolism and adipose tissue wasting (Molfino et al. 2010) and negatively influencing morbidity, mortality and patient's quality of life.

Cancer patients are at high risk of protein-energy malnutrition due to several symptoms (Barajas Galindo et al. 2017). Alterations in appetite are common among different types of cancer and include early satiety, nausea, vomiting and smell and taste alterations (Molfino et al. 2010; Barajas Galindo et al. 2017).

Weight loss and anorexia are key components of cachexia (Fearon et al. 2011), and novel evidence from experimental studies and clinical trials highlights the importance of characterizing the complexity of the disorders of appetite in cancer patients to identify more effective preventative strategies and therapeutic options (Laviano et al. 2017b).

Although the pathogenesis of cancer anorexia has been largely investigated in animal models, in cancer patients, the use of invasive techniques to study *in vivo* the function of central appetite-regulating areas, including the hypothalamus, is limited by technical difficulties and ethical considerations.

Often patients experience anorexia as a constant feeling of "wanting to eat but having no desire to eat." In some cases, loss of appetite is associated with the experience of feeling full quickly after eating a small amount of food or feeling "disgust" (food aversion) when eating specific meals (Hopkinson and Corner 2006).

In addition, there are other physical factors contributing to patients losing appetite for food, including fatigue, mouth ulcers, pain, nausea, difficulty with swallowing and gastrointestinal disturbance. Also, many of these symptoms may be attributable to treatment side effects (Cooper et al. 2015).

Moreover, appetite modifications during cancer are often associated with increased inflammatory response. Elevated inflammatory markers may be determined by the presence of cancer itself or by the effects of chemo-/radiotherapies.

PATHOPHYSIOLOGY OF ANOREXIA

There are multiple mechanisms beyond anorexia in cancer. The pathophysiology of cancer anorexia is complex and involves different domains influencing eating behavior. Limiting the assessment of cancer anorexia to questions investigating changes in appetite may limit the correct identification of the targets to address. During cancer, appetite is suppressed by the functional disruption of the neuronal pathways regulating physiological eating behavior (Nicolini et al. 2013).

Causes can be categorized as being due to peripheral or central mechanisms (Cooper et al. 2015; Barajas Galindo et al. 2017).

Peripherally, these can be due to (1) substances released from or by the tumor, that is, pro-inflammatory cytokines, lactate and peptides that modify food intake; (2) increased plasma tryptophan levels leading to increased central serotonin; (3) alterations of release of peripheral hormones that alter feeding, that is, ghrelin; (4) tumors causing dysphagia or altering gut function; or (5) tumors altering nutrients, that is, zinc deficiency. Moreover, as a peripheral mechanism, chemotherapy can alter taste perception and causes nausea, vomiting, mucositis and abdominal pain, leading to the loss of appetite (Cooper et al. 2015).

Central causes of anorexia include depression and pain. Within the central nervous system, tumors create a variety of alterations in neurotransmitters, neuropeptides and prostaglandins that modulate eating behavior (Cooper et al. 2015), and alterations in serotonin and corticotrophin-releasing factor (Fearon et al. 2011; Wallengren et al. 2013).

Under physiological conditions, the hypothalamus plays a relevant role in the control of appetite and food intake and in the regulation of energy expenditure (Molfino et al. 2010). It receives peripheral drives and transduces them into neuronal activities (Laviano et al. 2008). Within the arcuate nucleus, a relevant hypothalamic area for the regulation of energy expenditure, two different neuronal cells are involved in energy balance regulation. The first population of neurons synthesizes proopiomelanocortin (POMC), a polypeptide precursor molecule of smaller active peptides, the melanocortins, which exert anorexigenic effects (Abdel-Malek 2001; Cone 2005). The second subset of neurons expresses neuropeptide Y (NPY) and agouti-related protein (AgRP). Both AgRP and NPY highly stimulate appetite. Several hormones, such as insulin, ghrelin and leptin, reach NPY/AgRP and POMC neurons from the periphery, increasing or downregulating food intake (Laviano et al. 2008; Molfino et al. 2010). The melanocortin system plays a crucial role in the homeostasis of energy metabolism, starting with activation of POMC neurons, in specific conditions, and releasing melanocortins from POMC axon terminals leading to suppressed food intake and increased energy expenditure. Simultaneously, the activity of the arcuate AgRP/NPY system is suppressed (Laviano et al. 2008). Anorexia is related, at least in part, to dysfunction of the melanocortin system, consisting of hyperactivity of POMC neurons and decreased activity of NPY/AgRP neurons, leading to hypothalamic resistance to peripheral inputs signaling energy depletion (Laviano et al. 2008).

Anorexia in cancer and chronic diseases is associated with a derangement of physiological homeostatic feedback. In fact, when it is present, leptin levels are reduced, whereas ghrelin concentrations are elevated or normal, and consistent data show that selective melanocortin receptor antagonism modulates food intake and reduces wasting in experimental models of chronic diseases (Molfino et al. 2010).

Pathogenic mechanisms of anorexia in chronic diseases are related to the onset of neuroinflammation, which impairs the neurochemical control of energy homeostasis. Neuroinflammation mediates the progressive insensitivity of the hypothalamic neurons to the signals arising from peripheral tissues (Laviano et al. 2003). Thus, anorexigenic signals prevail on peripheral orexigenic mediators promoting the progressive depletion of energy stores and the catabolism of lean body mass and fat tissues, which lead to the clinical features of cachexia (Molfino et al. 2010).

Proinflammatory cytokines, such as interleukin (IL)-1, IL-6 and tumor necrosis factor-α (TNFα) from the periphery play a role in the pathogenesis of anorexia by specific mechanisms that act on the central nervous system (Molfino et al. 2010). Particularly, cytokines may induce the hypothalamic expression of the anorexigenic neurotransmitter serotonin.

Serotonin is a neurotransmitter that determines several behavioral and physiological processes, including energy balance, and plays a role in mediating satiety through its effects in the hypothalamus (Tecot 2007). Moreover, food intake reduction seems to be mediated by the activation of the POMC neurons, whose increased rate appears to be facilitated by serotonin (Tecot 2007).

Moreover, IL-1, which is produced by lymphocytes and macrophages, is the most potent anorexic cytokine, reducing the size, duration and frequency of meals but not the desire to eat (Laviano et al. 1996). Cytokines are a group of peptide hormones that generally act in a synergistic or antagonist cascade system to produce their effects stimulating immunoreactive nitric oxide synthase in the hypothalamus, suggesting a mechanism by which they alter central neuropeptides mediating the dysfunction of the melanocortin system (Gadek-Michalska et al. 2012); IL-1 can act directly crossing the blood-brain barrier or by activating ascending fibers of the vagal nerve to release IL-1 in the central nervous system. Peripheral infusion of IL-1 induces anorexia and raises brain tryptophan levels, thereby stimulating increased serotonin synthesis (Sato et al. 2003). Similarly, TNFα reduces food intake either peripherally or centrally (Torelli et al. 1999). Serotonin appears to mediate also the TNFα inhibitory effect on food intake (Langhans and Hrupka 1999).

On the contrary, older studies showed that IL-6, another inflammatory cytokine, does not play a role in cancer anorexia, not acting in reducing appetite or food intake (Strassmann et al. 1992). However, a more recent experimental study explored the connections between peripheral inflammation, anorexia and hypothalamic serotonin metabolism and signaling pathways and investigated the response of two hypothalamic neuronal cell lines to TNFα and IL-6 (Dwarkasing et al. 2016). Mice were injected with TNFα and IL-6 and showed decreased food intake, in association with altered expression of inflammation-related genes in the hypothalamus. In addition, hypothalamic serotonin turnover showed to be elevated (Dwarkasing et al. 2016). The results underline that peripheral inflammation reaches the hypothalamus where it affects hypothalamic serotoninergic metabolism associated with decreased food intake.

A number of studies have found that lactate is a potent anorexic agent (Barajas Galindo et al. 2017). Malignant tumors often have an increase in glycolysis associated with an increase in lactic dehydrogenase activity and lactate production, and lactate infusion decreased food intake in humans (Schultes et al. 2012).

Rossi Fanelli et al. found that plasma free tryptophan, the amino acid precursor of serotonin, was elevated in cancer patients with anorexia and that the ratio between free tryptophan/competing neutral amino acid was elevated in cancer patients with anorexia and early satiety compared with non-anorexic cancer patients and with controls (Rossi Fanelli et al. 1986). Another study showed that the surgical excision of tumors in cancer patients reduced the plasma tryptophan levels and anorexia (Cangiano et al. 1994). Tryptophan elevation, beyond its role as precursor of serotonin, may play a role in cancer-induced anorexia (Schultes et al. 2012).

All of these substances produced and released in periphery may also interact with the autonomic nervous system by informing the hypothalamic neurons on the metabolic and inflammatory status of peripheral tissues, and by transmitting central signals, which should be considered as the feedback response to this information (Laviano et al. 2008). The inflammation-induced modulation of the sympathetic nervous system may affect brain tryptophan concentrations, which are frequently involved in mediating anorexia-related symptoms. Also, central melanocortin agonists stimulate adipose tissue lipolysis and brown adipose tissue thermogenesis through the sympathetic nervous system (Brito et al. 2007). Indeed, therapies aimed at interfering with the activity of the vagus nerve may improve the metabolism of peripheral tissues, including reduced lipolysis and preserved basal metabolic rate (Lainscak et al. 2006).

As an example, in humans the administration of ghrelin improves anorexia, increases lean body mass and reduces sympathetic nerve activity (Nagaya et al. 2004, 2005; Molfino et al. 2010).

The characterization of the clinical and molecular pathophysiology of cancer anorexia may enhance the efficacy of preventive and therapeutic strategies.

Also, imaging techniques have been applied to the functional study of the neural correlates of cancer anorexia (Laviano et al. 2017a,b; Molfino et al. 2017). We recorded in anorexic and non-anorexic lung cancer patients and in healthy controls hypothalamic activation by functional magnetic resonance imaging (fMRI), before, immediately after the administration of an oral nutritional supplement and then after 15 minutes (Molfino et al. 2017). The grey of the hypothalamus and blood oxygen level dependent (BOLD) intensity were calculated and normalized for basal conditions. At all time points, anorexic patients showed lower hypothalamic activity compared with non-anorexic cancer patients and responded differently to oral challenges (Molfino et al. 2017). This supports the hypothesis that a central control of appetite dysregulation during cancer anorexia exists, before and after oral intake.

It is possible that the reduced interest in food, observed in cancer patients, may be secondary to impaired activation of hypothalamic feeding centers by visual cues (Laviano et al. 2017b). In this light, Sánchez-Lara et al. (2013) studied treatment-naïve anorexic and non-anorexic lung cancer patients. Data from fMRI based on BOLD signals were analyzed while the patients perceived pleasant and unpleasant food pictures. The non-anorexic patients demonstrated BOLD activation, comprising frontal brain regions in the premotor and the prefrontal cortices, only while watching unpleasant stimuli. The anorexic patients demonstrated no activation while watching the pleasant and unpleasant food pictures (Sánchez-Lara et al. 2013). This evidence highlights that anorexic cancer patients present a loss of activation in the brain regions associated with food stimuli processing. These results are consistent with experiences in the clinical environment, as patients describe themselves as not experiencing sensations of hunger or having appetite.

In cancer patients, changes in taste and smell occur frequently, either before starting anticancer therapies or as a side effect of chemo- and radiotherapy (Laviano et al. 2017b). They disrupt eating behavior by reducing global food intake and/or restricting intake only to specific foods, that is, meat aversion, determining impaired nutritional status. However, as a limit in clinical studies, there is not a gold standard assessment tool for taste and smell changes (Laviano et al. 2017b).

"NUMBERS" OF ANOREXIA

The prevalence of anorexia during chronic diseases is strongly related to the severity of the underlying disease.

Barajas Galindo et al. (2017) studied cancer patients to determine the prevalence of different appetite disorders and their influence on dietary intake, nutritional status and quality of life. Among 128 cancer patients, 61.7% presented changes in appetite, more common in women and with the presence of cachexia. Nevertheless, no significant effects were documented on energy or macronutrient intake among different appetite alterations.

A clinical study (Arezzo di Trifiletti et al. 2013), enrolling consecutive patients admitted to an internal medicine ward, utilized four appetite tools to assess the prevalence of anorexia. It significantly varied according to the diagnostic tool used. Except for visual analogue scale (VAS), all the tested tools identified patients with impaired nutritional and functional variables. This study further supports the concept that in clinical practice, disorders of appetite reflect different underlying mechanisms whose impacts on clinical outcome measures may differ.

Recently, Muscaritoli et al. (2017) conducted a prospective, observational study to investigate the prevalence of malnutrition in cancer patients at their first medical oncology visit. Appetite loss was evaluated with a two-step questionnaire, first to determine the presence of appetite loss using a modified version of the Functional Assessment of Anorexia-Cachexia Therapy (FAACT) questionnaire, and next to quantify it on the VAS of appetite. Based on FAACT scores, poor appetite was present in 41% of patients, with mean scores varying by tumor type and stage of disease.

According to FAACT score, patients with high gastrointestinal tract cancer resulted already anorexic in the non-metastatic phase. By contrast, all metastatic patients were anorexic based on the FAACT questionnaire. By VAS scoring, 44.5% of patients perceived appetite impairment. All patients in metastatic stage were anorexic based on the VAS.

In the last years, several reviews have documented existing evidence on cancer anorexia from perspectives of healthcare professionals and, also, beyond the biomedical perspective, with a specific focus on the psychosocial impact of anorexia and on quality of life (Muscaritoli et al. 2016; Wheelwright et al. 2016). The results revealed the multidimensional nature of cachexia, loss of appetite and weight loss experienced by patients and caregivers, which was not recognized and adequately managed by healthcare professionals. It underscores the need for increased awareness among physicians on this condition and its management (Muscaritoli et al. 2016; Wheelwright et al. 2016).

In conclusion, appetite disorders are highly prevalent among cancer patients at risk of malnutrition and have a definitive impact on nutritional status and quality of life. The coexistence of anorexia and early satiety represents the poorest condition. Most patients believe "not eating is dying," which is a symbol of progressive weakness and death. The correct identification of each kind of appetite alteration could allow a tailored treatment.

APPLICATIONS TO OTHER AREAS OF TERMINAL OR PALLIATIVE CARE

Appetite and weight loss occur frequently in cancer, and it is important to identify and correct any underlying issues for better management to improve patients' quality of life. Several studies, explored in this chapter, recognized different etiology due to peripheral or central mechanisms beyond anorexia in cancer.

Due to the potential implications of these mechanisms on treatment, further research and knowledge translation of symptom cluster research have been increasingly advocated for palliative care.

PRACTICAL METHODS

Tumor growth is associated with several neurochemical and metabolic modifications, which can lead to the onset of the loss of appetite, anorexia, severely impacting on the course of the underlying disease and on patient quality of life. However, the clinical relevance of anorexia is frequently underestimated, and treatments are often initiated during the advanced stages of the disease. The optimal therapeutic strategy for anorexic cancer patients should include changes in dietary habits, achieved via nutritional counseling, as well as a pharmacologic approach, aimed at interfering with peripheral or central mechanisms underlying anorexia. The possibility to improve the understanding of the influence that the tumor has on the host's metabolism may result in a greater awareness of its relevance among healthcare professionals involved in clinical management of cancer patients and in a better preservation of a better nutritional and metabolic status.

ETHICAL ISSUES

There are currently no ethical issues to be noted. Research on cancer anorexia focuses on exploring the extent and strength of symptoms and how they may negatively affect patients' quality of life and cancer treatment.

KEY FACTS: CANCER ANOREXIA

- Anorexia is a complex condition that may be often present among cancer patients.
- Anorexia represents a negative prognostic factor influencing weight loss, lean body mass catabolism and adipose tissue wasting.
- Anorexia has a definitive impact on patient's outcome by contributing to nutritional status and quality of life.

- It has been documented that anorexia, weight loss and malnutrition are common at cancer patients' first visit to a medical oncology center.
- There is an increasing need for awareness among physicians of anorexia and its management in cancer patients.

SUMMARY POINTS

- This chapter focuses on cancer anorexia which consists of reduction or loss of the desire to eat.
- Multiple causes are beyond anorexia in cancer, categorized in peripheral or central mechanisms.
- Pathogenic mechanisms of cancer anorexia are related to the onset of neuroinflammation.
- Changes in taste and smell, mucositis, nausea and vomiting occur frequently in cancer, contributing to loss of appetite and difficulties in eating.
- The prevalence of anorexia in cancer is strongly related to the severity of the underlying disease.

LIST OF ABBREVIATIONS

AgRP Agouti-Related Protein
BOLD Blood Oxygen Level Dependent
FAACT Functional Assessment of Anorexia-Cachexia Therapy
fMRI Functional MRI
IL Interleukin
NPY Neuropeptide Y
POMC Proopiomelanocortin
TNF Tumor Necrosis Factor
VAS Visual Analogue Scale

REFERENCES

Abdel-Malek, Z. A. 2001. Melanocortin receptors: Their functions and regulation by physiological agonists and antagonists. *Cellular and Molecular Life Sciences* 58:434–41.

Arezzo di Trifiletti, A., P. Misino, P. Giannantoni, B. Giannantoni, A. Cascino, L. Fazi, F. Rossi Fanelli and A. Laviano. 2013. Comparison of the performance of four different tools in diagnosing disease-associated anorexia and their relationship with nutritional, functional and clinical outcome measures in hospitalized patients. *Clinical Nutrition* 32:527–32.

Barajas Galindo, D. E. et al. 2017. Appetite disorders in cancer patients: Impact on nutritional status and quality of life. *Appetite* 114:23–7.

Brito, M. N. et al. 2007. Differential activation of the sympathetic innervation of adipose tissues by melanocortin receptor stimulation. *Endocrinology* 148:5339–47.

Cangiano, C., N. A. Brito, D. J. Baro, C. K. Song and T. J. Bartness. 1994. Cytokines, tryptophan and anorexia in cancer patients before and after surgical tumor ablation. *Anticancer Research* 14:1451–6.

Cone, R. D. 2005. Anatomy and regulation of the central melanocortin system. *Nature Neuroscience* 8:571–8.

Cooper, C., S. T. Burden, H. Cheng and Molassiotis A. 2015. Understanding and managing cancer-related weight loss and anorexia: Insights from a systematic review of qualitative research. *Journal of Cachexia Sarcopenia Muscle* 6:99–111.

Dwarkasing, J. T., R. F. Witkamp, M. V. Boekschoten, M. C. Ter Laak, M. S. Heins and K. van Norren. 2016. Increased hypothalamic serotonin turnover in inflammation-induced anorexia. *BMC Neuroscience* 17:26.

Fearon, K. et al. 2011. Definition and classification of cancer cachexia: An international consensus. *Lancet Oncology* 12:489–95.

Gadek-Michalska, A., J. Tadeusz, P. Rachwalska, J. Spyrka and J. Bugajski. 2012. Brain nitric oxide synthases in the interleukin-1β-induced activation of hypothalamic-pituitary-adrenal axis. *Pharmacological Reports* 64:1455–65.

Hopkinson, J. and J. Corner. 2006. Helping patients with advanced cancer live with concerns about eating: A challenge for palliative care professionals. *Journal of Pain and Symptom Management* 31:293–305.
Lainscak, M., I. Keber and S. D. Anker. 2006. Body composition changes in patients with systolic heart failure treated with beta-blockers: A pilot study. *International Journal of Cardiology* 106:319–22.
Langhans, W. and B. Hrupka. 1999. Interleukins and tumor necrosis factor as inhibitors of food intake. *Neuropeptides* 33:415–24.
Laviano, A., L. Di Lazzaro and M. I. T. D. Correia. 2017a. To feed or not to feed in ICU: Evidence based medicine versus physiology-based medicine. *Nutrition* 38:6–7.
Laviano, A., A. Inui, D. L. Marks, M. M. Meguid, C. Pichard, F. Rossi Fanelli and M. Seelaender. 2008. Neural control of the anorexia–cachexia syndrome. *American Journal of Physiology-Endocrinology and Metabolism* 295:1000–8.
Laviano, A., A. Koverech and M. Seelaender. 2017b. Assessing pathophysiology of cancer anorexia. *Current Opinion in Clinical Nutrition and Metabolic Care* 20:340–5.
Laviano, A., M. M. Meguid and F. Rossi-Fanelli. 2003. Cancer anorexia: Clinical implications, pathogenesis, and therapeutic strategies. *Lancet Oncology* 4:686–94.
Laviano, A., M. M. Meguid, Z.J. Yang, J. R. Gleason, C. Cangiano and F. Rossi Fanelli. 1996. Cracking the riddle of cancer anorexia. *Nutrition* 12:706–10.
Molfino, A., A. Iannace, M. C. Colaiacomo, A. Farcomeni, A. Emiliani, G. Gualdi, A. Laviano and F. Rossi Fanelli. 2017. Cancer anorexia: Hypothalamic activity and its association with inflammation and appetite-regulating peptides in lung cancer. *Journal of Cachexia Sarcopenia Muscle* 8:40–7.
Molfino, A., A. Laviano and F. Rossi Fanelli. 2010. Contribution of anorexia to tissue wasting in cachexia. *Current Opinion in Supportive and Palliative Care* 4:249–53.
Muscaritoli, M. et al. (PreMiO Study Group). 2017. Prevalence of malnutrition in patients at first medical oncology visit: The PreMiO study. *Oncotarget* 8:79884–96.
Muscaritoli, M., F. Rossi Fanelli and A. Molfino. 2016. Perspectives of health care professionals on cancer cachexia: Results from three global surveys. *Annals of Oncology* 27:2230–6.
Nagaya, N., T. Itoh, S. Murakami, H. Oya, M. Uematsu, K. Miyatake and K. Kangawa. 2005. Treatment of cachexia with ghrelin in patients with COPD. *Chest* 128:1187–93.
Nagaya, M., J. Moriya, Y. Yasumura, M. Uematsu, F. Ono, W. Shimizu, K. Ueno, M. Kitakaze, K. Miyatake and K. Kangawa. 2004. Effects of ghrelin administration on left ventricular function, exercise capacity, and muscle wasting in patients with chronic heart failure. *Circulation* 110:3674–9.
Nicolini, A., P. Ferrari, M. C. Masoni, M. Fini, S. Pagani, O. Giampietro and A. Carpi. 2013. Malnutrition anorexia and cachexia in cancer patients: A mini-review on pathogenesis and treatment. *Biomedicine and Pharmacotherapy* 67:807–17.
Rossi Fanelli, F., C. Cangiano, F. Ceci, R. Cellerino, F. Franchi, E. T. Menichetti, M. Muscaritoli and A. Cascino. 1986. Plasma tryptophan and anorexia in human cancer. *European Journal of Cancer and Clinical Oncology* 22:89–95.
Sato, T., A. Laviano, M. M. Meguid, C. Chen, F. Rossi-Fanelli and K. Hatakeyama. 2003. Involvement of plasma leptin, insulin and free tryptophan in cytokine-induced anorexia. *Clinical Nutrition* 22:139–46.
Sánchez-Lara, K., O. Arrieta, E. Pasaye, A. Laviano, R. E. Mercadillo, R. Sosa-Sánchez and N. Méndez-Sánchez. 2013. Brain activity correlated with food preferences: A functional study comparing advanced non-small cell lung cancer patients with and without anorexia. *Nutrition* 29:1013–9.
Schultes, B., S. M. Schmid, B. Wilms, K. Jauch-Chara, K. M. Oltmanns and M. Hallschmid. 2012. Lactate infusion during euglycemia but not hypoglycemia reduces subsequent food intake in healthy men. *Appetite* 58:818–21.
Strassmann, G., C. O. Jacob, R. Evans, D. Beall and M. Fong. 1992. Mechanisms of experimental cancer cachexia. Interaction between mononuclear phagocytes and colon-26 carcinoma and its relevance to IL-6-mediated cancer cachexia. *Journal of Immunology* 148:3674–8.
Tecot, L. H. 2007. Serotonin and the orchestration of energy balance. *Cell Metabolism* 6:352–61.
Torelli, G. F., M. M. Meguid, L. L. Moldawer, C. K. Edwards 3rd, H. J. Kim, J. L. Carter, A. Laviano and F. Rossi Fanelli. 1999. Use of recombinant human soluble TNF receptor in anorectic tumor-bearing rats. *American Journal of Physiology – Regulatory, Integrative and Comparative Physiology* 277:830–55.
Wallengren, O., K. Lundholm and I. Bosaeus. 2013. Diagnostic criteria of cancer cachexia: Relation to quality of life, exercise capacity and survival in unselected palliative care patients. *Supportive Care in Cancer* 21:1569–77.
Wheelwright, S., A. S. Darlington, J. B. Hopkinson, D. Fitzsimmons, A. White and C. D. Johnson. 2016. A systematic review to establish health-related quality of life domains for intervention targets in cancer cachexia. *BMJ Supportive and Palliative Care* 6:307–14.

Section IV

Cancer

19 Preoperative Nutrition Assessment and Optimization in the Cancer Patient

Shalana O'Brien, Allison Bruff, and Jeffrey M. Farma

CONTENTS

INTRODUCTION

Malnutrition is common with chronic illness, especially among those in the hospital, with 10%–50% of hospitalized patients meeting criteria for malnutrition. Surgery increases the risk of malnutrition due to increased metabolic demands and stress response. In one study, 13.7% of stomach cancer patients were malnourished preoperatively, which increased to 81.3% after curative resection. Increased age, preoperative weight loss, and open surgery increased these risks (Shim et al. 2013). Poor preoperative nutrition status worsens postoperative outcomes and increases rates of complications in many operations. This is also true for cancer patients and is a significant modifiable risk factor. Cancer patients have increased rates of preoperative malnutrition for numerous reasons. Cancer-related cachexia is a common cause of malnutrition due to the catabolic effect of cancer. Gastrointestinal (GI) motility, absorption, and function can be affected with GI cancers, dysphagia, or bowel obstructions. Nausea and emesis are common complications of numerous treatments, especially certain chemotherapeutic agents. Multiple procedures as part of their workup and evaluation, such as endoscopy, biopsy, and port placement, can result in patients being allowed nothing by mouth for several days at times. All of these issues are exacerbated by the problem of malnutrition. In this chapter we explore the surgical complications related to malnutrition, preoperative malnutrition screening tools, and potential interventions for malnutrition.

ASSESSMENT

Nutrition should be assessed by a registered dietician as a part of a multidisciplinary team managing the patient. The patient's care team should be aware of and monitor the patient's nutritional status, with assistance from any of the available assessment tools. Monitoring of the patient's weight, oral intake, and calorie counts is a starting point to the process. It is important to monitor appetite, taste change, dysphagia, weakness, nausea, pain, and mental status as these can all affect oral intake. Laboratory values including prealbumin, albumin, transferrin, and cholesterol can augment the clinical assessment, leading to a comprehensive view of the patient's nutritional status.

MALNUTRITION DEFINITION

Malnutrition in cancer patients is defined by a negative energy balance due to changes in metabolism, decreased intake, and systemic inflammation. Cancer-related malnutrition may also be described using terms such as sarcopenia and cachexia. Many screening tools exist for detecting malnutrition, but reliable indicators include weight loss greater than 10%, body mass index (BMI) less than 18.5, and albumin less than 3.5 g/dL (Table 19.1).

COMPLICATIONS OF MALNUTRITION

Malnutrition is associated with higher rates of postoperative complications in surgical patients. The degree of malnutrition is also correlated with the rates and severity of the complications. These complications include impaired healing, surgical site infections, increased length of stay, and increased mortality.

Wound healing impairment: In malnourished surgical patients wound healing is decreased. The phases of wound healing are affected and fibroblast proliferation, collagen synthesis, and angiogenesis are decreased (Norman et al. 2008).

Infections: Surgical site infections (SSIs) are common postoperative complications associated with significant morbidity and cost. Poor nutritional status is associated with increased rates of SSI in many types of cancer. Colorectal cancer patients in the National Surgical Quality Improvement Program (NSQIP) database with hypoalbuminemia have increased rates of superficial and deep SSIs (Hu et al. 2015). In addition, malnourished pancreatic cancer patients undergoing pancreaticoduodenectomy had significantly higher rates of SSI (Shinkawa et al. 2013).

Length of stay: Length of stay (LOS) is increased in those with poor nutrition. In GI cancers, increased length of stay has been correlated with increased preoperative weight loss, decreased preoperative albumin levels, and increased postoperative weight change (Garth et al. 2010). All three of these parameters are markers of poor nutritional status. The average LOS is increased by 40%–70% in malnourished patients compared to well-nourished patients (Norman et al. 2008). Severe malnutrition increases the length of stay even further.

TABLE 19.1
Postoperative Complications in Malnourished Patients

Complications of Malnutrition
Increased postoperative complications
Increased postoperative length of stay
Impaired wound healing
Increased mortality

Mortality: In multiple different cancers, nutritional status has been shown to be associated with mortality. Lung cancer patients who lived less than six months after diagnosis had decreased weight and nutritional laboratory values compared to patients who lived longer (Norman et al. 2008). In elderly gastric cancer patients treated with gastrectomy, those with low preoperative nutrition status had five-year overall survival that was 18% while patients with high preoperative nutrition had double the five-year overall survival at 36% (Sakurai et al. 2016).

SCORING SYSTEMS

Multiple scoring systems for the evaluation of nutritional status exist. We have chosen to provide an overview of the most commonly used scoring systems (Figures 19.1 and 19.2).

Scored Patient-Generated Subjective Global Assessment

The subjective global assessment scoring system was developed in the 1980s for use as a clinical tool to evaluate nutritional status (Detsky 1987). This scoring method was then modified in the 1990s for use in oncology patients and remains in frequent use today as the patient-generated subjective global assessment (PG-SGA) (Ottery 1996). This involves questions the patient answers about weight change, diet, GI symptoms, and functional status. The second half is an objective assessment

Scored Patient-Generated Subjective Global Assessment (PG-SGA)

History: Boxes 1 - 4 are designed to be completed by the patient.
[Boxes 1-4 are referred to as the PG-SGA Short Form (SF)]

Patient Identification Information

1. Weight *(See Worksheet 1)*

In summary of my current and recent weight:

I currently weigh about _____ pounds
I am about _____ feet _____ inches tall

One month ago I weighed about _____ pounds
Six months ago I weighed about _____ pounds

During the past two weeks my weight has:
☐ decreased (1) ☐ not changed (0) ☐ increased (0)

Box 1 ☐

2. Food intake: As compared to my normal intake, I would rate my food intake during the past month as
☐ unchanged (0)
☐ more than usual (0)
☐ less than usual (1)

I am now taking
☐ *normal food* but less than normal amount (1)
☐ little solid food (2)
☐ only liquids (3)
☐ only nutritional supplements (3)
☐ very little of anything (4)
☐ only tube feedings or only nutrition by vein (0) Box 2 ☐

3. Symptoms: I have had the following problems that have kept me from eating enough during the past two weeks (check all that apply)
☐ no problems eating (0)
☐ no appetite, just did not feel like eating (3)
☐ nausea (1)
☐ constipation (1)
☐ mouth sores (2)
☐ things taste funny or have no taste (1)
☐ problems swallowing (2)
☐ pain; where? (3) _______________
☐ other (1)** _______________
**Examples: depression, money, or dental problems
☐ vomiting (3)
☐ diarrhea (3)
☐ dry mouth (1)
☐ smells bother me (1)
☐ feel full quickly (1)
☐ fatigue (1)

Box 3 ☐

4. Activities and Function:
Over the past month, I would generally rate my activity as:
☐ normal with no limitations (0)
☐ not my normal self, but able to be up and about with fairly normal activities (1)
☐ not feeling up to most things, but in bed or chair less than half the day (2)
☐ able to do little activity and spend most of the day in bed or chair (3)
☐ pretty much bed ridden, rarely out of bed (3)

Box 4 ☐

The remainder of this form is to be completed by your doctor, nurse, dietitian, or therapist. Thank you.

Additive Score of Boxes 1-4 ☐ A

email: faithotterymdphd@aol.com or info@pt-global.org

FIGURE 19.1 Patient-generated subjective global assessment score (PG-SGA) tool for use to evaluate the nutritional status of patients. This tool utilizes weight, food intake, symptoms, activities and function, metabolic demand, and physical exam findings to assign a PG-SGA score. (With permission from Ottery, F. D. 1996. *Nutrition* 12 (1): S19.)

Scored Patient-Generated Subjective Global Assessment (PG-SGA)

Additive Score of Boxes 1-4 (See Side 1) ☐ A

Worksheet 1 – Scoring Weight Loss

To determine score, use 1-month weight data if available. Use 6-month data only if there is no 1-month weight data. Use points below to score weight change and add one extra point if patient has lost weight during the past 2 weeks. Enter total point score in Box 1 of PG-SGA.

Weight loss in 1 month	Points	Weight loss in 6 months
10% or greater	4	20% or greater
5-9.9%	3	10- 19.9%
3-4.9%	2	6- 9.9%
2-2.9%	1	2- 5.9%
0-1.9%	0	0- 1.9%

Numerical score from Worksheet 1 ☐

5. Worksheet 2 – Disease and its relation to nutritional requirements:

Score is derived by adding 1 point for each of the following conditions:

- ☐ Cancer
- ☐ Presence of decubitus, open wound or fistula
- ☐ AIDS
- ☐ Presence of trauma
- ☐ Pulmonary or cardiac cachexia
- ☐ Age greater than 65
- ☐ Chronic renal insufficiency

Other relevant diagnoses (specify) ______________________

Primary disease staging (circle if known or appropriate) I II III IV Other

Numerical score from Worksheet 2 ☐ B

6. Worksheet 3 – Metabolic Demand

Score for metabolic stress is determined by a number of variables known to increase protein & caloric needs. **Note:** Score fever intensity or duration, whichever is greater. The score is additive so that a patient who has a fever of 38.8 °C (3 points) for < 72 hrs (1 point) and who is on 10 mg of prednisone chronically (2 points) would have an additive score for this section of 5 points.

Stress	none (0)	low (1)	moderate (2)	high (3)
Fever	no fever	> 99 and < 101	≥ 101 and < 102	≥ 102 °F
Fever duration	no fever	< 72 hours	72 hours	> 72 hours
Corticosteroids	no corticosteroids	low dose (< 10 mg prednisone equivalents/day)	moderate dose (≥ 10 and < 30 mg prednisone equivalents/day)	high dose (≥ 30 mg prednisone equivalents/day)

Numerical score from Worksheet 3 ☐ C

7. Worksheet 4 – Physical Exam

Exam includes a subjective evaluation of 3 aspects of body composition: fat, muscle, & fluid. Since this is subjective, each aspect of the exam is rated for degree. Muscle deficit/loss impacts point score more than fat deficit/loss. Definition of categories: 0 = no abnormality, 1+ = mild, 2+ = moderate, 3+ = severe. Rating in these categories is *not* additive but are used to clinically assess the degree of deficit (or presence of excess fluid).

Muscle Status				
temples (temporalis muscle)	0	1+	2+	3+
clavicles (pectoralis & deltoids)	0	1+	2+	3+
shoulders (deltoids)	0	1+	2+	3+
interosseous muscles	0	1+	2+	3+
scapula (latissimus dorsi, trapezius, deltoids)	0	1+	2+	3+
thigh (quadriceps)	0	1+	2+	3+
calf (gastrocnemius)	0	1+	2+	3+
Global muscle status rating	**0**	**1+**	**2+**	**3+**

Fat Stores				
orbital fat pads	0	1+	2+	3+
triceps skin fold	0	1+	2+	3+
fat overlying lower ribs	0	1+	2+	3+
Global fat deficit rating	**0**	**1+**	**2+**	**3+**
Fluid status				
ankle edema	0	1+	2+	3+
sacral edema	0	1+	2+	3+
ascites	0	1+	2+	3+
Global fluid status rating	**0**	**1+**	**2+**	**3+**

Point score for the physical exam is determined by the overall subjective rating of the total body deficit. No deficit score = 0 points; Mild deficit score = 1 point; Moderate deficit score = 2 points; Severe deficit score = 3 points. **Again, muscle deficit/loss takes precedence over fat loss or fluid excess.**

Numerical Score for Worksheet 4 ☐ D

Total PG-SGA Score (**Total numerical score of A+B+C+D**) ☐

Clinician Signature ______________________ RD RN PA MD DO Other ________ Date ____________

Global PG-SGA Category Rating (Stage A, Stage B or Stage C) ☐

Worksheet 5 – PG-SGA Global Assessment Categories

Category	Stage A Well-nourished	Stage B Moderate/suspected malnutrition	Stage C Severely malnourished
Weight	No weight loss OR recent non-fluid wt gain	≤ 5% loss in 1 month (≤10% in 6 months) OR Progressive weight loss	> 5% loss in 1 month (>10% in 6 months) OR Progressive weight loss
Nutrient intake	No deficit OR Significant recent improvement	Definite decrease in intake	Severe deficit in intake
Nutrition Impact Symptoms (NIS)	None OR significant recent improvement allowing adequate intake	Presence of NIS (Box 3 of PG-SGA)	Presence of NIS (Box 3 of PG-SGA)
Functioning	No deficit OR Significant recent improvement	Moderate functional deficit OR Recent deterioration	Severe functional deficit OR Recent significant deterioration
Physical Exam	No deficit OR chronic deficit but with recent clinical improvement	Evidence of mild to moderate loss of muscle mass &/or muscle tone on palpation &/or loss of SQ fat	Obvious signs of malnutrition (e.g., severe loss muscle, fat, possible edema)

Nutritional Triage Recommendations: Additive score is used to define specific nutritional interventions including patient & family education, symptom management including pharmacologic intervention, and appropriate nutrient intervention (food, nutritional supplements, enteral, or parenteral triage).

First line nutrition intervention includes optimal symptom management.

Triage based on PG-SGA point score

- 0-1 No intervention required at this time. Re-assessment on routine and regular basis during treatment.
- 2-3 Patient & family education by dietitian, nurse, or other clinician with pharmacologic intervention as indicated by symptom survey (Box 3) and lab values as appropriate.
- 4-8 Requires intervention by dietitian, in conjunction with nurse or physician as indicated by symptoms (Box 3).
- ≥ 9 Indicates a critical need for improved symptom management and/or nutrient intervention options.

email: faithotterymdphd@aol.com or info@pt-global.org

FIGURE 19.2 Worksheets for use with the patient-generated subjective global assessment (PG-SGA) tool. These are used to score patient responses on weight loss, condition, metabolic stress, and physical exam findings. The findings are then used to assign a nutritional category of well-nourished, moderately malnourished/suspected malnutrition, or severely malnourished. (With permission from Ottery, F. D. 1996. *Nutrition* 12 (1): S19.)

based on weight loss, specific conditions, metabolic factors, and physical examination. The result is that patients are grouped into groups A, B, and C corresponding to well-nourished, moderately malnourished, and severely malnourished patients. Numerous studies have demonstrated its validity with a very high sensitivity up to 98% to detect malnutrition (Bauer et al. 2002).

Nutrition Risk Screening

An additional screening tool used to evaluate nutritional status of patients is the Nutritional Risk Screening (NRS-2002). This screening tool was developed in order to establish guidelines that would predict both the presence of an already malnourished state and also the risk of developing worsening nutritional status based on clinical disease severity. Patients are screened upon admission to the hospital by the admitting team. Questions range from assessment of nutritional status (current BMI on admission, weight loss in the last three months, and reduction of food intake) to severity of current disease. The final part of the screening tool combines scores from severity of malnourishment and severity of disease along with age adjustment to then determine if the patient is at high risk of malnourishment during hospitalization and requires intervention. Patients placed in the low-risk category are recommended to have weekly screenings (Kondrup et al. 2003) (Tables 19.2 and 19.3).

TABLE 19.2
Nutritional Risk Screening (NRS 2002) Screening Tool for Malnutrition Using Body Mass Index (BMI), Weight Loss, Decreased Intake and Illness as Parameters for Further Screening

Nutritional Risk Screening (NRS 2002)

Step 1: Initial screening	**Yes**	No
1 Is BMI <20.5 kg/m²?		
2 Has the patient lost weight within the last three months?		
3 Has the patient had reduced dietary intake in the last week?		
4 Is the patient severely ill? (e.g., in intensive therapy)		

Yes: If the answer is "Yes" to any question, the screening in Step 2 is performed.
No: If the answer is "No" to all questions, the patient is re-screening at weekly intervals. If the patient, for example, is scheduled for a major operation, a preventive nutritional care plan is considered to avoid the associated risk status.

Source: Adapted with permission from Kondrup, J. et al. 2003. *Clinical Nutrition* 22 (3): 321–336.

SCORING SYSTEM COMPARISON

Because no single screening tool has been shown to adequately assess nutritional status of patients, oncologists have sought to compare PG-SGA and NRS-2002 as a way to determine their efficacy. NRS-2002 has been recommended by the European Society for Clinical Nutrition and Metabolism (ESPEN) and PG-SGA by the American Dietetic Association. Ryu and Kim (2010) studied the nutritional status of gastric cancer patients before and at 6- and 12-month intervals after radical gastrectomy. They compared the relationship between the screening tools in addition to objective parameters such as BMI, mid-arm circumference, and serum albumin level. Both screening tools consistently identified patients as malnourished if they had a significant percentage of weight loss preoperatively. Additionally, in the six-month postoperative period, a strong correlation was found between the scoring tools and the objective measurements. The initial preoperative nutritional assessment had differing numbers of patients labeled as malnourished, but they concluded that a combination of PG-SGA, NRS-2002, and objective measurements must be used to adequately address the needs of the cancer patient.

Another comparison study found strong correlation between PG-SGA and NRS-2002 (Du et al. 2017). Patients with greater than 15 types of cancer were screened with both screening tools and had anthropometric and laboratory results documented. The incidence of malnutrition was found to be 86.3% by PG-SGA and 30.7% by NRS-2002, likely, as the authors claim, due to the fact that anthropometric measurements are included in the PG-SGA. They found a strong relationship between scores from SGA and scores from NRS-2002. However, in regard to albumin, a marker for nutritional status, PG-SGA had a higher sensitivity than NRS-2002, 93.78% to 43.13%, respectively. Due to this finding, the authors concluded that PG-SGA was the more appropriate screening tool for cancer patients.

INTERVENTIONS

Preoperative nutritional status can be augmented via multiple escalating approaches. Patients can be encouraged to increase their intake of food, especially protein-rich foods. Formal nutritional counseling offers more structured ongoing support to patients by a healthcare professional. Oral

TABLE 19.3
Nutritional Risk Screening (NRS 2002) Secondary Screening Tool for Malnutrition UsingDegree of Weight Loss, Degree of Decreased Food Intake, Body Mass Index (BMI), and Severity of Disease to Calculate a Score

Nutritional Risk Screening (NRS 2002)

Step 2: Final screening

Impaired nutritional status		**Severity of disease (~ increase in requirements)**	
Absent **Score 0**	Normal nutritional status	Absent **Score 0**	Normal nutritional requirements
Mild **Score 1**	Weight loss >5% in three months or food intake below 50%–75% of normal requirement in preceding week	Mild **Score 1**	Hip fracture, chronic patients, in particular with acute complications: cirrhosis, chronic obstructive pulmonary disease, chronic hemodialysis, diabetes, oncology
Moderate **Score 2**	Weight loss >5% in two months or BMI 18.5–20.5 + impaired general condition or food intake below 25%–60% of normal requirement in preceding week	Moderate **Score 2**	Major abdominal surgery, stroke, severe pneumonia, hematologic malignancy
Severe **Score 3**	Weight loss >5% in one month (>15% in three months) or BMI <18.5 + impaired general condition or food intake below 0%–25% of normal requirement in preceding week	Severe **Score 3**	Head injury, bone marrow transplantation, intensive care patients (APACHE >10)
Score:	+	**Score:**	**= Total score**
Age	if ≥70 years: add 1 to total score above	**= age-adjusted total score**	

Score ≥ 3: the patient is nutritionally at risk and a nutritional care plan is initiated.
Score < 3: weekly rescreening of the patient. If the patient, for example, is scheduled for a major operation, a preventive nutritional care plan is considered to avoid the associated risk status.

Source: Adapted with permission from Kondrup, J. et al. 2003. *Clinical Nutrition* 22 (3): 321–336.
Note: If this score is above three the patient is at risk, and a nutritional care plan should be initiated.

nutritional supplements are mixtures containing high levels of calories and protein and are available over the counter or via prescription. Medications such as appetite stimulants and prokinetics may be given to increase oral intake or gut motility. If nutritional needs are unable to be met via oral intake, and the remainder of the GI system is functioning, enteral nutrition may be given through an enteral access tube. Last, total parenteral nutrition (TPN) can be given if poor nutrition is due to intolerance of enteral feeds, malabsorption, or if enteral feeding is not an option due to GI tract blockage.

Immune-modulating enteral formulas or immune-enhancing diets contain supplements such as arginine, glutamine, omega-3 fatty acids, and additional antioxidants to improve immune cell function and wound healing, and reduce inflammation. These formulations are usually reserved for patients who are going through an acute stress state such as major elective surgery, trauma, burns, or prolonged intensive care unit ICU stay. However, there have been conflicting reports on their benefits. Studies have shown that nutrients such as arginine reduce pro-inflammatory cytokines such as IL-6 and TNF-α while promoting T-cell function. Arginine can also lead to increased nitric oxide especially in septic patients who metabolize arginine to nitric oxide or trauma patients who have increased arginine breakdown. Omega-3 fatty acids from fish oil modulate production of eicosanoids (prostaglandins, thromboxane) to help reduce tissue inflammation. Immune-enhancing diets formulas can have different composition of nutrients and can be tailored to the patient's disease severity and state (Gianotti et al. 2002; Marik and Zaloga 2010).

BENEFITS OF NUTRITIONAL SUPPORT

Supplementation boosts nutrition in surgical patients and is associated with better outcomes. A randomized controlled trial gave well-nourished patients with GI or abdominal cavity cancers a protein-rich hypercaloric drink for 14 days prior to surgery in addition to their regular diet. Body weight, albumin, total protein, transferrin, and total lymphocyte count decreased in the control group on measurement prior to surgery. The control group had 17 complications, while the interventional arm had 8 complications (Kabata et al. 2015). Another study tracked advanced pancreatic cancer patients who were evaluated by the SGA and received medical nutrition therapy by a registered dietician. Approximately 70% of study participants maintained or improved their nutritional status, proving the importance of the involvement of nutrition professionals (Vashi et al. 2015).

Immune-modulating diets have been shown to be beneficial for surgical patients. A randomized controlled trial studied the effects of preoperative immune-enhancing diets in patients with gastric carcinoma. Patients were given either a formula that contained arginine, RNA, and omega-3 fatty acids or an isocaloric formula for seven days prior to surgery. Postoperative complications such as infections (wound, respiratory, abdominal cavity), the need for antibiotics, and number of days with systemic inflammatory response were significantly lower in the intervention group. Length of stay and weight loss had no statistically significant change. While there was a decline in $CD4^{+}$T-cells in both groups, the rate of decline in the immune-enhancing diet group was less (Okamoto et al. 2009).

TIMING OF INTERVENTION

Benefits have been shown when immune-enhancing diets have been started both in the preoperative and postoperative stages (Hegazi et al. 2014). Due to the amount of time the nutrients require to take effect in the body, immune-enhancing formulas can be started in the preoperative phase for the cancer patient undergoing elective surgery and continued into the perioperative phase.

GUIDELINES

ESPEN guidelines recommend that all cancer patients be screened for malnutrition and those with a positive screen undergo a full evaluation. Nutritional intervention is recommended for all malnourished patients or those at risk. Protein intake should be at least 1–1.5 g/kg. Enteral nutrition is recommended if oral nutrition is inadequate and parenteral nutrition is recommended if enteral nutrition is inadequate (Arends et al. 2016). In surgical patients at high risk for malnutrition, nutritional supplementation is recommended preoperatively for 10–14 days. Elective surgical treatment should be postponed for those at high risk of malnutrition in order to allow preoperative supplementation. Total volume of fluid should not exceed 25–30 mL/kg daily and total sodium should be less than 1 mmol/kg daily. Fluid overload is common in cancer patients due to hormonal changes, decreased free water clearance, and decreased insensible losses with decreased activity. Fluid status should be monitored, and barring dehydration, fluids should be given conscientiously (Bozzetti 2015) (Figure 19.3).

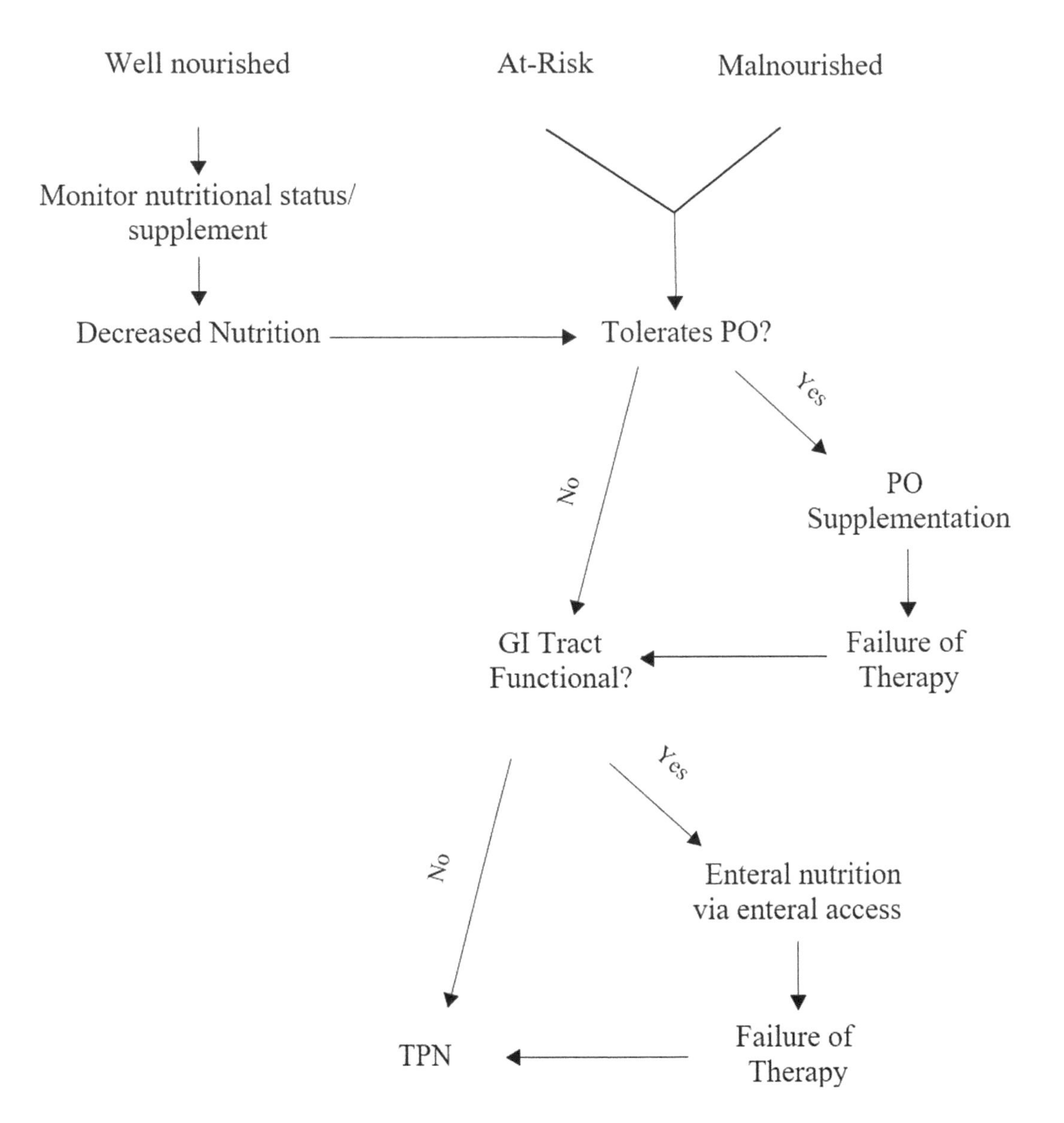

FIGURE 19.3 Decision algorithm for nutritional intervention in well-nourished, at-risk, and malnourished patients.

APPLICATIONS TO OTHER AREAS OF PALLIATIVE CARE

Poor preoperative nutritional status can increase rates of postoperative complications and complications may make a patient ineligible for or delay systemic therapy. Palliative chemotherapy and palliative radiation typically need to be postponed until a patient has recovered from a surgical procedure, and, therefore, avoiding complications is important for being eligible for other therapies. Complications and nutritional status also affect quality of life and pain, necessitating other treatment modalities and pain control.

ETHICAL PRINCIPLES

In the cancer and palliative care patient especially, we do not want to cause harm from surgical procedures. Complications that may not be as significant for a healthy individual can cause significant harm and decreased quality of life in the cancer patient. A well-nourished patient has a lower risk of complications, and for this reason we would recommend nutritional screening for all cancer patients, especially those undergoing surgery. However, the monetary costs of nutritional support should be weighed with the ethical principle of justice and ensuring that all patients will be able to receive support.

KEY FACTS: CANCER

- Cancer occurs when normal cells in the body grow abnormally, which can then spread and invade other areas of the body.
- The abnormal cells spread to distant parts of the body and grow, which is called metastasis.
- Cancer cells can develop in any tissue or organ in the body and are named after their original location.
- Cancer can be treated with chemotherapy, radiation, surgery, or a combination of the three.
- Cancer is the second leading cause of mortality in the United States after heart disease.
- For women, breast cancer is the most common newly diagnosed cancer.
- Prostate cancer is the most common newly diagnosed cancer for men.
- However, more men and women die from lung cancer each year than any other cancer in the United States.

SUMMARY POINTS

- Malnutrition is very common in cancer patients.
- All cancer patients should be screened for malnutrition.
- Numerous screening tools are effective for detecting malnutrition.
- Preoperative malnutrition is associated with increased length of stay, complications, and decreased survival.
- Nutrition can be augmented.
- Nutritional supplementation in surgical patients improves nutrition and decreases complications.
- Nutritional supplementation is recommended preoperatively for 10–14 days.

LIST OF ABBREVIATIONS

BMI Body Mass Index
ESPEN European Society for Clinical Nutrition and Metabolism
GI Gastrointestinal
LOS Length of Stay
NPO Nil Per Os
NRS Nutritional Risk Screening
PG-SGA Patient-Generated Subjective Global Assessment
SSI Surgical Site Infection
TPN Total Parenteral Nutrition

REFERENCES

Arends, J., P. Bachmann, V. Baracos, N. Barthelemy, H. Bertz, F. Bozzetti et al. 2016. ESPEN Guidelines on Nutrition in Cancer Patients. *Clinical Nutrition* 36 (1): 11–48.

Bauer, J., S. Capra, and M. Ferguson. 2002. Use of the Scored Patient-Generated Subjective Global Assessment (PG-SGA) as a Nutrition Assessment Tool in Patients with Cancer. *European Journal of Clinical Nutrition* 56 (8): 779–785.

Bozzetti, F. 2015. Tailoring the Nutritional Regimen in the Elderly Cancer Patient. *Nutrition* 31 (4): 612–614.

Detsky, A. S., J. R. McLaughlin, J. P. Baker, N. Johnston, S. Whittaker, R. A. Mendelson, and K. N. Jeejeebhoy. 1987. What Is Subjective Global Assessment of Nutritional Status? *Journal of Parenteral and Enteral Nutrition* 11 (1): 8–13.

Du, H., B. Liu, Y. Xie, J. Liu, Y. Wei, H. Hu, B. Luo, and Z. Li. 2017. Comparison of Different Methods for Nutrition Assessment in Patients with Tumors. *Oncology Letters* 14 (1): 165–170.

Garth, A. K., C. M. Newsome, N. Simmance, and T. C. Crowe. 2010. Nutritional Status, Nutrition Practices and Post-Operative Complications in Patients with Gastrointestinal Cancer. *Journal of Human Nutrition and Dietetics* 23 (4): 393–401.

Gianotti, L., M. Braga, L. Nespoli, G. Radaelli, A. Beneduce, and V. Di Carlo. 2002. A Randomized Controlled Trial of Preoperative Oral Supplementation with a Specialized Diet in Patients with Gastrointestinal Cancer. *Gastroenterology* 122 (7): 1763–1770.

Hegazi, R. A., D. S. Hustead, and D. C. Evans. 2014. Preoperative Standard Oral Nutrition Supplements vs Immunonutrition: Results of a Systematic Review and Meta-Analysis. *Journal of the American College of Surgeons* 219 (5): 1078–1087.

Hu, W., L. C. Cajas-Monson, S. Eisenstein, L. Parry, B. Cosman, and S. Ramamoorthy. 2015. Preoperative Malnutrition Assessments as Predictors of Postoperative Mortality and Morbidity in Colorectal Cancer: An Analysis of ACS-NSQIP. *Nutrition Journal* 14 (1): 91.

Kabata, P., T. Jastrzębski, M. Kąkol, K. Król, M. Bobowicz, A. Kosowska, and J. Jaśkiewicz. 2015. Preoperative Nutritional Support in Cancer Patients with no Clinical Signs of Malnutrition—Prospective Randomized Controlled Trial. *Supportive Care in Cancer* 23 (2): 365–370.

Kondrup, J., H. H. Rasmussen, O. Hamberg, and Z. Stanga. 2003. Nutritional Risk Screening (NRS 2002): A New Method Based on an Analysis of Controlled Clinical Trials. *Clinical Nutrition* 22 (3): 321–336.

Marik, P. E. and G. P. Zaloga. 2010. Immunonutrition in High-Risk Surgical Patients: A Systematic Review and Analysis of the Literature. *Journal of Parenteral and Enteral Nutrition* 34 (4): 378–386.

Norman, K., C. Pichard, H. Lochs, and M. Pirlich. 2008. Prognostic Impact of Disease-Related Malnutrition. *Clinical Nutrition* 27 (1): 5–15.

Okamoto, Y., K. Okano, K. Izuishi, H. Usuki, H. Wakabayashi, and Y. Suzuki. 2009. Attenuation of the Systemic Inflammatory Response and Infectious Complications after Gastrectomy with Preoperative Oral Arginine and [Omega]-3 Fatty Acids Supplemented Immunonutrition. *World Journal of Surgery* 33 (9): 1815.

Ottery, F. D. 1996. Definition of Standardized Nutritional Assessment and Interventional Pathways in Oncology. *Nutrition* 12 (1): S19.

Ryu, S. W. and I. H. Kim. 2010. Comparison of Different Nutritional Assessments in Detecting Malnutrition among Gastric Cancer Patients. *World Journal of Gastroenterology* 16 (26): 3310.

Sakurai, K., T. Tamura, T. Toyokawa, R. Amano, N. Kubo, H. Tanaka et al. 2016. Low Preoperative Prognostic Nutritional Index Predicts Poor Survival Post-Gastrectomy in Elderly Patients with Gastric Cancer. *Annals of Surgical Oncology* 23 (11): 3669–3676.

Shim, H., J. H. Cheong, K. Y. Lee, H. Lee, J. G. Lee, and S. H. Noh. 2013. Perioperative Nutritional Status Changes in Gastrointestinal Cancer Patients. *Yonsei Medical Journal* 54 (6): 1370–1376.

Shinkawa, H., S. Takemura, T. Uenishi, M. Sakae, K. Ohata, Y. Urata, K. Kaneda, A. Nozawa, and S. Kubo. 2013. Nutritional Risk Index as an Independent Predictive Factor for the Development of Surgical Site Infection after Pancreaticoduodenectomy. *Surgery Today* 43 (3): 276–283.

Vashi, P., B. Popiel, C. Lammersfeld, and D. Gupta. 2015. Outcomes of Systematic Nutritional Assessment and Medical Nutrition Therapy in Pancreatic Cancer. *Pancreas* 44 (5): 750–755.

20 Palliative Gastrojejunostomy and the Impact on Nutrition in Cancer

Dorotea Mutabdzic, Poornima B. Rao, and Jeffrey M. Farma

CONTENTS

INTRODUCTION

Gastric outlet obstruction (GOO) is typically manifest by the progressive inability to tolerate oral intake over the course of weeks to months. A patient will present with nausea and vomiting that becomes progressively more severe and ultimately results in a complete inability to tolerate anything by mouth.

Acute Presentation of Gastric Outlet Obstruction

The development of GOO or proximal gastrointestinal obstruction in a patient with a known background of advanced malignant disease portends a generally poor prognosis. Though reports in the literature have been variable, recent prospective observational studies report a median overall survival of approximately 64 days in patients who develop GOO secondary to unresected primary or metastatic cancer (Schmidt et al. 2009). Given the anticipated short duration of survival following the development of GOO, symptom relief and overall quality of life should be paramount in discussions of treatment options for patients. The performance status of the patient and the patient's capacity to undergo interventional procedures and, as necessary, repeat interventions should be considered. Various palliative surgical techniques have been employed and studied over the past two decades.

Occasionally, an acute clinical presentation may manifest. Patients present with severe dehydration as well as a hypochloremic, hypokalemic metabolic alkalosis related to chronic and refractory vomiting. The degree of malnutrition present is associated with the duration of obstructive symptoms and etiology of the obstruction. Because of the intimate anatomic associations within the upper gastrointestinal tract, an array of malignancies may cause the symptom complex that typifies GOO based on intrinsic or extrinsic (compressive) obstruction of the upper gastrointestinal tract. These include gastric cancer; gastrointestinal stromal tumors; the spectrum of periampullary malignancies including pancreatic, ampullary, duodenal and biliary cancers; and peritoneal carcinomatosis, generally related to gastric, pancreatic and gynecologic malignancies.

Clinical Presentation

The diagnosis of GOO is predominantly made clinically. Patient history including concomitant symptoms, such as weight loss, jaundice, abdominal pain and steatorrhea, may point to a specific etiology. Additional symptoms include eating restrictions and early satiety, dysphagia to solids and/or liquids, nausea and vomiting and gastroesophageal reflux (Table 20.1). Physical examination may point to a specific malignancy. The presence of a palpable abdominal mass and lymphadenopathy in the periumbilical or supraclavicular region may suggest locally advanced disease, as well as the presence of a gastric succession splash, and tympani in the left upper quadrant indicative of gastric dilation and stasis of gastric contents.

Diagnostic Evaluation

Diagnostic evaluation should consist of a complete evaluation for intestinal obstruction. Initial imaging studies include a chest x-ray and abdominal films (Figure 20.1). The presence of a large gastric bubble or dilated stomach and the absence of small bowel dilation or pathologic air-fluid levels suggest more proximal obstruction. Occasionally pneumobilia may be detected indicating duodenal obstruction distal to the ampulla of Vater. A measure of serum electrolytes, creatinine, complete blood count and coagulation profile should be performed. Intravenous access should be established and intravenous hydration as well as, electrolyte replacement should be promptly initiated. Nasogastric (NG) decompression and placement of a urinary bladder catheter will permit continual reassessment of fluid resuscitative efforts and determination of ongoing losses.

Ultimately, cross-sectional imaging with computed tomography or magnetic resonance imaging should be obtained to confirm the clinical diagnosis, and will allow for a more accurate determination of the presence of locally advanced or metastatic disease (Figure 20.2). Upper endoscopy will allow

TABLE 20.1
Common Signs and Symptoms of Gastric Outlet Obstruction

Nausea
Vomiting
Abdominal pain
Weight loss
Inability to tolerate oral intake
Dehydration with hypochloremic, hypokalemic metabolic alkalosis
Vitamins A, C, D, E, K and B12 deficiencies
Steatorrhea

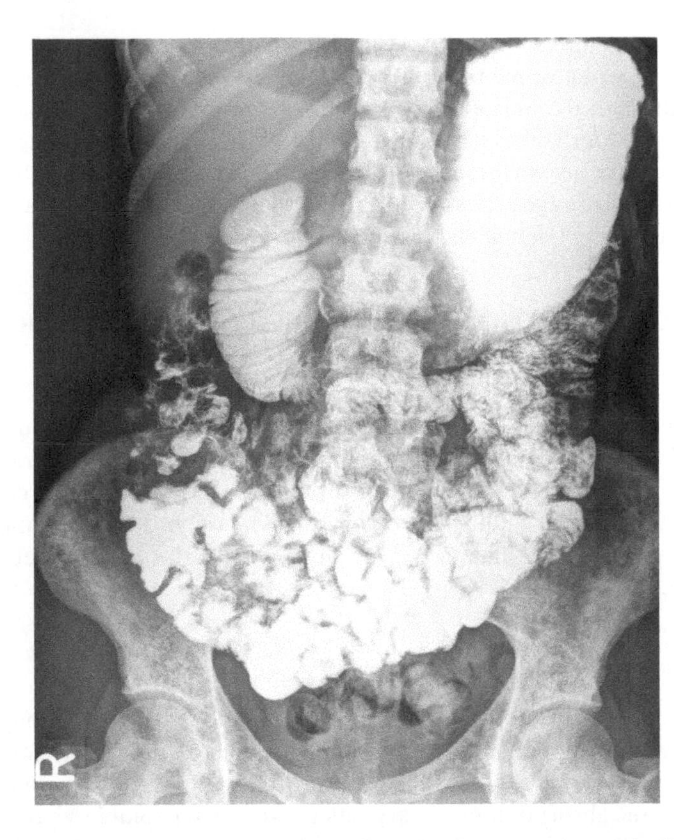

FIGURE 20.1 Upper gastrointestinal (UGI) series. UGI series demonstrating markedly distended stomach and proximal duodenum.

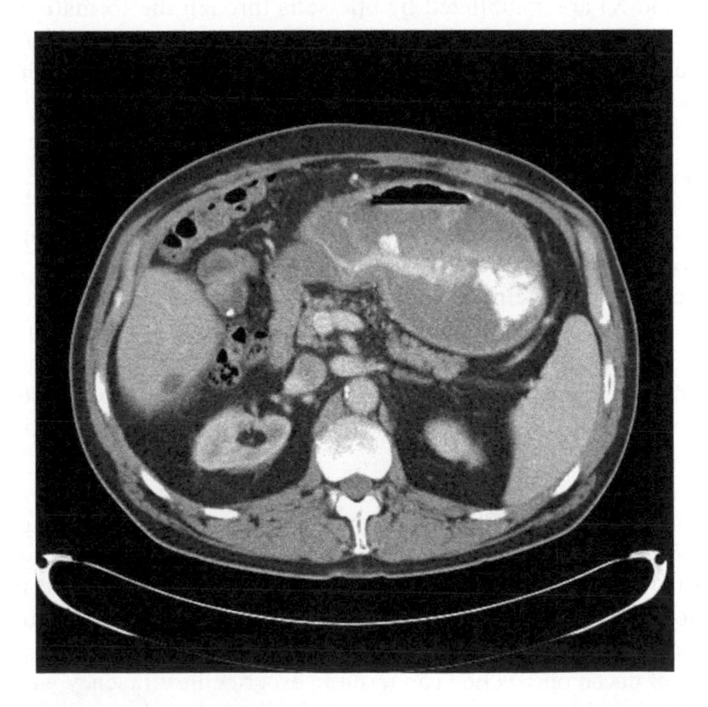

FIGURE 20.2 Gastric outlet obstruction. Computed tomography demonstrating dilated stomach with a narrowed duodenum due to progressive extrahepatic cholangiocarcinoma.

for direct intraluminal examination and determination of the presence of intrinsic versus extrinsic compression of the upper intestinal tract, as well as the exact location of obstruction. In addition, tissue biopsy for pathological evaluation and ultimately diagnosis can be performed. Clinical context will determine the need for additional testing. A history of prior surgical intervention for upper gastrointestinal cancer, the known presence of recurrent or metastatic disease or history of additional obstructive symptoms to suggest possibility of multilevel obstructive disease will necessitate additional diagnostic testing (Helton and Fisichella 2007).

NUTRITIONAL COMPLICATIONS OF GASTRIC OUTLET OBSTRUCTION

Proximal Gastric Outlet Obstruction

Proximal gastrointestinal obstruction results in multiple unique nutritional sequelae. With isolated obstruction at the level of the pylorus, the normal physiologic function of gastric secretion of acid and intrinsic factor will be impaired. The effects of this can be seen with decreased absorption of dietary iron and vitamin C from within the proximal small bowel. In addition, limited intrinsic factor leads to decreased absorption of vitamin B12 (cobalamin) from the terminal ileum and can lead to fatigue and anemia.

Duodenal and Biliary Obstruction

More distal duodenal obstruction can affect bile salt homeostasis. Though enterohepatic circulation of bile acids may be unaffected by duodenal obstruction, secretion often is, leading to obstruction of the biliary tree and bile secretion. The result is obstructive jaundice, which has implications on the absorption of dietary fats as well as fat-soluble vitamins. Bile salts are secreted into the duodenum in response to the presence of luminal fatty acids. Once luminal lipolysis has occurred, free long-chain and medium-chain fatty acids and fat-soluble vitamins (vitamin A, E, D and K) are solubilized by bile salts through the formation of micelles. The absence of bile salt secretion into the intestinal tract compromises this process, leading to fat-soluble vitamin deficiencies, as well as fatty acid malabsorption, which results in the collateral effect of secretory diarrhea.

Pancreatic Duct Obstruction

Similarly, isolated pancreatic duct obstruction can lead to a symptom complex of pancreatic insufficiency. The pancreas produces and secretes enzymes essential for the digestion and absorption of carbohydrates, proteins and fats. Though initiated with exposure to salivary amylase, carbohydrate digestion is propagated through exposure to pancreatic amylase. Pancreatic amylase converts complex carbohydrates into small oligosaccharides, which are presented to the intestinal brush border where the completion of digestion by way of specific disaccharidases occurs. This is followed by both active and passive absorption of the monosaccharide moieties, which are then used for nutrition.

Protein hydrolysis is initiated with mechanical dispersion in the oral cavity and gastric pepsin digestion in the stomach. Within the duodenum, endopeptidases produced by the pancreas hydrolyze bonds within polypeptide chains to permit the generation of oligopeptides. These may be further hydrolyzed into smaller di- or tri-peptides at the intestinal brush border, and then absorbed and utilized for nutrition. Fat absorption requires pancreatic lipase activity to generate free fatty acids from triglyceride moieties, which may then be solubilized and absorbed. Disruption in pancreatic function as a result of ductal obstruction can result in exocrine insufficiency with the consequence of malnutrition related to the inability to appropriately digest and absorb carbohydrates, proteins and fats.

Nutritional Deficiencies

The obvious nutritional issue as related to GOO and proximal duodenal obstruction is inadequate caloric intake and absorption. More subtle, however, is the progressive development of specific vitamin and mineral deficiencies. Patients with proximal duodenal obstruction often exhibit a profound deficiency in vitamin K that evolves with the progression of biliary obstruction. A significant coagulopathy results from inability to absorb vitamin K due to lack of bile salts within the intestinal lumen. Therefore, the ability to synthesize factors essential to both arms of the coagulation cascade is compromised. Recognition and treatment of this deficiency are essential prior to the performance of any invasive diagnostic or therapeutic procedures (Vander et al. 1990).

SURGICAL TECHNIQUES

Patients with periampullary malignancies are often found to have unresectable disease at the time of diagnosis. Bypass of the area of obstruction is the mainstay of therapy for GOO for the palliation of symptoms. This strategy may employ a combination of percutaneous, endoscopic and surgical techniques based on the clinical constellation of symptoms.

Gastrojejunostomy

Gastrojejunostomy remains the gold standard for palliation of symptoms of GOO; however, there has been a rapid evolution of bypass technique. Surgical bypass has been traditionally performed through an open technique (Figure 20.3). The precise technique of a surgical gastrojejunostomy has

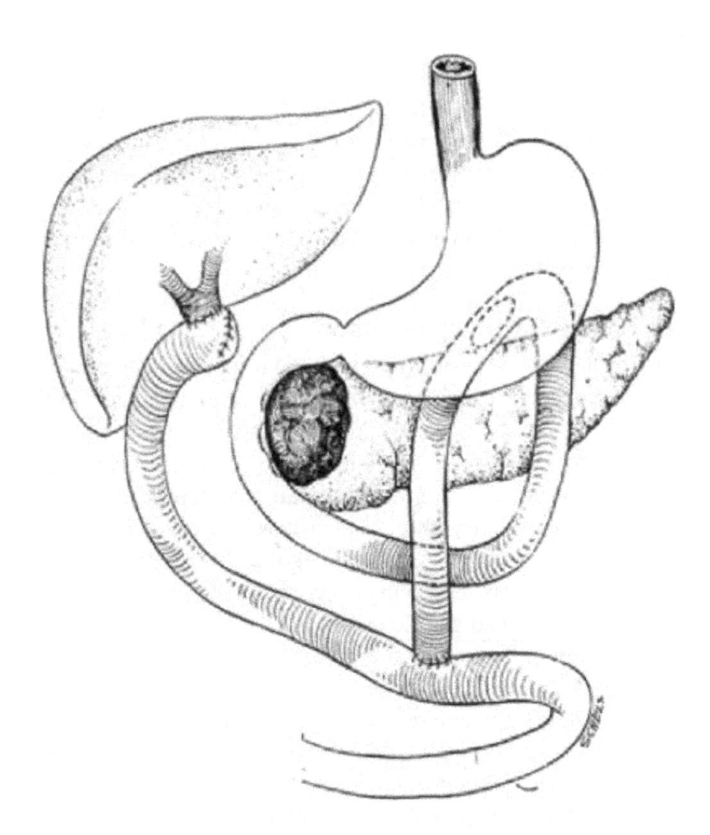

FIGURE 20.3 Combined gastrojejunostomy and hepaticojejunostomy. (From Scott, EN et al. 2009. *HPB* 11(2): 118–124, with permission.)

been described with permutations designed to minimize long-term complications associated with the procedure.

The results of surgical palliation for GOO are well defined in the literature. The results of a retrospective review reported from the Hopkins group have been validated by other centers in prospective studies. In high-volume centers, surgical biliary and gastric bypass for palliation of symptoms can be accomplished with low operative mortality – typically reported at less than 5%, and with an acceptable morbidity rate of less than 25%. In addition, palliative surgical procedures resulted in improved median survival of more than six months, compared with the generally accepted dismal prognosis of those who are not palliated (Sohn et al., 1999).

Loop anterior gastrojejunostomy creates an anastomosis between the stomach proximal to the area of obstruction and the antimesenteric aspect of the jejunum 15–25 cm distal to the ligament of Treitz, and thus distal to the level of obstruction. A two-layer hand-sewn side-to-side anastomosis is typically configured to create a luminal diameter of 5–7 cm in length. Described variations of this procedure include retrocolic retrogastric posterior loop gastrojejunostomy, antecolic retrogastric posterior loop gastrojejunostomy and antecolic antegastric anterior loop gastrojejunostomy. However, there is no consensus or data related to outcomes using these different techniques in the context of GOO. We know in the gastric bypass literature that antecolic gastrojejunostomy leads to a lower rate of internal hernia formation (Geubbels et al., 2015), although this complication may not be relevant to patients with GOO as internal hernias are a delayed complication of bypass surgery and associated with significant weight loss. More recent descriptions detail the use of surgical stapling devices for creation of the anastomosis, as well as using minimally invasive laparoscopic techniques. The bypass procedure does not require functional bowel division. The procedure is well suited for isolated GOO where the biliary and pancreatic duct systems remain patent.

Risks Associated with Gastrojejunostomy

As with any surgical procedure, there are risks of bleeding, infection and anastomotic leak. More specific to the gastrojejunostomy procedure are rates of delayed gastric emptying varying with technique and ranging from 2% to 31% (Doberneck and Berndt, 1987). There is frequent biliopancreatic drainage into the stomach leading to the possibility of bile reflux–induced gastritis. In addition, because of the direct transit of acidic gastric contents into the more distal and less buffered small bowel, anastomotic ulceration (a marginal ulcer) and bleeding within the efferent jejunal limb can occur (Lillemoe, 1998).

Partial Stomach-Partitioning Gastrojejunostomy

Several techniques have evolved in an effort to minimize the anatomic and physiologic consequences of the loop gastrojejunostomy and to limit postoperative symptoms related to the procedure, while at the same time avoiding the risks of a more radical operative resection in the setting of palliative treatment. Partial stomach-partitioning gastrojejunostomy was originally described in an Asian series. The technique adds partial division of the distal stomach while maintaining a tunnel of 2–3 cm in diameter along the lesser curvature. The gastrojejunostomy is performed to the stomach that is proximal to the partial transaction (Kaminishi et al., 1997). The theoretical advantage of the procedure is that it permits preferential emptying of gastric contents through the gastrojejunostomy, thereby minimizing the rate of delayed gastric emptying. This also allows for endoscopic access to the distal stomach and duodenum for potential endoscopic therapeutic maneuvers. In addition, the constant irritation of enteric contents on a tumor mass with the resultant ulceration and bleeding may be minimized by diversion of the enteral stream (Kwon and Lee, 2004). While this procedure is not as commonly performed, a meta-analysis in 2016 did suggest that partial stomach-partitioning gastrojejunostomy has a lower risk of delayed gastric emptying and has a decreased length of stay when compared to traditional gastrojejunostomy. There was no difference in other complications including operative time, total postoperative complications or time to oral intake (Arrangoiz et al., 2013; Arciero et al., 2006; Kubota et al., 2007; Kumagai et al., 2016).

Role of Prophylactic Gastrojejunostomy

The concept of prophylactic gastrojejunostomy in the context of upper gastrointestinal malignancy has been the subject of significant debate and investigation. Prophylactic gastrojejunostomy for advanced gastric cancer has not been studied presumably because if a gastric cancer is deemed unresectable, there is almost certainly an element of GOO. Initial reports on patients with unresectable pancreatic adenocarcinoma as determined by laparoscopic staging suggested that they seldom developed gastroduodenal obstruction that required therapeutic intervention. The rate of development of obstruction was determined to be less than 20%, and as a result, the performance of a laparotomy for creation of a gastrojejunal bypass with the risks associated with both in the context of unresectable cancer were determined to be too great to advocate in the setting of palliative therapy (Espat et al., 1999). Subsequent studies have demonstrated that the perioperative morbidity and mortality of gastrojejunostomy in the setting of unresectable pancreatic or periampullary cancer are relatively low. Of the patients whose biliary obstruction is treated with surgical bypass, approximately 20%–30% will go on to develop GOO as a result of either local tumor growth or the development of progressive metastatic disease if a gastric bypass is not performed concomitantly (Shyr et al., 2000; Sohn et al., 1999). Two meta-analyses including randomized and retrospective data have shown no difference in perioperative morbidity and mortality with significant reduction in long-term GOO. These studies suggest that patients who are found to have unresectable pancreatic or periampullary cancer should have prophylactic gastrojejunostomy at the time of the operation as it adds little perioperative risk and has significant benefit in preventing GOO (Gurusamy et al., 2013; Huser et al., 2009; Lillemoe et al., 1999; Van Heek et al., 2003).

Biliary Obstruction

Patients with disease known to be unresectable at the time of presentation and whose symptoms are related to biliary obstruction alone are often treated with endoscopic or percutaneous biliary decompressive procedures. Numerous studies have examined the efficacy of nonsurgical approaches to biliary obstruction in comparison to surgical palliative procedures in both prospective and retrospective fashion. The main advantage of stenting procedures is the ability to use an endoscopic or percutaneous approach with minimal impact to the patient. However, several problems may arise as a result of stent placement with respect to palliation of symptoms. Often, patients are subjected to repeat interventions to maintain stent patency and position, which when compromised can lead to repeat hospitalizations to manage stent-related complications and infections. Several retrospective studies and three randomized trials have suggested that there is no difference in periprocedural mortality and overall survival between endoscopic and surgical biliary decompression in patients with unresectable pancreatic cancer. One randomized trial showed improved overall survival for surgical decompression, but the number of patients in all of these studies was low (Poruk and Wolfgang, 2016).

Surgical decompression offers some advantages including a reduction in need for maintenance interventional procedures as well as fewer hospital readmissions, but is associated with increased early complications. In addition, both gastric outlet and biliary obstruction can be addressed at the same operation. Endoscopic decompression is associated with shorter length of stay and lower cost but with increased long-term complications (Poruk and Wolfgang, 2016). The recommendation of surgical bypass needs to be made in the context of patient-associated factors, which include anticipated survival (greater than six months), adequate performance status and patient suitability to tolerate general anesthesia with its associated risks.

Minimally Invasive Surgical Techniques

A more recent advancement in surgical palliation of upper gastrointestinal obstruction has been the utilization of laparoscopic techniques for unresectable advanced upper gastrointestinal malignant disease. The comparison of open versus laparoscopic surgical approaches to palliative gastrojejunostomy has yet to be the subject of randomized controlled analysis, though several retrospective analyses have been reported. Recent reports indicate that in expert hands, a laparoscopic gastrojejunostomy may be performed without significant difference in mean surgery time, operative blood loss, postoperative length of stay, median time to tolerate a regular diet and median survival in comparison to an open surgical approach, and may afford the patient early decreased postoperative pain (Bergamaschi et al., 1998; Guzman et al., 2009; Maeda et al., 2017; Navarra et al., 2006; Ojima et al., 2017).

Nonsurgical Options

The most recent development in palliative therapy for GOO has been the employment of self-expanding metal (SEMS) intraluminal stent technology. Stents are also evolving quickly with now both covered and uncovered stents being widely available. Many studies have evaluated the efficacy of stents at relieving GOO and have compared covered and uncovered stents. In systematic reviews comparing covered and uncovered stents, there has been no difference shown in terms of efficacy. However, use of covered stents has a higher incidence of stent migration and a lower incidence of stent obstruction (Minata et al., 2016; Pan et al., 2014). While stents are very effective at relieving GOO, they have a relatively high rate of complications such as migration or obstruction which require re-intervention. Re-intervention is almost always endoscopic rather than surgical.

Comparison between surgical gastrojejunostomy and endoscopic stenting has been the subject of intense review. The techniques have been compared head to head in randomized trials; however, patient numbers in all reported series have been small. There have been multiple meta-analyses of these studies including randomized and retrospective data. These have shown no difference in 30-day mortality, complication rates or survival when comparing surgical gastrojejunostomy and endoscopic stenting. However, endoscopic stenting has been shown to have shorter time to oral intake, shorter length of hospital stay and greater likelihood of tolerating oral intake (Jeurnink et al., 2007a,b; Ly et al., 2010; Minata et al., 2016; Mittal et al., 2004; Zheng et al., 2012). While a difference in rate of complications between the two groups has not been shown, the types of complications certainly are different (Minata et al., 2016).

Therefore, studies show that both endoscopic stenting and surgical gastrojejunostomy are effective and have similar complication rates. The advantage of endoscopic stenting is decreased length of hospital stay, shorter time to oral intake and not requiring general anesthesia. The advantage of surgical gastrojejunostomy is decreased need for re-intervention. Given the increasing ease of access to skilled endoscopists, the ability to perform the procedure with sedation rather than general anesthesia, and the faster recovery and time to oral intake, endoscopic stenting is likely to become increasingly utilized in this setting.

GUIDELINES

On initial presentation of patients with GOO, the mainstay of treatment includes palliation of symptoms, hydration, correction of electrolyte abnormalities and pain control. Our clinical pathway is demonstrated in Figure 20.4. We utilize endoscopy, radiographic imaging and biopsy techniques to determine the extent of malignancy, the potential for resection and the level of gastrointestinal obstruction. Early evaluation of nutritional status and consultation with nutritionist are imperative. All of these patients should also have consultation with the multidisciplinary team including palliative medicine to address and come up with the best individualized plan of treatment. If palliation of unresectable malignancy is the mainstay of care we determine the best treatment strategy by evaluating extent of disease, nutritional status, performance status, underlying malignancy and anticipated survival (Nakakura and Warren, 2007). Based on all of these criteria, and most importantly the patients' and families' specific palliative goals, we then proceed with either endoscopic, surgical or percutaneous treatment options.

ETHICAL ISSUES

As with all interventions the risks and benefits of the procedure must be fully discussed with the patients and their families. A multidisciplinary approach to these difficult situations helps to facilitate

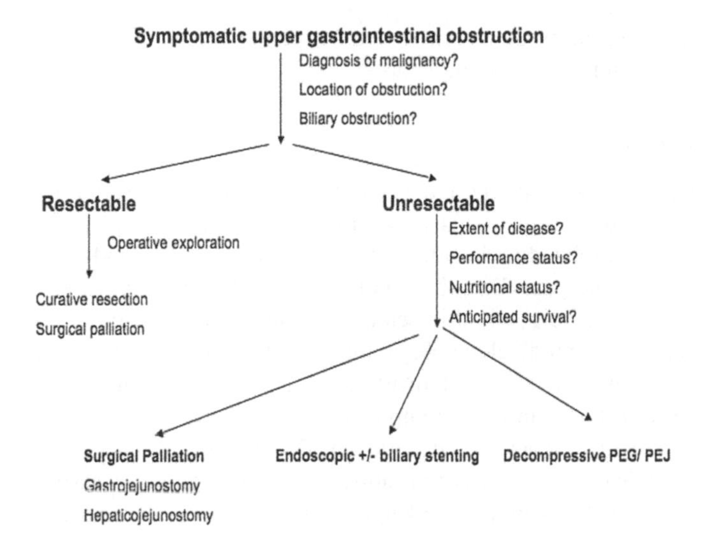

FIGURE 20.4 Management of gastric outlet obstruction. A proposed pathway to facilitate decision-making about management and evaluation of gastric outlet obstruction.

open discussions about reasonable goals of treatment. These treatments need to be individualized to the patient's desires and all the goals of palliation should be discussed and explored to determine the best course of action. If a patient has a more favourable prognosis and can tolerate surgical intervention, we feel that surgical gastrojejunostomy can offer a high success rate and durable palliation without need for multiple re-interventions. This determination is subjective and is based on experience, nutritional reserve, performance status and estimated life expectancy all in attempts to predict operative outcomes.

In patients who clinically appear unable to tolerate operative intervention, endoscopic stenting is likely to be successful and more easily tolerated than gastrojejunostomy. In either clinical scenario, a frank discussion with the patient and his/her caregivers needs to be held about prognosis and the anticipated course of disease so that realistic expectations can be set and discussion of end-of-life issues can take place earlier rather than later.

APPLICATION TO OTHER AREAS OF PALLIATIVE CARE

The advantages of palliative gastrojejunostomy include improving overall nutrition and giving patients who would otherwise no longer be able to eat the ability to do so. Eating is a social activity that greatly contributes to quality of life. In addition, palliative gastrojejunostomy may make patients eligible for other palliative treatments in the form of medications that can be given orally as opposed to injections, for example.

KEY FACTS: PALLIATIVE GASTROJEJUNOSTOMY

- Gastrojejunostomy is an operative procedure in which a connection is made between the stomach and the jejunum to allow ingested food to bypass a blockage caused by a tumor.
- Gastrojejunostomy can safely be performed either through a midline abdominal incision or laparoscopically in a minimally invasive approach.
- The connection between the stomach and the jejunum can be either sewn with sutures or made using a stapling device.
- Potential complications of gastrojejunostomy include bleeding, wound infection, anastomotic leak, anastomotic stricture and delayed gastric emptying.

- In the postoperative course, a patient's diet is typically slowly advanced and the patient is monitored closely for signs of complications.

SUMMARY POINTS

- Gastric outlet and biliary obstruction can arise due to upper gastrointestinal malignancies.
- Presentation includes severe nausea, vomiting, dehydration and abdominal pain with nutritional sequelae related to dehydration, vitamin deficiencies and malabsorption.
- Treatment must be individualized based on patient's desires and symptoms, performance status and life expectancy. A multidisciplinary team including surgery, gastroenterology, nutrition, social work, medical oncology and palliative medicine is imperative.
- Early evaluation of nutrition and institution of parenteral nutrition are necessary to maximize nutrition and minimize complications.
- Surgical bypass and endoscopic stenting offer equally high success rates and complication rates.
- Endoscopic stenting is more likely to require re-intervention but is associated with shorter time to oral intake and shorter hospital length of stay, and does not require general anesthesia.

A frank discussion should be held outlining the likely course of disease and setting realistic expectations early on.

LIST OF ABBREVIATIONS

CT Computed Tomography
GOO Gastric Outlet Obstruction
MRI Magnetic Resonance Imaging
NG Nasogastric Tube
PEG Percutaneous Endoscopic Gastrostomy
PEJ Percutaneous Endoscopic Jejunostomy
SEMS Self-Expanding Metal Stent

REFERENCES

Arciero, CA, Joseph, N, Watson, JC, Hoffman, JP. 2006. Partial stomach-partitioning gastrojejunostomy for malignant duodenal obstruction. *American Journal of Surgery* 191:428–432.

Arrangoiz, R, Papavasiliou, P, Singla, S, Siripurapu, V, Li, T, Watson, JC, Hoffman, JP, Farma, JM. 2013. Partial stomach-partitioning gastrojejunostomy and the success of this procedure in terms of palliation. *American Journal of Surgery* 206(3): 333–339.

Bergamaschi, R, Marvik, R, Thorensen, JE et al. 1998. Open versus laparoscopic gastrojejunostomy for palliation in advanced pancreatic cancer. *Surgery, Laparoscopy, and Endoscopy* 8:92.

Doberneck, RC, Berndt GA. 1987. Delayed gastric emptying after palliative gastrojejunostomy for carcinoma of the pancreas. *Archives of Surgery* 122: 827–9.

Espat, NJ, Brennan, MF, Conlon, KC. 1999. Patients with laparoscopically staged unresectable pancreatic adenocarcinoma do not require subsequent surgical biliary or gastric bypass. *Journal of the American College of Surgeons* 188: 649–55; discussion 655–7.

Geubbels, N, Lijftogt, N, Fiocco, M, van Leersum, NJ, Wouters, MW, de Brauw, LM. 2015. Meta-analysis of internal herniation after gastric bypass surgery. *British Journal of Surgery* 102(5): 451–460.

Gurusamy, KS, Kumar, S, Davidson, BR. 2013. Prophylactic gastrojejunostomy for unresectable periampullary carcinoma. *Cochrane Database of Systematic Reviews* 28(2): CD008533.

Guzman, EA, Dagis, A, Bening, L, Pigazzi, A. 2009. Laparoscopic gastrojejunostomy in patients with obstruction of the gastric outlet secondary to advanced malignancies. *American Surgeon* 75: 129–132.

Helton, WS, Fisichella, PM. 2007. *Intestinal Obstruction. In ACS Surgery Principles and Practice*, 6th edition. Ed. Souba WW, Fink, MP, Jurkovich, GJ et al. 514–533. New York: WebMD Professional Publishing.

Huser, N, Michalski, CW, Schuster, T, Friess, H, Kleeff, J. 2009. Systematic review and meta-analysis of prophylactic gastrojejunostomy for unresectable advanced pancreatic cancer. *British Journal of Surgery* 96(7): 711–719.

Jeurnink, SM, van Eijck, CHJ, Steyerberg, EW et al. 2007a. Stent versus gastrojejunostomy for palliation of gastric outlet obstruction: A systematic review. *BMC Gastroenterology* 7:18.

Jeurnink, SM, Steyerberg, EW, Van't Hof, G et al. 2007b. Gastrojejunostomy versus stent placement in patients with malignant gastric outlet obstruction: A comparison in 95 patients. *Journal of Surgical Oncology* 96: 389–396.

Kaminishi, M, Yamaguchi, H, Shimizu, N et al. 1997. Stomach-partitioning gastrojejunostomy for unresectable gastric carcinoma. *Archives of Surgery* 132: 184–7

Kubota, K, Kuroda, J, Origuchi, N et al. 2007. Stomach-partitioning gastrojejunostomy for gastroduodenal outlet obstruction. *Archives of Surgery* 141: 607–611.

Kumagai, K, Rouvelas, I, Ernberg, A et al. 2016. A systematic review and meta-analysis comparing partial stomach partitioning gastrojejunostomy versus conventional gastrojejunostomy for malignant gastroduodenal obstruction. *Langenbeck's Archives of Surgery* 401(6): 777–85.

Kwon, JJ, Lee, HG. 2004. Gastric partitioning gastrojejunostomy in unresectable distal gastric cancer patients. *World Journal of Surgery* 28: 365–368.

Lillemoe, KD. 1998. Palliative therapy for pancreatic cancer. *Surgical Oncology Clinics of North America* 7:199–216.

Lillemoe, KD, Cameron, JL, Hardacre, JM et al. 1999. Is prophylactic gastrojejunostomy indicated for unresectable periampullary cancer? A prospective randomized trial. *Annals of Surgery* 230:322–328; discussion 328–33.

Ly, J, O'Grady, G, Mittal, A, Plank, L, Windsor, JA. 2010. A systematic review of methods to palliate malignant gastric outlet obstruction. *Surgical Endoscopy* 24(2): 290–297.

Maeda, Y, Shinohara, T, Katayama, T, Minagawa, N, Sunahara, M, Nagatsu, A, Futakawa, N, Hamada, T. 2017. A laparoscopic approach is associated with decreased incidence of SSI in patients undergoing palliative surgery for malignant bowel obstruction. *International Journal of Surgery* 42: 90–94.

Minata, MK, Bernardo, WM, Rocha, RS, Morita, FH, Aquino, JC, Cheng, S, Zilberstein, B, Sakai, P, de Moura, EG. 2016. Stents and surgical interventions in the palliation of gastric outlet obstruction: A systematic review. *Endoscopy International Open* 4(11): E1158–E1170.

Mittal, A, Windsor, J, Woodfield, J et al. 2004. Matched study of three methods for palliation of malignant pyloroduodenal obstruction. *British Journal of Surgery* 91:205–209.

Nakakura, EK, Warren, RS. 2007. Palliative care for patients with advanced pancreatic and biliary cancers. *Surgical Oncology* 16:293–7.

Navarra, G, Musolino, C, Venneri, A et al. 2006. Palliative antecolic isoperistaltic gastrojejunostomy: A randomized controlled trial comparing open and laparoscopic approaches. *Surgical Endoscopy* 20:1831–4.

Ojima, T, Nakamori, M, Nakamura, M, Katsuda, M, Hayata, K, Yamaue, H. 2017. Laparoscopic gastrojejunostomy for patients with unresectable gastric cancer with gastric outlet obstruction. *Journal of Gastrointestinal Surgery* 21(8): 1220–1225.

Pan, YM, Pan, J, Guo, LK, Qiu, M, Zhang, JJ. 2014. Covered versus uncovered self-expandable metallic stents for palliation of malignant gastric outlet obstruction: A systematic review and meta-analysis. *BMC Gastroenterology* 14: 170.

Poruk, KE, Wolfgang, CL. 2016. Palliative management of unresectable pancreas cancer. *Surgical Oncology Clinics of North America* 25(2): 327–337.

Schmidt, C, Gerdes, H, Hawkins, W et al. 2009. A prospective observational study examining quality of life in patients with malignant gastric outlet obstruction. *American Journal of Surgery* 198: 92–99.

Shyr, Y, Su, C, Wu, C, Lui, W. 2000. Prospective study of gastric outlet obstruction in unresectable pancreatic adenocarcinoma. *World Journal of Surgery* 24: 60–65.

Sohn, TA, Lillemoe, KD, Cameron, JL et al. 1999. Surgical palliation of unresectable periampullary adenocarcinoma in the 1990s. *Journal of the American College of Surgeons* 188(6): 658–666.

Vander, AJ, Sherman, JH, Luciano, DS. 1990. *Human Physiology*. 5th edition. New York: McGraw-Hill.

Van Heek, NT, De Castro, SMM, van Eijck, CH et al. 2003. The need for a prophylactic gastrojejunostomy for unresectable periampullary cancer: A prospective randomized trial with special focus on assessment of quality of life. *Annals of Surgery* 238:894–902; discussion 902–905.

Zheng, B, Wang, X, Ma, B, Tian, J, Jiang, L, Yang, K. 2012. Endoscopic stenting versus gastrojejunostomy for palliation of malignant gastric outlet obstruction. *Digestive Endoscopy* 24(2): 71–78.

21 Nutritional Status and Relationship to Upper Gastrointestinal Symptoms in Patients with Advanced Cancer Receiving Palliative Care

Giacomo Bovio and Maria Luisa Fonte

CONTENTS

INTRODUCTION

According to the World Health Organisation (WHO) definition (2016), malnutrition refers to deficiencies, excesses or imbalances in a person's intake of energy and/or nutrients. The term *malnutrition* covers two broad groups of conditions. One is "undernutrition"—which includes underweight (low weight for age) and micronutrient deficiencies or insufficiencies (a lack of important vitamins and minerals). The other is overweight, obesity and diet-related noncommunicable diseases (such as heart disease, stroke, diabetes and cancer).

Patients with advanced cancer are often affected by malnutrition and nutritional issues. Approximately 80% of these patients show cancer cachexia with its characteristic weight loss, anorexia, alterations in metabolism, asthenia, reduced calorie intake, depletion of fat mass and serious muscle catabolism.

Cancer cachexia is a multifactorial syndrome in which there is loss of skeletal muscle mass unresponsive by conventional nutritional support and leads to progressive functional impairment. In this syndrome there is a negative protein and energy balance due to a variable combination of reduced food intake and abnormal metabolism.

The diagnostic criterion for cachexia is weight loss greater than 5% over the past six months, or weight loss greater than 2% in patients with body mass index (BMI) less than 20 kg/m^2, or depleted skeletal muscle mass (sarcopenia).

The European Palliative Care Research Collaborative (2011) has agreed that cachexia syndrome progresses through three distinct stages: precachexia, cachexia and refractory cachexia (Fearon et al. 2011).

Severity can be classified according to degree of depletion of energy stores and body protein (BMI) in combination with degree of ongoing weight loss.

Assessment of classification of cancer cachexia should include anorexia, catabolic status, muscle mass and strength, and functional and psychosocial impairment (Fearon et al. 2011).

Variation in terminology is found around the central concept of cancer-associated malnutrition (Jensen et al. 2010) or cachexia, but regardless of these different terms, the presence of reduced food intake and metabolic derangements (e.g., elevated resting metabolic rate, insulin resistance, lipolysis and proteolysis which aggravate weight loss and are provoked by systemic inflammation and catabolic factors) is consistently accepted.

It is important to underline that all the new terms have appeared in the oncology literature, including sarcopenia, precachexia and refractory cachexia, but are still at the level of proposed terms and cannot at this time be presented as operational (Arends, Bachmann, and Baracos 2017).

In this context, early nutritional assessment is particularly important when dealing with palliative care patients: an adequate nutritional approach could play a fundamental role in improving their quality of life (Table 21.1).

TABLE 21.1
Key Features of Cancer Cachexia Syndrome

1. It is a complex metabolic syndrome often affecting cancer patients.
2. It increases morbidity and mortality.
3. It is different from other secondary anorexia cachexia syndromes since it shows an increase in proinflammatory cytokines.
4. It alters carbohydrate metabolism (increased gluconeogenesis, glucose intolerance and insulin resistance), lipid metabolism (lipolysis activation, increased lipid mobilizing factor) and protein metabolism (increased turnover and proteolysis, increased acute phase proteins, increased proteolysis-inducing factor).
5. It entails weight loss, anorexia, fatigue and other associated symptoms such as impaired oral intake.

Malnutrition: Causes and Consequences

All malnutrition events can be ascribed to the following causes:

- Reduced food intake due to anorexia, nausea, dysphagia, etc.
- Loss of nutrients due to diarrhoea, malabsorption, vomiting, nephrotic syndrome, haemorrhage
- Increased nourishment needs due to surgical operations, sepsis
- Alterations in metabolism caused by neoplasia, such as for example hypermetabolism

Lack of nutrients at the cell level causes biochemical damage due to the alteration of the cell enzymatic systems; then functional damage follows, with either general symptoms such as asthenia, anorexia or specific symptoms; in the end, the damage becomes anatomical.

Malnutrition has serious consequences for all organs and systems.

APPLICATION TO OTHER AREAS OF PALLIATIVE CARE

The assessment of nutritional status is relevant for both home and hospital patients. Nutritional screening represents a basic tool to detect malnutrition and enables the setting up of all necessary measures in order to restore a correct nutritional status. Nutritional assessment should be performed at least once a week, and this is particularly important for malnourished patients.

The importance of a nutritional screening is supported by many articles that state that the correction of malnutrition involves positive effects such as an increase in life expectancy, a reduction in the length of hospitalization, a quicker recovery from ulcers and an improved quality of life.

Nutritional assessment is a prerequisite for taking any nutritional action and carrying out a successful monitoring of nutritional parameters, including an active control of any nutrition-related symptoms.

PRACTICAL PROCEDURES AND TECHNIQUES

There are many different parameters involved in nutritional assessment in clinical practice (weight, height, sex, subcutaneous fat thickness, laboratory analysis, etc.). Each parameter, however, does not by itself allow a correct diagnosis.

The clinical practice of the nutritional assessment usually covers the following issues: case history, dietary records, physical examination, anthropometric measurements and laboratory analysis.

Case History

This enables the assessment of the primitive tumour and any metastases, together with other contingent pathology and medical treatments. In palliative care patients, the assessment of appetite is of particular importance, and it is performed by means of numerical and visual rating scales.

Dietary Records

In order to evaluate food consumption and dietary habits, investigations are carried out by means of a set of recordings made either by qualified personnel or by the patients themselves. Investigation about food intake may cover either a short or a long period of time, possibly using special questionnaires where appropriate.

Food intake inadequacy is considered to be present when the patient cannot eat for more than a week or when the estimated energy intake is less than 60% of requirement for more than one or two weeks.

TABLE 21.2
Weight Classification in Relation to Body Mass Index (BMI)

BMI (kg/m^2)	Weight Classification
<18.5	Underweight
18.5–24.99	Normal weight
25.0–29.99	Overweight
≥ 30.0	Obese

The main evaluation tools are the following:

- *The 24-hour food recall*: This is a recording of food and beverage intake over the previous 24 hours.
- *Diet diaries*: These involve the collection of data based on specific instructions, made either by the patient or by the caregiver, enabling an assessment of serving size and frequencies. Recordings are to be made either over a week or over three non-consecutive days including one Sunday or public holiday.
- *Food frequency questionnaires*: These are usually associated with dietary history. They assess food intake over a day, a week or a longer period.
- *Dietary history*: The reconstruction of the patient's dietary history requires an interview in order to collect data about the food intake over the long term (Table 21.2).

Physical Examination

This is an evaluation of all those elements that may represent markers of malnutrition: measurement of fat mass and muscle mass, examination of the skin and its annexes, detection of pressure ulcers and oedemas.

Anthropometric Assessment

Body Weight

Body weight (BW) is the simplest anthropometric index giving rapid information about a patient's nutritional status. In palliative care units, it is not always easy to weigh patients, since they are often unable to stand. In this event, weighing chairs or hoisting systems are used. Any change in body composition implies a change in BW. When considering this parameter, however, attention should also be given to the actual extent of variation and to its duration in time. An unintentional weight loss greater than 10% over the previous six months is considered a sign of malnutrition and cachexia and implies reduced survival.

To make weight independent from height, the use of the BMI (weight, kg/height, m^2) was introduced (Table 21.3).

Body Height

The height of patients who are unable to stand can be estimated by measuring either their knee height, ulna length or demispan. The patient's height is then estimated by means of formulas and/or tables (Table 21.4).

Circumferences

Circumferences reflect nutritional status and body fat distribution. Arm circumference and waist and hip circumferences are usually measured. Waist and hip circumferences are rarely used in palliative care, whereas they are mostly considered in obese patients.

TABLE 21.3
Height Assessment in Bedridden Patients

Estimating Height (cm) from Knee Height	
Females	84.88 – (0.24 × age) + (1.83 × knee height)
Males	64.19 – (0.04 × age) + (2.02 × knee height)
Estimating Height (cm) from Demispan	
Females	(1.35 × demispan) + 60.1
Males	(1.40 × demispan) + 57.8

Source: Chumlea W.C., 1988. In *Athropometric Standardization Reference Manuals*, ed. T.G. Lohman, A.F. Roche and R. Martorell, Campaign: Human Kinetics Books; Bassey, E.J., 1986. *Annals of Human Biology*, 13:499–502.

Laboratory Analysis

Laboratory analysis is also needed when evaluating nutritional status: routine blood tests, urinalysis, nutrient levels, metabolic balances, immunological tests and functional tests.

The comparison of some laboratory data with data obtained from other nutritional investigations supplies important indexes enabling a further nutritional assessment (i.e., creatinine/height index).

TABLE 21.4
Dietary Record Methods

Methods	Advantages	Disadvantages
Diet diary	• Permits accurate estimates • Accurate method if patient is instructed by professional staff and/or feels deeply motivated	• Time consuming for the patient who must be committed to the task • Requires the patient to be instructed • Applicable only to educated patients • The patient, feeling monitored, might modify his/her dietary habits • High incidence of mistakes and/or incomplete data if compared to the 24-hour food recall
24-hour food recall	• Easy • Direct • Inexpensive • Needs a limited amount of time • Subject does not need to be instructed	• Since it is based on a single day it does not supply sufficient data to compensate for daily, seasonal and festivity variations • Overestimates small intakes and underestimates big intakes • 10% underestimating food consumption
Scale weighing	• Accurate method	• Highly time and personnel consuming • High financial costs • Not applicable when not taking meals at home
Food frequency questionnaires	• Fast and practical method • A survey considering the long period of time	• Diminished accuracy
Dietary history	It gives hints about the patient's overall diet	• Overestimating food consumption, particularly micronutrients • Time consuming

Plasma Proteins

The assessment of low plasma protein levels contributes to the nutritional assessment process, since an inadequate energy-protein intake may result in a decreased synthesis of proteins.

Serum albumin forms a large proportion of plasma proteins, and its reduction may be indicative of malnutrition. On account of both its long half-life (about 15–20 days) and its distribution (it is also found in the extracellular space), albumin does not represent an accurate index of malnutrition when malnutrition is not prolonged in time.

Transferrin is a ß-globulin for iron ion delivery with a half-life of 8–10 days. Since transferrin values are affected by specific pathological conditions and by iron deficiency, they are not an absolute index of malnutrition.

Prealbumin is a carrier of the thyroid hormone thyroxine with a half-life of about two days, and rapidly reflects malnutrition status by modifying its concentration. Its values may be affected by hyperthyroidism, acute infections and trauma.

Retinol-binding protein has a half-life of about 10 hours and carries vitamin A. It is filtered by glomerulus and reabsorbed by renal tubules, thus increasing its value then in the event of renal failure. The reduction in its plasma concentration is a reliable indicator of malnutrition.

The C-reactive protein (CRP) level is a blood marker of inflammation. An elevated CRP level has been associated with increased weight loss and decreased albumin concentration, quality of life, function and survival.

Laboratory Analysis to Assess Muscle Mass

Considering the extent of muscle wasting caused by malnutrition, the collection of creatinuria and 3-methylhistidine is particularly important.

Creatinuria is the end product of skeletal muscle creatinine catabolism. Its values are reliable when renal function is normal and if urine collection occurs after at least two days of creatinine-free diet. By matching the subject values with the corresponding sex/age % reference values, the creatinine/height index is obtained.

As 3-methylhistidine is an amino acid of the fibrillar proteins, its excretion follows the disruption of these proteins. It is a good indicator of muscle catabolism.

Nitrogen Balance

It is the measure of nitrogen output subtracted from nitrogen input, expressed in grams. A negative balance indicates an endogenous protein catabolism. Evaluation is made by distinguishing, respectively, a mild catabolism, range from −5 to −10, moderate −10/−15, serious when greater than −15. The main input of nitrogen comes from diet proteins. Nitrogen output occurs through the excretion of urine and faeces and via the skin.

Immunological Tests

The association between malnutrition and immune system alterations has been widely ascertained. The principal tests used are total lymphocyte counts, T-helper lymphocyte counts and complement fraction 3. Results must be carefully evaluated since alterations in the immune system may also be due to pathologies such as cirrhosis of the liver or renal failure or to drug therapies (steroids, immunosuppressors, etc.).

Functional Tests

Appropriate tests may concern the immune system, capillary and red blood cell fragility, prothrombin time, platelet aggregation, respiratory and muscle function assessment.

There is the possibility, however, of interferences not strictly related to nutrition.

Biochemical analysis in nutritional assessment also includes vitamins, minerals and trace elements.

Hand grip strength (HGS) is an assessment tool of muscle function in clinical settings. A systematic review of HGS as a nutritional marker (Norman et al. 2010) suggests that this measure would be a good indicator of nutrition status. The review also highlights the potential monitoring capabilities of

HGS to detect improvements in nutritional status following supplementation. HGS proved to have a high test and re-test reliability, as well as high inter-rater reliability (Mathiowetz et al. 1985).

Nutritional Screening Tools

Subjective global assessment (SGA) consists of a questionnaire enabling an easy approach to nutritional assessment. It has a first section dealing with medical history and a second section concerning physical examination.

Patients are thus divided into three categories: well nourished, mildly moderately malnourished and severely malnourished.

Thoresen et al. (2002), in a palliative setting, compared SGA results with results obtained from an objective method and they found a high correlation. SGA can be employed in patients receiving palliative care as an easy tool for nutritional assessment.

American Society for Parenteral and Enteral Nutrition guidelines (August and Huhmann 2009) for patients receiving anticancer treatment and for those undergoing haematopoietic cell transplantation, recommend patient-generated subjective global assessment (PG-SGA), SGA and nutritional risk index (NRI) as nutritional assessment tests. The PG-SGA is an adaptation of the SGA. NRI includes measurement of albumin and data on habitual and measured weight.

Other nutritional assessment methods are nutritional risk screening (NRS) and Malnutrition Universal Screening Tool (MUST). Both consider BMI, unintentional weight loss, food intake, clinical condition and/or administered treatment, and classify the risk of malnutrition.

Mini Nutritional Assessment (MNA) is applied to the elderly. It entails anthropometric, general, dietary and subjective assessment and classifies patients as "at risk of malnutrition" or "malnourished." A study (Slaviero et al. 2003) conducted in patients with advanced cancer receiving palliative chemotherapy has ascertained an association between baseline history of weight loss, CRP and MNA score.

ESPEN guidelines (Kondrup et al. 2003) recommend MUST, NRS and MNA for the elderly.

Bauer et al. (2002) verified that PG-SGA is equally effective compared to SGA when assessing the nutritional status of cancer patients in acute-care medical facilities.

The ESPEN expert group suggested three key steps to update nutritional care for cancer patients: screen all patients with cancer for nutritional risk early in the course of their care, regardless of BMI and weight history; expand nutrition-related assessment practices to include measures of anorexia, body composition, inflammatory biomarkers, resting energy expenditure and physical function; use multimodal nutritional interventions with individualized plans, including care focused on increasing nutritional intake, lessening inflammation and hypermetabolic stress, and increasing physical activity (Arends, Baracos and Bertz 2017).

Human Body Composition

Body composition is modified by physiological (age, sex and physical activity), pathological and nutritional issues. Malnutrition affects body composition by diminishing fat and fat-free mass. In addition, malnutrition can alter intra- and extra-cellular volume, and its negative impact on the availability of both ATP and creatine phosphate can compromise the sodium-potassium exchange mechanisms and, consequently, the overall balance of electrolytes.

Hence, the role of body composition data collection should be considered when investigating nutritional status.

Body Composition Measurement Techniques

The main body composition measurement techniques are the following: measurement of the thickness of the subcutaneous fat using a body caliper, bioelectrical impedance analysis (BIA), dual-energy x-ray absorptiometry (DEXA), imaging techniques (ultrasound, computed tomography [CT] and magnetic resonance imaging [MRI] scans) and total body potassium measurement.

TABLE 21.5
Plasma Proteins

Protein	Half-Life	Causes of Alterations	Specificity
Transferrin	8 days	↓ pregnancy, chronic infections, liver cirrhosis etc. ↑ Iron deficiency	Low
Albumin	15–19 days	↓Kwashiorkor, serious organic depletion, malabsorption, liver pathologies, nephropathies, etc.	Low
Pre-albumin	1–2 days	Thyroxine availability	Good
Retinol-binding protein	10 hours	Retinol levels: ↓protein-energy malnutrition	Good

The measurement of the thickness of the subcutaneous fat using a body caliper is an easy, inexpensive and quick method of estimating body fat mass. In clinical practice the following skinfolds are measured: triceps, biceps, iliac crest and subscapular skinfold.

The average of three consecutive measurements should be considered.

Durnin and Womersley (1974) provided a table that makes it possible to quantify the total body fat mass from the sum of the four skinfolds.

The triceps skinfold (Tsf) is important since, together with AC, it gives the arm circumference (AMC) and arm muscle area (AMA).

BIA is a non-invasive technique based on the principle of electrical conduction being different through the different body districts on account of the different amount of water and electrolytes. It measures whole-body impedance, the opposition of the body to alternating current consisting of two components: resistance (R) and reactance (Xc). Resistance is the decrease in voltage reflecting conductivity through ionic solutions. Reactance is the delay in the flow of current measured as a phase shift, reflecting dielectric properties, that is, capacitance, of cell membranes and tissue interfaces.

Over the past years, the BIA application to assess the health status and to predict the outcome of therapy in cancer patients has been studied to some extent. The most commonly used parameter was the phase angle since it incorporates the two directly measured values of resistance and reactance without any further requirement of data derivation.

DEXA considers the body's absorption of photons when irradiated by x-rays at two different energy levels. It is used to evaluate bone mineral density. At present, it is considered as the most reliable body composition assessment technique.

Imaging techniques, such as CT and MRI scanning, assess body fat mass distribution. Ultrasound scans measure the thickness of subcutaneous fat and visceral fat. These techniques are of limited use in clinical practice due to high costs (Table 21.5).

ASPECTS OF NUTRITIONAL STATUS IN PALLIATIVE CARE

There are not many works at present concerning the nutritional evaluation of palliative care patients. The following data refer either to specific studies of nutritional evaluation or to studies aimed at evaluating the effectiveness of artificial nutrition and covering palliative care patients, too.

A Norwegian study of 46 patients (Thoresen et al., 2002), comparing SGA adequacy opposed to traditional methods of nutritional assessment in palliative care patients, showed that 24 patients (52%) had a weight loss greater than 10%. Mean BMI was 23 ± 4.9 kg/m^2. Thirteen patients (28%) had Tsf below the fifth percentile, while 10 patients (22%) had a mid-arm muscular circumference below the fifth percentile.

Albumin and prealbumin were below the normal range in 15 (33%) and in 35 patients (76%), respectively.

A study (Sarhill et al., 2003) was completed on 352 patients with metastatic tumour referrals to a palliative medicine program. Weight loss was detected in 307 patients with 71% showing a weight loss greater than 10% compared to healthy state body weight. BMI showed no alterations due probably to the previous presence of obesity in most patients. Eight-three percent of patients had hypophagia. The authors recorded a reduced energy intake (EI) and body composition alterations: 51% of patients showed a reduction in fat mass (measured by Tsf) and 30% had a reduced AMA. Median albumin was 3.2 g/dL. Sixty-six percent of patients were hypoalbuminemic. Of 50 patients 74% had a high CRP.

In another study (Hutton et al., 2006), 151 patients recruited from a regional cancer centre and palliative care program showed a mean EI of 1610 ± 686 kcal/day, a mean EI/kg/BW of 25.1 ± 10. EI < 34 Kcal/kg/BW/day was assessed in 81% of patients. EI was balanced in proteins (16.3% ± 5.3; 1 ± 0.4 g/kg BW), carbohydrates (55.0 ± 8.5%) and fat (29.7 ± 7.2%). Mean weight loss was 12.7 ± 14.6%.

Out of 144 palliative care patients on a free diet (Bovio et al., 2008), 72/128 patients (56%) reported a weight loss greater than 10%. Tsf and AMA were below the fifth percentile in 23% (33 patients) and in 47% (68 patients), respectively. Mean EI was 1337 ± 578 Kcal/day and was lower than calculated mean resting energy expenditure (REE) (1347 ± 213). Fifty-two percent of patients (75 patients) had EI lower than their REE. Mean EI/kg/BW was 22.56 ± 11. EI was regularly distributed in proteins (15.4 ± 4.8%; 0.88 ± 0.4 g/kg/BW), carbohydrates (52.4 ± 11.6%) and lipids (28.8 ± 9.3%), but 27% of patients (39 patients) were taking less than 0.6 g/proteins/kg/BW/day. Serum prealbumin, serum transferrin and serum albumin were below normal, respectively, in 74%, 74% and 76% of the patients.

Further data on the nutritional assessment of palliative care patients can be found in works about the impact of artificial nutrition on survival, nutritional status and quality of life.

The nutritional risk status and the nutritional support of 621 cancer patients admitted to palliative home care services were investigated by telephone interviews (Orrevall et al., 2009). This showed that 302/593 patients (51%) had a weight loss greater than 10% compared to healthy state body weight. Mean BMI in 596 patients was 22 ± 4 kg/m^2. BMI was less than 18.5 kg/m^2 in 15% of patients. According to a modified NRS-2002 the number of patients at nutritional risk was 419 (68%).

In 2004, Lundholm et al. evaluated 309 patients divided into two groups. One group was receiving cyclooxygenase inhibitors and recombinant erythropoietin; the other group, as well as being treated pharmacologically with the same medications, was also receiving nutritional support. Neither group was being administered any specific cancer therapy due to absence of efficacy. Pretreatment weight loss percentage was 10 ± 1 in the nutritional support and 9 ± 1 in the control group. EI was 1686 ± 56 in the nutritional support group and 1774 ± 49 Kcal in the control group, whereas serum albumin was, respectively, 33 ± 0.4 and 34 ± 0.4 g/L in the nutritional support and in the control group.

Slaviero et al. (2003) considered 73 patients with advanced cancer before palliative chemotherapy treatment with docetaxel and vinorelbine. The aim of the study was to evaluate the relationship between anthropometric, biochemical data and MNA. Nine patients (12%) had weight loss greater than 10%, and six patients (8%) had BMI less than 20 kg/m^2. MNA data showed that 9 patients (12%) were malnourished and 47 (64%) were at nutritional risk. Median albumin and prealbumin were 37.5 g/L and 0.22 mg/L, respectively.

Pironi et al. (1997) studied 164 patients receiving only palliative care. All patients were administered home artificial nutrition (HAN) (135 by enteral and 29 by parenteral nutrition). The aim of the study was to estimate the utilization rate and to evaluate the efficacy of HAN in preventing death from cachexia and in improving patients' performance status. During the study, 18 patients were readmitted to the hospital for palliative radiation or chemotherapy. One hundred thirty-five patients (82%) showed protein-energy malnutrition. Protein-energy malnutrition was diagnosed when BMI was less than 20 in males and less than 19 kg/m^2 in females or when there was a weight loss greater than 10% during the previous six months.

From this work BMI data can also be collected. BMI, after the first month of HAN, was 19 ± 2.7 kg/m^2 in 13 patients, increasing their Karnofsky performance status (KPS) score; 20.9 ± 2.6 kg/m^2 in 19 patients, decreasing their KPS score and 19.5 ± 3.6 kg/m^2 in 132 patients with unmodified KPS.

Bozzetti et al. (2002) studied 69 patients to assess the impact of home parenteral nutrition (HPN) on nutritional status, quality of life and survival. Thirty-six patients (52%) were administered a second- or third-line chemotherapy. This study includes data on the nutritional status assessed before the administration of nutritional therapy. In particular, 56 patients (81%) had weight loss greater than 10%; median serum albumin was 3.3 g/dL; lymphocyte count 1150 cells/mm^3 and serum transferrin 189 mg/dL.

The benefits and risks of nutritional interventions have to be balanced mostly in patients with advanced disease (Arends, Bachmann and Baracos 2017).

Only a few papers have been published recently about nutritional intervention efficacy in palliative care patients. Recently Theilla et al. (2018) suggest that HPN is an important palliative therapy for patients with advanced cancer: 35% out of 153 patients survived for six months, 27% for one year, 18.9% for two years and 3.9% for seven years, then HPN is a relevant therapy for patients with advanced cancer.

In patients with malignant esophageal obstruction, enteral feeding by tube and patients with esophageal stenting had longer median survival, higher calorie intake, higher serum albumin and shorter hospital stay than patients with nil per os (Yang et al. 2015) (Table 21.6).

RELATIONSHIP BETWEEN NUTRITIONAL STATUS AND UPPER GASTROINTESTINAL SYMPTOMS

Yavutzsen et al. (2009) have recently conducted a survey by administering to 95 palliative care patients a 22-item questionnaire aimed at assessing the degree of anorexia and the prevalence of other gastrointestinal symptoms. The severity of weight loss did not influence the prevalence of gastrointestinal symptoms; the most severe anorexia emerged in patients with the highest weight loss. Mean Eastern Cooperative Oncology Group Performance Status (ECOG-PS) was 1.9 ± 1.1.

Another study (Bovio et al. 2009), conducted on 143 palliative care patients with mean ECOG-PS 3.1 ± 0.49, showed an association between the different symptoms of the upper gastrointestinal system and malnutrition parameters. In particular, xerostomia, anorexia and dysphagia for solids showed a higher occurrence in patients with $EI < REE$, whereas dysphagia for liquids mostly affected patients experiencing a weight loss.

EI was lower in patients with xerostomia, nausea, dysphagia for liquids and solids, dysgeusia, hypogeusia and vomiting if compared to patients unaffected by these same symptoms. Patients with anorexia, nausea, dysphagia for solids and liquids showed a higher weight loss compared to that of patients unaffected by these same symptoms, whereas patients with anorexia and hypogeusia showed a lower BMI.

In 105 patients receiving palliative care, those with lung and stomach cancer had the most evidence of malnutrition and higher prevalence of upper gastrointestinal symptoms than patients with colon, liver and breast cancer (Bovio et al. 2014).

ETHICAL ISSUES

The nutritional assessment of palliative care patients should be considered whenever the administration of an adequate nutritional therapy may result in an improved quality of life and performance status. The nutritional assessment of palliative care patients is to be considered ethical and professionally correct even when artificial nutrition is inapplicable.

TABLE 21.6
Nutritional Facts in Patients Receiving Palliative Care

Author	Patients	Weight Loss	Body Mass Index (BMI)	Energy Intake	Body Composition	Other
Thoresen et al. (2002)	46	52% with weight loss >10%; mean weight loss 15 ± 12.3%	23 ± 4.9 kg/m^2		28% had Tsf <5th percentile; 22% had MAMC <5th percentile	Albumin reduced in 15 patients (33%); prealbumin reduced in 35 patients (76%)
Sarhill et al. (2003)	352	71% of 307 patients with weight loss >10%	Median BMI: 23.6 kg/m^2	83% of patients with hypophagia	51% with severe fat deficiency; 30% with significant muscle mass reduction	Increased C-reactive protein in 74%; median albumin: 3.2 g/dL
Hutton et al. (2006)	151	Mean weight loss 12.7 ± 14.6%	23.4 ± 5 kg/m^2	1610 ± 686 kcal/day; 25.1 ± 10 kcal/kg/body weight; proteins 1 ± 0.4 g/kg/day		
Bovio et al. (2008)	144	56% with weight loss >10%; mean weight loss 11.32 ± 11%	22.4 ± 4.2 kg/m^2	1337 ± 578 kcal/day; 22.6 ± 11 kcal/kg/body weight; proteins 0.88 ± 0.4 g/kg/day	23% with Tsf <5th percentile; 47% with arm muscle area <5th percentile	Prealbumin low in 74%; transferrin low in 74%; albumin low in 76%; mean serum albumin 3.1 ± 0.5 g/dL
Orreval et al. (2009)	621	51% with weight loss >10%	22 ± 4 kg/m^2			68% nutritionally at risk
Lundholm et al. (2004)	309	Weight loss 10 ± 1% in nutritional support group and 9 ± 1 in the control group		1686 ± 56 in the nutritional support group and 1,774 ± 49 kcal/day in the control group		Mean serum albumin 33 ± 0.4 in nutritional support and 34 ± 0.4 g/L in control group

(Continued)

TABLE 21.6 (*Continued*)
Nutritional Facts in Patients Receiving Palliative Care

Author	Patients	Weight Loss	Body Mass Index (BMI)	Energy Intake	Body Composition	Other
Slaviero et al. (2003)	73 patients before palliative chemotherapy	9 patients (12%) with weight loss >10%	6 patients (8%) with BMI < 20 kg/m^2			9 patients (12%) malnourished and 47 (64%) at nutritional risk; median albumin and prealbumin were, respectively, 37.5 g/L and 0.22 mg/L
Pironi et al. (1997)	164 patients in home artificial nutrition		19 ± 2.7 kg/m^2 in 13 patients; 20.9 ± 2.6 in 19 patients; 19.5 ± 3.6 in 132 patients			135 patients (82%) with protein energy malnutrition
Bozzetti et al. (2002)	69 patients in home parenteral nutrition	56 patients (81%) with weight loss >10%				Median serum albumin: 3.3 g/dL; median lymphocyte count 1150 cells/mm^3; median serum transferrin 189 mg/dL

Note: Results are expressed as mean ± standard Deviation.
Abbreviations: MAMC, mid-arm muscular circumference; Tsf = triceps skinfold.

KEY FACTS

- Malnutrition affects about 80% of advanced cancer patients.
- Cancer cachexia is a multifactorial syndrome characterised by skeletal muscle mass loss, unresponsive to conventional nutritional support. It leads to progressive functional impairment.
- Malnutrition limits therapy efficacy, quality of life and survival.
- Early nutritional status screening and intervention have positive effects on quality of life for both home and hospital patients.
- Upper gastrointestinal symptoms are associated with malnutrition.

SUMMARY POINTS

- Weight loss, anorexia, alterations in metabolism, asthenia, reduced calorie intake, depletion of fat mass and serious muscle catabolism are the main aspects of malnutrition.
- Nutritional assessment usually covers the following issues: case history, dietary records, physical examination, anthropometric measurements and laboratory analysis.
- The main nutritional screening tools are subjective global assessment, nutritional risk screening, Malnutrition Universal Screening Tool and Mini Nutritional Assessment.
- The benefits and risks of nutritional interventions have to be balanced mostly in patients with advanced disease.
- Recent literature suggests that HPN is an important palliative therapy for patients with advanced cancer.
- The nutritional assessment of palliative care patients is to be considered ethical and professionally correct even when artificial nutrition is inapplicable.

LIST OF ABBREVIATIONS

AC	Arm Circumference
AMA	Arm Muscle Area
AMC	Arm Muscle Circumference
ASPEN	American Society for Parenteral and Enteral Nutrition
BIA	Bioelectrical Impedance Analysis
BW	Body Weight
CRP	C-reactive protein
DEXA	Dual Energy X-Ray Absorptiometry
ECOG-PS	Eastern Cooperative Oncology Group Performance Status
EI	Energy Intake
ESPEN	European Society for Clinical Nutrition and Metabolism
HAN	Home Artificial Nutrition
HGS	Hand Grip Strength
HPN	Home Parenteral Nutrition
KPS	Karnofsky Performance Status
MNA	Mini Nutritional Assessment
MUST	Malnutrition Universal Screening Tool
NRI	Nutritional Risk Index
NRS	Nutritional Risk Screening
PG-SGA	Patient-Generated Subjective Global Assessment
REE	Resting Energy Expenditure
SGA	Subjective Global Assessment
Tsf	Triceps Skinfold

REFERENCES

Arends J., Bachmann, P., and Baracos, V., 2017. ESPEN guidelines on nutrition in cancer patients. *Clinical Nutrition*, 36:11–48.

Arends, J., Baracos, V., and Bertz, H., 2017. ESPEN expert group recommendations for action against cancer-related malnutrition. *Clinical Nutrition*, 36:1187–96.

August, D.A. and Huhmann M.B., 2009. American Society for Parenteral and Enteral Nutrition (A.S.P.E.N.) Board of Directors. A.S.P.E.N. clinical guidelines: nutrition support therapy during adult anticancer treatment and in hematopoietic cell transplantation. *Journal of Parenteral and Enteral Nutrition*, 33:472–500.

Bassey, E.J., 1986. Demi-span as a measure of skeletal size. *Annals of Human Biology*, 13:499–502.

Bauer, J., Capra, S. and Ferguson M., 2002. Use of the scored Patient-Generated Subjective Global Assessment (PG-SGA) as a nutrition assessment tool in patients with cancer. *European Journal of Clinical Nutrition*, 56:779–85.

Bovio, G., Bettaglio, R. and Bonetti G., 2008. Evaluation of nutritional status and dietary intake in patients with advanced cancer on palliative care. *Minerva Gastroenterologica e Dietologica*, 54:243–50.

Bovio, G., Montagna, G., and Bariani C., 2009. Upper gastrointestinal symptoms in patients with advanced cancer:Relationship to nutritional and performance status. *Supportive Care in Cancer*, 17:1317–24.

Bovio, G., Fonte, M.L., and Baiardi, P., 2014. Prevalence of upper gastrointestinal symptoms and their influence on nutritional state and performance status in patients with different primary tumors receiving palliative care. *American Journal of Hospice and Palliative Care*, 31:20–6.

Bozzetti, F., Cozzaglio, L. and Biganzoli E., 2002. Quality of life and length of survival in advanced cancer patients on home parenteral nutrition. *Clinical Nutrition*, 21:281–88.

Chumlea W.C., 1988. Methods of Nutritional Anthropometric Assessment for Special Groups. In *Athropometric Standardization Reference Manuals*, ed. T.G. Lohman, A.F. Roche and R. Martorell, Campaign: Human Kinetics Books.

Durnin, J.V.G.A., Womersley J., 1974. Body fat assessed from total body density and its estimation from skinfold thickness: Measurements on 481 men and women aged from 16 to 72 years. *British Journal of Nutrition*, 32:77–97.

The European Palliative Care Research Collaborative. 2011. Available at: http://www.cancercachexia.com/literature-watch/43_clinical-practice-guidelines-on-cancer-cachexia-in-advanced-cancer

Fearon, K., Strasser, F., and Anker S.D., 2011. Definition and classification of cancer cachexia: An international consensus. *Lancet Oncology* 12:489–95.

Hutton, J.L., Martin, L., and Field C.J., 2006. Dietary patterns in patients with advanced cancer: Implications for anorexia-cachexia therapy. *American Journal of Clinical Nutrition*, 84:1163–70.

Jensen, G.L., Mirtallo, J., and Compher C., 2010. Adult starvation and disease-related malnutrition: A proposal for etiology based diagnosis in the clinical practice setting from the international consensus guideline committee. *Journal of Parenteral and Enteral Nutrition* 34:156–9.

Kondrup, J., Allison, S.P. and Elia M., 2003. ESPEN guidelines for nutrition screening 2002. *Clinical Nutrition*, 22:415–21.

Lundholm, K., Daneryd, P., and Bosaeus I., 2004. Palliative nutritional intervention in addition to cyclooxygenase and erythropoietin treatment for patients with malignant disease: Effects on survival, metabolism, and function. *Cancer* 100:1967–77.

Mathiowetz, V., Kashman, N., and Volland, G., 1985. Grip and pinch strength: Normative data for adults. *Archives of Physical Medicine and Rehabilitation*, 66:69–74.

Norman, K., Stobaus, N., and Gonzalez, M.C., 2010. Hand grip strength: Outcome predictor and marker of nutritional status. *Clinical Nutrition*, 30:135–42.

Orrevall, Y., Tishelman, C. and Permert J., 2009. Nutritional support and risk status among cancer patients in palliative home care services. *Supportive Care in Cancer*, 17:153–61.

Pironi, L., Ruggeri, E. and Tanneberger S., 1997. Home artificial nutrition in advanced cancer. *Journal of the Royal Society of Medicine*, 90:597–603.

Sarhill, N., Mahmoud, F. and Walsh D., 2003. Evaluation of nutritional status in advanced metastatic cancer. *Supportive Care in Cancer*, 11:652–59.

Slaviero, K.A., Read, J.A. and Clarke S.J., 2003. Baseline nutritional assessment in advanced cancer patients receiving palliative chemotherapy. *Nutrition and Cancer*, 46:148–57.

Theilla, M., Cohen, J., and Kagan, I., 2018. Home parenteral nutrition for advanced cancer patients: Contributes to survival? *Nutrition*, 54:197–200.

Thoresen, L., Fjeldstad, I. and Krogstad K., 2002. Nutritional status of patients with advanced cancer: The value of using the subjective global assessment of nutritional status as a screening tool. *Palliative Medicine*, 16:33–42.

Yang, C.W., Lin, H.H., and Hsieh, T.Y., 2015. Palliative enteral feeding for patients with malignant esophageal obstruction: A retrospective study. *BMC Palliative Care*, 14:58.

Yavuzsen, T., Walsh, D. and Davis M.P., 2009. Components of the anorexia-cachexia syndrome: Gastrointestinal symptom correlates of cancer anorexia. *Supportive Care in Cancer*, 17:1531–41.

22 Nutrition and Palliative Surgery for Head and Neck Cancer

Takeshi Shinozaki

CONTENTS

INTRODUCTION

ADVANCED HEAD AND NECK CANCER

Each year, head and neck cancer (HNC) affects up to 600,000 people worldwide (Ferlay et al. 2010). In Japan, there were an estimated 29,200 new cases of HNC and 9,209 deaths due to HNC, which accounted for approximately 4% and 3% of all cancers, respectively (Foundation for Promotion of Cancer Research 2012). Many patients have advanced disease at diagnosis, and their prognosis remains poor despite the emergence of new therapeutic options over the last few decades (Bonner et al. 2006; Lorch et al. 2011; Machiels et al. 2015; Vermorken et al. 2007, 2008). Intensive treatment, which is said to be at "the upper limit of human tolerance" (Corry et al. 2010), has generated problems such as acute and late treatment-related toxicity (Murphy and Deng 2015; Ringash et al. 2015). In general, patients with incurable HNC have one or more of the following specific symptoms (Ledeboer et al. 2006; Lin et al. 2011; Sesterhenn et al. 2015; Suarez-Cunqueiro et al. 2008; Talmi et al. 1995, 1997): (1) functional symptoms associated with eating, speaking, and breathing caused by the anatomical location of the tumor (e.g., dysphagia and dyspnea); (2) late toxicity and comorbidity from previous treatment (e.g., aphonia and xerostomia); (3) complications from medical devices (e.g., feeding tube and tracheostomy cannula); and (4) symptoms caused by a fungating tumor (e.g., cosmetic change, malodor, and bleeding). These symptoms substantially reduce quality of life (QOL) as well as physical functioning.

Most of these symptoms are caused by locoregional lesions. Visceral metastasis is less frequent in HNC than in other cancers (Lokker et al. 2013). Therefore, predicting prognosis accurately is often difficult because lung, liver, or kidney function might remain intact, even if locoregional lesions impair respiration and consciousness.

As HNC progresses, it may cause airway obstruction, esophageal obstruction, and aspiration. Oncologists evaluate a patient and determine whether any curative treatment is possible, but for some patients, curative surgery, radiotherapy, chemotherapy, and other treatments are not indicated. For such patients, the airway might need to be controlled with a tracheostomy tube, and nutrition might need to be provided through a gastrostomy tube or a central venous catheter (Vassilopoulos et al. 1998) (Figure 22.1). Percutaneous endoscopic gastrostomy is useful for treating obstructions of the upper digestive tract. For information on tracheostomy and gastrostomy, please refer to pertinent textbooks.

Nutrition and Quality of Life

Such invasive procedures for controlling the airway and providing nutrition can markedly decrease a patient's QOL, and many patients wish to maintain oral intake for as long as possible. Furthermore, conditions that decrease QOL can continue for more than a year when the function of vital organs, such as the lungs and liver, is not impaired. When patients with advanced cancer of the thoracic esophagus have difficulty swallowing, they have been treated with stents, lasers, and an argon plasma coagulator (Bancewicz 1999; Kubba and Krasner 2000). Stent placement in the thoracic esophagus is an established procedure, although complications can occur (Bancewicz 1999; Bethge and Vakil 2001). However, stent placement in the lower pharynx and cervical esophagus is difficult because of anatomical problems (Kubba and Krasner 2000). Bethge and Vakil reported complications in five of seven cases of stent placement in patients with cancer of the cervical esophagus (Bethge and Vakil 2001), and Moses and Wong found difficulties in the use of self-expanding metal stents in the cervical esophagus but still suggested that this approach may be useful (Moses and Wong 2002). Other reports have suggested that palliative surgery may be appropriate for selected patients (Azuren et al. 1997; Gentile et al. 1999).

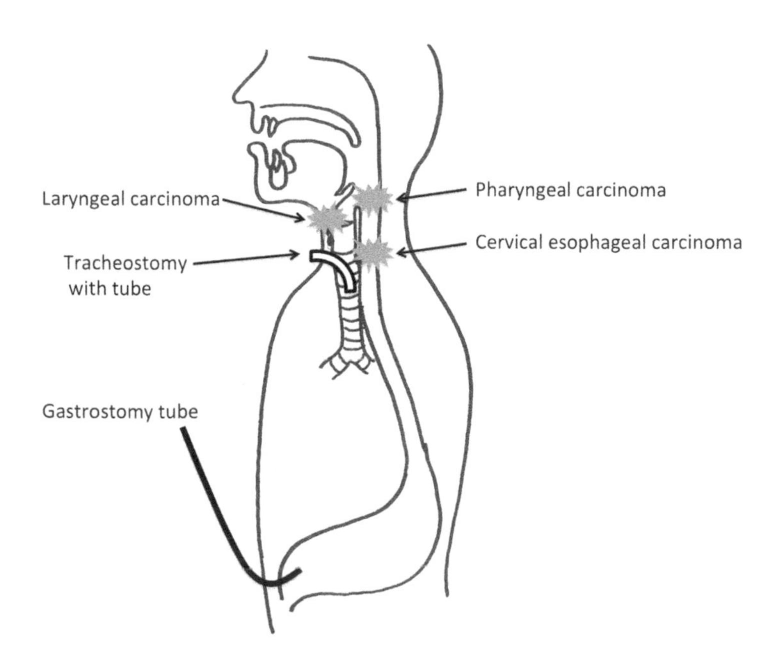

FIGURE 22.1 Problems caused by head and neck cancer. Head and neck cancer causes airway and esophageal obstruction, which may necessitate tracheostomy and gastrostomy.

APPLICATIONS IN OTHER AREAS OF TERMINAL OR PALLIATIVE CARE

The airway takes priority over other areas. Sedation becomes necessary when the oncologist cannot keep a patient's airway open. The medical staff must consider the negative effects on the airway of dysphagia, aspiration, tracheostomy, and a nasogastric tube.

PRACTICAL METHODS AND TECHNIQUES

Palliative Surgery

In total pharyngolaryngoesophagectomy (TPLE), after the larynx, hypopharynx, and cervical esophagus have been excised, the food passage is reconstructed with a free jejunum flap, and a permanent tracheostoma is prepared (Figure 22.2). Resection of the larynx permanently disables phonation by means of the vocal cords, but the permanent tracheostoma enables tube-free airway control. The ability to intake food orally is restored by reconstructing a pathway from the pharynx to the upper gastrointestinal tract. Tumor ulceration, bleeding, and foul odors tend to decrease QOL (Azuren et al. 1997). TPLE may control bleeding, pain, and odors from the primary lesion. In contrast, a well-prepared permanent tracheostoma causes no such problems, and restoration of oral intake ability maintains the pleasure of eating. Therefore, TPLE markedly improves QOL and increases the chances that the patient can be cared for at home (Shinozaki et al. 2007). Many palliative surgeries, such as bypass surgery, have been reported for the treatment of obstruction caused by cancers of the digestive tract.

Complications and Hospitalization

In our hospital, complications of TPLE were evaluated in 269 patients. Additional operations were performed within one month after surgery for 33 patients because of thrombosis or fistulae (12.3%). Six patients (2.2%) died within one month after surgery. Balloon dilation was required to treat postoperative stenosis in 27 patients (10.0%). The mean duration of hospitalization was 22.5 days, and oral intake started an average of 13.7 days after surgery (Sarukawa et al. 2006). Feuer et al.

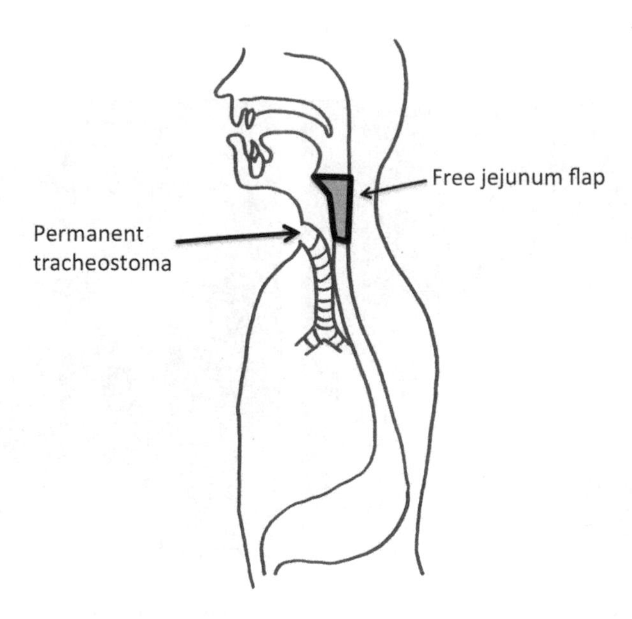

FIGURE 22.2 Diagram of total pharyngolaryngoesophagectomy. The food passage is reconstructed with a free jejunum flap, and a permanent tracheostoma is prepared.

reviewed 22 reports of palliative surgery for obstruction of the lower digestive tract and found mortality rates within 30 days after surgery of 5%–32% (Feuer et al. 1999).

Case 1

A 69-year-old man was admitted to our hospital after T4N2cM0 cancer of the cervical esophagus was diagnosed (Figure 22.3). Central venous nutrition was started because the patient had difficulty with oral food intake but wished to see it improve. Because the tumor had invaded a vertebra, we recommended palliative surgery. TPLE aimed at improving oral intake was performed on October 28. Chemotherapy was not administered because of the patient's poor general condition. The operation lasted 11 hours 10 minutes, and the volume of blood loss was 727 mL. However, the tumor that had invaded the vertebra could not be completely removed. Oral intake was started on postoperative day (POD) 9 and was maintained for 138 days (Figure 22.4). Bougienage was performed on PODs 44 and 121 to dilate the constriction of the jejunoesophageal anastomosis. Irradiation with 70 Gy was started on POD 21. The patient was satisfied with the results of surgery but died on POD 198 of hyposthenia due to growth of the primary tumor.

Case 2

The patient was a 73-year-old man who visited a physician in September and was found to have cancer of the cervical esophagus. An initial examination at our hospital was performed on October 9. Irradiation (60 Gy) and concomitant chemotherapy with cisplatin and 5-fluorouracil were started, but the cancer continued to progress. Oral intake became impossible on December 12 owing to aspiration, and percutaneous endoscopic gastrostomy was performed on December 27. In March 2002 the patient expressed his wish to regain oral intake ability, but at that time radical surgery was considered impossible because of multiple lymph node metastases. TPLE was performed on May 20 with the aim of restoring oral intake ability. Only the primary lesion was excised; neck dissection was not performed. The operation lasted 5 hours 23 minutes, and the volume of blood loss was 240 mL. On the same day, an additional operation was performed to remove an arterial thrombus in the region of anastomosis. Oral intake was started on POD 7 and was maintained for 199 days. Ingestion of steamed rice was possible for a certain period, but the diet mostly consisted of porridge.

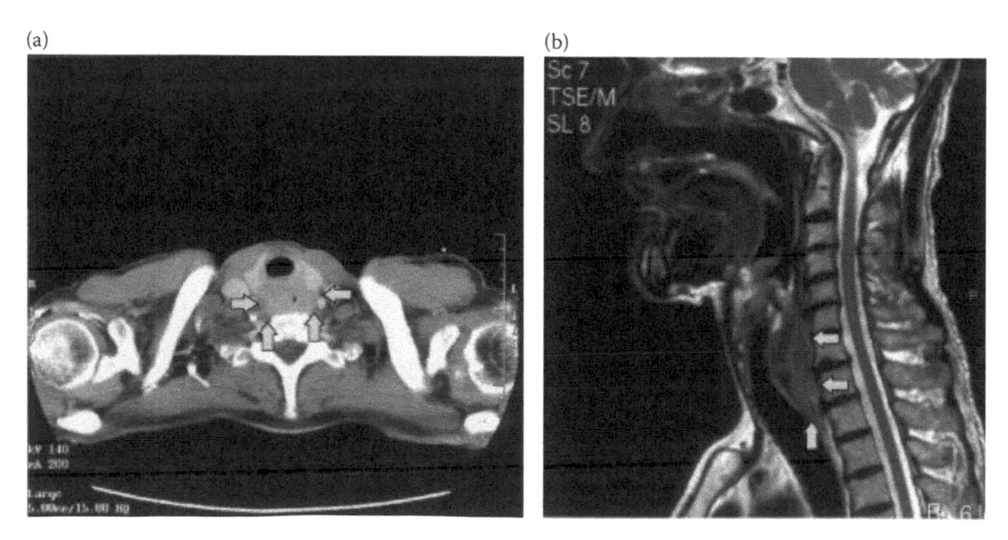

FIGURE 22.3 Enhanced computed tomography (a) and magnetic resonance imaging (T2) (b) of patient 1. Cervical esophageal cancer invaded the vertebra. Prevertebral invasion is evaluated, which is not an indication to undergo curative operation.

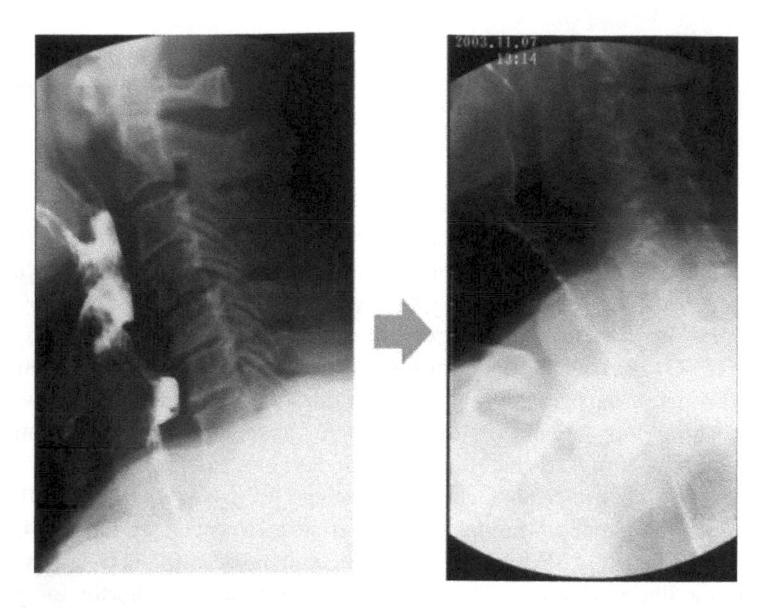

FIGURE 22.4 Videofluoroscopy of patient 1. Preoperative (left) and postoperative (right) images. Pharyngeal clearance was improved after the operation.

Because the patient could eat his favorite foods after some time, he was satisfied with the results of the surgery. He died on POD 269.

Indication

TPLE is an invasive procedure, and deaths may occur in the perioperative period. Of the 269 patients who underwent TPLE at our hospital, 6 (2.2%) died within one month. TPLE requires preoperative and postoperative hospital management and has corresponding associated costs (Kubba and Krasner 2000). This has led to doubts regarding the value of TPLE for patients who cannot undergo radical therapy or for patients in the terminal stage of cancer. Some argue that invasive surgery that cannot achieve complete resolution is not recommended. Surgical treatment should aim to improve symptoms, minimize postoperative complications, and shorten the duration of hospitalization. The indications for surgery should be determined on the basis of an overall evaluation of patient satisfaction and potential risks.

The decision to perform palliative therapy may also depend on current trends and local culture. Until a decade ago, inpatients of palliative care wards in Japan who had laryngeal cancer did not receive tracheotomy for airway obstruction, and some Japanese physicians still believe that palliative surgery or chemotherapy should not be performed for patients with advanced cancer. Furthermore, patients who do not want invasive surgery or blood transfusions may not agree to palliative TPLE. Evaluation of QOL is also very difficult because QOL varies among cultures and cannot be measured with a single scale. Thus, the issue of whether to perform palliative surgery requires further consideration of the beliefs and wishes of patients and other persons concerned (Blazeby et al. 2000). The proficiency of each medical facility should also be taken into account, because morbidity and mortality rates vary among facilities. Maximizing QOL by minimizing morbidity and mortality rates is the goal of palliative TPLE. Treatment should be performed only after patients have received an adequate explanation of possible complications and have given their informed consent (Vandeweyer et al. 2000).

Palliative TPLE is not appropriate for all patients with incurable cancer who wish to maintain oral intake. However, QOL was markedly improved following TPLE in the two patients described here. Both patients were satisfied with the outcomes of the surgery.

Palliative TPLE may be appropriate for selected patients, depending on the location and speed of advancement of lesions, their general condition, and living environment, and in accordance with their wishes and religious and personal beliefs.

Benefit of Gastrostomy

We conducted a multicenter, prospective, observational study to examine QOL and functional status in terminally ill HNC patients. Enteral feeding was required by 53 (73.6%) of 72 patients at baseline and by 43 patients (59.7%) just before death. Oral feeding was possible for 22 (30.6%) of patients at baseline but in only 17 patients (23.6%) just before death. For patients fed through a percutaneous gastrostomy tube (PEG), the time between study enrollment and death was significantly shorter than for patients fed through a nasogastric tube. Median duration of hospitalization was significantly shorter for gastrostomy-fed patients (21 days) than for nasogastric tube–fed patients (64 days, $P < 0.05$, Wilcoxon rank-sum test) (Figure 22.5) (Shinoaki et al. 2017).

Eating is one of the most important factors influencing QOL. We hypothesized that QOL differs among patients receiving nutrition through different routes. However, we did not find a significant difference in EORTC QLQ-C15-PAL between PEG-fed and nasogastric tube–fed patients. However, in this study, the median period of hospitalization was significantly shorter for gastrostomy-fed patients than for nasogastric tube–fed patients (21 versus 64 days). Although artificial nutrition in terminally ill cancer patients is controversial (Good et al. 2008; Raijmakers et al. 2011), this difference might reflect the fact that patients with a PEG tube were able to receive nutrition and medications as long as possible before hospitalization. In other words, patients without a PEG tube may have been hospitalized earlier due to malnutrition than patients with a PEG tube. This is a hypothesis raised by the results of this study, which require confirmation in a future study.

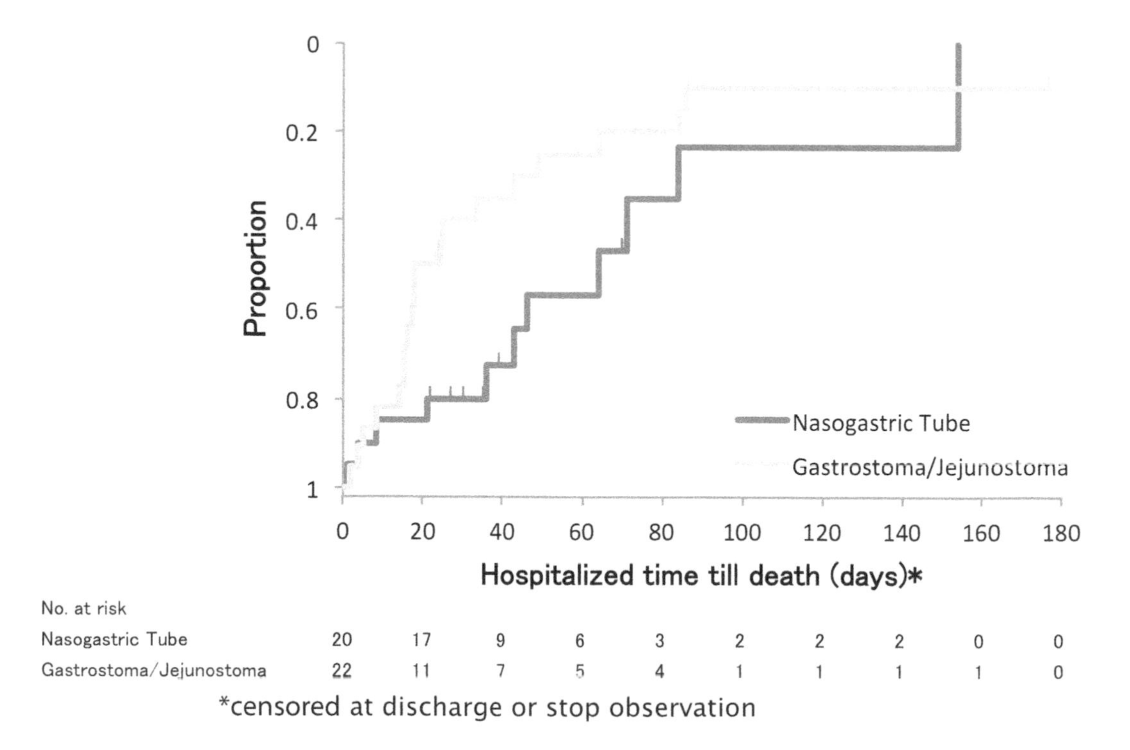

FIGURE 22.5 Duration of hospitalization until death. In patients fed through a percutaneous gastrostomy tube, the length of time between hospitalization and death was significantly shorter than in patients fed through a nasogastric tube.

ETHICAL ISSUES

As mentioned, the decision to perform palliative TPLE may also depend on current trends and local culture. Palliative surgery may be appropriate for selected patients on the basis of the location and speed of advancement of lesions, their general condition, and living environment, and in accordance with their wishes and religious and personal beliefs.

KEY FACTS

- Head and neck cancer is often accompanied by airway and nutrition problems.
- The airway is controlled with an inserted tracheotomy tube.
- These procedures markedly decrease patients' quality of life.
- The route of nutritional intake might be predictive for the duration of the hospital stay.

SUMMARY POINTS

- As head and neck cancer progresses, it often causes airway and esophageal obstruction, which may necessitate tracheostomy, gastrostomy, or central venous nutrition.
- In total pharyngolaryngoesophagectomy, the food passage is reconstructed with a free jejunum flap, and a permanent tracheostoma is prepared.
- Two patients who underwent total pharyngolaryngoesophagectomy were satisfied with the outcomes of the surgery.
- This palliative surgery may be appropriate for selected patients on the basis of the location and speed of advancement of lesions, their general condition, and living environment, in accordance with their wishes and religious and personal beliefs.
- The route of nutritional intake (nasogastric tube versus percutaneous gastric tube) might be predictive of the duration of hospital stay.

LIST OF ABBREVIATIONS

HNC Head and Neck Cancer
POD Postoperative Day
QOL Quality of Life
TPLE Total Pharyngolaryngoesophagectomy

REFERENCES

Azuren DJ, Go LS, Kirkland ML: Palliative gastric transposition following pharyngolaryngoesophagectomy. *Am Surg* 63:410–413, 1997.

Bancewicz J: Palliation in oesophageal neoplasia. *Ann R Coll Surg Engl* 81:382–386, 1999.

Bethge N, Vakil N: A prospective trial of a new self-expanding plastic stent for malignant esophageal obstruction. *Am J Gastroenterol* 96:1350–1354, 2001.

Blazeby JM, Alderson D, Farndon JR: Quality of life in patients with oesophageal cancer. *Rec Results Cancer Res* 155:193–204, 2000.

Bonner JA, Harari PM, Giralt J et al.: Radiotherapy plus cetuximab for squamous-cell carcinoma of the head and neck. *N Engl J Med* 354:567–78, 2006.

Corry J, Peters LJ, Rischin D: Optimising the therapeutic ratio in head and neck cancer. *Lancet Oncol* 11:287–91, 2010.

Ferlay J, Shin H-R, Bray F et al.: Estimates of worldwide burden of cancer in 2008: GLOBOCAN 2008 [Internet]. *Int J Cancer* 127:2893–2917, 2010.

Feuer DJ, Broadley KE, Shepherd JH: Systematic review of surgery in malignant bowel obstruction in advanced gynecological and gastrointestinal cancer. *Gynecol Oncol* 75:313–322, 1999.

Gentile M, Cecere C, Elia S: Palliative surgical treatment of thoracic esophageal cancer. *Minerva Chir* 54:835–842, 1999.

Good P, Cavenagh J, Mather M et al.: Medically assisted nutrition for palliative care in adult patients. *Cochrane Database Syst Rev* 4: CD006274, 2008.

Kubba AK, Krasner N: An update in the palliative management of malignant dysphagia. *Eur J Surg Oncol* 26:116–129, 2000.

Ledeboer QCP, Van der Velden L-A, De Boer MF et al.: Palliative care for head and neck cancer patients in general practice. *Acta Otolaryngol* 126:975–80, 2006.

Lin Y-L, Lin I-C, Liou J-C: Symptom patterns of patients with head and neck cancer in a palliative care unit. *J Palliat Med* 14:556–9, 2011.

Lokker ME, Offerman MPJ, van der Velden L-A et al.: Symptoms of patients with incurable head and neck cancer: Prevalence and impact on daily functioning. *Head Neck* 35:868–76, 2013.

Lorch JH, Goloubeva O, Haddad RI et al.: Induction chemotherapy with cisplatin and fluorouracil alone or in combination with docetaxel in locally advanced squamous-cell cancer of the head and neck: Long-term results of the TAX 324 randomised phase 3 trial. *Lancet Oncol* 12:153–9, 2011.

Machiels J-PH, Haddad RI, Fayette J et al.: Afatinib versus methotrexate as second-line treatment in patients with recurrent or metastatic squamous-cell carcinoma of the head and neck progressing on or after platinum-based therapy (LUX-Head & Neck 1): An open-label, randomised phase 3 trial. *Lancet Oncol* 2045:1–12, 2015.

Moses FM, Wong RK: Stents for esophageal disease. *Curr Treat Options Gastroenterol* 5:63–71, 2002.

Murphy BA, Deng J: Advances in supportive care for late effects of head and neck cancer. *J Clin Oncol* 33:3314–3321, 2015.

Raijmakers NJH, van Zuylen L, Costantini M et al.: Artificial nutrition and hydration in the last week of life in cancer patients. A systematic literature review of practices and effects. *Ann Oncol* 22:1478–86, 2011.

Ringash J: Survivorship and quality of life in head and neck cancer. *J Clin Oncol* 33, 2015.

Sarukawa S, Sakuraba M, Kimata Y: Standardization of free jejunum transfer after total pharyngolaryngoesophagectomy. *Laryngoscope* 116:976–981, 2006.

Sesterhenn AM, Folz BJ, Bieker M et al.: End-of-life care for terminal head and neck cancer patients. *Cancer Nurs* 31:E40–6, 2015.

Shinozaki T, Ebihara M, Iwase S et al.: Quality of life and functional status of terminally ill head and neck cancer patients: A nation-wide, prospective observational study at tertiary cancer centers in Japan. *Jpn J Clin Oncol* 47(1):47–53, 2017.

Shinozaki T, Hayashi R, Yamazaki M: Palliative total pharyngo-laryngo-esophagectomy. *Auris Nasus Larynx*, 34:561–4, 2007.

Suarez-Cunqueiro M-M, Schramm A, Schoen R et al.: Speech and swallowing impairment after treatment for oral and oropharyngeal cancer. *Arch Otolaryngol Head Neck Surg* 134:1299–304, 2008.

Talmi YP, Roth Y, Waller A et al.: Care of the terminal head and neck cancer patient in the hospice setting. *Laryngoscope* 105:315–8, 1995.

Talmi YP, Waller A, Bercovici M et al.: Pain experienced by patients with terminal head and neck carcinoma. *Cancer* 80:1117–23, 1997.

Vandeweyer E, Urbain FC, Andry G: Reconstructive surgical techniques after palliative tumor excision. *Rev Med Brux* 21:423–428, 2000.

Vassilopoulos PP, Filopoulos E, Kelessis N: Competent gastrostomy for patients with head and neck cancer. *Support Care Cancer* 1:479–481, 1998.

Vermorken JB, Mesia R, Rivera F et al.: Platinum-based chemotherapy plus cetuximab in head and neck cancer. *N Engl J Med* 359:1116–27, 2008.

Vermorken JB, Remenar E, van Herpen C et al.: Cisplatin, fluorouracil, and docetaxel in unresectable head and neck cancer. *N Engl J Med* 357:1695–704, 2007.

23 Position of Appetite and Nausea in Symptom Clusters in Palliative Radiation Therapy

Selina Chow, Vithusha Ganesh, Carlo DeAngelis, Caitlin Yee, Henry Lam, Akanksha Kulshreshtha, and Edward Chow

CONTENTS

INTRODUCTION

Cancer patients undoubtedly experience a variety of symptoms associated with their pathology and its treatment. A symptom is defined as a "subjective experience reflecting the biopsychosocial functioning, sensations, or cognition of an individual" (Dodd et al. 2001). Symptoms are multidimensional and can include a patient's perception of prevalence, intensity and distress (Chow et al. 2007). Patients undergoing treatment for advanced cancer experience an array of symptoms which, due to common etiology or causal relationships, can present in clinically significant clusters.

Symptom clusters research in advanced cancer is complicated due to several variables that can confound the symptom experience. Subjective reports of symptom distress can be confounded by long-term experience with the disease, presence of multiple symptoms, duration of disease experience or any other perceptual disorders (Chow et al. 2007; Fan et al. 2007). The "partial mediation model" (Beck et al. 2005) alludes to the complexity in understanding dynamics of symptom concurrence in advanced cancer. The model explains how two symptoms can influence each other indirectly through effects on a common symptom. For instance, pain could affect sleep and indirectly influence subjective reports of fatigue (Beck et al. 2005).

Analyses of causal factors underlying commonly observed symptoms in advanced cancer could provide the theoretical framework for correlations between symptoms in a cluster. Nausea and vomiting are frequently observed in advanced cancer. While nausea is an unpleasant subjective feeling of wanting to vomit, vomiting is the forceful expulsion of gastric contents (Lagman et al. 2005). Metabolic abnormalities, brain metastases, chemotherapy, radiation therapy (RT), constipation and certain medications (i.e., opioids or antibiotics) can dispose a patient to develop nausea and vomiting. Emotional distress (for instance, anxiety and fear) and pain can also stimulate the development of nausea. Nausea and vomiting centres in the medulla have been hypothesized to share common afferent neural pathways (Lagman et al. 2005), which may explain their concurrence in advanced cancer patients (Walsh and Rybicki 2006). Prioritization of certain symptoms by patients can increase the possibility of those symptoms being relieved through clinical intervention. This hypothesis was confirmed for some physical symptoms, such as pain and constipation. However, symptom prioritization had little influence over the alleviation of subjective symptoms such as nausea, fatigue, physical function, role function and activity (Stromgren et al. 2002).

Symptom clusters may be useful in more quickly identifying and treating the underlying pathology that is to blame for the symptoms that invariably present. The importance of including quality of life (QOL) and symptoms as a component of palliative treatment assessment was emphasized by Tannock (1987), who wrote, "When cure is elusive, it is time to start treating the patient and not the tumor."

KEY FEATURES OF SYMPTOM CLUSTERS

What Are They?

- Symptoms rarely occur in isolation, especially in the case of advanced cancer patients. Past reporting indicates that cancer patients experience an average of 11–13 concurrent symptoms. These symptoms are a consequence of the disease and/or the associated treatment (Barsevick et al. 2006).
- They could also have a significant effect on patients' physical, emotional and cognitive sense of well-being.
- Systematic attention to the occurrence of multiple symptoms in cancer patients identified the presence of symptom "clusters."
- Dodd et al. (2001) were among the first to coin the term *symptom clusters* in their research in pain, fatigue and sleep disturbances. They described symptom clusters as having the presence of three or more concurrent related symptoms that may or may not have a common etiology. The suggested strength of these relationships was not specified in the study, nor was the amount of time that all symptoms within a cluster must be present to be considered one.
- Kim et al. (2005) described symptom clusters as two or more related symptoms that occur together, form a stable group, and are relatively independent of other clusters. They also described symptom clusters as affecting disease course, treatment, function, QOL or prognosis, all of which differ from the summation of individual symptoms. The available literature additionally suggests that at least 75% of the symptoms within the cluster, including the most prevalent symptom must be present in order for a patient to be considered as experiencing the cluster.
- Additionally, Miakowski et al. (2004) defined symptom clusters as sharing a common etiology in each individual cluster and having a common variance.

Why Are They Useful?

- Cancer patients report experiencing multiple symptoms, and these predict changes in patient function, treatment failures and post-therapeutic outcomes.

- Many of the earlier clinical studies focused on treating the dimensions of individual symptoms, rather than the multiple symptoms presented by most patients. While studying individual symptoms advanced the understanding of isolated symptoms, this may have explained why single-symptom treatment did not necessarily improve QOL.
- There are new avenues in symptom management and palliative care due to research in symptom clusters, as well as an increased awareness of symptom clusters due to significant research on the influence of concurrent symptoms on patient outcomes.
- This research will be valuable in patient cancer treatment, especially in aiding symptom management and increasing the understanding of disease pathophysiology (Walsh and Rybicki, 2006).

TOOLS USED IN SYMPTOM CLUSTER RESEARCH

The majority of symptom cluster studies in the oncology setting have utilized common assessment tools including the M.D. Anderson Symptom Inventory (MDASI), the Symptom Distress Scale (SDS), and the Edmonton Symptom Assessment System (ESAS). All three instruments assess nausea and lack of appetite. Analytic methodology has also yet to be standardized in symptom cluster research. Factor analyses are most frequently used in this area of research to identify up to four symptom clusters (Kim and Abraham 2008).

In the studies discussed in further detail in this chapter, the ESAS, Spitzer Quality of Life Index (SQLI) and Functional Living Index–Emesis (FLIE) were used. The ESAS is a validated 11-point scale in the cancer population, assessing nine frequently observed symptoms (pain, fatigue, nausea, depression, anxiety, drowsiness, appetite, sense of well-being and shortness of breath) with a rating from 0 to 10 (0 = absence of symptom, 10 = worst possible symptom) (Bruera et al. 1991). The SQLI assesses QOL based on five domains: activity, daily living, health, support and outlook. Each item is scored on a three-point scale from zero to two, with zero being the worst and two the best, yielding a total score ranging from 0 to 10 (Hird et al. 2010). The FLIE is a validated nausea- and vomiting-specific QOL tool to assess the impact of nausea and vomiting on physical activities, social and emotional function, and ability to enjoy meals. This 18-item tool, with half of the items for nausea and the other half for vomiting, has a possible summary score ranging from 18 to 126, where lower scores indicate an increased negative impact on a patient's QOL (Poon et al. 2015).

Three statistical procedures were also utilized: the exploratory factor analysis (EFA), principal component analysis (PCA), and hierarchical cluster analysis (HCA). There is no standard methodology in symptom cluster research, and several other analyses have been used in the literature, aside from the aforementioned three (Kim et al. 2013).

RADIATION-INDUCED NAUSEA/VOMITING

Palliative RT is an established treatment for a variety of malignancies, whether given alone or as a combinatory component with surgery or chemotherapy (Feyer et al. 2005). As palliative interventions are unlikely to lead to prolonged survival and significant tumour regression, QOL and reducing patient symptomology become a more meaningful endpoint when compared with the traditional endpoints, such as survival times and local control. Thus, the therapeutic benefits of treatment must also take into consideration the degree of tolerable side effects.

Approximately one-third of patients undergoing RT experience radiation-induced nausea and vomiting (RINV) (Feyer et al. 2005). There tends to be a distinct pattern of RINV, with an asymptomatic latent period lasting approximately 40–90 minutes, followed by an acute nausea and/or vomiting period of about six to eight hours. Following the acute period is the recovery period. Although these symptoms are usually less severe and less frequent with RT than with chemotherapy, they may still be distressing for a large proportion of RT patients. Thus, this can lead to unplanned interruptions in radiation treatment if the symptoms are prolonged and/or severe. In addition, persistent nausea and vomiting throughout RT may cause dehydration, electrolyte imbalance and malnutrition, further impinging patients' QOL.

RINV has been reported to occur more frequently in patients who receive total-body or half-body irradiation, as well as those who receive radiation to the upper abdomen (Feyer et al. 2005). Other factors that influence radiation-induced emesis are the dose and fractionation given, and patient characteristics (e.g., age, sex, previous nausea and vomiting, etc.). Emesis also increases proportionally with irradiation volume, emphasizing the importance of field size. Increased severity and duration of nausea or vomiting may lead to loss of appetite and/or weight loss.

NAUSEA/VOMITING IN SYMPTOM CLUSTERS

Symptom clusters consisting of loss of appetite and emesis have been identified in the palliative patient population at large. Results from one PCA conducted on ESAS data from initial consultations across several oncology palliative care clinics at their centre, Cheung et al. (2009) identified a cluster containing nausea, decreased appetite, dyspnea, fatigue and drowsiness. This particular cluster accounted for 45% of the total variance and demonstrated high internal reliability, with a Cronbach's alpha coefficient of 0.76. Due to the implications of nausea, decreased appetite, fatigue and drowsiness in cancer-related anorexia-cachexia, the authors suggested the involvement of the syndrome in the etiology of the cluster. Similar findings were observed in several other studies. In a systematic review of symptom clustering in patients with advanced cancer, nausea-appetite loss was found to be one of the four most common clusters, reported by 13 studies (Dong et al. 2014).

The impact of RT on the patient experience may be reflected in symptom cluster research specific to this treatment setting. Similar to the study conducted by Cheung et al., baseline clusters containing nausea and loss of appetite in patients at a palliative RT clinic were produced by both the PCA (nausea, lack of appetite and dyspnea) and EFA (nausea, lack of appetite, tiredness, drowsiness, well-being, pain and dyspnea) (Ganesh et al. 2017). Fan et al. (2007) demonstrated a similar recurring relationship between nausea and lack of appetite in patients before and following RT. In a PCA of ESAS scores from 1,296 palliative patients with various sites of metastases, the group observed that nausea and lack of appetite consistently clustered together from baseline to the end of their follow-up period at 12 weeks' post-radiation. Lack of appetite and nausea also clustered together in both the EFA and HCA methods in a re-analysis of the same dataset (Chen et al. 2012) (Table 23.1).

The following studies have also been conducted with groups of patients with specific disease characteristics.

Bone Metastases

Bone metastases are a frequent complication of cancer. Symptomatic bone metastases can cause patients significant pain and functional interference. Studies have demonstrated pain relief in 60%–70% of patients, as well as stabilization or improvement of QOL with palliative RT (McDonald et al. 2014). RT to bone metastases in the lower abdominal and pelvic region carries a risk of RINV, as serotonin released by damaged gastrointestinal (GI) mucosa acts on receptor cells on afferent neurons and signals an emetic response in the brain (Dennis et al. 2012; Salvo et al. 2012).

In our previous study, the primary objective was to study whether bone pain "clusters" with any other symptoms in 518 patients with bone metastases before and after RT. The secondary objective was to compare and contrast the cluster patterns in responders and non-responders to RT. Three symptom clusters were found using a PCA on patient responses to the ESAS at 1, 2, 4, 8 and 12 weeks post-treatment (Figure 23.1). Shortness of breath, nausea and poor appetite clustered together in the third cluster (Chow et al. 2007). Khan et al. (2012) conducted a re-analysis of the same dataset with the EFA and HCA (Table 23.2). The HCA and PCA methods both found an identical cluster 1

TABLE 23.1
Summary of Symptom Clusters in Patients Receiving Palliative Radiation Therapy

	Baseline			One-Week Follow-Up			Two-Week Follow-Up			Four-Week Follow-Up			Eight-Week Follow-Up			Twelve-Week Follow-Up		
Symptom	**PCA**	**EFA**	**HCA**	**PCA**	**EFA**	**HCA**	**PCA**	**EFA**	**HCA**	**PCA**	**EFA**	**HCA**	**PCA**	**EFA**	**HCA**	**PCA**	**EFA**	**HCA**
Depression	Δ	Δ	Δ	Δ	Δ	Δ	Δ	Δ	Δ	Δ	Δ	Δ	Δ	Δ	Δ	Δ	Δ	Δ
Anxiety	Δ	Δ	Δ	Δ	Δ	Δ	Δ	Δ	Δ	Δ	Δ	Δ	Δ	Δ	Δ	Δ	Δ	Δ
Fatigue	O	O	O	O	O	O	O	O	O	O	O	O	O	O	O	O	O	O
Drowsiness	O	O	O	O	O	O	O	O	O	O	O	O	O	O	O	O	O	O
Pain	X	O	X	X	O	X	X	O	O	O	O	–	Δ	Δ	Δ	O	O	O
Nausea	X	O	X	X	O	X	X	O	O	O	O	O	O	O	O	Δ	O	Δ
Poor appetite	X	O	X	X	O	X	X	O	O	O	O	O	O	O	O	Δ	O	Δ
Dyspnea	O	O	O	O	O	O	O	O	–	O	O	O	O	O	–	Δ	O	–
Poor well-being	X	O	X	Δ	Δ	Δ	Δ	Δ	Δ	Δ	Δ	Δ	Δ	Δ	Δ	Δ	O	Δ

Source: Reproduced from Chen E et al. 2012. *Journal of Pain and Symptom Management*, 44(1):23–32.

Note: Symptoms with corresponding symbols indicate they were in the same cluster. Dashes indicate the symptom was not present in any clusters.

Abbreviations: EFA, exploratory factor analysis; HCA, hierarchical cluster analysis; PCA, principal component analysis.

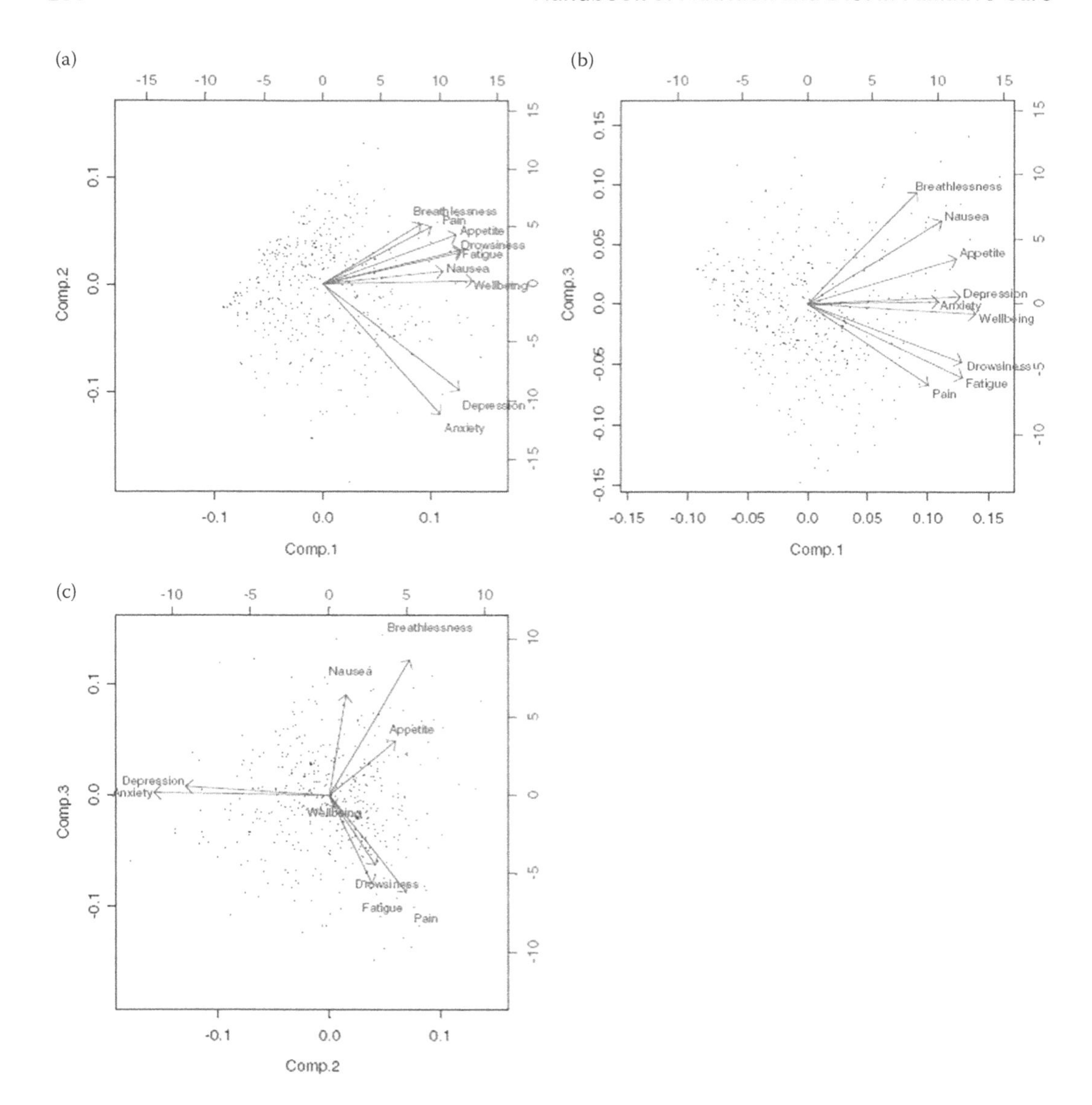

FIGURE 23.1 Biplot among three principal components or clusters in bone metastases patients following radiation therapy. Biplot depicting the planes of a three-dimensional model. The arrows of longer length and closer proximity suggest a higher correlation between symptoms. The cluster was represented in all biplots, but was best evidenced in (c) as all three clusters were evident in the biplot between components 2 and 3. Clusters 2 and 3 were clear in the biplots in (a) and (b). A principal component analysis with varimax rotation was used to transform a number of observed variables into a smaller number of variables (called principal components). (Reproduced from Chow E et al. 2007. *Support Care Cancer*, 15(9):1035–43.)

at baseline, consisting of pain, fatigue, nausea, drowsiness, poor appetite, sense of well-being and dyspnea. At one week following palliative RT, PCA and HCA identified identical symptom clusters, one of which consisted of pain, nausea and poor appetite. EFA grouped fatigue, drowsiness, pain, poor appetite and dyspnea into cluster 2. At the two-week follow-up, PCA and HCA once again derived identical clusters. Cluster 1 included depression, anxiety, nausea, poor appetite, and well-being. EFA's two clusters were composed of fatigue, drowsiness, pain, poor appetite, and dyspnea; and depression, anxiety, nausea and sense of well-being. At the four-week follow-up, EFA and HCA both distinguished a cluster with fatigue, drowsiness, pain, nausea and poor appetite. PCA

TABLE 23.2
Summary of Symptom Clusters in Patients Receiving Palliative Radiation Therapy for Bone Metastases

	Baseline ($n = 518$)			One-Week Follow-Up ($n = 272$)			Two-Week Follow-Up ($n = 297$)			Four-Week Follow-Up ($n = 231$)			Eight-Week Follow-Up ($n = 231$)			Twelve-Week Follow-Up ($n = 193$)		
Symptom	**PCA**	**EFA**	**HCA**	**PCA**	**EFA**	**HCA**	**PCA**	**EFA**	**HCA**	**PCA**	**EFA**	**HCA**	**PCA**	**EFA**	**HCA**	**PCA**	**EFA**	**HCA**
Depression	Δ	Δ	Δ	Δ	Δ	Δ	Δ	Δ	Δ	Δ	Δ	Δ	Δ	–	Δ	Δ	Δ	Δ
Anxiety	Δ	Δ	Δ	Δ	Δ	Δ	Δ	Δ	Δ	Δ	Δ	Δ	Δ	–	Δ	Δ	Δ	Δ
Fatigue	O	O	O	O	O	O	O	O	O	O	O	O	Δ	–	O	O	O	O
Drowsiness	O	O	O	O	O	O	O	O	O	O	O	O	O	–	O	O	O	O
Pain	O	O	O	X	O	X	O	O	O	Δ	O	O	Δ	–	Δ	O	O	O
Nausea	X	O	X	X	Δ	X	Δ	Δ	Δ	O	O	O	O	–	O	X	O	X
Poor appetite	X	O	X	X	O	X	Δ	O	Δ	O	O	O	Δ	–	Δ	Δ	O	Δ
Dyspnea	X	O	X	O	O	O	–	O	–	–	Δ	–	–	–	–	X	O	X
Poor well-being	O	O	O	Δ	Δ	Δ	Δ	Δ	Δ	Δ	Δ	Δ	Δ	–	Δ	Δ	Δ	Δ

Source: Reproduced from Khan L et al. 2012. *World Journal of Oncology*, 3(1):23–32.

Note: Symptoms with corresponding symbols indicate they were in the same cluster. Dashes indicate the symptom was not present in any clusters.

Abbreviations: EFA, exploratory factor analysis; HCA, hierarchical cluster analysis; PCA, principal component analysis.

identified a similar cluster, excluding pain. At eight weeks following treatment, EFA did not identify any symptom clusters. PCA identified two clusters, one composed of drowsiness and nausea, and the other of depression, anxiety, fatigue, pain, poor appetite and well-being. Similar clusters were identified using HCA. Cluster 1 using HCA included fatigue, drowsiness and nausea. Cluster 2 consisted of depression, anxiety, pain, poor appetite and well-being. At the 12-week follow-up, PCA and HCA identified three identical clusters. Cluster 1 was composed of depression, anxiety, poor appetite and well-being. Cluster 3 consisted of nausea and dyspnea. EFA distinguished cluster 2 with fatigue, drowsiness, pain, nausea, poor appetite and dyspnea.

Brain Metastases

Despite the brain being another common site of metastases, afflicting up to 20% of patients with cancer, prognosis remains poor for patients with disease in the brain (Lin and DeAngelis, 2015). A rapid deterioration in patient function is usually expected following diagnosis, with potential devastating effects to social, physical and mental capabilities. Whole brain RT (WBRT) is considered a standard treatment for patients with multiple metastases; whereas stereotactic radiosurgery is recommended for oligometastatic disease. Surgical resection with or without post-operative WBRT is considered for larger masses. A common symptom of this type of metastases, nausea and vomiting can also be a consequence of cerebral edema induced by RT. Other supportive measures such as corticosteroids or antiepileptic medications may be prescribed.

We examined if symptom clusters in patients with brain metastases existed and whether (if present) they changed following WBRT (Chow et al. 2008). Over a period of three years, 170 patients received WBRT. The ESAS was administered at baseline (prior to WBRT), and at 1, 2, 4, 8 and 12 weeks following WBRT. Nausea and poor appetite clustered together, along with poor sense of well-being at baseline. Poor appetite, along with fatigue and drowsiness, were also found to have a significant overall trend of increasing symptom distress over time. Those same three symptoms also revealed worse symptom distress scoring at 12-week follow-up compared with baseline.

A second study by Hird et al. (2010) explored symptom clusters in cancer patients with brain metastases using the SQLI, along with a study-made questionnaire consisting of 17 brain metastases-specific symptoms items (scored as none, mild, moderate or severe). These 17 items included headache, weakness, memory loss, confusion, dizziness, trouble concentrating, decreased alertness, imbalance problems, seizures, speech difficulty, vision problems, problems with smell, hearing or tingling, numbness, fatigue, personality change and nausea and vomiting. Patients in this study completed these two QOL assessments at baseline, and at one-, two-, and three-month follow-up following WBRT. Responses to the SQLI were analyzed using the PCA to identify symptom clusters. The same dataset was later re-analyzed using the EFA and HCA methods in a separate study (Khan et al. 2013).

At baseline, approximately 24% and 21% of patients rated nausea and vomiting, respectively, as mild, moderate or severe (Hird et al. 2010). At each follow-up and across all three analyses, nausea and vomiting consistently clustered together, although the constituents of each symptom cluster changed over time (Table 23.3). The initial study found that by employing an instrument more focused on patients with brain metastases, more symptom clusters were identified (Hird et al. 2010). However, a limitation in investigating the relationship of symptom clusters and WBRT is the absence of a control group in these two studies.

Few studies in this area of research have aimed to find clinically relevant responses, such as QOL outcomes. If WBRT were indeed beneficial in relieving symptoms experienced by patients with brain metastases, the prevalence of a symptom cluster would be expected to diminish. However, this was clearly not the case, as three symptom clusters still appeared at 12 weeks in our study (Chow et al. 2007). In fact, the strength of the internal consistencies of the clusters seemed to strengthen during the 12-week period. The shift of symptoms and increase in cluster strength at 12 weeks may be the result of a changing patient population due to attrition, volatility of a symptom experience in each patient, the effect of WBRT or due to the deterioration of the patients.

TABLE 23.3
Summary of Symptom Clusters in Patients Receiving Whole Brain Radiation Therapy for Brain Metastases

	Baseline			One-Month Follow-Up			Two-Month Follow-Up			Three-Month Follow-Up		
	PCA	EFA	HCA	PCA	EFA	HCA	PCA	EFA	HCA	PCA	EFA	HCA
Headache	X	X	X	X	X	X	X	X	O	X	O	X
Weakness	O	Δ	O	Δ	Δ	O	Δ	Δ	Δ	Δ	Δ	Δ
Memory loss	O	O	O	O	O	O	O	O	X	O	O	O
Confusion	O	O	O	O	O	O	O	O	X	O	O	O
Dizziness	X	O	X	X	Δ	X	X	X	O	X	X	X
Trouble concentrating	O	O	O	O	O	O	O	O	X	O	O	O
Decreased alertness	O	O	O	O	O	O	O	O	O	Δ	O	Δ
Imbalance problems	O	O	O	O	O	O	X	X	O	O	O	O
Seizures	Δ	Δ	Δ	Δ	Δ	Δ	X	X	O	Δ	Δ	Δ
Speech difficulty	Δ	X	Δ	O	O	O	Δ	O	X	O	T	O
Vision problems	O	Δ	O	O	O	O	Δ	Δ	Δ	X	X	X
Problems with smell/hearing/tingling	O	O	Δ	X	Δ	X	X	X	O	O	O	O
Numbness	Δ	Δ	Δ	Δ	Δ	Δ	Δ	Δ	Δ	Δ	Δ	Δ
Fatigue	O	O	O	O	O	O	Δ	Δ	Δ	X	X	X
Personality change	Δ	O	Δ	O	O	O	O	O	X	O	T	O
Nausea	X	X	X	X	X	X	T	T	X	X	X	X
Vomiting	X	X	X	X	X	X	T	T	X	X	X	X

Source: Reproduced from Khan L et al. 2013. *Supportive Care in Cancer*, 21:467–73.
Note: Symptoms with corresponding symbols indicate they were in the same cluster. Dashes indicate the symptom was not present in any clusters.
Abbreviations: EFA, exploratory factor analysis; HCA, hierarchical cluster analysis; PCA, principal component analysis.

Gastrointestinal Cancers

The most significant factor in emetogenic risk for patients receiving radiation is anatomical site, with treatment to the upper abdomen carrying a 60%–90% risk of RINV and treatment to the lower abdomen carrying a 30%–60% risk. Patients with GI cancer are typically radiated in this area. Dong et al. (2016) observed that appetite clustered with nausea and vomiting in patients receiving various therapies for colorectal cancer.

Analyzing symptom clusters in FLIE data from 86 GI patients receiving curative or palliative RT with a PCA, Poon et al. (2015) observed strong correlations at all follow-up intervals between nausea's effect on patients' ability to make meals and its effect on patients' willingness to spend time with family or friends. These results highlight other ways in which nausea may indirectly impact diet (e.g., meal preparation).

APPLICATIONS TO OTHER AREAS OF PALLIATIVE CARE

Several studies explored in this chapter reported nausea, vomiting and lack of appetite to be prevalent in patients at baseline, preceding any RT. Clustering of these symptoms in palliative patient populations has been well noted in the literature, irrespective of therapies used (Cheung et al. 2009). Emesis and weight loss concern clinicians of patients with advanced malignant and non-malignant disease alike (Collis and Mather, 2015).

Recognizing that certain symptoms tend to occur concurrently allows for better management to improve patients' QOL. The knowledge that certain symptoms share a common etiology or are consequential of one another may better facilitate the development and prescription of therapies, while limiting poly-pharmacy and its associated toxicities (Kirkova et al. 2010). Due to these potential implications on treatment, further research and knowledge translation of symptom cluster research has been increasingly advocated for palliative care (Bennion and Molassiotis 2013).

GUIDELINES

Clustering of emesis and loss of appetite in patients receiving palliative RT provides further support for the management of RINV. Patients receiving RT with emetic risk should be offered anti-emetics, as outlined in evidence-based guidelines released by the Multinational Association of Supportive Care in Cancer/European Society for Medical Oncology (MASCC/ESMO) (Aapro et al. 2016).

As far as clinical practice is concerned, symptom clusters, much like the expected symptoms of a given syndrome, may be useful in more quickly identifying and treating the underlying pathology that is to blame for the symptoms that invariably present.

Symptoms within a cluster may or may not have the same origin, and symptoms must have stronger relationships within the same cluster than with symptoms in other clusters. There is still substantial debate concerning a universal working definition of symptom clusters. A lack of consensus on a symptom assessment tool and statistical methodology is a limitation in the extrapolation of findings and generalization of symptom clusters from various studies.

Cancer patients report experiencing multiple symptoms, and these predict changes in patient function, treatment failures and post-therapeutic outcomes. They may have an adverse effect on patient outcomes and have synergistic effects as a predictor of patient morbidity. Adoption of objective measures of symptom presence and severity, administered by trained nurses or physicians, could eliminate problems associated with a subjective self-report questionnaire. It is important to recognize cancer symptoms as dynamic constructs, to understand the comprehensive character of the disease process and potentially improve symptom assessment and management.

When the intent of radiation is palliation, the effect that it has on QOL and symptom distress should be considered. Further investigation is warranted to determine the validity of the clusters. Investigation of symptom clusters in brain metastases should also take into account the steroid dose, given that symptoms such as loss of appetite, lethargy and breathlessness may be directly affected by steroid use.

Symptom clusters in advanced cancer may be specific to the type of cancer, treatment or a combination of factors. Thus, assessment tools specifically designed and validated for a particular cancer population are preferred over a general questionnaire to ensure the extraction of symptom clusters that are relevant to the specific symptomology of that cancer. Future research should focus on physiological mechanisms underlying the expression of symptom clusters specific to advanced cancer.

ETHICAL ISSUES

There are currently no ethical issues to be noted. Symptom cluster research focuses on exploring the extent and strength to which symptoms can occur together, and thus capturing how concurrent symptoms may negatively affect patients' QOL.

KEY FACTS

- As a consequence of their treatment and/or disease, patients with advanced cancer can experience a multitude of symptoms which can occur concurrently in clusters.
- Symptoms in these clusters may be related to one another through causal relationships or common etiology.
- Radiation-induced nausea/vomiting may lead to electrolyte imbalances, dehydration, malnutrition, weight loss and weakness.
- Nausea and loss of appetite often clustered together at baseline and during many of the follow-ups for bone metastases patients.
- Nausea may also indirectly impact diet in palliative patients through impairing patients' ability to make meals, and their willingness to spend time with family/friends.
- In order to prevent treatment-induced nausea/vomiting, physicians should follow the appropriate antiemetic regimens outlined by clinical guidelines.

SUMMARY POINTS

- It is important to monitor how symptom clusters observed in a palliative cancer population change over time, to establish a definite relationship between symptoms within a cluster and to provide information on the effectiveness of management strategies commonly employed to treat or contain the cancer.
- Symptom clusters in advanced cancer may be specific to the type of cancer, treatment or a combination of both factors.
- Radiation-induced nausea/vomiting, which happens in one-third of patients, may impinge on patients' quality of life due to problems such as electrolyte imbalances, dehydration, malnutrition, weight loss and weakness.
- Following radiation therapy for bone metastases, nausea and loss of appetite often clustered together during many of the follow-ups for bone metastases patients.
- Brain metastases patients who received palliative radiation therapy had the symptoms of nausea and vomiting consistently clustering together at each follow-up. These were just 2 of the 17 brain metastases-specific symptoms that consistently remained together, suggesting whole brain radiation therapy was not able to weaken the clusters and perhaps not able to improve quality of life.

ACKNOWLEDGEMENTS

We thank the generous support of Bratty Family Fund, Michael and Karyn Goldstein Cancer Research Fund, Joey and Mary Furfari Cancer Research Fund, Pulenzas Cancer Research Fund, Joseph and Silvana Melara Cancer Research Fund, and Ofelia Cancer Research Fund.

REFERENCES

Aapro M, Gralla RJ, Herrstedt J, Molassiotis A, Roila F. 2016. MASCC/ESMO antiemetic guideline. Retrieved August 4, 2017 from: http://www.mascc.org/assets/Guidelines-Tools/mascc_antiemetic_guidelines_english_2016_v, 1.

Barsevick A, Whitmer K, Nail LM et al. 2006. Symptom cluster research: Conceptual, design, measurement, and analysis issues. *Journal of Pain and Symptom Management*, 31(1):85–95.

Beck SL, Dudley WN, Barsevick A. 2005. Pain, sleep, disturbance, and fatigue in patients with cancer: Using a mediation model to test a symptom cluster. *Oncology Nursing Forum*, 32(3):542.

Bennion AE, Molassiotis A. 2013. Qualitative research into the symptom experiences of adult cancer patients after treatments: A systematic review and meta-analysis. *Supportive Care in Cancer*, 21(1):9–25.

Bruera E, Kuehn N, Miller MJ, Selmser P, Macmillan K. 1991. The Edmonton Symptom Assessment System (ESAS): A simple method for the assessment of palliative care patients. *Journal of Palliative Care*, 7(2):6–9.

Chen E, Nguyen J, Khan L et al. 2012. Symptom clusters in patients with advanced cancer: A reanalysis comparing different statistical methods. *Journal of Pain and Symptom Management*, 44(1):23–32.

Cheung WY, Le LW, Zimmermann C. 2009. Symptom clusters in patients with advanced cancers. *Supportive Care in Cancer*, 17(9):1223–30.

Chow E, Fan G, Hadi S, Filipczak L. 2007. Symptom clusters in cancer patients with bone metastases. *Support Care Cancer*, 15(9):1035–43.

Chow E, Fan G, Hadi S et al. 2008. Symptom clusters in cancer patients with brain metastases. *Journal of Clinical Oncology*, 20:76–82.

Collis E, Mather H. 2015. Nausea and vomiting in palliative care. *British Medical Journal*, 351:h6249.

Dennis K, Zhang L, Lutz S et al. 2012. International patterns of practice in the management of radiation therapy-induced nausea and vomiting. *International Journal of Radiation Oncology Biology Physics*, 84(1):49–60.

Dodd MJ, Miakowski C, Paul SM. 2001. Symptom clusters and their effect on the functional status of patients with cancer. *Oncology Nursing Forum*, 28:465–70.

Dong ST, Butow PN, Costa DSJ et al. 2014. Symptom clusters in patients with advanced cancer: A systematic review of observational studies. *Journal of Pain and Symptom Management*, 48(3):411–48.

Dong ST, Costa DS, Butow PN et al. 2016. Symptom clusters in advanced cancer patients: An empirical comparison of statistical methods and the impact on quality of life. *Journal of Pain and Symptom Management*, 51(1):88–98.

Fan G, Hadi S, Chow E. 2007. Symptom clusters in patients with advanced-stage caner referred for palliative radiation therapy in an outpatient setting. *Support Cancer Therapy*, 4:157–162.

Feyer P, Maranzano E, Molassiotis A et al. 2005. Radiotherapy-induced nausea and vomiting (RINV): Antiemetic guidelines. *Support Care Cancer*, 13(2):122–8.

Ganesh V, Zhang L, Chan S et al. 2017. An update in symptom clusters using the Edmonton Symptom Assessment System in a palliative radiotherapy clinic. *Supportive Care in Cancer*, 25:3321–7.

Hird A, Wong J, Zhang L et al. 2010. Exploration of symptom clusters within cancer patients with brain metastases using the Spitzer Quality of Life Index. *Supportive Care in Cancer*, 18(3):335–42.

Khan L, Cramarossa G, Chen E et al. 2012. Symptom clusters using the Edmonton Symptom Assessment System in patients with bone metastases: A reanalysis comparing different statistical methods. *World Journal of Oncology*, 3(1):23–32.

Khan L, Cramarossa G, Lemke M et al. 2013. Symptom clusters using the Spitzer Quality of Life Index in patients with brain metastases – A reanalysis comparing different statistical methods. *Supportive Care in Cancer*, 21:467–73.

Kim HJ, McGuire DB, Tulman L et al. 2005. Symptom clusters: Concept analysis and clinical implications for cancer nursing. *Cancer Nursing*, 28:270–84.

Kim HJ, Abraham IL. 2008. Statistical approaches to modeling symptom clusters in cancer patients. *Cancer Nursing*, 31(5):E1–10.

Kim HJ, Abraham I, Malone PS. 2013. Analytical methods and issues for symptom cluster research in oncology. *Current Opinion in Supportive Palliative Care*, 7:45–53.

Kirkova J, Walsh D, Aktas A, Davis MP. 2010. Cancer symptom clusters: Old concept but new data. *American Journal of Hospice and Palliative Care*, 27(4):282–8.

Lagman RL, Davis MP, LeGrand SB, Walsh D. 2005. Common symptoms in advanced cancer. *Surgical Clinics of North America*, 85(2):237–55.

Lin X, DeAngelis LM. 2015. Treatment of brain metastases. *Journal of Clinical Oncology*, 33(30):3475–84.

McDonald R, Chow E, Rowbottom L et al. 2014. Quality of life after palliative radiotherapy in bone metastases: A literature review. *Journal of Bone Oncology*, 4(1):24–31.

Miakowski C, Dodd M, Lee K. 2004. Symptom clusters: The new frontier in symptom management research. *Journal of the National Cancer Institute Monographs*, 32:17–21.

Poon M, Dennis K, DeAngelis C et al. 2015. Symptom clusters of gastrointestinal cancer patients undergoing radiotherapy using the Functional Living Index-Emesis (FLIE) quality-of-life tool. *Supportive Care in Cancer*, 23(9):2589–98.

Salvo N, Doble B, Khan L et al. 2012. Prophylaxis of radiation-induced nausea and vomiting using 5-hydroxytryptamine-3 serotonin receptor antagonists: A systematic review of randomized trials. *International Journal of Radiation Oncology Biology Physics*, 82(1):408–17.

Stromgen AS, Goldschmidt D, Groenvold M et al. 2002. Self-assessment in cancer patients referred to palliative care: A study of feasibility and symptom epidemiology. *Cancer*, 94(2):512–7.

Tannock IF. 1987. Treating the patient, not just the cancer. *New England Journal of Medicine*, 317:1534–5.

Walsh D, Rybicki L. 2006. Symptom clustering in advanced cancer. *Supportive Care in Cancer*, 14:831–6.

24 Vitamin Deficiency in Patients with Terminal Cancer

Renata Gorska and Dominic J. Harrington

CONTENTS

INTRODUCTION

We are entirely dependent on dietary and other exogenous sources of vitamins to satisfy our requirements. A suboptimal supply of these nutrients disturbs metabolic networks and has a wide variety of repercussions. The first half of the twentieth century was the golden age for the identification and characterisation of vitamins, discoveries that originated from the detailed investigation of pathological changes induced by severe deficient states. Sensitive laboratory-based assays for the direct measurements of vitamin blood levels were subsequently developed, and applied to the further study of vitamins in health and disease. Although the determination of circulatory levels gives a good indication of current body stores/dietary exposure for some vitamins, greater insight can often be gained when these assays are used in combination with functional biomarkers that directly reflect status within target tissues.

CHALLENGES FACED BY PATIENTS WITH TERMINAL CANCER

In addition to poor dietary intake, surgical and nonsurgical interventions used for the treatment of cancer can induce vitamin deficiencies. The absorption of vitamins is reliant on the gastrointestinal tract; interventions that compromise the functionality of this system diminish bioavailability. Radiation therapy can cause damage to the gastrointestinal mucosa, while chemotherapy regimes may impair epithelial cell function (Figure 24.1). Malabsorption as a consequence of diarrhoea is an added complication associated with chemotherapy (Davila and Bresalier 2008; Stein, Voigt, and Jordan 2010).

In some patients, demand for a specific vitamin may exceed an apparently adequate dietary intake. For example, radiation therapy and chemotherapy increase free radical formation, potentially leading to the greater utilisation of vitamins with antioxidant properties (Jonas et al. 2000). Deficient states can also arise through the sequestering of nutrients to support tumour progression. Drug hepatotoxicity (Davila and Bresalier 2008) provides an additional challenge by impeding the utilisation of some vitamins despite replete tissue stores, leading to the development of functional deficient states.

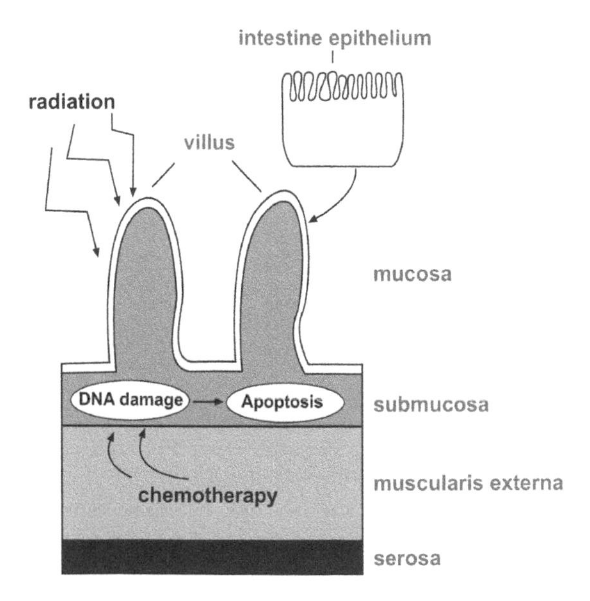

FIGURE 24.1 Structure of the small intestinal wall and effects of chemotherapy and radiation. Chemotherapy and radiation therapy may severely damage the intestinal mucosa, impeding micronutrient absorption.

FAT-SOLUBLE VITAMINS

Fat-soluble vitamins are absorbed from the proximal intestine and dependent on bile and pancreatic juice secretion for solubilisation (Figure 24.2). Any condition causing the prolonged intestinal malabsorption of fat will lead to a secondary deficiency of fat-soluble vitamins. Deficient states lead to the depletion of tissue stores and are indicated by a decrease in circulatory levels long before pathological changes develop. Sensitive assays for all four fat-soluble vitamin groups are available (Table 24.1).

VITAMIN A

Vitamin A is a generic term for compounds with retinol activity, for example, various aldehyde (retinal), alcohol (retinol) and acid (retinoic acid) forms. The main circulatory form is retinol bound to retinol-binding protein. Vitamin A is required for physiological processes that include vision, maintenance of mucosal barriers, haematopoiesis, bone development and immunocompetence (Ball 2004).

Recently absorbed retinol is transported to hepatic stellate cells for storage as retinyl esters. The mobilisation of these stores to counter dietary restriction or malabsorption is sufficient to maintain circulatory levels and satisfy metabolic demand for several months. The vitamin A status of patients with terminal cancer has not been widely studied. Retinoids have been used in therapy in survivors of breast cancer, hepatocellular carcinoma and head and neck cancers. Recent evidence shows that vitamin A is a valuable therapeutic and chemopreventive agent (Okuno et al. 2004; Bunaciu and Yen 2015).

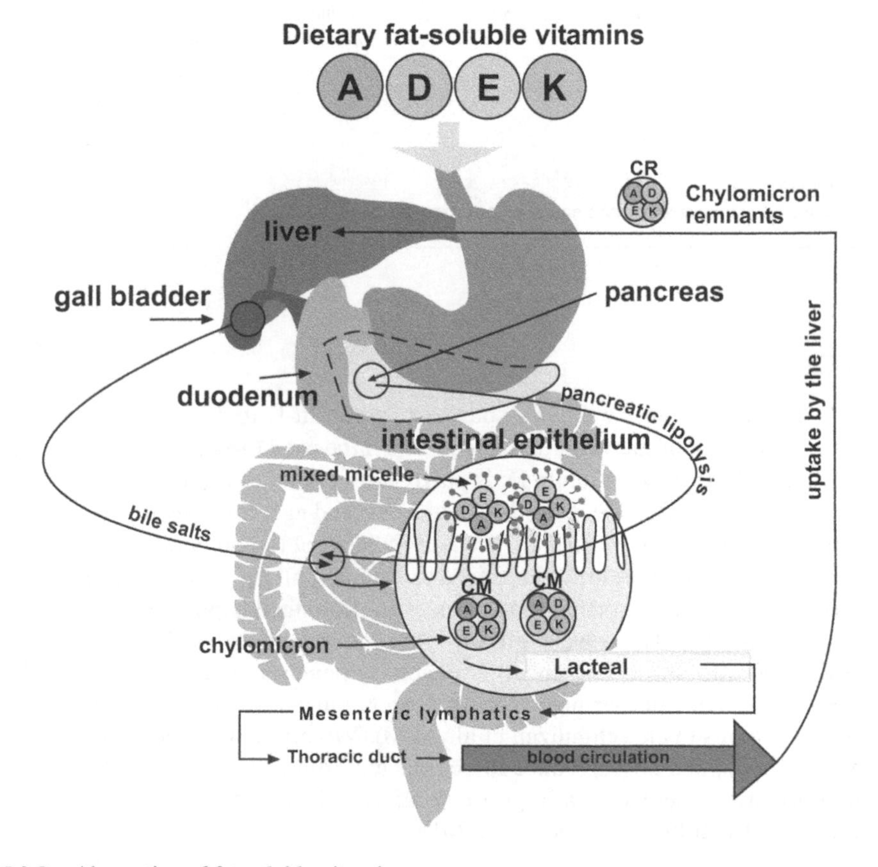

FIGURE 24.2 Absorption of fat-soluble vitamins.

TABLE 24.1
Fat-Soluble Vitamins

	Major Functions	Recommended Daily Allowance (RDA)[a]	Effects of Deficiency	Laboratory Test Available
Vitamin A	Vision, reproduction, growth and development, cellular differentiation, immune function	900 μg/day	Night-blindness, keratomalacia, impaired mucus secretion	Plasma retinol, plasma retinol/retinol-binding protein molar ratio, fasting plasma retinyl esters
Vitamin D	Regulation of calcium and phosphate blood levels, bone mineralisation control of cell proliferation and differentiation modulation of immune system	5 μg/day[b]	Impaired bone mineralisation, osteomalacia	Plasma 25-hydroxycholecalciferol, plasma 25-hydroxyergocalciferol
Vitamin E	Antioxidant, maintain nervous system	15 mg/day	Neurological disorders, haemolytic anaemia	Plasma α-tocopherol
Vitamin K	Coenzyme for a vitamin K–dependent carboxylase, blood coagulation bone metabolism	120 μg/day[b]	Bleeding, osteoporosis, coronary heart disease	Plasma phulloquinone (vitamin K_1), des-carboxy-prothrombin (PIVKA-II), undercarboxylated osteocalcin (ucOC), osteocalcin, urinary vitamin K metabolites, urinary γ-carboxyglutamic acid (Gla)

[a] RDA in adult male.
[b] Adequate intake (AI) is indicated because no RDA can be established.

VITAMIN D

The patient's dependence on the dietary sources of vitamin D to satisfy physiological need is dependent on the amount of the vitamin that can be synthesised through exposure to sunlight. In turn, production of 25-hydroxy-vitamin D_3 is partly a function of the patient's skin pigmentation (darker pigmentation less effective at northern latitudes) and age, since the thinning of the skin on the elderly patient diminishes epidermal 7-dehydrocolesterol (its precursor) (Holick, Matsuoka, and Wortsman 1989). Brief periods of exposure to bright sunlight generate sufficient vitamin D in white patients, although at northern latitudes even prolonged exposure will bring no benefit during the winter months. The wavelength of light required to convert 7-dehydrocholesterol to previtamin D_3 (290–315 nm, UV-B range) is unable to penetrate glass (Ball 2004). Vitamin D supplementation showed improvement in pain scores, muscle weakness and quality of life in prostate cancer patients (Van Veldhuizen et al. 2000). Vitamin D treatment in palliative cancer patients may reduce opioid doses, reduce infections and improve quality of life (Bergman et al. 2015). This pilot study has led to a large randomised, placebo controlled study; it started in November 2017 and will finish in December 2019.

VITAMIN E

Vitamin E is a generic term for a group of tocopherols and tocotrienols. α-Tocopherol is most commonly studied because it is stored by the body, and deficient states can be reversed using this vitamin. α-Tocopherol is an antioxidant with a role in the preservation of cell membranes and may protect against oxidative stress. Ninety percent of α-tocopherol is stored in adipose tissue; these reserves are released slowly during dietary restriction to buffer vitamin E status (Blatt, Leonard, and Traber 2001). A decrease in dietary α-tocopherol intake or malabsorption is not reflected by a corresponding decrease in circulatory levels for approximately one month.

Many studies have implicated suboptimal vitamin E status with the development of several cancers. Vitamin E deficiency leads to erythrocyte haemolysis and the development of neurological disorders. Plasma levels of vitamin E were not compromised in male patients with colorectal tumours (Saygili et al. 2003). Of interest, however, vitamin E supplementation has been shown to have a neuroprotective effect in patients treated with cisplatin chemotherapy (Pace et al. 2010). Vitamins A and E and their combinations have been tried in patients with cancer being treated with chemotherapy, and/or with radiation therapy. Recent analysis demonstrated that vitamin A and E topical application had performed better on oral mucositis than systemic administration (Chaitanya et al. 2017).

VITAMIN K

Vitamin K is a cofactor for γ-glutamyl carboxylase, which catalyses the post-translational modification of specific peptide-bound glutamate residues into γ-carboxyglutamate in vitamin K–dependent proteins. The liver synthesises seven vitamin K–dependent proteins that have a crucial role in blood coagulation (factors II, VII, IX and X; proteins C, S and Z). Extrahepatic vitamin K–dependent proteins (osteocalcin, matrix Gla protein, Gas6 and periostin) are implicated in bone formation, mineralisation, regulation and repair. The most abundant forms of vitamin K are phylloquinone (vitamin K_1), which is present in plants and accounts for ~90% of dietary vitamin K intake; and the menaquinones (vitamins K_2), which are of bacterial origin.

In the United Kingdom, the daily dietary vitamin K reference value is 1 μg/kg, an intake that is regarded as adequate with respect to maintenance of normal coagulation function.

An inadequate supply of vitamin K prevents the optimal γ-carboxylation of vitamin K–dependent proteins. These proteins lack functionality and are referred to as protein-induced vitamin K absence (PIVKAs). The measurement of PIVKA-II (undercarboxylated factor II) is a functional indicator of vitamin K status, since PIVKA-II is not detectable at appreciable concentrations in the circulation of healthy adults. The prothrombin time (or international normalised ratio [INR]) is a poor indicator of vitamin K status (Suttie 1992). Hepatic stores of vitamin K_1 are rapidly (less than three days) depleted during dietary restriction (Usui et al. 1990).

The vitamin K concentration in plasma shows a linear correlation with triglyceride in acute-phase response, similarly to other lipid-soluble vitamins such as vitamin A and E. Plasma phylloquinone concentrations in patients with critical illness should therefore be interpreted with caution and expressed as the plasma phylloquinone:triglyceride ratio (Azharuddin et al. 2007). The susceptibility of patients with cancer to vitamin K deficiency has been highlighted in two studies. In the first, autologous bone marrow transplantation was linked with a rapid fall in circulatory levels of vitamin K_1 (Elston et al. 1995). In the second study, very low serum vitamin K_1 concentrations were present in a fifth of palliative care patients suggesting poor tissue stores 1 (Harrington et al. 2008). A precarious vitamin K status was confirmed by elevated levels of PIVKA-II in 78% of patients recruited to this study. In the prospective cohort study, higher intakes of menaquinones were reported to be associated with common forms of cancer including prostate, lung, breast and colorectal. Dietary intake of menaquinones was nonsignificantly inversely associated with overall cancer incidence, and the association was stronger for cancer mortality. There was no association with phylloquinone intake (Nimptsch et al. 2010).

WATER-SOLUBLE VITAMINS

Water-soluble vitamins have a wide array of functions (Table 24.2). With the notable exception of vitamin B_{12} only limited the quantities of water-soluble vitamins are stored within tissue. To facilitate absorption across the enterocytes, vitamin-specific membrane transport processes have evolved within the small intestine (Figure 24.3).

VITAMIN C (ASCORBIC ACID)

Early signs of vitamin C deficiency include general fatigue, anorexia and depression. Severe deficiency leads to scurvy, which is characterised by capillary bleeding, perifollicular haemorrhage, gingivitis and poor wound healing. Scurvy develops within one to three months of absolute dietary vitamin C restriction, when the body pool size falls below 300 mg (normal pool size ~1500 mg).

Low circulatory levels of vitamin C are common in patients with advanced cancer (Saygili et al. 2003) and an association with prognosis has been described (Mayland, Bennett, and Allan 2005). The incidence of vitamin C deficiency in critically ill patients has also been investigated (Schorah et al. 1996; Alexandrescu, Dasanu, and Kauffman 2009). Several recent studies have shown that oral and intravenous supplementation in terminal cancer patients relieve a number of cancer and chemotherapy-related symptoms, such as fatigue, insomnia, loss of appetite, nausea and pain (Carr, Vissers, and Cook 2014; Mochamat et al. 2017).

FOLATE (VITAMIN B_9)

Folate has an array of biological functions that include the production of purine and pyrimidine nucleotides for DNA synthesis and repair, and the regulation of gene expression through the synthesis of the methyl group donator S-adenosylmethionine (SAM) (Ball 2004).

Patients with advanced cancer develop folate deficiency for several reasons: inadequate dietary intake sustained over a period of one to four months; malabsorption; exposure to folate-antagonists; and the sequestering of folate by tumour cells. A deficient state can also be induced through vitamin B_{12} deficiency, whereby folate is trapped as methyl derivatives leading to a shortage of nomethylated forms to support DNA and RNA synthesis (Figure 24.4).

Through its DNA repair function, folate is considered to be protective against the initial development of cancer; however, existing tumours are dependent on the availability of folate to support rapid growth and propagation. It is for this reason that folate antagonists are widely used as chemotherapeutic agents to retard tumour cell proliferation.

Folate status is typically assessed by measurement of serum folate levels. This has the disadvantage of only providing an insight into folate intake during the preceding few days. Since the folate content of erythrocytes is fixed at erythropoiesis, red cell–based folate assays reflect mean status over 100–120 days (the time that red cells circulate). Both of these assays report the sum of many different types of folate and are unable to differentiate between the various circulatory forms. Many factors influence the spectrum of folates present in the circulation, including common methylenetetrahydrofolate reductase polymorphisms and vitamin B_{12} or B_2 deficiency (Pfeiffer et al. 2004). This can lead to misinterpretation when assays of vitamin total folate are utilised. Circulatory levels of homocysteine are a functional marker of folate status. 5-Methyltetrahydrofolate, the most abundant form of folate, is an essential methyl donor for the methionine synthase and vitamin B_{12}–mediated conversion of homocysteine to methionine. Circulatory levels of patient homocysteine >15 μmol/L are consistent with folate and/or vitamin

TABLE 24.2
Water-Soluble Vitamins

	Major Functions	Recommended Daily Allowance (RDA)[a]	Effects of Deficiency	Laboratory Test Available
Vitamin B_1 (Thiamine)	Coenzyme in the metabolism of carbohydrates and branched-chain amino acids	1.2 mg/day	Beriberi, Wernicke-Korsakoff syndrome, confusion, cardiac failure, nerve membrane disorder	Thiamine diphosphate, erythrocyte transketolase index (early marker of thiamine deficiency), α-keto acids in urine
Vitamin B_2 (Riboflavin)	Coenzyme in numerous redox reactions	1.3 mg/day	No severe specific deficiency syndrome; impacts on vitamin B_3, B_6, B_9; cheilosis, angular stomatitis	Riboflavin, flavin adenine dinucleotide (FAD), flavin mononucleotide (FMN), erythrocyte glutathione reductase activity
Vitamin B_3 (Niacin)	NAD and NADP act as acceptor or donor of electrons for redox reactions	16 mg/day	Pellagra: dermatitis, diarrhoea, dementia	Urinary excretion of N'-methyl-nicotinamide, N′-methyl-2-pyridone-5-carboxamide, no reliable blood test available
Vitamin B_5 (Pantothenic acid)	Needed for formation of coenzyme A, is essential for the metabolism of carbohydrates, fats and proteins	5 mg/day[b]	No severe specific deficiency syndrome, painful peripheral neuropathy	Urine pantothenic acid
Vitamin B_6 (Pyridoxine)	Amino acids metabolism, glycogen phosphorylase (release of glucose from stored glycogen); in brain – synthesis of the neurotransmitter, serotonin from the amino acid, tryptophan, dopamine; niacin formation – critical reaction in the synthesis of niacin from tryptophan; hormone function	1.3 mg/day	Irritability, depression, confusion, inflammation of the tongue, sores or ulcers of the mount, ulcers of the skin at the corners of the mouth	Pyridoxal 5-phosphate (PLP), urinary excretion of 4-pyridoxic acid
Vitamin B_7 (Biotin)	Enzyme cofactor, prosthetic group for four carboxylase enzymes; synthesis of fatty acids, amino acids and glucose, energy metabolism, excretion metabolism of by-products from protein metabolism, maintenance of healthy hair, toenails and fingernails	30 μg/day	Very rare, hair loss, scaly red rash around the eyes, nose, mouth and genital area, neurological disorders	Biotin, 3-hydroxyisovaleric acid and 3-hydroxyisovaleryl carnitine, biotinylated 3-methylcrotonyl-CoA carboxylase (holo-MCC), propionyl-CoA carboxylase (holo-PCC)

(*Continued*)

TABLE 24.2 (*Continued*)
Water-Soluble Vitamins

	Major Functions	Recommended Daily Allowance (RDA)[a]	Effects of Deficiency	Laboratory Test Available
Vitamin B_9 (Folate)	One-carbon metabolism of nucleic acids and amino acids	400 μg/day	Megaloblastic anaemia, fatigue, palpitations	Red blood cell folate(s), serum folate(s), plasma 5-methyltetrahydrofolate, homocysteine
Vitamin B_{12} (Cyanocobalamin)	Coenzyme for methionine synthase, coenzyme for metabolism of methylmalonate to succinate (coenzyme L-methylmalonylcoenzyme A mutase)	2.4 μg/day	Megaloblastic anemia, pernicious anaemia, gastrointestinal lesions, neurological damage	Serum B_{12}, methylmalonic acid (MMA), urine MMA, holotranscobalamin (TC), homocysteine
Vitamin C (Ascorbic acid)	Controlling redox potential within cells, hydroxylation reactions, formation of collagen, required to maintain iron in the reduced state, reduces potentially carcinogenic free radicals to non-radical form	90 mg/day	Scurvy, failure of wound healing, anaemia	Ascorbic acid, dehydroascorbic acid, urine dipstick test, ascorbate present in leucocytes

[a] RDA in adult male.
[b] Nutrients indicate adequate intake (AI) because no RDA can be established.

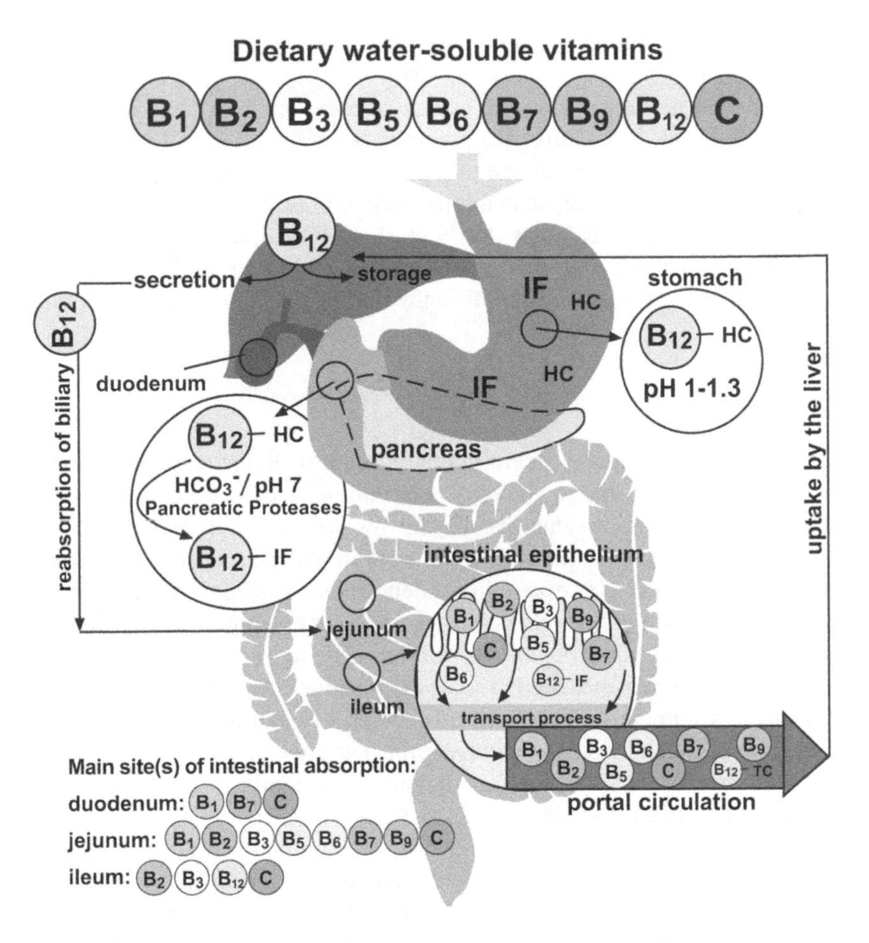

FIGURE 24.3 Absorption of water-soluble vitamins with particular reference to vitamin B_{12}. (HC, holohaptocorrin; IF, intrinsic factor; TC holotranscobalamin.)

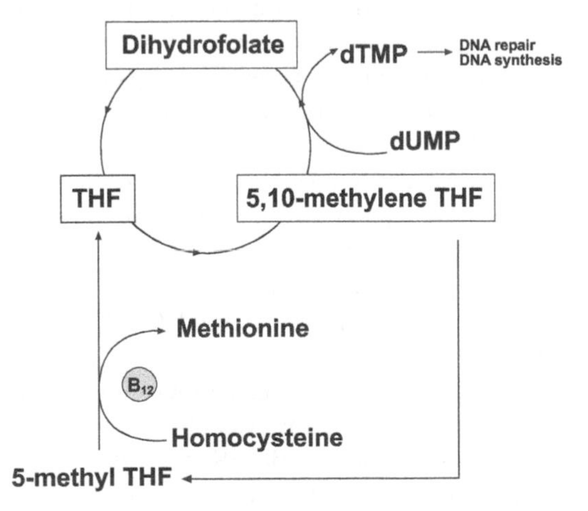

FIGURE 24.4 Interrelation between folate, vitamin B_{12} and homocysteine metabolism. Vitamin B_{12} is required for the conversion of 5-methyl THF to 5,10-methylene THF and the metabolism of homocysteine to methionine. (B_{12}, vitamin B_{12}; dTMP, deoxythymidine monophosphate; dUMP, deoxyuridine monophosphate; THF, tetrahydrofolate.)

B_{12} deficiency provided the patient has good renal function (functional tests for vitamin B_{12} status is outlined in Section 26.3.3).

The correction of folate deficiency with excessive doses of folic acid, an artificial chemical analogue of folate, is of concern. Unlike the naturally occurring dietary folates, folic acid is fully oxidised and unsubstituted. The conversion of folic acid to its physiological form is dependent on dihydrofolate reductase. When the capacity of this enzyme (~400 μg/d) is exceeded, unmetabolised folic acid accumulates in the circulation (Kelly et al. 1997). Circulatory folic acid is associated with decreased natural killer cytotoxicity (Troen et al. 2006). In addition, the masking of the haematological symptoms of vitamin B_{12} deficiency that may lead to neurological damage is well known.

VITAMIN B_{12}

Vitamin structure B_{12} has the largest and most complicated structure of all vitamins. In the centre of this structure is a cobalt ion; hence, the term "cobalamin" is used for any compound possessing vitamin B_{12} activity. Vitamin B_{12} is synthesised by microorganisms and enters the food chain in food of animal origin. Deficient states induced by poor dietary intake (i.e., vegetarian or vegan chain diets) take up to 20 years to manifest. However, clinical deficiencies as a consequence of abnormalities in one of the multiple steps that regulate cobalamin absorption or enterohepatic circulation present more rapidly (approximately two years) (Figure 24.3). Ultimately, intestinal uptake of vitamin B_{12} takes place in the ileum by a receptor-mediated process that includes the calcium-dependent binding of a vitamin B_{12}/intrinsic factor complex, whereby this complex is translocated through the enterocytes to the portal circulation and bound to transcobalamin. The cobalamin-saturated form is referred to as holotranscobalamin (holoTC), whereas apo-holotranscobalamin refers to the unsaturated form (Ermens, Vlasveld, and Lindemans 2003).

The measurement of serum levels of vitamin B_{12} is commonly used as a marker of vitamin B_{12} status. It is often not widely appreciated that circulatory vitamin B_{12} is predominately bound to two proteins and that "front-line" laboratory assays do not discriminate between these forms. Although ~80% of vitamin B_{12} is carried by haptocorrin (holohaptocorrin, abbreviated as HC), extrahepatic cellular receptors have not been described. HoloTC facilitates receptor-mediated uptake of cobalamin therein to all cells. Circulatory levels of HC decline slowly in response to the onset of a deficient state, typically taking three to six years to fall below the lower limit of most assay reference ranges. Circulatory levels of holoTC fall quickly and give an early indication of deficiency, although in assays that cannot discriminate between these two forms this decline is masked by the more abundant HC. Deficiency of vitamin B_{12} is common in patients with serum levels within the reference range and can be revealed by measuring holoTC, methylmalonic acid assay (MMA) and/or homocysteine (Harrington 2017).

In humans the functions of two enzymes are dependent on vitamin B_{12}: methylmalonyl-CoA mutase and methionine synthase. Methylmalonyl-CoA mutase vitamin converts methylmalonyl-CoA to succinyl-CoA. When the supply of of vitamin B_{12} is suboptimal, this reaction cannot proceed, leading to the increased formation of methylmalonic acid.

Methionine synthase is folate mediated and essential for the synthesis of methionine from homocysteine (Section 26.3.2).

Functional vitamin B_{12} deficiency is common in patients with advanced malignancy. Improvement in chemotheraphy-induced peripheral neuropathy was observed in patients with both functional vitamin B_{12} deficiency and neurologic abnormalities (Schloss et al. 2015; Solomon 2016). In over 50% of patients with hepatocellular carcinoma, elevated levels of HC are found, most likely as a result of diminished clearance by the liver (Ermens et al. 2003). In other cancers, breast, pancreatic, stomach and colon, large increases in both unsaturated TC and HC are occasionally seen. Elevated serum vitamin B_{12} levels and their relation to C-reactive protein have been evaluated as a predictive factor of prognosis (Kelly, White, and Stone 2007). Other studies suggested that carcinoid tumours are associated with the development of pernicious anaemia (Rybalov and Kotler 2002). In patients with advanced colorectal cancer treated with chemotherapy, serum levels of vitamin B_{12}, folate and homocysteine were satisfactory pre- and post-therapy. Interestingly, patients with subclinically low vitamin B_{12} prior to treatment had greater survival than patients with higher values (Bystrom et al. 2009).

VITAMIN B_6

Pyridoxal and the phosphate ester derivative pyridoxal 5′-phosphate account for 75%–80% of the circulatory forms of vitamin B_6. Vitamin B_6 deficiency has been implicated in the development of diseases affected by steroid hormones, including prostate and breast cancers. An inverse association between dietary vitamin B_6 intake and risk for colorectal adenoma or cancer has also been reported (Wei et al. 2005). Few studies have investigated the vitamin B_6 status of terminally ill patients with cancer. No deterioration in status was seen in patients with advanced breast cancer treated with megestrol acetate or tamoxifen (Schrijver et al. 1987). Recent data from the prospective study in women with breast cancer during chemotherapy showed that even though there was adequate intake during the treatment, it was not enough to ensure adequacy after the end of chemotherapy for vitamins B_6 and B_1 (Custódio et al. 2016).

THIAMINE (VITAMIN B_1)

Syndromes caused by thiamine deficiency include beriberi and Wernicke-Korsakoff syndrome. Thiamine has two primary functions: α-keto acid decarboxylation (carbohydrate metabolism) and transketolation (pentose phosphate pathway).

Low plasma thiamine levels are common and are associated with increased mortality in patients in intensive care units (Donnino et al. 2010). Thiamine deficiency is also well described in patients with advanced cancer (Barbato and Rodriguez 1994). In particular, thiamine deficiency presents in patients with rapidly growing malignancies. To support rapid growth and proliferation, tumour cells require large amounts of energy, which in part is derived from the anaerobic breakdown of glucose to ATP. The pentose phosphate pathway is important in glucose metabolism, with transketolase an integral enzyme for the nonoxidative synthesis of 5-carbon sugars. Thiamine is metabolised to thiamine pyrophosphate, the cofactor of transketolase. The upregulation of transketolase activity during tumour progression has been widely reported.

Transketolase activity is decreased in thiamine deficiency and is used as an early marker of decreasing thiamine status. Thiamine supplementation is common in cancer patients, although concerns have been raised that in some cases this has the propensity to accelerate tumour growth (Comin-Anduix et al. 2001). Macleod (2000) presented a case study of a terminally ill cancer patient who developed thiamine-related Wernicke encephalopathy, despite apparently adequate dietary intake.

RIBOFLAVIN (VITAMIN B_2)

Riboflavin is a component of coenzymes flavin mononucleotide (FMN) and flavin adenine dinucleotide (FAD), and is involved in the metabolism of several other vitamins (vitamin B_6, niacin and folate). Interaction between folate and riboflavin in patients with colorectal and cervical cancer showed that increased plasma riboflavin levels were associated with decreased plasma homocysteine levels (Powers 2005). The study by Custódio et al. (2016) in women with breast cancer showed that despite no significant change in niacin and riboflavin intake during the treatment, a high prevalence of deficiency for niacin and riboflavin (60%) was observed after administration of the last cycle of chemotherapy.

NIACIN (VITAMIN B_3)

Niacin (nicotinic acid) deficiency or pellagra is a result of an inadequate dietary intake of niacin or tryptophan. Niacin can be synthesised from tryptophan, a reaction that is reliant on vitamins B_2, and B_6. In the context of cancer, studies on niacin deficiency have focused mainly on the risk of cancer rather than status in terminally ill patients.

BIOTIN (VITAMIN B_7)

Biotin is a cofactor to many enzymatic reactions involved in metabolism of lipid proteins and carbohydrates. Biotin deficiency is exceedingly rare, but can develop after three to four weeks of dietary restriction or through malabsorption.

PANTOTHENIC ACID (VITAMIN B_5)

Deficiencies of this vitamin are exceptionally rare and have not been widely studied in cancer patients.

PRACTICAL METHODS AND TECHNIQUES

Fat-Soluble Vitamins

Vitamin A

Retinol is measured in serum/plasma most commonly by high-performance liquid chromatography (HPLC). The typical reference range is 1.4–3.8 μmol/L.

Vitamin D

Serum based on vitamin chromatographic $D_3 + D_2$ is predominately measured by competitive immunoassays or methods based on chromatographic separation (HPLC, liquid chromatography-mass spectrometry [LC-MS/MS]). Typical reference limits are as follows: optimal status 50–200 nmol/L; insufficiency 30–50 nmol/L; severe deficiency <30 nmol/L.

Vitamin E

α-Tocopherol is most commonly measured in serum/plasma by HPLC. The typical reference range is 11.6–41.8 μmol/L. Levels of α-tocopherol correlate with cholesterol and hence are often expressed as the α-tocopherol-cholesterol ratio (reference range >2.22).

Vitamin K

Phylloquinone is measured in serum/plasma by HPLC or LC-MS/MS. The typical reference range is 0.33–3.44 nmol/L. Hepatic functional status is assessed by PIVKA-II measurement by enzyme-linked immunosorbent assay (ELISA) or chemiluminescent microparticle immunoassay.

Water-Soluble Vitamins

Vitamin C

Vitamin C (ascorbic acid) is measured in plasma by various techniques (e.g, HPLC). The typical reference range is 22–85 μmol/L.

Folate

Folate status is assessed by measurement in serum (short-term indicator) and red blood cells (mean status over ~120 days). The typical reference range is serum 7–36 nmol/L, red cell 408–1700 nmol/L. Functional status is partly indicated by homocysteine levels (<15 μmol/L).

Vitamin B_{12}

Various methodologies are available: chemical, microbiological or immunoassay. Serum cobalamin concentration is often determined by automated immunoassays. The typical reference range is 250–900 ng/L. Functional status is indicated by holotranscobalamin (marketed as "active B12") (holoTC <25 pmol/L are classified as deficient) and MMA levels (280 nmol/L cut-off applied to patients younger than 65 years old with good renal function; cut-off of >360 nmol/L applied to patients older than 65 years).

Vitamin B_6

Direct methods include determination of pyridoxal-5′-phosphate in whole blood. The typical reference range is 35.2–110.1 nmol/L, and ethylenediaminetetraacetic acid (EDTA) plasma measured by HPLC is 14.6–72.9 nmol/L.

Thiamine (Vitamin B_1)

Whole blood levels are determined by HPLC. The typical reference range is 66.5–200 nmol/L. Functional status is indicated by erythrocyte transketolase activity.

Riboflavin (Vitamin B_2)

Direct methods include the determination of FAD and FMN in whole blood by HPLC. The typical reference range (FAD) is 120–160 nmol/L.

Niacin (Vitamin B_3)

Urinary excretion of metabolites, N-methyl-nicotinamide and N-methyl-2-pyridone-5-carboxamide are used to assess niacin status. Nicotinamide adenine dinucleotide (NAD+) and nicotinamide adenine dinucleotide phosphate (NADP+) concentrations and their ratio in red blood cells may be sensitive and reliable status indicators. A ratio of erythrocyte NAD to NADP <1.0 may identify subjects at risk of developing deficiency.

Biotin (Vitamin B_7)

Biotin is measured in serum/plasma by microbiological methods, avidin-binding assays, determination of biotin excretion and 3-hydroisovaleric acid. Typical serum concentrations are in the range of 100–400 μmol/L.

Pantothenic Acid (Vitamin B_5)

Typical blood levels are in the range of 0.9–1.5 μmol/L. Status can be deduced from urinary pantothenate excretion.

KEY FACTS: VITAMIN DEFICIENCY IN PATIENTS WITH TERMINAL CANCER

- Vitamins are chemically diverse.
- The impact of terminal cancer on status is greater for some vitamins than it is for others.
- Deficient states develop at very different rates (from a few days to several years).
- Vitamin status can be monitored with a variety of laboratory-based assays long before pathological changes manifest.
- Stages of vitamin deficiency (B_{12}, folate, vitamin K) are illustrated in Figure 24.5.

Key Points:

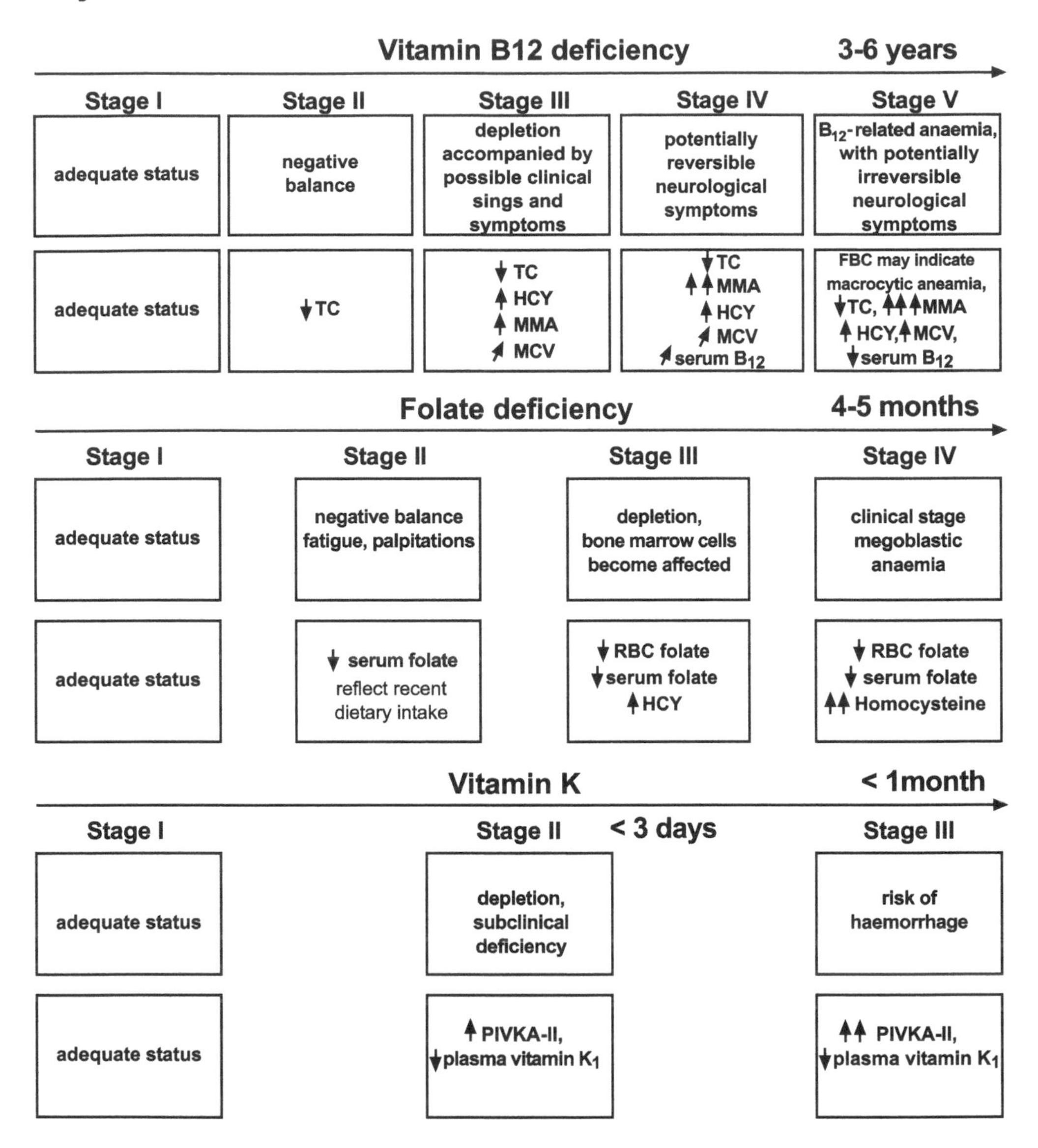

FIGURE 24.5 Stages of depletion for vitamin B_{12}, folate and vitamin K. For each vitamin the stages of deficiency are shown and available laboratory tests indicated. (FBC, full blood count; HCY, homocysteine; MCV, mean corpuscular volume; MMA, methylmalonic acid; PIVKA-II, des-carboxy-prothrombin; RBC, red blood cell; TC, holotranscobalamin.)

SUMMARY POINTS

- Vitamins are required to support many metabolic networks.
- Vitamin deficiencies are common in patients with terminal cancer as a consequence of anorexia, and the use of treatment regimes that induce nausea and a loss of appetite.
- Vitamin deficiencies in patients with terminal cancer can result from surgical interventions, and impaired gastrointestinal function following chemotherapy and radiation therapy.
- Laboratory tests are widely available to identify deficient states and monitor the efficacy of nutritional support.

- A high proportion of patients with terminal cancer are unlikely to maintain an adequate vitamin status without nutritional support. It must, however, be recognised that some vitamins are required for the growth and proliferation of tumour cells.

LIST OF ABBREVIATIONS

FAD	Flavin Adenine Dinucleotide
FBC	Full Blood Count
FMN	Flavin Mononucleotide
HC	Holohaptocorrin
HCY	Homocysteine
IF	Intrinsic Factor
INR	International Normalised Ratio
MCV	Mean Corpuscular Volume
MMA	Methylmalonic Acid
NAD	Nicotinamide Adenine Dinucleotide
NADP	Nicotinamide Adenine Dinucleotide Phosphate
PIVKAs	Protein Induced by Vitamin K Absence (or Antagonism)
PIVKA-II	des-Carboxy-prothrombin
RBC	Red Blood Cell
SAM	S-adenosylmethionine
TC	Holotranscobalamin II
ucOC	Undercarboxylated Osteocalcin

ACKNOWLEDGEMENTS

The authors gratefully acknowledge our colleagues Agata Sobczyńska-Malefora and Kieran Voong from the Human Nutristasis Unit. We also thank Viapath and Guy's and St. Thomas' NHS Foundation Trust for their continued support.

REFERENCES

Alexandrescu, D. T., C. A. Dasanu, and C. L. Kauffman. 2009. Acute scurvy during treatment with interleukin-2. *Clinical and Experimental Dermatology* 34:811–14.

Azharuddin, M. K., D. St J. O'Reilly, A. Gray, and D. Talwar. 2007. HPLC method for plasma vitamin K1: Effect of plasma triglyceride and acute-phase response on circulating concentrations. *Clinical Chemistry* 53:1706–13.

Ball, G. F. M. 2004. *Vitamins. Their Role in the Human Body.* Oxford, UK: Blackwell.

Barbato, M., and P. J. Rodriguez. 1994. Thiamine deficiency in patients admitted to a palliative care unit. *Palliative Medicine* 8:320–24.

Bergman, P., S. Sperneder, J. Höijer, J. Bergqvist, and L. Björkhem-Bergman. 2015. Low vitamin D levels are associated with higher opioid dose in palliative cancer patients – Results from an observational study in Sweden edited by K. Ikeda. *PLOS ONE* 10:e0128223.

Blatt, D. H., S. W. Leonard, and M. G. Traber. 2001. Vitamin E kinetics and the function of tocopherol regulatory proteins. *Nutrition* 17:799–805.

Bunaciu, Rodica P. and Andrew Yen. 2015. Retinoid chemoprevention: Who can benefit? *Current Pharmacology Reports* 1:391–400.

Bystrom, P., K. Bjorkegren, A. Larsson, L. Johansson, and A. Berglund. 2009. Serum vitamin B12 and folate status among patients with chemotherapy treatment for advanced colorectal cancer. *Upsala Journal of Medical Sciences* 114:160–64.

Carr, A. C., M. C. M. Vissers, and J. S. Cook. 2014. The effect of intravenous vitamin C on cancer- and chemotherapy-related fatigue and quality of life. *Frontiers in Oncology* 4:283.

Chaitanya, N. C. et al. 2017. Role of vitamin E and vitamin A in oral mucositis induced by cancer chemo/radiotherapy- a meta-analysis. *Journal of Clinical and Diagnostic Research JCDR* 11: ZE06–ZE09.

Comin-Anduix, B., J. Boren, S. Martinez et al. 2001. The effect of thiamine supplementation on tumour proliferation: A metabolic control analysis study. *European Journal of Biochemistry* 268:4177–82.
Custódio, I. D. D. et al. 2016. Impact of chemotherapy on diet and nutritional status of women with breast cancer: A prospective study. *PLOS ONE* 11:e0157113.
Davila, M., and R. S. Bresalier. 2008. Gastrointestinal complications of oncologic therapy. *Nature Clinical Practice Gastroenterology and Hepatology* 5:682–96.
Donnino, M. W. et al. 2010. Thiamine deficiency in critically ill patients with sepsis. *Journal of Critical Care* 25:576–81.
Elston, T. N., J. M. Dudley, M. J. Shearer, and S. A. Schey. 1995. Vitamin K prophylaxis in high-dose chemotherapy. *Lancet* 345:1245.
Ermens, A. A. M., L. T. Vlasveld, and J. Lindemans. 2003. Significance of elevated cobalamin (vitamin B12) levels in blood. *Clinical Biochemistry* 36:585–90.
Harrington, D. J. 2017. Laboratory assessment of Vitamin B 12 Status. *Journal of Clinical Pathology* 70:168–73.
Harrington, D. J., H. Western, C. Seton-Jones, S. Rangarajan, T. Beynon, and M. J. Shearer. 2008. A study of the prevalence of vitamin K deficiency in patients with cancer referred to a hospital palliative care team and its association with abnormal haemostasis. *Journal of Clinical Pathology* 61:537–40.
Holick, M. F., L. Y. Matsuoka, and J. Wortsman. 1989. Age, vitamin-D, and solar ultraviolet. *Lancet 2* 8671: 1104–5.
Jonas, C. R., A. B. Puckett, D. P. Jones et al. 2000. Plasma antioxidant status after high-dose chemotherapy: A randomized trial of parenteral nutrition in bone marrow transplantation patients. *American Journal of Clinical Nutrition* 72:181–89.
Kelly, P., J. McPartlin, M. Goggins, D. G. Weir, and J. M. Scott. 1997. Unmetabolized folic acid in serum: Acute studies in subjects consuming fortified food and supplements. *American Journal of Clinical Nutrition* 65:1790–95.
Kelly, L., S. White, and P. C. Stone. 2007. The B-12/CRP index as a simple prognostic indicator in patients with advanced cancer: A confirmatory study. *Annals of Oncology* 18:1395–99.
Macleod, A. D. 2000. Wernicke's encephalopathy and terminal cancer: Case report. *Palliative Medicine* 14:217–18.
Mayland, C. R., M. I. Bennett, and K. Allan. 2005. Vitamin C deficiency in cancer patients. *Palliative Medicine* 19:17–20.
Mochamat et al. 2017. A systematic review on the role of vitamins, minerals, proteins, and other supplements for the treatment of cachexia in cancer: A European Palliative Care Research Centre Cachexia Project. *Journal of Cachexia, Sarcopenia and Muscle* 8:25–39.
Nimptsch, K., S. Rohrmann, R. Kaaks, and J. Linseisen. 2010. Dietary vitamin K intake in relation to cancer incidence and mortality: Results from the Heidelberg Cohort of the European Prospective Investigation into Cancer and Nutrition (EPIC-Heidelberg). *American Journal of Clinical Nutrition* 91:1348–58.
Okuno, M., S. Kojima, R. Matsushima-Nishiwaki et al. 2004. Retinoids in cancer chemoprevention. *Current Cancer Drug Targets* 4:285–98.
Pace, A. et al. 2010. Vitamin E neuroprotection for cisplatin neuropathy: A randomized, placebo-controlled trial. *Neurology* 74:762–66.
Pfeiffer, C. M., Z. Fazili, L. Mccoy, M. Zhang, and E. W. Gunter. 2004. Determination of folate vitamers in human serum by stable-isotope-dilution tandem mass spectrometry and comparison with radioassay and microbiologic assay. *Clinical Chemistry* 50:423–32.
Powers, H. J. 2005. Interaction among folate, riboflavin, genotype, and cancer, with reference to colorectal and cervical cancer. *Journal of Nutrition* 135:2960S–66S.
Rybalov, S., and D. P. Kotler. 2002. Gastric carcinoids in a patient with pernicious anemia and familial adenomatous polyposis. *Journal of Clinical Gastroenterology* 35:249–52.
Saygili, E. I., D. Konukoglu, C. Papila, and T. Akcay. 2003. Levels of plasma vitamin E, vitamin C, TBARS, and cholesterol in male patients with colorectal tumors. *Biochemistry-Moscow* 68:325–28.
Schloss, Janet M., Maree Colosimo, Caroline Airey, and Luis Vitetta. 2015. Chemotherapy-induced peripheral neuropathy (CIPN) and vitamin B12 deficiency. Supportive care in cancer. *Official Journal of the Multinational Association of Supportive Care in Cancer* 23:1843–50.
Schorah, C. J., C. Downing, A. Piripitsi et al. 1996. Total vitamin C, ascorbic acid, and dehydroascorbic acid concentrations in plasma of critically ill patients. *American Journal of Clinical Nutrition* 63:760–65.
Schrijver, J., J. Alexieva Figusch, N. van Breederode, and H. A. van Gilse. 1987. Investigations on the nutritional status of advanced breast cancer patients. The influence of long-term treatment with megestrol acetate of tamoxifen. *Nutrition and Cancer* 10:231–45.
Suttie, J. W. 1992. Vitamin K and human nutrition. *Journal of the American Dietetic Association* 92:585–90.

Solomon, L. R. 2016. Functional vitamin B12 deficiency in advanced malignancy: Implications for the management of neuropathy and neuropathic pain. *Supportive Care in Cancer* 24:3489–94.

Stein, A., W. Voigt, and K. Jordan. 2010. Chemotherapy-induced diarrhea: Pathophysiology, frequency and guideline-based management. *Therapeutic Advances in Medical Oncology* 2:51–63.

Troen, A. M., B. Mitchell, B. Sorensen et al. 2006. Unmetabolized folic acid in plasma is associated with reduced natural killer cell cytotoxicity among postmenopausal women. *Journal of Nutrition* 136:189–94.

Usui, Y., H. Tanimura, N. Nishimura, N. Kobayashi, T. Okanoue, and K. Ozawa. 1990. Vitamin K concentrations in the plasma and liver of surgical patients. *American Journal of Clinical Nutrition* 51:846–52.

Van Veldhuizen, P. J., S. A. Taylor, S. Williamson, and B. M. Drees. 2000. Treatment of vitamin D deficiency in patients with metastatic prostate cancer may improve bone pain and muscle strength. *Journal of Urology* 163:187–90.

Wei, E. K., E. Giovannucci, J. Selhub, C. S. Fuchs, S. E. Hankinson, and J. Ma. 2005. Plasma vitamin B-6 and the risk of colorectal cancer and adenoma in women. *Journal of the National Cancer Institute* 97:684–92.

25 Childhood Leukemia, Malnutrition, and Mortality as Components of Palliative Care

Juan Manuel Mejía-Aranguré, Elva Jiménez-Hernández, María Salome Anaya-Florez, and Juan Carlos Núñez-Enríquez

CONTENTS

INTRODUCTION

Leukemia is the most common type of cancer in children around the globe. This disease is characterized by an abnormal oligoclonal proliferation of immature lymphoid or myeloid precursors that progressively replace the bone marrow (BM) of normal cells. Then, the neoplastic cells spread through the circulation and may invade various organs and tissues such as the lymph nodes, liver, spleen, central nervous system (CNS), among others (Greenlee et al. 2000; Mwirigi, Dillon, and Raj 2017).

Leukemias are classified as acute or chronic. Approximately 97% correspond to acute leukemias (ALs). Of these, 80%–85% are acute lymphoblastic leukemias (ALLs), and the remaining 10%–15% are of myeloid origin (acute myoblastic leukemia [AML]) (Gurney et al. 1995).

ALL incidence rates vary among populations. In developed countries, this is 25–30 cases per million children under 15 years of age displaying a peak incidence between the ages of two and five years (Ross et al. 1994; Gurney et al. 1995; Swensen et al. 1997; Ries, Kosary, and Hankey 1999; Margolin, Steuber, and Poplack 2006). In recent years, an increase in the incidence of ALL has been reported, mainly for the Hispanic population residing in the United States. Notably, Mexico has one of the highest incidence rates for this disease reported worldwide (Pérez-Saldivar et al. 2011; Bhojwani, Yang, and Pui 2015).

Despite advancements in the knowledge, biology, and treatment of ALs, currently, they represent the leading cause of disease-related deaths during childhood in developing countries. Approximately 90% of children with ALL from developed countries are alive five years after diagnosis confirmation (Pui and Evans 2013). These achievements have been attributed to the use of multiagent chemotherapy, administration of CNS-directed therapy, blood transfusions, use of the correct antibiotic, minimal residual disease detection, and treatment based on specific molecular features; while in developing countries, the five-year survival rate is not higher than 65%.

It is well known that deaths from ALL are mainly due to relapses, disease progression, and treatment-related complications such as severe infections, bleeding, specific organ toxicities, etc. (Pui 2010).

NUTRITIONAL STATUS IN CHILDREN WITH LEUKEMIA

Children with leukemia are particularly vulnerable to malnutrition, due to their high nutrient requirement due to disease, their treatment, and growth and development needs during childhood (Han-Markey 2000; Jaime-Pérez et al. 2008; Tazi et al. 2008).

The prevalence and degree of malnutrition depend mainly on the stage of the disease (Bauer, Jürgens, and Frühwald 2011). In AL children, negative consequences of malnutrition are prolonged hospitalizations, toxicity related to treatment, reduced response to antitumor treatment, poor quality of life, and bad outcomes (Van Cutsem and Arends 2005).

Leukemia patients often reduce their food intake due to the systemic effect of the disease, psychological conditions, adverse effects of the treatment, nutrients metabolism alterations, and the lower energy expenditure due to prolonged rest.

Likewise, several substances produced directly or indirectly by the neoplasm, such as pro-inflammatory cytokines, have been implicated in the pathogenesis of malnutrition and in the development of cachexia associated with cancer (Paccagnella, Morassutti, and Rosti 2011). In addition, it is well recognized that an inadequate nutritional status may be a factor that affects the immune function, and the metabolism of drugs used in chemotherapy (Caccialanza et al. 2016).

The nutritional status of AL children may change during chemotherapy phases. Chemotherapy drugs cause adverse effects such as dysgeusia with aversion to food, alteration in the absorption and metabolism of nutrients, as well as complications such as gastrointestinal toxicity (nausea, vomiting, mucositis, diarrhea, constipation, and xerostomia), hepatotoxicity, nephrotoxicity, infections, and alterations in the emotional and psychological states of the child. All of these factors play an important role in the etiology of malnutrition (Paccagnella, Morassutti, and Rosti 2011).

Malnutrition also includes circumstances of high-energy supply resulting in over-nutrition with an increase in adipose tissue (overweight/obesity). Although malnutrition has been defined or described in many ways, there is no consensus regarding a specific definition to identify children at risk (Hunger et al. 2012).

The World Health Organization (WHO) recommends the weight-for-height index to investigate the nutritional status of children and adolescents (Butte, Garza, and de Onis 2007). Moreover, it has been proposed that a loss in body weight of 5% or more constitutes acute malnutrition, and a value of weight-for-age below the fifth percentile may reflect chronic malnutrition (Smith, Stevens, and Booth 1991). However, to date, there is no gold standard for evaluating nutritional status in children, and height and weight measurements may be useful for assessing nutritional status in leukemia patients. Particularly, for children living in developing countries, it has been recommended to use other anthropometric indicators such as the mid-upper arm circumference (MUAC), triceps-skinfold thickness (TSFC), and serum albumin (SA).

Physiopathology of Malnutrition in Children with Cancer

Many biological mechanisms have been postulated as involved in the development of malnutrition in children with leukemia. They include (1) complex interactions between energy and metabolism of the substrate, (2) hormonal and inflammatory components, and (3) alterations of the metabolic compartments (Skipworth et al. 2007).

In animal models, pro-inflammatory cytokines such as interleukin (IL)-1α, IL-1β, IL-6, tumor necrosis factor (TNF)-α, interferon (IFN)-γ have been shown to be released by neoplastic cells or by cells of the immune or stromal system of children with cancer, in combination with other mediators, which affect food intake and energy expenditure, resulting in the well-known clinical cancer-cachexia syndrome (Tisdale 2009).

It is evident that energy deficit and metabolic abnormalities play an important role in the progression of cachexia syndrome observed in children with leukemia. This is due to (1) increased nutrient requirements; (2) loss of energy caused by frequent gastrointestinal dysfunction secondary to chemotherapy-induced toxicity; (3) excessive use of energy as a result of the use of aggressive multi-regimen chemotherapy schemes; (4) metabolic and hormonal alterations; (5) stress caused by uncontrolled pain or unavoidable procedures such as bone marrow aspiration, blood samples, application of intrathecal chemotherapies and lumbar punctures; and finally, (6) the high prevalence of appetite disorders and changes in taste due to xerostomia caused by chemotherapy (Skipworth et al. 2007).

Prevalence of Nutritional Alterations in Children with Acute Leukemia

The prevalence of nutritional alterations (NAs) in patients with AL varies depending on the time of the disease in which it is evaluated, as well as the socioeconomic level of the population studied, the different diagnostic techniques used, the individual variability, the chemotherapy regimen, and the definition used.

NAs vary from malnutrition to obesity.

When only the weight adjusted by the age of the patient is used, it should be considered as an unspecific parameter to assess the nutritional status, because it varies with the state of hydration and the tumor burden (Rogers 2014).

Therefore, in low-income countries, the most feasible and recommended anthropometric measurements are the MUAC, TSFC, and SA, as demonstrated for the Central American group Asociación de Hemato-Oncología Pediátrica de Centro América (AHOPCA) (Sala et al. 2012).

Undernutrition

Yazbeck et al. reported a prevalence of 25.5% for undernutrition in childhood ALL at the time of diagnosis [30]. Reilly et al. noted a prevalence of 7% in patients classified as standard-risk ALL ($n = 1019$) (Yazbeck et al. 2016).

In Mexico, the prevalence of undernutrition is very variable, for example, Jaime-Pérez et al. (2008) investigated the nutritional status of 102 children with ALL in northern Mexico, most were well nourished and had a normal body composition (Jaime-Pérez et al. 2008). Rivera-Luna et al. (2008) conducted a study in 100 children with ALL and reported that undernutrition grade 1 occurred in 24% of patients, grade 2 in 8%, and grade 3 in 1% (Rivera-Luna et al. 2008). More recently, the Mexican Inter-Institutional Group for the Identification of the Causes of Childhood Leukemia (MIGICCL) published the results of a multicenter study that included 794 children with ALL using different anthropometric indicators to classify the nutritional status of patients at the time of diagnosis. In this study, the prevalence of undernutrition was ~5.6% by using measurements such as the weight/height, height/age, and body mass index age adjusted by the sex of the patient and subsequent comparison with WHO and Centers for Disease Control and Prevention 2000 growth charts (Martín-Trejo et al. 2017).

Overweight and Obesity

It is important to mention that obesity has been described among survivors of ALL, especially those who have received cranial irradiation (Veringa et al. 2012). Although there are studies such as those by Hassan, Lin, and Torno (2013), who studied 132 children survivors of ALL who did not receive cranial radiation and observed that 69/132 (52.3%) children were overweight or obese at the end of treatment and remained the same after two years of surveillance (Hassan, Lin, and Torno 2013). In recent years, an increased prevalence of overweight and obesity has been noted worldwide, and children with leukemia are not an exception to this.

EFFECTS OF NUTRITIONAL STATUS

Prognosis of Children with Acute Leukemia

Although malnutrition is frequently cited as an indicator of poor prognosis in pediatric patients with leukemia (Yazbeck et al. 2016), it is not a component considered in the clinical trials conducted in these children. Malnutrition has been used indiscriminately between protein-energy malnutrition, and the other spectrum—patients who are overweight or obese.

In recent studies, overweight and obesity have been associated with a poor prognosis in leukemia children; they are more likely to persist with minimal residual disease (MRD) (Orgel, Tucci, et al. 2014) and display shorter event-free survival (EFS) (Borowitz et al. 2003; Borowitz et al. 2008; Orgel, Tucci, et al. 2014).

A biological link between obesity and leukemia treatment response has been identified. There is evidence that adipocytes can interact with neoplastic cells to promote invasion, proliferation, and drug resistance (Pramanik et al. 2013). Adipocytes secrete numerous factors intervening in proliferation, migration, and metastasis, such as insulin-like growth factor (IGF-1), leptin, platelet-derived growth factor, metalloproteinase 11, IL-6, and stromal cell-derived factor-1α (SDF-1α) (Roberts, Dive, and Renehan 2010). Some of these also contribute to the strong association observed among obesity, relapse, and mortality (Ehsanipour et al. 2013).

The presence of adipocytes in *in vitro* and *in vivo* studies markedly reduces the efficacy of some chemotherapeutic agents used in childhood leukemia treatment (vincristine, dexamethasone, asparaginase, and daunorubicin) (Behan et al. 2009; Pramanik et al. 2013; Ehsanipour et al. 2013). Obese patients receive high doses of chemotherapy agents that later contribute to failure in post-induction treatment. They are vulnerable to develop toxicity in organs such as the pancreas, liver, kidney, among others (Orgel, Sposto, et al. 2014).

Chemotherapy-Related Toxicity

A significant proportion of deaths observed in children with leukemia is caused by chemotherapy toxicity. During treatment, severe and acute adverse effects may affect different organs. The most common are the opportunistic infections, mucositis, central or peripheral neuropathy, osteonecrosis, thromboembolism, sinusoidal obstruction syndrome, endocrinopathies (adrenal insufficiency, hyperglycemia), nephrotoxicity, hypersensitivity, pancreatitis, and L-asparaginase-induced hyperlipidemia (Schmiegelow et al. 2017). Gastrointestinal toxicity occurs in up to 40% after the application of anti-metabolites or drugs that cause DNA damage. The main manifestation is mucositis with alteration in the intake and absorption of nutrients and the subsequent loss of weight (Yang, Hu, and Xu 2012).

Conversely, significant weight gain is seen in 15%–40% of children with ALL, reflecting corticosteroid exposure and reduced physical activity, with insulin resistance, hyperglycemia, and prediabetes, which could indicate the need to modify the diet and therapy with insulin (Chow et al. 2013).

Obesity is considered a late adverse effect of ALL treatment in survivors (Hassan, Lin, and Torno 2013). Although the pathophysiology of radiation exposure in the hypothalamic-pituitary-adrenal axis is not very clear, it is known that hypothalamic centers are responsible for regulating satiety, hunger, and energy balance. The alteration in insulin and leptin signaling may contribute to obesity of hypothalamic origin. Although radiation can contribute to several hormonal deficiencies of the pituitary gland, there is evidence that growth hormone is the most sensitive to this effect (Iughetti et al. 2012). Growth hormone deficiency can cause a decrease in body mass, increase the percentage of body fat, alter the metabolism of lipoproteins, increase peripheral resistance to insulin, and decrease glucose tolerance. Several studies have shown a dose-response effect of cranial irradiation, with an increased risk of obesity with radiation doses of 20–30 Gy (Brouwer et al. 2012). Other studies have shown that even low doses of radiation (18–20 Gy) can predispose to obesity (Odame et al. 1994).

Treatment Response

Undernutrition has been reported as a negative prognostic factor in children with leukemia. It has been associated with an increase in morbidity and with low disease-free survival (DFS) rates due to the development of severe infections, hemorrhages and treatment abandonment. In a study conducted in Pribnow et al. (2017), 67% of children with cancer were undernourished at the moment of diagnosis, and 92.2% of them developed morbidities during the first 90 days after treatment initiation. Undernutrition was associated with severe infections as the first cause of mortality ($p = 0.033$) (Pribnow et al. 2017). The impact of obesity is not trivial; a meta-analysis found that obesity at diagnosis is an indicator of poor prognosis in children with leukemia, with an increase of up to a 35% mortality risk (Orgel et al. 2016).

Early Mortality

Although several prognostic factors have been identified to be useful for stratifying the risk of early mortality in children with leukemia, other factors such as race, poverty, and malnutrition remain controversial (Martín-Trejo et al. 2017). In developed countries, early mortality occurs in 1%–5% of ALL children (Bazrafshan 2017), while for AML it is higher. The D-COG (Dutch Childhood Oncology Group) reported that early death occurs in approximately 13.1% of AML patients (Slats et al. 2005). The most common causes are infections (mainly bacterial), hemorrhage, and septic shock (Slats et al. 2005; Bazrafshan 2017). These causes are similar to those reported in developing countries, with the difference that early mortality occurs at often much higher rates. Early deaths percentages in some developing countries are as follows: El Salvador 12.5% (Gupta et al. 2009), India 17% (Advani et al. 1999), Cairo 19.2% (Hafez et al. 2016), and Mexico 7%–16.6% (Lopez-Facundo NA, Talavera-Piña

2008; Jiménez-Hernández et al. 2015). In a recent Mexican study by Martín-Trejo et al. (2017), an association between malnutrition and early mortality was not observed (Martín-Trejo et al. 2017). However, in a previous Mexican case-control study conducted by Mejía-Aranguré et al., it was found that children with malnutrition at the time of diagnosis were 2.5 times more likely to die during early phases of treatment compared to children without malnutrition (Mejía-Aranguré et al. 1999).

For many years, oncological research has focused on survival and mortality. However, there are very few studies reporting state-of-the-art palliative care and quality of life in childhood AL survivors (Zeltzer et al. 2008).

About 15%–20% of patients with ALL suffer from relapses and are treated with salvage chemotherapy, which consists of intensive chemotherapy, often including irradiation to the CNS and/or hematopoietic transplant. The cure rates of these patients rarely reach 37% (Einsiedel et al. 2005). In addition, survivors are at risk of late adverse effects and second neoplasms (Michel et al. 2010). The late effects observed most frequently are cardiac, endocrine, neurological, renal, and visual system effects which lead the patient to a poor quality of life (Goldsby et al. 2010). The Childhood Cancer Survivor Study (CCSS) group conducted a 25-year follow-up study among survivors of ALL. Cumulative mortality was 13% at 25 years after diagnosis. The main causes of death were relapses ($n = 483$) and second neoplasms ($n = 89$) (Mody et al. 2008).

CHEMOTHERAPY-REFRACTORY LEUKEMIA AND END OF LIFE

Chemotherapy-refractory leukemia (CRL) is defined as the failure to achieve complete remission after one or two cycles of induction chemotherapy. Failure to primary induction is rare in ALL and occurs in only 2%–3% of the patients (Joyce et al. 2013), while in AML, it occurs between 7% and 20% of the cases (Zwaan et al. 2015).

In a meta-analysis of 14 cooperative groups, 1,041 patients were analyzed in a follow-up period of 10 years; overall survival was 32% (Schrappe et al. 2012). In comparison, 71%–93% of patients with ALL who achieved complete remission then reached second remission. Therefore, those who do not respond to the treatment of the first relapse or subsequent relapses are also considered recurrent or with secondary refractory leukemia and are susceptible to palliative care provision (Ko et al. 2010).

For AML with contemporary treatments 80%–90% reach complete remission, and long-term survival on average is 50%. Of patients who achieve complete remission, 30%–40% suffer from relapse; after recurrence, survival is very poor, between 21% and 33%, and these patients have need for palliative care (Rubnitz et al. 2007; Zwaan et al. 2015).

The prognostic factors associated with the risk of recurrent or refractory leukemia are (a) the time relapsed between achievement of the first remission to relapse, (b) the site of relapse (isolated bone marrow relapse), and (c) specific cytogenetic alterations (BCR-ABL1, MLL-AF4, etc.). The prognosis of patients with an early isolated bone marrow relapse is poor, with overall five-year survival rates of 13% (Dalle et al. 2005). In the study by Rubnitz et al., they reported factors associated with AML refractoriness, such as (a) male gender ($p = 0.005$), (b) M5 and M7 morphology ($p = 0.001$), and (c) the time between diagnosis confirmation and recurrence ($p = 0.041$) (Rubnitz et al. 2007).

APPLICATIONS TO OTHER AREAS OF TERMINAL OR PALLIATIVE CARE

Palliative care includes those measures provided to cancer patients to alleviate the secondary symptoms either to the side effects of the chemotherapy or to those produced by the progression of the disease in order to ameliorate suffering.

The last period in the life of a child suffering from cancer is of crucial importance, not only for the child, but also for the child's parents and other family members. The way the child dies will remain in the memory of the child's parents forever.

Multiple problems in the management of the child who is dying may arise in this last phase. Then, the goal of therapy must be centered on maintaining comfort and support for the child and the family, so care should be extended in different areas to achieve physical, psychological, social, and spiritual well-being. All this is the responsibility of the healthcare team (Weaver et al. 2015).

ETHICAL ISSUES

The American Academy of Pediatrics (AAP) advocates for an integrated and interdisciplinary approach to competent and compassionate care: "in which the components of palliative care are offered at the time of diagnosis and are continued during the course of the disease, regardless of the result." (Care 2000) Likewise, the Worldwide Palliative Care Alliance (WPCA) recognizes the importance of integrating palliative care as a human right for children, even in health system environments with limited resources, for which it requires global collaboration for an evidence-based and resource-efficient approach to best practice standards for the early integration of palliative care for children and their families (Stephen 2014).

PRACTICAL METHODS ON PALLIATIVE CARE PROVISION

The needs for palliative care of children with cancer depend largely on the type of tumor and the location. However, little is known about the needs of children with hematological malignancies such as leukemias, since a good number of publications deal with the needs of children with solid tumors. Likewise, the literature lacks prospective studies to describe the symptoms that could affect quality of life, as well as determination of the best way to develop effective palliative care strategies in these patients (Harris 2004).

The child with leukemia requires a greater demand for palliative care, from diagnosis, during treatment, and at the end of life. In each haemato-oncological unit, a multidisciplinary palliative care team must be available to provide comprehensive care to the child and the child's family members to reduce prolonged stays, unintended hospital readmissions, and visits to emergency services, since they become a major problem.

Collins and colleagues used the Memorial Symptom Assessment Scale in 160 children with cancer from 10 to 18 years, where it was reported that the most common symptoms (35%) were lack of energy, pain, drowsiness, nausea, cough, lack of appetite, and psychological symptoms (sadness, nervousness, worry, and irritability).

The most distressing symptoms in patients with leukemia were difficulty swallowing, ulcers in the mouth, pain, and insomnia (Collins et al. 2000). The palliative care of children with acute leukemia consists of transfusions of blood components in a timely manner, antibiotic prophylaxis, antifungal, pain medications, antineoplastic chemotherapy to reduce tumor burden, cranial radiation therapy when CNS infiltration exists, nutritional and emotional support, among other therapies.

PALLIATIVE CHEMOTHERAPY

In patients with refractory leukemia, palliative chemotherapy (PC) can be chosen, administering chemotherapy at doses not toxic to maintain as much as possible the control of symptoms caused by progression of the disease. In this regard, it has been reported that the use of PC can be effective to produce a decrease in tumor burden at a level that is enough to alleviate symptoms, but which, unfortunately, is not optimal to cure. These medications must be chosen considering the conditions of the patient to produce minimal toxicity. Some medications used for palliative chemotherapy in children with ALL include vincristine on a weekly basis, oral prednisone, and 6-mercaptopurine daily. For AML, cytarabine is used at low doses. All this is done with frequent monitoring of the hematological parameters and physical examination to detect the presence of toxic effects in a timely manner, and if necessary, to modify the dose, or suspend it (Armstrong-Dailey, Zarbock Goltzer, and Zarbock 1993).

PALLIATIVE RADIOTHERAPY

Palliative radiotherapy (PR) is a well-established modality for palliating the symptoms of local or metastatic advanced cancer in adult patients (Loblaw et al. 2012). However, in pediatrics there is little information about its use. Some of the pediatric studies have evaluated the role of PR in the management of incurable pediatric neoplasms, the majority of patients included are those with solid tumors, and only a very small number are patients with leukemias. In a study conducted by Bhasker et al., PR was used in patients with chloromas due to AML (Bhasker, Bajpai, and Turaka 2008). Rahn included seven patients with leukemia (Rahn et al. 2015); likewise, Varma used PR in six patients with leukemia (Varma, Friedman, and Stavas 2017). In 50% of patients in these studies, a complete response was achieved, and the other achieved only partial response of the symptoms that motivated the use of PR. In general, it was well tolerated, so the authors recommend the use of this to alleviate some symptoms associated with refractory leukemia in children (Lo et al. 2015; Bhasker, Bajpai, and Turaka 2008; Rahn et al. 2015; Varma, Friedman, and Stavas 2017).

NUTRITIONAL SUPPORT OF THE END-STAGE LEUKEMIA PEDIATRIC PATIENT

The most important is the anorexia-cachexia syndrome, anemia, or deterioration of the general state that can be the direct cause of death.

Nutrient Administration Routes and Indications

The choice of nutrition administration route relies on the patient´s clinical condition. Ideally, the oral route is preferred taking into account the presentation of food to stimulate appetite and the consistency to improve digestion and absorption according to symptoms. When the oral route is not possible, enteral nutrition should be used, which may be intragastric (nasogastric tube or gastrostomy) or transpyloric (nasoduodenal, nasojejunal, or jejunostomy).

Importantly, enteral nutrition is contraindicated in severe clinical conditions like intestinal perforation, bleeding from the digestive tract, intestinal ischemia, malabsorption syndrome, and high-output gastrointestinal fistulas. In these cases, total parenteral nutrition (TPN) can be considered. However, TPN is an invasive therapy with multiple complications and should be a consensual decision by the palliative care team and parents (Arends et al. 2017; O'Hara 2017).

Taking into Account Preferences of Patients

- Provide food according to the patient's preference and when the patient wants, offering food frequently every three or four hours, in an attractive presentation, with different consistency and flavors, providing easy-to-handle foods with high calorie content in small portions and a variety of menus.
- Encourage the consumption of protein foods such as white meat, fish, egg, etc.
- Take care of the environment and foster the company of the family.
- Avoid foods that produce flatulence and those that are very spicy and with strong odors (O'Hara 2017).

Management of Cachexia

- Cachexia is a condition suffered by the patient due to the involuntary loss of weight and muscle mass.
- A nutritional assessment should be made taking into account the clinical history, including the analysis of caloric intake, pharmacological treatment, physical examination, subjective global

assessment, anthropometric assessment, and biochemical parameters (pre-albumin, retinol transporter protein, transferrin, nitrogen balance, creatinine index, and total lymphocyte count).

- Patients should be specifically questioned not only about the presence of anorexia, but also early satiety, xerostomia, nausea, diarrhea, and constipation.
- *Recommendations for early satiety*: Feed in small portions and more frequently, low-fat foods and preferably without insoluble fiber.
- *Xerostomy*: Increase the administration of soft, liquid, and cold foods. Do not give dry food.
- *Nausea*: Start dry, low-fat foods, break up food, do not administer acidic juices, keep the patient seated after feeding, do not mix cold and hot foods.
- *Diarrhea*: Offer oral hydration salts, liquids, and an astringent diet.
- *Constipation*: Increase the administration of liquids and foods rich in insoluble fiber (Eberhardie 2002; Bazzan et al. 2013; Owens et al. 2013; O'Hara 2017; Arends et al. 2017).

Ensure an Adequate Amount of Calories

To ensure an adequate amount of calories, the diet should cover the needs of the patient, with crushed diets of high nutritional value, such as porridges, purées, or pudding.

Some nutritional supplements by the oral route can be used. They are classified in different ways according to their clinical use (complete formulation or incomplete formulation), to their energy density and protein content, to the presence of specific nutrients directed to the treatment of special pathologies, or according to its form of presentation.

The schedule of administration of the supplement should be agreed on with the patient and family so that it does not affect the normal consumption of natural foods. In fact, when supplements are prescribed as a complement and not as "oral or enteral nutrition," they should be administered at times that do not interfere with the main meals, in small doses throughout the day.

Reduce Intake of Foods Associated with Cancer Recurrence

As far as possible, the diet should try to reduce foods that are associated with cancer recurrence, such as refined sugars, sweets, industrialized juices, soft drinks, fried foods, and junk foods that have few nutrients, and foods rich in omega-6 fatty acids which increase the inflammatory response and are a risk factor for cancer (O'Hara 2017).

Avoid Foods that Promote Inflammation and Oxidative Stress

It is well recognized that red meat is pro-inflammatory and pro-carcinogenic, so it is suggested that it be reduced from the diet of palliative care patients. However, it is important to ensure that patients continue to receive nutrients commonly found in meats such as iron, vitamin B, and essential amino acids (Bazzan et al. 2013).

Also, as recommended, patients with end-stage leukemia must not eat foods such as red meat high in fat or meats prepared certain ways, such as smoked (sausages), due to the presence of nitrates, nitrites, and heterocyclic aromatic amines. Carcinogens such as aromatic heterocyclic amines are formed after extensive heating (>180°C).

Moreover, avoid sodium nitrite (used as a colored fixative in meat), together with secondary amines of meat proteins that produce nitrosamines that are carcinogenic (Mosby et al. 2012).

Food Supplements Related to the Prevention and Recurrence of Cancer

Prolonged breastfeeding is the ideal food for prevention and for avoiding recurrence of cancer in the infant. Likewise, those foods based on plants, including fruits, vegetables, and whole grains, a favorable ratio of omega-6 and omega-3 polyunsaturated fatty acids, and the consumption of fish have a protective effect against cancer.

While there are many benefits of eating well, the data are controversial on whether diet alone can prevent the reappearance of certain cancers. However, there is strong evidence that a plant-based diet reduces the risk of cancer in general. Plant foods contain antioxidants such as beta-carotene, lycopene, and vitamins A, C, and E, which protect cells from free radicals (Bazzan et al. 2013).

Probiotics and Prebiotics

Prebiotics are non-digestible compounds in foods that produce beneficial effects on the host, selectively stimulating the growth and activity of the microbiota.

Prebiotics include inulin and fructose-oligosaccharides, found in artichokes, asparagus, bananas, chicory, garlic, leeks, oats, onions, soybeans, and wheat.

Probiotics with live microorganisms that exert a beneficial effect on host health are not pathogenic nor toxic and should be free of adverse effects. Probiotics may be beneficial in diarrhea due to chemotherapy or radiotherapy, but their use is questioned in immunocompromised patients due to the risk of bacteremia, and the doses and time of treatment with probiotics are not well established until date.

Both prebiotics and probiotics are important to maintain intestinal health, and this symbiosis maintains a balance in the host-diet microbiota. A change in one of these factors triggers a disease state (Bazzan et al. 2013; Owens et al. 2013; Watsky et al. 2014; Sendrós Madroño 2016; O'Hara 2017; Arends et al. 2017).

Omega-3 Fatty Acids

Omega-3 polyunsaturated fatty acids, such as α-linoleic acid, eicosapentaenoic acid, and docosahexaenoic acid, that stimulate the anti-inflammatory response, act by inhibiting the production of pro-inflammatory cytokines and reducing tumor cachexia. It is suggested that reducing omega-6 intake and increasing the intake of omega-3 fatty acids could be beneficial in reducing fatigue in patients with cancer.

Omega-3 fatty acids have beneficial effects on the neuronal damage. For example, a high consumption of polyunsaturated fatty acids rich in omega-3, which has its origin mainly in fish, inhibits tumor promotion (Bazzan et al. 2013). Some foods rich in omega-3 are fish (mackerel, salmon, tuna, herring, sardines, hake, caviar, anchovies, and oysters) and seeds such as flaxseed and walnuts.

Vitamin D Supplementation

Vitamin D is obtained from food and activated by exposure to the sun. It is very important to maintain bone health, since it fixes calcium and phosphorus; it also intervenes in other tissues, especially in the immune system. In recent years, there has been a growing emphasis on the importance of maintaining adequate levels of vitamin D to help maintain overall health and immune function. Similarly, it is recommended to maintain adequate levels of vitamin D in patients with advanced cancer and undergoing palliative care.

The vitamin D receptors are found in almost every cell of the body; therefore, vitamin D can regulate proliferation, differentiation, and apoptosis. It is usually measured by means of an active metabolite of vitamin D (levels of 25-dihydroxyvitamin D); if the normal values or equal to 30 nanograms/mL, insufficiency levels below 15 ng/mL, and a deficiency lower than 10 ng/mL. Toxic levels greater than 150 ng/mL are considered.

Vitamin D deficiency, prematurity, and malnutrition are common pathologies that negatively influence bone turnover (Watsky et al. 2014).

Multivitamins and Antioxidants

There are studies that explore the link between cancer and inflammation. The inflammation itself is associated with high levels of oxidative stress that can damage most of the body's tissues and genetic material that can ultimately lead to the formation of cancer. Oxidative stress decreases mainly vitamin C, vitamin E, and selenium. In recent years, a large number of studies have attributed a protective effect to polyphenols and foods containing these compounds (e.g., cereals, coffee, dark chocolate, plants, tea, or vegetables) against the development and spread of cancer, when they are used as chemopreventive agents. The mechanism of action of these polyphenols is probably based on antioxidant activity (Bazzan et al. 2013).

KEY FACTS

- Childhood leukemia and palliative care are closely related.
- Nutritional status in children with acute leukemia is of importance to take into account.
- Nutritional status has been reported to affect the prognosis of children with leukemia.
- Chemotherapy-related toxicity is one of the main obstacles to achieve cure rates in children with leukemia from developing countries.
- Nutritional support of the end-stage leukemia pediatric patient is mandatory.

SUMMARY POINTS

- Childhood leukemia mortality is high in developing countries.
- Relapse, refractoriness, and treatment toxicity are the main causes of mortality.
- Leukemia children are vulnerable to suffer from malnutrition.
- Malnutrition is associated with higher mortality rates in children with leukemia.
- Nutritional support is a key element in the treatment of leukemia.
- Multiple causes trigger alteration in the nutritional status of children with end-stage leukemia.
- Palliative care and nutritional support help to provide the physiological requirements but are also for the social, cultural, and psychological benefit and the well-being of the patient with leukemia.

LIST OF ABBREVIATIONS

95% CI	95% Confidence Interval
AAP	American Academy of Pediatrics
AHOPCA	Central American Group
AL	Acute Leukemias
ALL	Acute Lymphoblastic Leukemia
AML	Acute Myeloblastic Leukemia
BM	Bone Marrow
CCSS	Childhood Cancer Survivor Study
CDC	Center for Disease Control
CMC	Chronic Medical Conditions
CNS	Central Nervous System
CRL	Chemotherapy-Refractory Leukemia
D-COG	Dutch Childhood Oncology Group
IL	Interleukins
MIGICCL	Mexican Inter-Institutional Group for the Identification of the Causes of Childhood Leukemia
MUAC	Mid-Upper Arm Circumference
NA	Nutritional Alterations
OR	Odds Ratio
PC	Palliative Chemotherapy

PR	Palliative Radiotherapy
SA	Serum Albumin
TPN	Total Parenteral Nutrition
TSFC	Triceps Skinfold Thickness
WAPC	World Alliance of Palliative Care
WHO	World Health Organization

REFERENCES

Advani, S, S Pai, D Venzon, M Adde, PK Kurkure, CN Nair, B Sirohi et al. 1999. Acute Lymphoblastic Leukemia in India: An Analysis of Prognostic Factors Using a Single Treatment Regimen. 10 (2): 167–76.

Arends, J, P Bachmann, V Baracos, N Barthelemy, H Bertz, F Bozzetti, K Fearon et al. 2017. ESPEN Guidelines on Nutrition in Cancer Patients. *Clinical Nutrition* 36 (1): 11–48.

Armstrong-Dailey, A, SZ Goltzer, and SF Zarbock. 1993. *Hospice Care for Children*. Oxford: Oxford University Press.

Bauer, J, H Jürgens, and MC Frühwald. 2011. Important Aspects of Nutrition in Children with Cancer. *Advances in Nutrition* 2 (2): 67–77.

Bazrafshan, A. 2017. The Etiology of Early Mortality in Pediatric Acute Leukemia. *Journal of Cancer Science and Therapy* 9 12 (Suppl.).

Bazzan, AJ, AB Newberg, WC Cho, and DA Monti. 2013. Diet and Nutrition in Cancer Survivorship and Palliative Care. *Evidence-Based Complementary and Alternative Medicine* 2013 (October): 917647.

Behan, JW, JP Yun, MP Proektor, EA Ehsanipour, A Arutyunyan, AS Moses, VI Avramis et al. 2009. Adipocytes Impair Leukemia Treatment in Mice. 69 (19): 7867–74.

Bhasker, S, V Bajpai, and A Turaka. 2008. Palliative Radiotherapy in Paediatric Malignancies. *Singapore Medical Journal* 49 (12): 998–1001.

Bhojwani, D, JJ Yang, and C-H Pui. 2015. Biology of Childhood Acute Lymphoblastic Leukemia. *Pediatric Clinics of North America* 62 (1): 47–60.

Borowitz, MJ, DJ Pullen, JJ Shuster, D Viswanatha, K Montgomery, CL Willman, and B Camitta. 2003. Minimal Residual Disease Detection in Childhood Precursor–B-Cell Acute Lymphoblastic Leukemia: Relation to Other Risk Factors. A Children's Oncology Group Study. *Leukemia* 17 (8): 1566–72.

Borowitz, MJ, M Devidas, SP Hunger, WP Bowman, AJ Carroll, WL Carroll, S Linda et al. 2008. Clinical Significance of Minimal Residual Disease in Childhood Acute Lymphoblastic Leukemia and Its Relationship to Other Prognostic Factors: A Children's Oncology Group Study. *Blood* 111 (12): 5477–85.

Brouwer, CAJ, JA Gietema, JM Vonk, WJE Tissing, HM Boezen, N Zwart, and A Postma. 2012. Body Mass Index and Annual Increase of Body Mass Index in Long-Term Childhood Cancer Survivors; Relationship to Treatment. *Supportive Care in Cancer* 20 (2): 311–18.

Butte, NF, C Garza, and M de Onis. 2007. Evaluation of the Feasibility of International Growth Standards for School-Aged Children and Adolescents. *Journal of Nutrition* 137 (1): 153–57.

Caccialanza, R, P Pedrazzoli, E Cereda, C Gavazzi, C Pinto, A Paccagnella, GD Beretta, M Nardi, A Laviano, and V Zagonel. 2016. Nutritional Support in Cancer Patients: A Position Paper from the Italian Society of Medical Oncology (AIOM) and the Italian Society of Artificial Nutrition and Metabolism (SINPE). *Journal of Cancer* 7 (2): 131–35.

Care, Committee on Bioethics and Committee on Hospital. 2000. American Academy of Pediatrics. Committee on Bioethics and Committee on Hospital Care. Palliative Care for Children. *Pediatrics* 106 (2 Pt 1): 351–57.

Chow, EJ, C Pihoker, DL Friedman, SJ Lee, JS McCune, C Wharton, CL Roth, and KS Baker. 2013. Glucocorticoids and Insulin Resistance in Children with Acute Lymphoblastic Leukemia. *Pediatric Blood and Cancer* 60 (4): 621–26.

Collins, JJ, ME Byrnes, IJ Dunkel, J Lapin, T Nadel, HT Thaler, T Polyak, B Rapkin, and RK Portenoy. 2000. The Measurement of Symptoms in Children with Cancer. *Journal of Pain and Symptom Management* 19 (5): 363–77.

Cutsem, EV and J Arends. 2005. The Causes and Consequences of Cancer-Associated Malnutrition. *European Journal of Oncology Nursing* 9 Suppl 2 (January): S51–63.

Dalle, J-H, A Moghrabi, P Rousseau, J-M Leclerc, S Barrette, ML Bernstein, J Champagne et al. 2005. Second Induction in Pediatric Patients with Recurrent Acute Lymphoid Leukemia Using DFCI-ALL Protocols. *Journal of Pediatric Hematology/Oncology* 27 (2): 73–79.

Eberhardie, C. 2002. Nutrition Support in Palliative Care. *Nursing Standard* 17 (2): 47–52; quiz 54-5.
Ehsanipour, EA, X Sheng, JW Behan, X Wang, A Butturini, VI Avramis, and SD Mittelman. 2013. Adipocytes Cause Leukemia Cell Resistance to L-Asparaginase via Release of Glutamine. *Cancer Research* 73 (10): 2998–3006.
Einsiedel, HG, A von Stackelberg, R Hartmann, R Fengler, M Schrappe, G Janka-Schaub, G Mann et al. 2005. Long-Term Outcome in Children with Relapsed ALL by Risk-Stratified Salvage Therapy: Results of Trial Acute Lymphoblastic Leukemia-Relapse Study of the Berlin-Frankfurt-Münster Group 87. *Journal of Clinical Oncology* 23 (31): 7942–50.
Goldsby, RE, Q Liu, PC Nathan, DC Bowers, A Yeaton-Massey, SH Raber, D Hill et al. 2010. Late-Occurring Neurologic Sequelae in Adult Survivors of Childhood Acute Lymphoblastic Leukemia: A Report from the Childhood Cancer Survivor Study. *Journal of Clinical Oncology* 28 (2): 324–31.
Greenlee, RT, T Murray, S Bolden, and PA Wingo. 2000. Cancer Statistics, 2000. *CA: A Cancer Journal for Clinicians* 50 (1): 7–33.
Gupta, S, M Bonilla, SL Fuentes, M Caniza, SC Howard, R Barr, ML Greenberg, R Ribeiro, and L Sung. 2009. Incidence and Predictors of Treatment-Related Mortality in Paediatric Acute Leukaemia in El Salvador. *British Journal of Cancer* 100 (7): 1026–31.
Gurney, JG, RK Severson, S Davis, and LL Robison. 1995. Incidence of Cancer in Children in the United States. Sex-, Race-, and 1-Year Age-Specific Rates by Histologic Type. *Cancer* 75 (8): 2186–95.
Hafez, HA, R Solaiman, D Bilal, and LM Shalaby. 2016. Early Deaths in Pediatric Acute Leukemia; A Challenge in Developing Countries. *Blood* 128 (22): 5160.
Han-Markey, T. 2000. Nutritional Considerations in Pediatric Oncology. *Seminars in Oncology Nursing* 16 (2): 146–51.
Harris, MB. 2004. Palliative Care in Children with Cancer: Which Child and When? *Journal of the National Cancer Institute Monographs* 2004 (32): 144–49.
Hassan, M, CH. Lin, and L Torno. 2013. Risk Factors for Obesity and Time Frame of Weight Gain in Non-Irradiated Survivors of Pediatric Acute Lymphoblastic Leukemia. *Journal of Cancer Therapy* 4 (1): 124–32.
Hunger, SP, X Lu, M Devidas, BM Camitta, PS Gaynon, NJ Winick, GH Reaman, and WL Carroll. 2012. Improved Survival for Children and Adolescents with Acute Lymphoblastic Leukemia between 1990 and 2005: A Report from the Children's Oncology Group. *Journal of Clinical Oncology* 30 (14): 1663–69.
Iughetti, L, P Bruzzi, B Predieri, and P Paolucci. 2012. Obesity in Patients with Acute Lymphoblastic Leukemia in Childhood. *Italian Journal of Pediatrics* 38 (1): 4.
Jaime-Pérez, JC, O González-Llano, JL Herrera-Garza, H Gutiérrez-Aguirre, E Vázquez-Garza, and D Gómez-Almaguer. 2008. Assessment of Nutritional Status in Children with Acute Lymphoblastic Leukemia in Northern México: A 5-Year Experience. *Pediatric Blood and Cancer* 50 (S2): 506–8.
Jiménez-Hernández, E, EZ Jaimes-Reyes, J Arellano-Galindo, X García-Jiménez, HM Tiznado-García, MT Dueñas-González, OM Villegas et al. 2015. Survival of Mexican Children with Acute Lymphoblastic Leukaemia under Treatment with the Protocol from the Dana-Farber Cancer Institute 00-01. *BioMed Research International* 2015 (January): 9 pp.
Joyce, MJ, BH Pollock, M Devidas, GR Buchanan, and B Camitta. 2013. Chemotherapy for Initial Induction Failures in Childhood Acute Lymphoblastic Leukemia: A Children's Oncology Group Study (POG 8764). *Journal of Pediatric Hematology/Oncology* 35 (1): 32–35.
Ko, RH, L Ji, P Barnette, B Bostrom, R Hutchinson, E Raetz, NL Seibel et al. 2010. Outcome of Patients Treated for Relapsed or Refractory Acute Lymphoblastic Leukemia: A Therapeutic Advances in Childhood Leukemia Consortium Study. *Journal of Clinical Oncology* 28 (4): 648–54.
Lo, SS-M, S Ryu, EL Chang, N Galanopoulos, J Jones, EY Kim, CD Kubicky et al. 2015. ACR Appropriateness Criteria® Metastatic Epidural Spinal Cord Compression and Recurrent Spinal Metastasis. *Journal of Palliative Medicine* 18 (7): 573–84.
Loblaw, DA, G Mitera, M Ford, and NJ Laperriere. 2012. A 2011 Updated Systematic Review and Clinical Practice Guideline for the Management of Malignant Extradural Spinal Cord Compression. *International Journal of Radiation Oncology, Biology, Physics* 84 (2): 312–17.
Lopez-Facundo NA, Talavera-Piña JO, Tejocote-Romero I. 2008. Mortalidad Temprana En Niños Con LLA En Un País En Vías de Desarrollo; Factores Asociados Con El Pronóstico. *Gamo* 7 (1): 93–101.
Margolin, JF, CP Steuber, and DG Poplack. 2006. Acute Lymphocytic Leukemia. In *Principles and Practice of Pediatric Oncology*, edited by PA Pizzo and DG Poplack, 5th ed., 538–90. Philadelphia: JB Lippincott.
Martín-Trejo, JA, JC Núñez-Enríquez, A Fajardo-Gutiérrez, A Medina-Sansón, J Flores-Lujano, E Jiménez-Hernández, R Amador-Sanchez et al. 2017. Early Mortality in Children with Acute Lymphoblastic Leukemia in a Developing Country: The Role of Malnutrition at Diagnosis. A Multicenter Cohort MIGICCL Study. *Leukemia and Lymphoma* 58 (4): 898–908.

Mejía-Aranguré, JM, A Fajardo-Gutiérrez, NI Reyes-Ruíz, R Bernáldez-Ríos, AM Mejía-Domínguez, S Navarrete-Navarro, and MC Martínez-García. 1999. Malnutrition in Childhood Lymphoblastic Leukemia: A Predictor of Early Mortality during the Induction-to-Remission Phase of the Treatment. *Archives of Medical Research* 30 (2): 150–53.

Michel, G, CE Rebholz, NX von der Weid, E Bergstraesser, and CE Kuehni. 2010. Psychological Distress in Adult Survivors of Childhood Cancer: The Swiss Childhood Cancer Survivor Study. *Journal of Clinical Oncology* 28 (10): 1740–48.

Mody, R, S Li, DC Dover, S Sallan, W Leisenring, KC Oeffinger, Y Yasui, LL Robison, and JP Neglia. 2008. Twenty-Five-Year Follow-up among Survivors of Childhood Acute Lymphoblastic Leukemia: A Report from the Childhood Cancer Survivor Study. *Blood* 111 (12): 5515–23.

Mosby, TT, M Cosgrove, S Sarkardei, KL Platt, and B Kaina. 2012. Nutrition in Adult and Childhood Cancer: Role of Carcinogens and Anti-Carcinogens. *Anticancer Research* 32 (10): 4171–92.

Mwirigi, A, R Dillon and K Raj. 2017. Acute Leukaemia. *Medicine* 45 (5): 280–86.

Odame, I, JJ Reilly, BE Gibson, and MD Donaldson. 1994. Patterns of Obesity in Boys and Girls after Treatment for Acute Lymphoblastic Leukaemia. *Archives of Disease in Childhood* 71 (2): 147–49.

O'Hara, PD. 2017. The Management of Nutrition in Palliative Care. *Links to Health and Social Care* 2 (1): 21–38.

Orgel, E, JM Genkinger, D Aggarwal, L Sung, M Nieder, and EJ Ladas. 2016. Association of Body Mass Index and Survival in Pediatric Leukemia: A Meta-Analysis. *American Journal of Clinical Nutrition* 103 (3): 808–17.

Orgel, E, R Sposto, J Malvar, NL Seibel, E Ladas, PS Gaynon, and DR Freyer. 2014. Impact on Survival and Toxicity by Duration of Weight Extremes during Treatment for Pediatric Acute Lymphoblastic Leukemia: A Report from the Children's Oncology Group. *Journal of Clinical Oncology* 32 (13): 1331–37.

Orgel, E, J Tucci, W Alhushki, J Malvar, R Sposto, CH Fu, DR Freyer, H Abdel-Azim, and SD Mittelman. 2014. Obesity Is Associated with Residual Leukemia Following Induction Therapy for Childhood B-Precursor Acute Lymphoblastic Leukemia. *Blood* 124 (26): 3932–38.

Owens, JL, SJ Hanson, JA McArthur, and TA Mikhailov. 2013. The Need for Evidence Based Nutritional Guidelines for Pediatric Acute Lymphoblastic Leukemia Patients: Acute and Long-Term Following Treatment. *Nutrients* 5 (11): 4333–46.

Paccagnella, A, I Morassutti, and G Rosti. 2011. Nutritional Intervention for Improving Treatment Tolerance in Cancer Patients. *Current Opinion in Oncology* 23 (4): 322–30.

Pérez-Saldivar, ML, A Fajardo-Gutiérrez, R Bernáldez-Ríos, A Martínez-Avalos, A Medina-Sanson, L Espinosa-Hernández, J de Diego Flores-Chapa et al. 2011. Childhood Acute Leukemias Are Frequent in Mexico City: Descriptive Epidemiology. *BMC Cancer* 11 (1): 355.

Pramanik, R, X Sheng, B Ichihara, N Heisterkamp, and SD Mittelman. 2013. Adipose Tissue Attracts and Protects Acute Lymphoblastic Leukemia Cells from Chemotherapy. *Leukemia Research* 37 (5): 503–9.

Pribnow, AK, R Ortiz, LF Báez, L Mendieta, and S Luna-Fineman. 2017. Effects of Malnutrition on Treatment-Related Morbidity and Survival of Children with Cancer in Nicaragua. *Pediatric Blood and Cancer* 64 (11): e26590.

Pui, C-H. 2010. Chapter 93. Acute Lymphoblastic Leukemia. In *Williams Hematology*, edited by MA Lichtman, TJ Kipps, U Seligsohn, K Kaushansky, and JT Prchal, 8th ed. New York: McGraw-Hill.

Pui, C-H and WE Evans. 2013. A 50-Year Journey to Cure Childhood Acute Lymphoblastic Leukemia. *Seminars in Hematology* 50 (3): 185–96.

Rahn, DA, AJ Mundt, JD Murphy, D Schiff, J Adams, and KT Murphy. 2015. Clinical Outcomes of Palliative Radiation Therapy for Children. *Practical Radiation Oncology* 5 (3): 183–87.

Ries, LA, CL Kosary, and BF Hankey. 1999. *SEER Cancer Statistics Review, 1973–1996*. Bethesda, MD: National Cancer Institute.

Rivera-Luna, R, A Olaya-Vargas, M Velásquez-Aviña, S Frenk, R Cárdenas-Cardós, C Leal-Leal, O Pérez-González, and A Martínez-Avalos. 2008. Early Death in Children with Acute Lymphoblastic Leukemia: Does Malnutrition Play a Role? *Pediatric Hematology and Oncology* 25 (1): 17–26.

Roberts, DL, C Dive, and AG Renehan. 2010. Biological Mechanisms Linking Obesity and Cancer Risk: New Perspectives. *Annual Review of Medicine* 61 (1): 301–16.

Rogers, PCJ. 2014. Nutritional Status as a Prognostic Indicator for Pediatric Malignancies. *Journal of Clinical Oncology* 32 (13): 1293–94.

Ross, JA, SM Davies, JD Potter, and LL Robison. 1994. Epidemiology of Childhood Leukemia, with a Focus on Infants. *Epidemiologic Reviews* 16 (2): 243–72.

Rubnitz, JE, BI Razzouk, S Lensing, S Pounds, C-H Pui, and RC Ribeiro. 2007. Prognostic Factors and Outcome of Recurrence in Childhood Acute Myeloid Leukemia. *Cancer* 109 (1): 157–63.

Sala, A, E Rossi, F Antillon, AL Ana Lucia Molina, T de Maselli, M Bonilla, A Hernandez et al. 2012. Nutritional Status at Diagnosis Is Related to Clinical Outcomes in Children and Adolescents with Cancer: A Perspective from Central America. *European Journal of Cancer (Oxford, England: 1990)* 48 (2): 243–52. Schrappe, M, SP Hunger, C-H Pui, V Saha, PS Gaynon, A Baruchel, V Conter et al. 2012. Outcomes after Induction Failure in Childhood Acute Lymphoblastic Leukemia. *New England Journal of Medicine* 366 (15): 1371–81.

Sendrós Madroño, JM. 2016. Aspectos Dietoterapéuticos En Situaciones Especiales Del Paciente Oncológico. Prebióticos y Probióticos, ¿tienen Cabida En La Terapia Nutricional Del Paciente Oncológico? *Nutrición Hospitalaria* 33 (1).

Schmiegelow, K, K Müller, SS Mogensen, PR Mogensen, BO Wolthers, UK Stoltze, R Tuckuviene, and T Frandsen. 2017. Non-infectious chemotherapy-associated acute toxicities during childhood acute lymphoblastic leukemia therapy. *F1000Res* 6444, doi: 10.12688/f1000research.10768.1. eCollection 2017.

Skipworth, RJE, GD Stewart, CHC Dejong, T Preston, and KCH Fearon. 2007. Pathophysiology of Cancer Cachexia: Much More than Host-Tumour Interaction? *Clinical Nutrition* 26 (6): 667–76.

Slats, AM, RM Egeler, A van der Does-van den Berg, C Korbijn, K Hählen, WA Kamps, AJP Veerman, and CM Zwaan. 2005. Causes of Death – Other than Progressive Leukemia – in Childhood Acute Lymphoblastic (ALL) and Myeloid Leukemia (AML): The Dutch Childhood Oncology Group Experience. *Leukemia* 19 (4): 537–44.

Smith, DE, MC Stevens, and IW Booth. 1991. Malnutrition at Diagnosis of Malignancy in Childhood: Common but Mostly Missed. *European Journal of Pediatrics* 150 (5): 318–22.

Stephen, RC. 2014. *Global Atlas of Palliative Care at End of Life*. Worldwide Palliative Care Alliance. World Health Organization. https://www.who.int/nmh/Global_Atlas_of_Palliative_Care.pdf. (accessed March 25, 2019).

Swensen, AR, JA Ross, RK Severson, BH Pollock, and LL Robison. 1997. The Age Peak in Childhood Acute Lymphoblastic Leukemia: Exploring the Potential Relationship with Socioeconomic Status. *Cancer* 79 (10): 2045–51.

Tazi, I, Z Hidane, S Zafad, M Harif, S Benchekroun, and R Ribeiro. 2008. Nutritional Status at Diagnosis of Children with Malignancies in Casablanca. *Pediatric Blood and Cancer* 51 (4): 495–98.

Tisdale, MJ. 2009. Mechanisms of Cancer Cachexia. *Physiological Reviews* 89 (2): 381–410.

Varma, S, DL Friedman, and M J. Stavas. 2017. The Role of Radiation Therapy in Palliative Care of Children with Advanced Cancer: Clinical Outcomes and Patterns of Care. *Pediatric Blood and Cancer* 64 (5): e26359.

Veringa, SJE, E van Dulmen-den Broeder, GJL Kaspers, and MA Veening. 2012. Blood Pressure and Body Composition in Long-Term Survivors of Childhood Acute Lymphoblastic Leukemia. *Pediatric Blood and Cancer* 58 (2): 278–82.

Watsky, MA, LD Carbone, Q An, C Cheng, EA Lovorn, MM Hudson, C-H Pui, and SC Kaste. 2014. Bone Turnover in Long-Term Survivors of Childhood Acute Lymphoblastic Leukemia. *Pediatric Blood and Cancer* 61 (8): 1451–56.

Weaver, MS, KE Heinze, KP Kelly, L Wiener, RL Casey, CJ Bell, J Wolfe, AM Garee, A Watson, and PS Hinds. 2015. Palliative Care as a Standard of Care in Pediatric Oncology. *Pediatric Blood and Cancer* 62 (S5): S829–33.

Yang, L, X Hu, and L Xu. 2012. Impact of Methylenetetrahydrofolate Reductase (MTHFR) Polymorphisms on Methotrexate-Induced Toxicities in Acute Lymphoblastic Leukemia: A Meta-Analysis. *Tumor Biology* 33 (5): 1445–54.

Yazbeck, N, L Samia, R Saab, MR Abboud, H Solh, and S Muwakkit. 2016. Effect of Malnutrition at Diagnosis on Clinical Outcomes of Children with Acute Lymphoblastic Leukemia. *Journal of Pediatric Hematology/Oncology* 38 (2): 107–10.

Zeltzer, LK, Q Lu, W Leisenring, JCI Tsao, C Recklitis, G Armstrong, AC Mertens, LL Robison, and KK Ness. 2008. Psychosocial Outcomes and Health-Related Quality of Life in Adult Childhood Cancer Survivors: A Report from the Childhood Cancer Survivor Study. *Cancer Epidemiology, Biomarkers and Prevention* 17 (2): 435–46.

Zwaan, CM, EA Kolb, D Reinhardt, J Abrahamsson, S Adachi, R Aplenc, ESJM De Bont et al. 2015. Collaborative Efforts Driving Progress in Pediatric Acute Myeloid Leukemia. *Journal of Clinical Oncology* 33 (27): 2949–62.

26 Eating-Related Distress in Terminally Ill Cancer Patients and Their Family Members

Koji Amano and Tatsuya Morita

CONTENTS

INTRODUCTION

Despite the great advances in research made in the last two decades, there is still a lack of understanding regarding the pathophysiology of cancer cachexia and its negative impact on patients and their family members, particularly with relation to feeding and nutrition. It has been acknowledged that in advanced cancer patients the involuntary loss of skeletal muscle mass and body weight are often caused by reductions in food intake due to cancer cachexia and are linked to the deterioration of nutritional status, performance status, treatment outcomes, survival, and quality of life. In addition, cancer cachexia affects not only patients, but also their family members, who travel with patients on their "cancer journey" (Evans et al. 2008; Bozzetti and Mariani 2009; Tisdale 2009; Fearon et al. 2011; Fearon et al. 2012; Laviano et al. 2012). Thus, a large number of advanced cancer patients and their family members suffer from psychosocial issues caused by cancer cachexia, of which eating-related distress (ERD) is one of the most representative (Strasser et al. 2007; Hopkinson et al. 2011; Oberholzer et al. 2013; Reid 2014; Hopkinson 2014; Cooper et al. 2015; Hopkinson 2016; Amano et al. 2016a,c; Amano et al. 2018; Wheelwright et al. 2016). The prevalence of ERD and the need for nutritional support in advanced cancer patients and their family members might be greater than medical staff think, particularly when patients become unable to consume sufficient nourishment orally and the negative impact of cancer cachexia becomes apparent (Amano et al. 2016a,c; Amano et al. 2018). Therefore, there is a need to address the psychosocial burdens associated with cancer cachexia, especially ERD, in both patients and their family members. However, the tools for evaluating ERD and the palliative care strategies for these disorders are not sufficiently developed.

CACHEXIA-ANOREXIA SYNDROME IN ADVANCED CANCER PATIENTS

Cancer cachexia is defined as a multifactorial syndrome involving the ongoing loss of skeletal muscle mass (with or without the loss of fat mass) that cannot be fully reversed by conventional nutritional support and leads to progressive functional impairment. Its pathophysiology is characterized by a negative protein and energy balance driven by a combination of reduced food intake and abnormal metabolism (Fearon et al. 2011). In addition, there is growing evidence that systemic chronic inflammation plays an important role in the mechanisms responsible for cancer cachexia and that inflammatory mediators, for example, proinflammatory cytokines and C-reactive protein (CRP), contribute to reduced food intake; abnormal metabolism; and a variety of symptoms, including anorexia, fatigue, and weight loss (Evans et al. 2008; Bozzetti and Mariani 2009; Tisdale 2009; Fearon et al. 2011; Fearon et al. 2012; Laviano et al. 2012; Amano et al. 2016b; Amano et al. 2017). Thus, it is important to assess all advanced cancer patients for reduced food intake and abnormal metabolism, manage their symptoms by suppressing chronic inflammation with multimodal treatments, and monitor their plasma CRP levels.

According to the consensus among international experts, there are three distinct stages of cancer cachexia: pre-cachexia, cachexia, and refractory cachexia (Fearon et al. 2011). The psychosocial burdens experienced by patients and their family members can change across the three stages of cancer cachexia, particularly from cachexia to refractory cachexia. Thus, in terms of the psychosocial burdens associated with cancer cachexia, palliative care that is tailored to the stage of each patient's disease is required.

MECHANISMS RESPONSIBLE FOR EATING-RELATED DISTRESS IN ADVANCED CANCER PATIENTS

As mentioned, the vast majority of advanced cancer patients suffer from reduced food intake and weight loss due to cancer cachexia, which are hard to prevent/alleviate using standard treatments. In particular, weight loss will inevitably occur despite caloric supplementation in patients with cancer cachexia. Furthermore, a retrospective study conducted at a cancer cachexia clinic indicated that most patients who experienced involuntary weight loss had three or more uncontrolled nutritional impact symptoms (NIS); that is, nausea, vomiting, constipation, diarrhea, dysgeusia, dysosmia, xerostomia, difficulty chewing, dysphagia, severe pain, dyspnea, anxiety, and/or depression (Del Fabbro et al. 2011). Indeed, previous studies indicated that a number of various types of ERD seen in advanced cancer patients are caused by a gap between reality and expectations (Hopkinson et al. 2011; Hopkinson 2014; Hopkinson 2016). This phenomenon is called the "Calman gap," which is also observed in types of distress associated with other symptoms, for example, pain and fatigue (Calman 1984).

A systematic review reported that the main causes of psychosocial burdens in advanced cancer patients are a lack of knowledge about cancer cachexia, unsuccessful attempts by patients to increase their body weight, and the expected occurrence of death (Oberholzer et al. 2013). Furthermore, in a small survey of advanced cancer patients conducted in an inpatient hospice in Japan, most of the patients, 28 of 37 (76%), had unmet general needs that could have been satisfied by medical staff with specific knowledge of nutritional therapy for cancer cachexia. Specific support, such as "attention to patients' ERD" and "an explanation of the reasons for anorexia and weight loss," was needed by more than half of the 28 patients who had unmet general needs (Amano et al. 2016a).

A review reported that ERD can escalate or de-escalate depending on patients' coping strategies (Oberholzer et al. 2013). In the previously mentioned survey, of the 19 ERD-related items the four most common belonged to the "coping strategies" group, and the fifth most common item belonged to the "mechanisms originating from the patients themselves" group. It also suggested that patients had strong concerns over "appetite loss," "an inability to eat," and "weight loss" and that "hopelessness," "fretting," and "a shortage of information" aggravated their distress (Amano et al. 2016a).

MECHANISMS RESPONSIBLE FOR EATING-RELATED DISTRESS IN FAMILY MEMBERS

Cancer cachexia impacts not only on advanced cancer patients, but also on their family members, as the patients start to exhibit reduced food intake and weight loss due to cancer cachexia. In qualitative studies investigating the ERD experienced by the family members of advanced cancer patients, the subjects' responses to the declining food intake and weight loss of patients were classified into three separate sub-processes: "fighting back," "letting nature take its course," or "waffling," with the latter referring to vacillating between the first two patterns (McClement et al. 2003; McClement et al. 2004). A systematic review reported that the five extracted themes in family members of advanced cancer patients were "impact on everyday life," "taking charge," "need for outside help," "conflict with patient," and "emotions" (Wheelwright et al. 2016). In a survey of bereaved family members conducted in inpatient hospices in Japan, the five most common of the 19 ERD-related items were categorized as "fighting back," and the sixth item was classified as "letting nature take its course" (Amano et al. 2016c). Thus, the "fighting back" sub-process can cause distress among family members.

The latter study also revealed that greater than 70% of family members of advanced cancer patients stated that such patients require nutritional support, and greater than 40% would like to receive a sufficient explanation about the reasons for the patient's weight loss. Explanatory factor analysis of ERD identified the following four domains: (factor 1) "feeling that family members forced the patient to eat to avoid death," (factor 2) "feeling that family members made great efforts to help the patient eat," (factor 3) "feeling that eating was a cause of conflict between the patient and family members," and (factor 4) "feeling that correct information was insufficient." Multivariate logistic regression analysis identified being a patient's spouse, fair/poor mental status among family members, factor 1, and factor 4 as independent determinants of major depression in bereaved family members. Insufficient care for ERD among family members, especially spouses with weakened mental statuses, might be associated with major depression among family members after the patient's death (Amano et al. 2016c). In a mixed methods study of male patients with advanced cancer and their female partners in Switzerland, the patients' partners expressed feelings of deep concern, frustration, and insufficiency with the patients and described the innovative efforts they had made to prepare appealing food (Strasser et al. 2007). These findings are consistent with a review in which the main causes of the psychosocial burdens experienced by the family members of cancer patients were found to be a lack of knowledge about cancer cachexia, unsuccessful attempts to increase the patient's body weight, and expected occurrence of the patient's death (Oberholzer et al. 2013). The negative impacts of cancer cachexia often affect cooking at home, couples' daily eating habits, and spousal relationships, and female partners tend to suffer from deeper distress than male partners (Strasser et al. 2007; Hopkinson 2014; Wheelwright et al. 2016).

CONFLICTS OVER FOOD BETWEEN ADVANCED CANCER PATIENTS AND THEIR FAMILY MEMBERS

Previous qualitative studies of advanced cancer patients and their family members suggested that reductions in the patient's dietary intake frequently became a source of conflict among patients and their family members in both inpatient and outpatient units (Holden 1991; Addington-Hall and McCarthy 1995; Oi-Ling et al. 2005; Hopkinson et al. 2008; Reid et al. 2009; Wheelwright et al. 2016). These conflicts tend to cause ERD in advanced cancer patients and their family members. In such cases, patients eat not because they want food, but because they want to satisfy their family members, who are encouraging them to eat. Family members often experience feelings of rejection when food is refused by patients. Thus, patients often choose social isolation or lie to their family members to avoid conflicts, but family members also feel guilty when they argue over patients' lack of dietary intake (Addington-Hall and McCarthy 1995; Reid et al. 2009; Wheelwright et al. 2016). Changes in food preferences and eating habits can also cause conflicts between patients and family members because they fail to see weight loss as an inevitable consequence of cancer cachexia. In addition, family members unintentionally place unnecessary pressure on patients to eat. While patients often feel dejected and harassed because of this pressure, their family members also suffer. Contrary to family members' intentions, their approach to such eating problems can become a barrier to food intake (Hopkinson et al. 2008; Reid et al. 2009; Wheelwright et al. 2016). Moreover, anorexia is one of the most distressing symptoms encountered in the last week of life in advanced cancer patients, but the family members of patients did not rate it as important (Oi-Ling et al. 2005). A qualitative study suggested that the perspectives of patients might not necessarily be shared by their family members and that weight loss in the patient was indeed a source of conflict within the family (Holden 1991).

In the previously mentioned mixed methods study of male patients and their female partners, it was suggested that the patients' partners were more concerned about the patients' weight loss than the patients themselves and that the patients felt more pressure to eat from their partners than they estimated (Strasser et al. 2007). In a small survey of advanced cancer patients, experience of conflicts over food was the item that exhibited the lowest frequency (5.5%) among the 19 ERD-related items, and the perceived need for intervention in such conflicts was low (18%) (Amano et al. 2016a). In a survey of bereaved family members, experience of conflicts over food exhibited one of the lowest frequencies (7.8%) among the 19 ERD-related items, while the perceived need for intervention in such conflicts was moderate (27.8%) (Amano et al. 2016c). It seems that overt emotional conflicts over food between patients and their family members seldom occur in inpatient hospices despite family members' covert distress.

TOOLS FOR EVALUATING EATING-RELATED DISTRESS

To the best of our knowledge, there is no validated tool for evaluating ERD among advanced cancer patients and their family members. Therefore, ad hoc questionnaires for both advanced cancer patients and their family members have been preliminarily developed, in which items were adopted from two quantitative studies (Amano et al. 2016a,c) (Tables 26.1 and 26.2). However, the development of further validated tools for evaluating ERD among advanced cancer patients and their family members is strongly needed in the near future.

APPLICATIONS TO OTHER AREAS OF TERMINAL OR PALLIATIVE CARE

Cachexia affects a wide spectrum of patients with end-stage chronic diseases, including acquired immune deficiency syndrome, chronic obstructive pulmonary disease, heart failure, renal failure, and rheumatoid arthritis. Although there are common mechanisms of wasting in each of these diseases, there are many unique aspects that are too complex to summarize in a single passage. Additionally, in comparison with advanced cancer, other chronic diseases have different dynamics, and patient decline may be slower. Therefore, it may be difficult to apply practical methods and techniques of palliative care for ERD used for advanced cancer patients to those with other chronic diseases.

PRACTICAL METHODS AND TECHNIQUES OF PALLIATIVE CARE FOR EATING-RELATED DISTRESS

As far as we know, there are no data from randomized controlled trials about palliative care for ERD among advanced cancer patients and their family members. However, some reviews have suggested that supportive, communicative, and educational interventions reduce the psychosocial burdens placed on patients and their family members by cancer cachexia (Hopkinson et al. 2011; Oberholzer et al. 2013; Hopkinson 2014; Reid 2014; Cooper et al. 2015; Wheelwright et al. 2016). In a survey of advanced cancer patients, many of the subjects stated that more attention should have been paid to their ERD and that they needed an explanation about the causes of cancer

TABLE 26.1
Questionnaire about Eating-Related Distress of Advanced Cancer Patients

	No	Seldom	Sometimes	Frequently	Always
Distress Originating from the Feelings of Patients					
Although I know that I have to eat enough, I cannot do that.	1	2	3	4	5
I want attention to be paid to my eating-related distress.	1	2	3	4	5
I do not know why I cannot eat enough.	1	2	3	4	5
I feel that a lack of nutrition makes my condition worse.	1	2	3	4	5
Distress Originating from Coping Strategies					
I wonder what kinds of food I can eat.	1	2	3	4	5
I wonder which nutrients I should preferentially consume.	1	2	3	4	5
I wonder how I can eat more.	1	2	3	4	5
I feel that more medical support about my daily diet is needed.	1	2	3	4	5
Distress Originating from the Relationship Between Patients and Their Families					
I am burdened by the meals that my family kindly serves me.	1	2	3	4	5
I have experienced conflict about my meals with my family.	1	2	3	4	5
I feel that I disregard the kindness that my family shows by making my meals.	1	2	3	4	5
I feel sad because I cannot enjoy dinner with my family.	1	2	3	4	5

Note: There is no validated tool for evaluating eating-related distress among advanced cancer patients. Therefore, the ad hoc questionnaire for them has been preliminarily developed.

cachexia (Amano et al. 2016a). In a survey of bereaved family members, half of the subjects wanted information about the negative impact of cancer cachexia on patients (Amano et al. 2016c). Furthermore, the need for nutritional support seems to be high among patients with cancer cachexia and their family members (Amano et al. 2016a,c; Amano et al. 2018). A mixed methods study carried out in the United Kingdom indicated that an intervention involving the provision of information, reassurance, and support for self-management had a positive effect on the lives of the family members of advanced cancer patients, for example, it improved their weight- and eating-related distress (Hopkinson et al. 2013). These results support the suggestions of the abovementioned reviews.

In addition, the results of the two previously mentioned surveys indicated that overt emotional conflicts over food between patients and their family members seldom occur in inpatient hospices (Amano et al. 2016a,c), while other qualitative studies indicated that ERD associated with conflicts over food might be real and serious problems for cancer patients and their family members (Holden 1991; Addington-Hall and McCarthy 1995; Oi-Ling et al. 2005; Hopkinson et al. 2008; Reid et al. 2009; Wheelwright et al. 2016). We can support patients and their family members in conflicts over food by drawing on our own experiences of families who have found effective ways of managing such conflicts. Sharing this experience can help to demonstrate that disagreements over food can be temporary and provide ideas that enable patients and their family members to see new ways of managing their problems (Hopkinson et al. 2008). In cases involving cancer cachexia, we should pay careful attention to conflicts over food and give appropriate explanations to family members as well as patients.

Finally, since cancer cachexia is a multifactorial syndrome, multimodal treatments, such as nutritional support, exercise therapy, and pharmacotherapy, are considered to be required (Evans et al. 2008; Bozzetti and Mariani 2009; Tisdale 2009; Fearon et al. 2011; Fearon et al. 2012; Laviano et al. 2012). If these treatments reduce the negative impact of cachexia on advanced cancer

TABLE 26.2
Questionnaire about Eating-Related Distress of Family Members of Advanced Cancer Patients

	No	Seldom	Sometimes	Frequently	Always
Distress Originating from the Feelings of Family Members Themselves					
Although I know that I have to help the patient eat enough, I cannot do that.	1	2	3	4	5
I want attention to be paid to my distress about the patient's eating.	1	2	3	4	5
I do not know why the patient cannot eat enough.	1	2	3	4	5
I feel that a lack of nutrition makes the patient's condition worse.	1	2	3	4	5
Distress Originating from Coping Strategies					
I wonder what kinds of food the patient can eat.	1	2	3	4	5
I wonder which nutrients the patient should preferentially consume.	1	2	3	4	5
I wonder how the patient can eat more.	1	2	3	4	5
I feel that more medical support about the patient's daily diet is needed.	1	2	3	4	5
Distress Originating from the Relationship Between Patients and Their Family Members					
I feel that the patient is burdened by the meals that I kindly serve him/her.	1	2	3	4	5
I have experienced conflict about the patient's meals with him/her.	1	2	3	4	5
I feel that the patient disregards the kindness that I show by making his/her meals.	1	2	3	4	5
I feel sad because the patient cannot enjoy dinner with me.	1	2	3	4	5

Note: There is no validated tool for evaluating eating-related distress among family members of advanced cancer patients. Therefore, the ad hoc questionnaire for family members has been preliminarily developed.

patients, the psychosocial burdens, including ERD, placed on patients and their family members might be alleviated. Therefore, if possible, multimodal treatments, the suppression of chronic inflammation, and evaluations of plasma CRP levels should be employed in cases of advanced cancer, even in the palliative care setting. Importantly, palliative care for ERD among patients and their family members needs to be tailored to the degree of cancer cachexia. In particular, patients with refractory cachexia might suffer the greatest ERD due to the ineffectiveness of multimodal treatments.

In summary, medical staff should (1) pay attention to ERD among advanced cancer patients and their family members, (2) appreciate the efforts such individuals make to cope, (3) manage conflicts over food among advanced cancer patients and their family members, (4) explain the mechanisms responsible for cancer cachexia and ERD as simply as possible, and (5) give optimal advice on how patients and their family members can cope with cancer cachexia. This strategy can help to alleviate the ERD experienced by advanced cancer patients and their family members.

ETHICAL ISSUES

Nutritional support, exercise therapy, and pharmacotherapy are essential for treating cancer cachexia. Nutritional treatment is an important component of nutritional support, as is the palliation of NIS and nutritional counseling, according to the European Society for Clinical Nutrition and Metabolism (ESPEN) guidelines on nutrition in cancer patients. However, the evidence supporting the advice suggested in these guidelines is weak (Arends et al. 2017). In addition, the guidelines state that nutritional support, especially artificial nutrition and hydration (ANH), is unlikely to provide any benefit for most cancer patients with very advanced disease (Arends et al. 2017). The ESPEN guidelines on the ethical aspects of ANH suggest that decisions on ANH have to consider social, cultural, emotional, and existential factors, as well as patients' spiritual and ethnic backgrounds and needs (Druml et al. 2016). Small amounts of food might have significant effects on terminally ill cancer patients and their family members and could contribute to improving their sense of well-being, autonomy, and dignity.

KEY FACTS: EATING-RELATED DISTRESS DUE TO CANCER CACHEXIA

- Cancer cachexia is defined as a multifactorial syndrome involving the ongoing loss of skeletal muscle mass that can be partially but not entirely reversed by conventional nutritional support.
- Loss of skeletal muscle mass leads to progressive functional impairment, increased chemotherapy toxicity, poor quality of life, and high mortality in advanced cancer patients.
- Systemic chronic inflammation plays an important role in the mechanisms responsible for cancer cachexia and contributes to a variety of symptoms, including anorexia, reduced food intake, and weight loss.
- As no effective medical intervention completely reverses cancer cachexia, nutritional support remains a mainstay of cancer cachexia treatment.
- A large number of advanced cancer patients and their family members suffer from psychosocial issues caused by cancer cachexia, of which eating-related distress is one of the most representative.

SUMMARY POINTS

- Management strategies for cancer cachexia should address not only patients' physical problems, but also the psychosocial burdens, including eating-related distress, experienced by patients and their family members.
- If multimodal treatments reduce the negative impact of cachexia on advanced cancer patients, the psychosocial burdens, including eating-related distress, placed on patients and their family members might be alleviated.
- The main causes of eating-related distress experienced by patients with cancer cachexia and their family members are a lack of knowledge about cachexia, unsuccessful attempts to increase body weight, expected occurrence of the patient's death, and conflicts over food between them.
- Supportive, communicative, and educational interventions would alleviate eating-related distress of patients with cancer cachexia and their family members.
- Palliative care for eating-related distress experienced by advanced cancer patients and their family members needs to be tailored to the severity of the patient's cachexia, especially in cases of refractory cachexia.

LIST OF ABBREVIATIONS

ANH	Artificial Nutrition and Hydration
CRP	C-Reactive Protein
ERD	Eating-Related Distress
ESPEN	The European Society for Clinical Nutrition and Metabolism
NIS	Nutritional Impact Symptoms

REFERENCES

Addington-Hall, J., M. McCarthy. 1995. Dying from cancer: Results of a national population-based investigation. *Palliat Med* 9: 295–305.

Amano, K., I. Maeda, T. Morita, M. Baba, T. Miura, T. Hama, I. Mori et al. 2017. C-reactive protein, symptoms and activity of daily living in patients with advanced cancer receiving palliative care. *J Cachexia Sarcopenia Muscle* 8(3): 457–465.

Amano, K., I. Maeda, T. Morita, R. Tatara, H. Katayama, T. Uno, I. Takagi. 2016a. Need for nutritional support, eating-related distress and experience of terminally ill cancer patients: A survey in an inpatient hospice. *BMJ Support Palliat Care* 6(3): 373–376.

Amano, K., I. Maeda, T. Morita, T. Miura, S. Inoue, M. Ikenaga, Y. Matsumoto et al. 2016b. Clinical implications of C-reactive protein as a prognostic marker in advanced cancer patients in palliative care settings. *J Pain Symptom Manage* 51(5): 860–867.

Amano, K., I. Maeda, T. Morita, Y. Okajima, T. Hama, M. Aoyama, Y. Kizawa et al. 2016c. Eating-related distress and need for nutritional support of families of advanced cancer patients: A nationwide survey of bereaved family members. *J Cachexia Sarcopenia Muscle* 7(5): 527–534.

Amano, K., T. Morita, J. Miyamoto, T. Uno, H. Katayama, R. Tatara. 2018. Perception of need for nutritional support in advanced cancer patients with cachexia: A survey in palliative care settings. *Support Care Cancer* 26: 2793–2799.

Arends, J., P. Bachmann, V. Baracos, N. Barthelemy, H. Bertz, F. Bozzetti, K. Fearon et al. 2017. ESPEN guidelines on nutrition in cancer patients. *Clin Nutr* 36: 11–48.

Bozzetti, F., L. Mariani. 2009. Defining and classifying cancer cachexia: A proposal by the SCRINIO Working Group. *JPEN J Parenter Enteral Nutr* 33: 361–367.

Calman, KC. 1984. Quality of life in cancer patients – A hypothesis. *J Med Ethics* 10: 124–127.

Cooper, C., ST. Burden, H. Cheng, A. Molassiotis. 2015. Understanding and managing cancer-related weight loss and anorexia: Insights from a systematic review of qualitative research. *J Cachexia Sarcopenia Muscle* 6: 99–111.

Del Fabbro, E., D. Hui, S. Dalal, R. Dev, ZI. Nooruddin, E. Bruera. 2011. Clinical outcomes and contributors to weight loss in a cancer cachexia clinic. *J Palliat Med* 14(9): 1004–1008.

Druml, C., PE. Ballmer, W. Druml, F. Oehmichen, A. Shenkin, P. Singer, P. Soeters et al. 2016. ESPEN guideline on ethical aspects of artificial nutrition and hydration. *Clin Nutr* 35: 545–556.

Evans, WJ., JE. Morley, J. Argilés, C. Bales, V. Baracos, D. Guttridge, A. Jatoi et al. 2008. Cachexia: A new definition. *Clin Nutr* 27: 793–799.

Fearon, K., DJ. Glass, DC. Guttridge. 2012. Cancer cachexia: Mediators, signaling, and metabolic pathways. *Cell Metabolism* 16(2): 153–166.

Fearon, K., F. Strasser, SD. Anker, I. Bosaeus, E. Bruera, RL. Fainsinger, A. Jatoi et al. 2011. Definition and classification of cancer cachexia: An international consensus. *Lancet Oncol* 12: 489–495.

Holden, CM. 1991. Anorexia in the terminally ill cancer patient: The emotional impact on the patient and family. *Hosp J* 7(3): 73–84.

Hopkinson, JB. 2014. Psychosocial impact of cancer cachexia. *J Cachexia Sarcopenia Muscle* 5(2): 89–94.

Hopkinson, JB. 2016. Food connections: A qualitative exploratory study of weight- and eating-related distress in families affected by advanced cancer. *Eur J Oncol Nurs* 20: 87–96.

Hopkinson, JB., DN. Wright, C. Foster. 2008. Management of weight loss and anorexia. *Annals of Oncology* 19(7): 289–293.

Hopkinson, JB., DR. Fenlon, CL. Foster. 2013. Outcomes of a nurse-delivered psychosocial intervention for weight- and eating-related distress in family carers of patients with advanced cancer. *Int J Palliat Nurs* 19(3): 116–123.

Hopkinson, JB., I. Okamoto, JM. Addington-Hall. 2011. What to eat when off treatment and living with involuntary weight loss and cancer: A systematic search and narrative review. *Support Care Cancer* 19(1): 1–17.

Laviano, A., M. Seelaender, S. Rianda, R. Silverio, F. Rossi Fanelli. 2012. Neuroinflammation: A contributing factor to the pathogenesis of cancer cachexia. *Crit Rev Oncog* 17(3): 247–251.

McClement, S., L. Degner, M. Harlos. 2003. Family beliefs regarding the nutritional care of a terminally ill relative: A qualitative study. *J Palliat Med* 6(5): 737–748.

McClement, SE., LF. Degner, M. Harlos. 2004. Family responses to declining intake and weight loss in a terminally ill relative. Part 1: Fighting back. *J Palliat Care* 20(2): 93–100.

Oberholzer, R., JB. Hopkinson, K. Baumann, A. Omlin, S. Kaasa, KC. Fearon, F. Strasser. 2013. Psychosocial effects of cancer cachexia: A systematic literature search and qualitative analysis. *J Pain Symptom Manage* 46(1): 77–95.

Oi-Ling, K., DT. Man-Wah, DN. Kam-Hung. 2005. Symptom distress as rated by advanced cancer patients, caregivers and physicians in the last week of life. *Palliative Medicine* 19(3): 228–233.
Reid, J. 2014. Psychosocial, educational and communicative interventions for patients with cachexia and their family carers. *Curr Opin Support Palliat Care* 8(4): 334–338.
Reid, J., H. McKenna, D. Fitzsimons, T. McCance. 2009. The experience of cancer cachexia: A qualitative study of advanced cancer patients and their family members. *Int J Nurs Stud* 46(5): 606–616.
Strasser, F., J. Binswanger, T. Cemy, A. Kesserlring. 2007. Fighting a losing battle: Eating-related distress of men with advanced cancer and their female partners. A mixed-methods study. *Palliat Med* 21(2): 129–137.
Tisdale, MJ. 2009. Mechanisms of cancer cachexia. *Physiol Rev* 89(2): 381–410.
Wheelwright, S., AS. Darlington, JB. Hopkinson, D. Fitzsimmons, C. Johnson. 2016. A systematic review and thematic synthesis of quality of life in the informal carers of cancer patients with cachexia. *Palliat Med* 30(2): 149–160.

Section V

Non-Cancer Conditions and Pharmacological Aspects

27 Nutrition and Appetite Regulation in Children and Adolescents with End-Stage Renal Failure

Kai-Dietrich Nüsken and Jörg Dötsch

CONTENTS

INTRODUCTION

The nutritional situation of patients with end-stage renal disease (ESRD) is very heterogeneous. There is no uniform "kidney diet": The demand of nutrients and fluid varies greatly, depending on age (infants, children, adolescents, adults), current body composition, mode of dialysis, underlying disease, concomitant diseases and residual diuresis. Many patients show an imbalance of energy homeostasis, characterized by increased energy consumption and a concomitant lack of appetite because of a uremia-induced, disturbed appetite regulation. Acute life-threatening conditions may occur in case of excessive hyperhydration and hyperkalemia. The most important aims of nutritional modifications are prevention of hyperhydration and cachexia and also adiposity, electrolyte disorders, disturbed bone metabolism and cardiovascular complications. In pediatric patients, it is most important to achieve an adequate growth and development. Guidelines on nutrition in renal failure are available from the National Kidney Foundation of the United States (NKF 2000, 2003, 2007, 2009) and the European Dialysis and Transplant Nurses Association/European Renal Care Association (EDTNA/ERCA 2009).

It is the objective of this chapter to review the pathophysiological changes of appetite and nutrition in end-stage renal failure with a special focus on children and adolescents.

APPETITE REGULATION

Normal Appetite Regulation

Hunger, appetite and satiety are regulated by complex mechanisms including peripheral endocrine and neuronal signals as well as cognition, perception and learned behavior. The information is mainly integrated at the hypothalamus and brainstem. Under physiological conditions, data about energy consumption and availability from currently ingested food as well as energy stores are used to maintain energy homeostasis and body weight. Dysregulation may result either in cachexia or adiposity. Hunger is a motivational state leading to acquisition and intake of food. Appetite is a similar state, but it emerges without a clear energy deficiency and with a more important role of palatability. Concerning satiety, one has to differentiate between preresorptive and postresorptive satiety. Preresorptive satiety is achieved 10–15 minutes after a meal, before any nutrients have been resorbed, and influences meal size. Mechanisms include signals from stretch- and chemo-receptors via the vagal nerve projecting to the brainstem and hormonal anorexigenic signals (Schwartz et al. 2000). Postresorptive satiety is achieved thereafter and is responsible for the interval between two meals. Mechanisms include afferent vagal nerve fibers, triggered both by portal glucosensors and by hepatic sensors of fatty acid oxidation, as well as hormonal signals. An important short- to medium-term regulator is the orexigenic hormone ghrelin (Wren et al. 2001). A very powerful medium- to long-term regulator is the anorexigenic hormone leptin (Halaas et al. 1995). The acetylated form of ghrelin (acyl-ghrelin) and leptin have opposing effects on hypothalamic nuclei, which control appetite and energy consumption. In the past, the ventromedial hypothalamus (VMN) was considered the satiety center, and the lateral hypothalamus (LHA) was considered the hunger center. However, current research showed that hypothalamic appetite regulation is more complex.

Dysregulation of Appetite in End-Stage Renal Disease

Leptin and Ghrelin

Leptin is a 16.7 kDa peptide hormone that is predominantly produced by adipocytes (Halaas et al. 1995). The anorexigenic effect of leptin was shown in rodents and man (Klein et al. 1996). Leptin reaches the hypothalamus via a saturable transport mechanism across the blood-brain barrier (Dötsch et al. 2005) and binds to its transmembrane receptor mainly in the arcuate nucleus (ARC) and the VMN. Leptin decreases food intake by stimulation of neurons which contain the anorexigenic peptide α-melanocyte-stimulating hormone, which then stimulates the melanocortin receptor 4, and by inhibition of neurons which contain the orexigenic peptides neuropeptide Y (NPY) and agouti-related peptide (AGRP). Additionally, leptin increases energy consumption via the paraventricular nucleus by elevating the concentrations of thyrotropin-releasing hormone and corticotropin-releasing hormone. Consequently, leptin induces a negative energy balance. In ESRD, circulating leptin concentrations are elevated (Besbas et al. 2003). Leptin is not sufficiently cleared by hemodialysis (HD), but significantly eliminated by peritoneal dialysis (PD) (Dötsch et al. 2005). Leptin knockout mice (ob/ob mice) do not show decreased food intake and do not develop uremic loss of body weight after subtotal nephrectomy, but the similarly uremic control group does. This hints at a role of hyperleptinemia in uremic inappetence (Cheung et al. 2005).

Ghrelin is a 3.24 kDa peptide hormone that is mainly secreted by the stomach (Wren et al. 2001). The orexigenic effect of ghrelin is mediated by its acetylated form (acyl-ghrelin), whereas desacyl-ghrelin and obestatin (a further product of the ghrelin gene) mediate anorexigenic effects (Naufel et al. 2010). It binds to its receptor mainly in the ARC and LHA. Acyl-ghrelin increases food intake by stimulating NPY and AGRP neurons and prevents reduction of food intake mediated by leptin (Nakazato et al. 2001). Total ghrelin, desacyl-ghrelin and obestatin concentrations are elevated in children with ESRD (Nüsken et al. 2004; Dötsch et al. 2005; Arbeiter et al. 2009; Monzani et al. 2017). As desacyl-ghrelin and obestatin inversely correlate with body mass index-standard deviation score (BMI-SDS) and/or weight SDS, they have been proposed as markers of nutritional status in children with ESRD (Monzani et al. 2017). Elevated total ghrelin concentrations are not contradictory to inappetence in ESRD, because only concentrations of desacyl-ghrelin, but not acyl-ghrelin, are increased (Büscher et al. 2010; Naufel et al. 2010).

In summary, leptin and acyl-ghrelin are antagonists in the context of appetite regulation and may play a role in the development of malnutrition in ESRD (Figure 27.1). As leptin is not eliminated

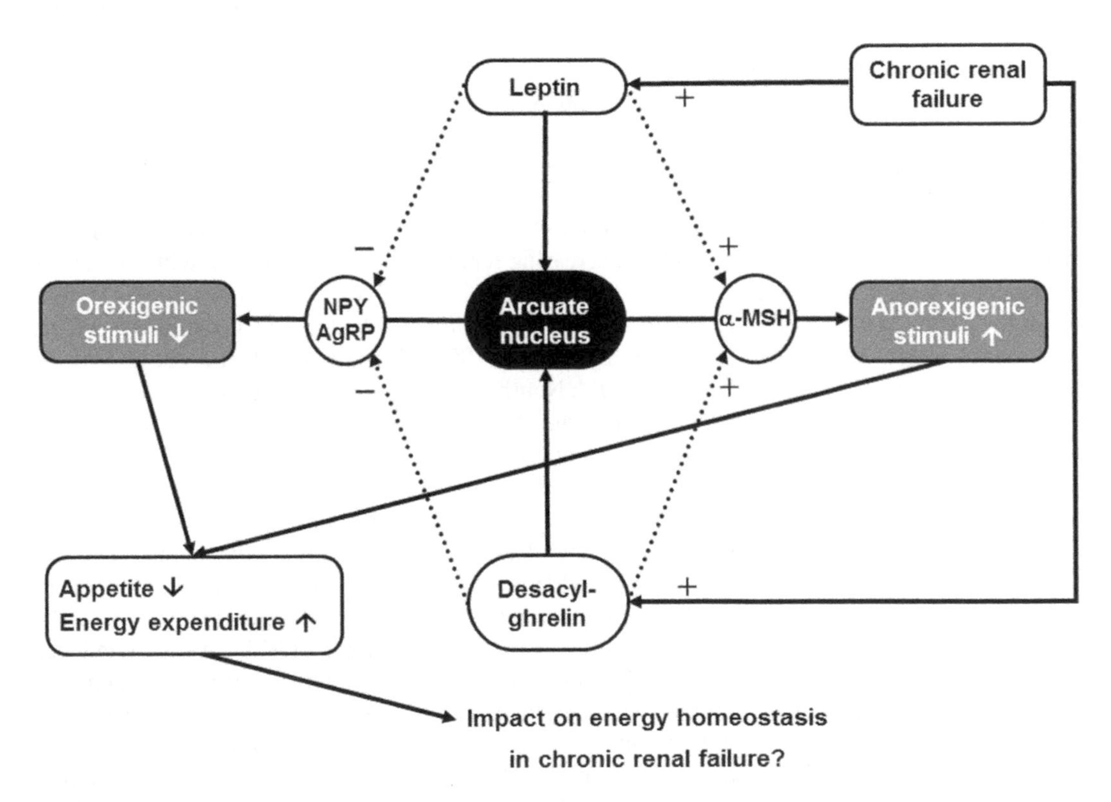

FIGURE 27.1 Postulated regulation of the leptin-ghrelin system in patients with chronic renal failure. (*Abbreviations:* AgRP, agouti-related peptide; α-MSH, alpha-melanocyte-stimulating hormone; NPY, neuropeptide Y.) (Adapted from Dötsch, J. et al., *Pediatr Nephrol*, 2005. 20(6): p. 701–6.)

and ghrelin is significantly cleared by HD, both may contribute to uremic loss of appetite in hemodialysis patients. Elevated desacyl-ghrelin combined with normal acyl-ghrelin concentrations may also contribute to inappetence. However, it is still not absolutely clear to which extent the hormones contribute to weight loss of dialysis patients (Gunta and Mak 2013). A therapeutic method to effectively eliminate leptin is not available so far, although high-flux dialysis filters, hemodiafiltration (HDF), as well as peritoneal dialysis show a certain clearance of leptin. With respect to ghrelin, there has been one promising therapeutic intervention in a group of 12 adult malnourished dialysis patients some years ago. Acyl-ghrelin was administered subcutaneously for one week and considerably increased energy balance (Ashby et al. 2009). Further research is needed to clarify the significance of leptin and ghrelin dysregulation in ESRD children and associated therapeutic options.

Uremia

Uremia describes the accumulation of a multitude of substances that are normally excreted by the kidneys. Apart from well-known parameters like urea or creatinine and the hormones previously depicted, many substances are unidentified (Chazot 2009). Sufficient elimination of uremic toxins by dialysis has been shown to be of major importance, as it is associated with improved clinical outcome and growth (Fischbach et al. 2010). Complications of uremia that contribute to inappetence include nausea, gastric emptying delay, peptic ulcers and *Helicobacter pylori* infections. A loss of taste also may contribute to reduced nutrient intake in patients with ESRD (Armstrong et al. 2010). Consequently, the intake of protein and energy progressively decreases with deteriorating renal function. On the molecular level, amino acid imbalance increases the transport of free tryptophan across the blood-brain barrier, creating a hyperserotoninergic state resulting in activation of the anorexigenic melanocortin receptor 4. Accumulating inflammatory cytokines also suppress appetite. Hemodialysis supports the inflammatory state because of recurring contact to extrinsic, potentially allergenic surfaces. Peritoneal dialysis leads to distension of the abdomen and an increased glucose load, which both are satiety signals (Rees and Shaw 2007; Chazot 2009).

PROTEIN ENERGY WASTING

Protein energy wasting (PEW) is defined as a loss of somatic and circulating body protein mass and energy reserves (Fouque et al. 2008). Decreasing renal function is associated with decreasing muscle mass in children (Foster et al. 2011; Oliveira et al. 2017). PEW is caused by multiple factors, strongly associated with morbidity and mortality, and highly prevalent in ESRD patients including children (Nydegger et al. 2007; Dukkipati and Kopple 2009; Kalantar-Zadeh et al. 2011; Castillo et al. 2012; Mak et al. 2012; Abraham et al. 2014; Nourbakhsh et al. 2014; Oliveira et al. 2017). Thus, PEW is a major risk factor for an adverse outcome of patients. Protein-energy malnutrition (PEM) is an inadequately low nutrient intake and an important part of PEW. Further factors contributing to PEW are inflammation, dialysate nutrient losses, metabolic acidosis and endocrine disorders. Additionally, concomitant diseases affect energy homeostasis. Cachexia is the result of severe PEW (Dukkipati and Kopple 2009; Abraham et al. 2014; Nourbakhsh et al. 2014; Oliveira et al. 2017).

There are four different criteria to diagnose PEW in adults. First, patients have low serum levels of albumin, prealbumin or cholesterol. Second, a reduced BMI, a reduced percentage of body fat or an unintended loss of body weight over three to six months indicate PEW. Third, a reduced muscle mass and an ongoing reduction of 5% muscle mass in three months or 10% in six months is pathologic. Last, an inadequate protein or energy intake relative to the individual's nutritional needs (PEM) is an important factor. Common findings when PEM is present is a protein intake less than 0.8 g/kg/d and an energy intake less than 25 kcal/kg/d (Fouque et al. 2008; Dukkipati and Kopple 2009). For children, an extended definition of PEW including short stature or poor growth has been proposed because it is more closely associated with clinical outcome and avoids underestimation of the prevalence of PEW (Abraham et al. 2014). The importance of PEM is underlined by studies showing that PEM was associated with increased mortality in children (Wong et al. 2000) and that adequate protein intake (defined as greater than 60% of the prescribed amount) was associated with decreased mortality rates (Mehta et al. 2015). In the following the different factors contributing to PEW are discussed.

Inflammation

Inflammation in ESRD is caused by multiple factors, including uremia, dialysis and the underlying disease. Inflammation leads to inappetence and increased energy consumption (Dukkipati and Kopple 2009). Chronic hyperleptinemia is associated with increased inflammation and blood pressure as well as atherosclerosis, muscle wasting and increased mortality (Gunta and Mak 2013). ESRD patients with a state of inflammation show further elevated leptin serum concentrations. The combination of all symptoms is called the *malnutrition-inflammation-atherosclerosis syndrome*. Concomitant diseases associated with inflammation are infected vascular access sites or catheters, peritonitis, systemic infections, vasculitis, diabetes mellitus, stroke, myocardial infarction, peripheral vascular ischemia, insufficient kidney grafts, impure dialysate and other factors (Dukkipati and Kopple 2009). Not only leptin, but also other pro-inflammatory cytokines like TNFα or interleukin-6 are elevated in ESRD patients (Mak et al. 2006). Ghrelin, on the other hand, could mediate anti-inflammatory and blood pressure lowering effects if its concentrations were sufficient (Gunta and Mak 2013).

Dialysate Nutrient Losses

Varying amounts of nutrients are lost into the dialysate. The most important among them are amino acids, peptides, proteins, water-soluble vitamins and minerals. The mode of dialysis significantly affects the amount and type of nutrients lost. Hemodialysis (HD) patients may lose up to 10 g of amino acids during a single dialysis session, but very low amounts of proteins because the membranes used preferably eliminate small molecules. However, HD patients may lose a significant amount of proteins due to dialysis-associated blood loss.

Peritoneal dialysis (PD) patients lose about 15 g total protein into the dialysate per day. In severe peritonitis or patients with a high peritonea transport rate, the protein loss is even higher. Loss of amino acids is about 3.5 g/d in PD patients. Water-soluble vitamins and electrolytes are lost into dialysate in both HD and PD patients (Dukkipati and Kopple 2009).

Metabolic Acidosis

Acidosis contributes to PEW because it induces protein catabolism (Lim et al. 1998). Especially HD patients are exposed to recurring academia before dialysis, whereas PD patients undergo continuous dialysis with sodium bicarbonate buffered solutions. Tubular bicarbonate loss may occur in patients with residual diuresis.

Endocrine Disorders and Concomitant Diseases

Endocrine disorders contributing to PEW in ESRD patients include resistance to insulin, especially in diabetic patients (Dukkipati and Kopple 2009), as well as resistance to growth hormone and to insulin-like growth factor I, which is highly important for growth in children (Blum et al. 1991; Rees and Jones 2013).

NUTRITION AND DIET

In adults, nutrition affects body weight, body composition and the development of chronic diseases. In infants, children and adolescents, nutrition is important for linear growth, neuro-cognitive development and sexual development (puberty). Deficits in linear growth and neurological development acquired during infancy may persist throughout life. The correct diet is an essential part of the treatment plan in all ESRD patients. Prior to nutritional therapy, the nutritional status, eating behaviour, metabolic status and electrolyte status have to be assessed. Macronutrient (fat, carbohydrate, protein and fiber), micronutrient (vitamins, minerals) and fluid intake have to be adjusted to the individual needs of a patient. The aims of nutritional therapy are to minimize the sequelae and complications of kidney failure, to maintain normal body composition in adults and to ensure an optimal development in children (Rees and Jones 2013).

In the following the general aspects of nutrition and diet are described before the different age groups are discussed in detail.

General Aspects of Nutrition and Diet in End-Stage Renal Failure

Calories, Protein and Body Weight

Cachectic patients are at high risk for complications and death. To maintain not only body weight but a healthy body composition, the supply of energy and protein has to be increased in many hemodialysis patients. Patients should weigh themselves every day and keep a diary on body weight and nutritional intake. However, the prevalence of obesity increases even among hemodialysis patients. Obese patients often show a severely altered body composition, with reduced muscle mass, reduced amount of functional tissues and a concomitantly high fat mass. These patients represent a high-risk group for cardiovascular complications, which are the major cause of death in HD patients (Bonthuis et al. 2013; Ku et al. 2016). Achieving and maintaining a healthy body weight by supply of an individually needed amount of energy, as well as maintaining a healthy body composition and immune system by supply of a sufficient amount of proteins is crucial for an optimal quality of life (NKF 2000; EDTNA/ERCA 2009).

Sodium and Fluids

There are plenty of sodium-rich nutrients in Western diets. Sodium induces thirst, leading to fluid intake and fluid retention. In oligo-anuric patients, excess fluid results in edema of the skin and lungs as well as pleural, pericardial and abdominal effusions. Furthermore, hypertension is promoted, with the possibility of concomitant cardiac hypertrophy, cardiac insufficiency, vascular damage, cerebral hemorrhage and death. The patient can recognize sudden weight gain and realize hyperhydration by daily weighing. The daily amount of sodium and fluid has to be individually determined for each patient. Loss of food palatability due to reduced salt can be compensated for by herbs and spices (NKF 2000; EDTNA/ERCA 2009).

Phosphorus and Calcium

Large amounts of phosphorus are typically found in dairy products, nuts, peanuts, legumes, mushrooms, cocoa, cola, meat and chocolate. Hyperphosphatemia results in secondary hyperparathyroidism and renal osteodystrophy. Calcium-phosphorous crystals accumulate in blood vessels as vascular plaques, and in heart, joints, muscles and skin, resulting in coronary heart disease, stroke and other complications. Reduction of nutritional phosphorus is the most important measure to avoid renal osteodystrophy and cardiovascular complications by calcium-phosphorus plaques. Additionally, administration of phosphate binding medication and vitamin D is recommended (NKF 2000; EDTNA/ERCA 2009). Vitamin D is supplemented by medication containing either cholecalciferol (inactive), 1-hydroxycholecalciferol (activated in the liver) or 1,25-dihydroxycholecalciferol (active vitamin D). Target organs of vitamin D are the intestines, the parathyroid, where it suppresses parathyroid hormone, the bone and the kidney. Adequate calcium phosphate metabolism has to be assessed by regular measurement of parathyroid hormone, calcium, phosphate and bone density (Wesseling-Perry and Salusky 2013).

Potassium

Excessive hyperkalemia is a life-threatening condition, because electromechanical dissociation and cardiac arrest may occur. Nutritional potassium reduction is absolutely necessary and life-saving. Large amounts of potassium are typically found in bananas, potatoes, oranges, tomatoes, legumes, certain fruit juices, chocolate, milk, yoghurt and protein-rich foods (NKF 2000; EDTNA/ERCA 2009).

Vitamins and Minerals

Eating a wide variety of foods is recommended to provide the body with vitamins and minerals. As dietary limitations reduce the variety of food and dialysis results in loss of vitamins and minerals in ESRD patients, supplementation of vitamins may be necessary. As described, adequate control of vitamin D and phosphate is essential to avoid renal osteodystrophy (NKF 2000; EDTNA/ERCA 2009). Iron is an essential component for treatment of renal anemia (Atkinson and Warady 2018). Additionally, deficiencies of folate, vitamin B12, carnitine, vitamin C and copper may contribute to renal anemia and have to be compensated (Bamgbola and Kaskel 2005; Calo et al. 2012; Lazarchick 2012; Raimann et al. 2013; Atkinson and Warady 2018). Control of selenium and zinc also is recommended because of their crucial roles in immunity and cell metabolism (Rucker et al. 2010).

INFANTS

In contrast to adults, who have to ingest as much energy as they consume to keep energy homeostasis and body weight, children need additional nutrients for growth and development. Birth weight usually doubles within four to five months and triples within 12 months. However, energy stores are small, so infants are endangered by fast decompensation in case of nutrient deficiency. In severe renal failure, an individually optimized nutrition is a clue for survival and adequate development. The courses of height, weight and BMI have to be continuously evaluated by percentile charts. The volume of drunken milk and the drinking pattern have to be recorded. The intake of energy, protein and electrolytes, especially sodium, potassium, calcium and phosphorus, has to be calculated. The individual status of protein metabolism, electrolytes, acid-base metabolism, bone metabolism and hematopoesis has to be assessed by laboratory measurements (Rees and Shaw 2007; NKF 2009).

In most cases, the baseline intake of energy and protein in infants with terminal renal failure is not sufficient. Restoration of normal protein and energy intake plus compensation for dialytic losses is recommended (see Tables 27.1–27.4 for dietary recommendations). In case of insufficient weight gain due to limited oral intake, tube feeding has to be performed (Rees and Shaw 2007; Foster et al. 2012). Sodium has to be supplemented in many patients, especially when kidney dysplasia or urogenital abnormalities are present. Hyperkalemia often is present, but hypokalemia also is possible. Acidosis and dysregulation of calcium-phosphate-metabolism need to be corrected. To treat renal anemia, iron supplementation is needed in addition to erythropoietin. The demand of fluid varies greatly and depends on daily urine volume, course of body weight, presence of edemas and blood pressure. In most cases, residual diuresis is present, so the fluid volume ingested by breastfeeding, infant milk or as special formula milk is eliminated by the kidney. Electrolyte disorders often can be controlled by modification of intake or excretion, respectively. Vitamins and trace element intake should be normalized (see Table 27.5 for dietary recommendations). In children with dialysis, it is suggested to apply water-soluble vitamin supplements. Severe, but not excessive uremia is present in many cases. As a result, dialysis often is not needed for survival. In the first year of life, the most important aim of all therapeutic efforts in an infant with ESRD is to achieve survival and adequate development without dialysis whenever possible. Dialysis is difficult and may frequently cause complications. However, dialysis is feasible in the first year of life and inevitably needed in case of conservatively uncontrollable hyperhydration, hyperkalemia as well as clinical symptoms of uremia including abnormal fatigue and limited consciousness, but also nausea and malnutrition, resulting in persistent failure to thrive.

TABLE 27.1
Equations to Estimate Energy Requirements in Children at Healthy Weights

Age	Estimated Energy Requirement (kcal/d) = Total Energy Expenditure + Energy Deposition
0–3 months	EER = [89 × weight (kg) − 100] + 175
4–6 months	EER = [89 × weight (kg) − 100] + 56
7–12 months	EER = [89 × weight (kg) − 100] + 22
13–35 months	EER = [89 × weight (kg) − 100] + 20
3–8 years	Boys: EER = 88.5–61.9 × age (y) + PA × [26.7 × weight (kg) + 903 × height (m)] + 20
	Girls: EER = 135.3–30.8 × age (y) + PA × [10 × weight (kg) + 934 × height (m)] + 20
9–18 years	Boys: EER = 88.5–61.9 × age (y) + PA × [26.7 × weight (kg) + 903 × height (m)] + 25
	Girls: EER = 135.3–30.8 × age (y) + PA × [10 × weight (kg) + 934 × height (m)] + 25

Source: From National Kidney Foundation – Kidney Disease Outcome Quality Initiative (NKF-KDOQI). *Am J Kidney Dis*, 2009. 53(3 Suppl 2): p. S1–123.

Abbreviations: EER, estimated energy requirement; PA, physical activity coefficient.

TABLE 27.2
Physical Activity (PA) Coefficients for Determination of Energy Requirements in Children Aged 3–18 Years

	Level of Physical Activity			
Gender	Sedentary	Low Active	Active	Very Active
	Typical activities of daily living (ADLs) only	ADL + 30–60 min of daily moderate activity (e.g., walking at 5–7 km/h)	ADL + ≥60 min of daily moderate activity	ADL + ≥60 min of daily moderate activity + an additional 60 min of vigorous activity or 120 min of moderate activity
Boys	1.0	1.13	1.26	1.42
Girls	1.0	1.16	1.31	1.56

Source: From National Kidney Foundation – Kidney Disease Outcome Quality Initiative (NKF-KDOQI). *Am J Kidney Dis*, 2009. 53(3 Suppl 2): p. S1–123.

TABLE 27.3
Acceptable Macronutrient Distribution Ranges

Macronutrient	Children 1–3 years (%)	Children 4–18 years (%)
Carbohydrate	45–65	45–65
Fat	30–40	25–35
Protein	5–20	10–30

Source: From National Kidney Foundation – Kidney Disease Outcome Quality Initiative (NKF-KDOQI). *Am J Kidney Dis*, 2009. 53(3 Suppl 2): p. S1–123.

Children

From the age of 12 months onwards, it is recommended to begin dialysis in all children with ESRD because of a clear benefit for the patient's growth and development. Peritoneal dialysis is applied in almost all patients up to an age of 10 years. Hemodialysis is predominantly used in adolescents (see Section "Adolescents"). At the start of dialysis, nutrition has to be adapted (see Tables 27.1–27.5 for recommendations). Although being less uremic after initiation of dialysis, major problems of

TABLE 27.4
Recommended Dietary Protein Intake in Children with End-Stage Renal Failure

	Age	DRI (g/kg/d)	DRI for HD (g/kg/d)[a]	DRI for PD (g/kg/d)[b]
Infants	0–6 months	1.5	1.6	1.8
	7–12 months	1.2	1.3	1.5
Children	1–3 years	1.05	1.15	1.3
	4–13 years	0.95	1.05	1.1
Adolescents	14–18 years	0.85	0.95	1.0

Source: From National Kidney Foundation – Kidney Disease Outcome Quality Initiative (NKF-KDOQI). *Am J Kidney Dis*, 2009. 53(3 Suppl 2): p. S1–123.

Abbreviation: DRI, dietary reference intake.

[a] DRI + 0.1 g/kg/d to compensate for dialytic losses.

[b] DRI + 0.15–0.3 g/kg/d depending on patient age to compensate for peritoneal losses.

TABLE 27.5
Dietary Reference Intake: Recommended Dietary Allowance (RDA) and Adequate Intake (AI)

	Infants		Children		Males		Females	
	0–6 months	7–12 months	1–3 years	4–8 years	9–13 years	14–18 years	9–13 years	14–18 years
Vitamin A (μg/d)	400	500	**300**	**400**	**600**	**900**	**600**	**700**
Vitamin C (mg/d)	40	50	**15**	**25**	**45**	**75**	**45**	**65**
Vitamin E (mg/d)	4	5	**6**	**7**	**11**	**15**	**11**	**15**
Vitamin K (μg/d)	2.0	2.5	**30**	**55**	**60**	**75**	**60**	**75**
Thiamin (mg/d)	0.2	0.3	**0.5**	**0.6**	**0.9**	**1.2**	**0.9**	**1.0**
Riboflavin (mg/d)	0.3	0.4	**0.5**	**0.6**	**0.9**	**1.3**	**0.9**	**1.0**
Niacin (mg/d; NE)	2[a]	4	**6**	**8**	**12**	**16**	**12**	**14**
Vitamin B6 (mg/d)	0.1	0.3	**0.5**	**0.6**	**1.0**	**1.3**	**1.0**	**1.2**
Folate (μg/d)	65	80	**150**	**200**	**300**	**400**	**300**	**400**
Vitamin B12 (μg/d)	0.4	0.5	**0.9**	**1.2**	**1.8**	**2.4**	**1.8**	**2.4**
Pantothenic acid (mg/d)	1.7	1.8	**2**	**3**	**4**	**5**	**4**	**5**
Biotin (μg/d)	5	6	**8**	**12**	**20**	**25**	**20**	**25**
Copper (μg/d)	200	220	**340**	**440**	**700**	**890**	**700**	**890**
Selenium (μg/d)	15	20	**20**	**30**	**40**	**55**	**40**	**55**
Zinc (mg/d)	2	3	**3**	**5**	**8**	**11**	**8**	**9**

Source: From National Kidney Foundation – Kidney Disease Outcome Quality Initiative (NKF-KDOQI). *Am J Kidney Dis*, 2009. 53(3 Suppl 2): p. S1–123.

Note: RDAs are in bold type; AIs are in ordinary type.

[a] As preformed niacin, not niacin equivalents (NE) for this age group.

young children with PD are loss of appetite and nausea because of continuous glucose resorption and distension of the abdomen. A considerable number of patients cannot be nourished orally and need tube feeding. Nutrient loss, especially protein loss to the dialysate because of a high peritoneal surface area, and hyperphosphatemia followed by hyperparathyroidism and renal osteodystrophy are significant issues. Hyperkalemia in PD patients is less common than in HD patients, but still of high relevance because of potentially life-threatening hyperkalemia. Food for the typical patient has to be rich in calories, rich in proteins, poor in phosphorus and poor in potassium. Vitamins and trace elements have to be normalized.

Adolescents

In adolescents, most patients prefer hemodialysis. One reason certainly is that adolescents worry about stigmatizing effects of the peritoneal dialysis catheter more than small children. In addition, peritoneal dialysis is considered to interfere more with "normal everyday life" of adolescents than hemodialysis. A significant number of the patients are oligo-anuric. However, the major problem with adolescents in puberty is malcompliance. As HD is a discontinuous method, the patients are threatened by decompensation before dialysis. Significant issues are excessive hyperhydration, leading to severe cardiovascular complications, and hyperkalemia resulting in cardiac arrhythmia and arrest. An elevated calcium phosphate product promotes atherosclerosis. Uremic toxins promote inappetence and uremia. Consequently, the patients are trained to assess their state of hydration by weighing and blood pressure measurement, to identify food that contains high amounts of potassium and phosphorus and to pay attention to a sufficient caloric intake (see Tables 27.1–27.5 for dietary recommendations). Fluid intake has to be restricted in oligo-anuric patients, food poor in potassium and phosphorus is mandatory for all patients. Because of potential malcompliance, parameters have to be checked frequently and periodic training is necessary. Unhealthy diet and associated obesity is a common issue in adolescents (Chen et al. 2017). Intradialytic parenteral nutrition is an option to improve nutritional status in case of PEW (Dukkipati et al. 2010).

APPLICATIONS TO OTHER AREAS OF TERMINAL OR PALLIATIVE CARE

The majority of patients in palliative care are threatened by kidney failure. Secondary kidney failure may occur in case of reduced kidney perfusion, for example, in patients with severe cardiac insufficiency or severe dehydration because of insufficient fluid intake or increased fluid loss. Recurrent urinary tract infections, nephrolithiasis, urinary obstructions, proteinuria, diabetes mellitus, arterial hypertension and cardiovascular disease are major risk factors contributing to kidney failure. Moreover, cancer may be associated with infiltration of the kidneys or chemotherapy-induced kidney damage.

PRACTICAL METHODS AND TECHNIQUES

Training of patients and their parents is mandatory. It has to be clarified unambiguously that dialysis, intake of medication and an adequate intake of fluid, potassium, phosphorus, protein and energy are essential for development, quality of life and survival. Therefore, main educational contents are practical application of dialysis, information on medication, assessment of hydration by weighing and blood pressure measurement, as well as identification, preparation and intake of appropriate food.

GUIDELINES

Guidelines on nutrition in renal failure are available from the NKF (2000, 2003, 2007, 2009) and the EDTNA/ERCA (2009).

ETHICAL ISSUES

In most pediatric patients, ESRD is not a condition of palliative care, but maximum therapy is applied. Most patients gain a good quality of life, receive a kidney graft after some years of dialysis, and survive until adulthood. However, in some cases, dialysis and transplantation may still be impossible, or maximum therapy may be linked to multiple complications and a poor quality of life. In these cases, consultation of a specialized pediatric ethics committee is desirable to discuss the various options with the parents and, if possible, the patient, and make decisions mutually after careful consideration.

KEY FACTS: RENAL FAILURE

- The physiological balance of water and electrolytes, the elimination of water-soluble toxins, blood pressure control, red blood cells regeneration and normal bone density all rely on normal kidney function.
- End-stage renal disease is incompatible with life unless the kidney function is replaced.
- Fluid overload may finally result in high blood pressure, heart failure and brain bleeding.
- Potassium overload may finally result in cardiac arrest.
- Reduced bone density may lead to fractures and abnormal growth.
- In addition to dialysis therapy, renal replacement therapy requires drug therapy and nutritional modifications.
- Nutritional modifications generally include reduced intake of potassium and phosphorus, and an individually optimized intake of fluid, protein and energy.
- End-stage renal disease in children may lead to impaired growth and development which can be improved by optimized renal replacement therapy (ideally renal transplantation) in combination with nutrition therapy (most importantly, the avoidance of protein energy wasting).
- An optimal combination of dialysis, drug therapy and nutrition is life saving and can largely normalize growth, cognitive and pubertal development.

SUMMARY POINTS

- End-stage renal failure substantially interferes with the major regulators of appetite and energy expenditure, namely leptin and ghrelin.
- Loss of appetite, waste of important nutrients by dialysis and chronic inflammation promote a state of catabolism in patients with end-stage renal failure.
- In infants, children and adolescents the underlying disease and varying age requirements determine the nature of nutritional dysregulation as well as the resulting management of the patients.
- Guidelines on nutrition in renal failure are available from the National Kidney Foundation of the United States (NKF 2000, 2003, 2007, 2009) and the European Dialysis and Transplant Nurses Association/European Renal Care Association (EDTNA/ERCA 2009).

LIST OF ABBREVIATIONS

AGRP Agouti-Related Peptide
ARC Arcuate Nucleus
α-MSH Alpha-Melanocyte-Stimulating Hormone
BMI Body Mass Index
EDTNA European Dialysis and Transplant Nurses Association
ERCA European Renal Care Association

ESRD	End-Stage Renal Disease
HD	Hemodialysis
KDOQI	Kidney Disease Outcomes Quality Initiative
LHA	Lateral Hypothalamic Area
NKF	National Kidney Foundation
NPY	Neuropeptide Y
PD	Peritoneal Dialysis
PEM	Protein Energy Malnutrition
PEW	Protein Energy Wasting
VMN	Ventromedial Hypothalamus

REFERENCES

Abraham, A.G. et al., Protein energy wasting in children with chronic kidney disease. *Pediatr Nephrol*, 2014. 29(7): p. 1231–8.

Arbeiter, A.K. et al., Ghrelin and other appetite-regulating hormones in paediatric patients with chronic renal failure during dialysis and following kidney transplantation. *Nephrol Dial Transplant*, 2009. 24(2): p. 643–6.

Armstrong, J.E. et al., Smell and taste function in children with chronic kidney disease. *Pediatr Nephrol*, 2010. 25(8): p. 1497–504.

Ashby, D.R. et al., Sustained appetite improvement in malnourished dialysis patients by daily ghrelin treatment. *Kidney Int*, 2009. 76(2): p. 199–206.

Atkinson, M.A. and B.A. Warady, Anemia in chronic kidney disease. *Pediatr Nephrol*, 2018. 33(2): p. 227–238.

Bamgbola, O.F. and F. Kaskel, Role of folate deficiency on erythropoietin resistance in pediatric and adolescent patients on chronic dialysis. *Pediatr Nephrol*, 2005. 20(11): p. 1622–9.

Besbas, N. et al., Relationship of leptin and insulin-like growth factor I to nutritional status in hemodialyzed children. *Pediatr Nephrol*, 2003. 18(12): p. 1255–9.

Blum, W.F. et al., Growth hormone resistance and inhibition of somatomedin activity by excess of insulin-like growth factor binding protein in uraemia. *Pediatr Nephrol*, 1991. 5(4): p. 539–44.

Bonthuis, M. et al., Underweight, overweight and obesity in paediatric dialysis and renal transplant patients. *Nephrol Dial Transplant*, 2013. 28(Suppl 4): p. iv195–iv204.

Büscher, A.K. et al., Alterations in appetite-regulating hormones influence protein-energy wasting in pediatric patients with chronic kidney disease. *Pediatr Nephrol*, 2010. 25(11): p. 2295–301.

Calo, L.A. et al., L carnitine in hemodialysis patients. *Hemodial Int*, 2012. 16(3): p. 428–34.

Castillo, A. et al., Nutritional status and clinical outcome of children on continuous renal replacement therapy: A prospective observational study. *BMC Nephrol*, 2012. 13: p. 125.

Chazot, C., Why are chronic kidney disease patients anorexic and what can be done about it? *Semin Nephrol*, 2009. 29(1): p. 15–23.

Chen, W. et al., Dietary sources of energy and nutrient intake among children and adolescents with chronic kidney disease. *Pediatr Nephrol*, 2017. 32(7): p. 1233–1241.

Cheung, W. et al., Role of leptin and melanocortin signaling in uremia-associated cachexia. *J Clin Invest*, 2005. 115(6): p. 1659–65.

Dötsch, J. et al., Alterations of leptin and ghrelin serum concentrations in renal disease: Simple epiphenomena? *Pediatr Nephrol*, 2005. 20(6): p. 701–6.

Dukkipati, R. and J.D. Kopple, Causes and prevention of protein-energy wasting in chronic kidney failure. *Semin Nephrol*, 2009. 29(1): p. 39–49.

Dukkipati, R., K. Kalantar-Zadeh, and J.D. Kopple, Is there a role for intradialytic parenteral nutrition? A review of the evidence. *Am J Kidney Dis*, 2010. 55(2): p. 352–64.

European Dialysis and Transplant Nurses Association/European Renal Care Association (EDTNA/ERCA), European guidelines for the nutritional care of adult renal patients. *EDTNA/ERCA*, 2009. J1: p. 22–46.

Fischbach, M. et al., Daily on line haemodiafiltration promotes catch-up growth in children on chronic dialysis. *Nephrol Dial Transplant*, 2010. 25(3): p. 867–73.

Foster, B.J. et al., Association of chronic kidney disease with muscle deficits in children. *J Am Soc Nephrol*, 2011. 22(2): p. 377–86.

Foster, B.J., L. McCauley, and R.H. Mak, Nutrition in infants and very young children with chronic kidney disease. *Pediatr Nephrol*, 2012. 27(9): p. 1427–39.

Fouque, D. et al., A proposed nomenclature and diagnostic criteria for protein-energy wasting in acute and chronic kidney disease. *Kidney Int*, 2008. 73(4): p. 391–8.

Gunta, S.S. and R.H. Mak, Ghrelin and leptin pathophysiology in chronic kidney disease. *Pediatr Nephrol*, 2013. 28(4): p. 611–6.

Halaas, J.L. et al., Weight-reducing effects of the plasma protein encoded by the obese gene. *Science*, 1995. 269(5223): p. 543–6.

Kalantar-Zadeh, K. et al., Diets and enteral supplements for improving outcomes in chronic kidney disease. *Nat Rev Nephrol*, 2011. 7(7): p. 369–84.

Klein, S. et al., Adipose tissue leptin production and plasma leptin kinetics in humans. *Diabetes*, 1996. 45(7): p. 984–7.

Ku, E. et al., Association of body mass index with patient-centered outcomes in children with ESRD. *J Am Soc Nephrol*, 2016. 27(2): p. 551–8.

Lazarchick, J., Update on anemia and neutropenia in copper deficiency. *Curr Opin Hematol*, 2012. 19(1): p. 58–60.

Lim, V.S., K.E. Yarasheski, and M.J. Flanigan, The effect of uraemia, acidosis, and dialysis treatment on protein metabolism: A longitudinal leucine kinetic study. *Nephrol Dial Transplant*, 1998. 13(7): p. 1723–30.

Mak, R.H. et al., Mechanisms of disease: Cytokine and adipokine signaling in uremic cachexia. *Nat Clin Pract Nephrol*, 2006. 2(9): p. 527–34.

Mak, R.H. et al., Cachexia and protein-energy wasting in children with chronic kidney disease. *Pediatr Nephrol*, 2012. 27(2): p. 173–81.

Mehta, N.M. et al., Adequate enteral protein intake is inversely associated with 60-d mortality in critically ill children: A multicenter, prospective, cohort study. *Am J Clin Nutr*, 2015. 102(1): p. 199–206.

Monzani, A. et al., Unacylated ghrelin and obestatin: Promising biomarkers of protein energy wasting in children with chronic kidney disease. *Pediatr Nephrol*, 2018. 33(4): p. 661–672.

Nakazato, M. et al., A role for ghrelin in the central regulation of feeding. *Nature*, 2001. 409(6817): p. 194–8.

National Kidney Foundation, Clinical practice guidelines for nutrition in chronic renal failure. Kidney Disease Outcomes Quality Initiative, National Kidney Foundation. *Am J Kidney Dis*, 2000. 35(6 Suppl 2): p. S1–140.

National Kidney Foundation, K/DOQI clinical practice guidelines for bone metabolism and disease in chronic kidney disease. *Am J Kidney Dis*, 2003. 42(4 Suppl 3): p. S1–201.

National Kidney Foundation, KDOQI clinical practice guidelines and clinical practice recommendations for diabetes and chronic kidney disease. *Am J Kidney Dis*, 2007. 49(2 Suppl 2): p. S12–154.

National Kidney Foundation, KDOQI clinical practice guideline for nutrition in children with CKD: 2008 update. *Am J Kidney Dis*, 2009. 53(3 Suppl 2): p. S1–123.

Naufel, M.F. et al., Plasma levels of acylated and total ghrelin in pediatric patients with chronic kidney disease. *Pediatr Nephrol*, 2010. 25(12): p. 2477–82.

Nourbakhsh, N., C.M. Rhee, and K. Kalantar-Zadeh, Protein-energy wasting and uremic failure to thrive in children with chronic kidney disease: They are not small adults. *Pediatr Nephrol*, 2014. 29(12): p. 2249–52.

Nüsken, K.D. et al., Effect of renal failure and dialysis on circulating ghrelin concentration in children. *Nephrol Dial Transplant*, 2004. 19(8): p. 2156–7.

Nydegger, A. et al., Body composition of children with chronic and end-stage renal failure. *J Paediatr Child Health*, 2007. 43(11): p. 740–5.

Oliveira, E.A. et al., Muscle wasting in chronic kidney disease. *Pediatr Nephrol*, 2018. 33(5): p. 789–98.

Raimann, J.G. et al., Is vitamin C intake too low in dialysis patients? *Semin Dial*, 2013. 26(1): p. 1–5.

Rees, L. and H. Jones, Nutritional management and growth in children with chronic kidney disease. *Pediatr Nephrol*, 2013. 28(4): p. 527–36.

Rees, L. and V. Shaw, Nutrition in children with CRF and on dialysis. *Pediatr Nephrol*, 2007. 22(10): p. 1689–702.

Rucker, D., R. Thadhani, and M. Tonelli, Trace element status in hemodialysis patients. *Semin Dial*, 2010. 23(4): p. 389–95.

Schwartz, M.W. et al., Central nervous system control of food intake. *Nature*, 2000. 404(6778): p. 661–71.

Wesseling-Perry, K. and I.B. Salusky, Chronic kidney disease: Mineral and bone disorder in children. *Semin Nephrol*, 2013. 33(2): p. 169–79.

Wong, C.S. et al., Anthropometric measures and risk of death in children with end-stage renal disease. *Am J Kidney Dis*, 2000. 36(4): p. 811–9.

Wren, A.M. et al., Ghrelin enhances appetite and increases food intake in humans. *J Clin Endocrinol Metab*, 2001. 86(12): p. 5992.

28 Linking Food Supplementation and Palliative Care in HIV

Keiron A. Audain

CONTENTS

INTRODUCTION

Human immuno-deficiency virus (HIV)/acquired immune deficiency syndrome (AIDS) remains a significant cause of mortality and morbidity in the world. Despite a global decline in the number of new infections, an estimated 5,000 adults and children are infected with HIV every day (UNAIDS 2017). As of 2016, 36.7 million people worldwide were living with HIV (UNAIDS 2017). Of this total, approximately 64% were in Sub-Saharan Africa, which remains the epicentre of the epidemic (UNAIDS 2017).

Despite efforts from related institutions, only 46% of adults and 49% of children had access to antiretroviral therapy (ART) in 2015 (UNAIDS 2015). During an HIV infection, ART can help stimulate appetite; improve gut health, thus reducing malabsorption; and reduce bouts of diarrhoea (Audain et al. 2015). Thus, in the absence of ART, the risk of undernutrition is increased. Undernourished individuals are at an increased risk of opportunistic infections due to a weakened immune system, hence furthering the progression of HIV (Audain et al. 2015).

A primary characteristic of AIDS is rapid weight loss; referred to as wasting. HIV-associated wasting has traditionally been attributed to intestinal inflammation, which is believed to be mitigated by both ART and management of opportunistic infections. As a result, less research emphasis has been placed on the clinical benefit of food security on AIDS recovery.

FOOD INSECURITY

The HIV epidemic has exacerbated food insecurity, particularly in Sub-Saharan Africa; owing to its debilitating impact on regional, national and household agricultural productivity (Singer et al. 2015). Food insecurity in turn has a negative impact on ART adherence. Insufficient food to match the increased appetite associated with ART is one of the primary reasons persons living with HIV/AIDS (PLWHA) default from their treatment regimen (Singer et al. 2015). This has been the key argument for food supplementation to be fully integrated into HIV palliative care, alongside ART. Undernourished PLWHA are between two and six times more likely to die within the first six months of initiating ART (UNAID 2015).

UNDERNUTRITION

A combination of HIV and undernutrition in an individual leads to a myriad of micronutrient deficiencies that can hinder immune functions and exacerbate HIV progression (Audain et al. 2015). Undernutrition in PLWHA can stem from a reduction in food consumption, with a key contributing factor being a poor appetite. Such can result from an inability to chew or swallow (e.g., due to esophageal candidiasis) or a lack of desire to eat due to nausea and/or depression (Suttajit 2007). Even when food is consumed, nutrient malabsorption can occur due to opportunistic infections, intestinal damage and other metabolic disorders (Colecraft 2008). The major consequence of a poor appetite and malabsorption is moderate to severe acute malnutrition, which is characterised by wasting (Figure 28.1).

APPLICATIONS TO OTHER AREAS OF PALLIATIVE CARE

An early World Health Organization (WHO) definition of palliative medicine is "the study and management of patients with active, progressive, far advanced disease for whom the prognosis is limited and the focus of care is the quality of life" (WHO 1990). This definition emphasized the idea that palliative care is reserved for the final stages of disease. More recently, it has been defined as "an approach that improves the quality of life of patients and their families facing the problem associated with life-threatening illness, through the prevention and relief of suffering by means of early identification and impeccable assessment and treatment of pain and other problems—physical, psychosocial, and spiritual" (WHO 2017), which implies that care can be provided as early as possible along the course of the chronic illness.

Given the chronic nature of HIV/AIDS, palliative care is offered to individuals at any clinical stage of the disease. Individuals are affected by a range of conditions throughout the course of HIV's progression, including those related to adverse treatment effects, opportunistic infections, or the virus itself. Some of these include diarrhoea, constipation, appetite loss, general fatigue, dyspnea, chronic pain, weight loss, depression, insomnia, coughing, nausea and vomiting (Herce and Flick 2015).

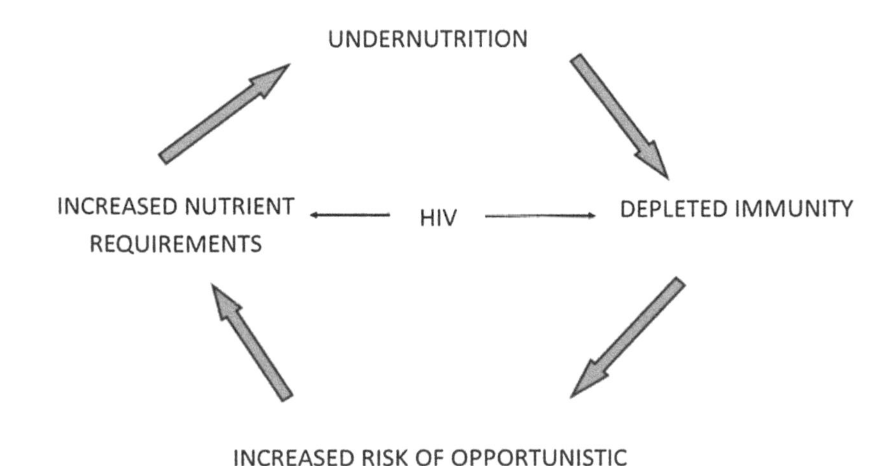

FIGURE 28.1 The HIV-undernutrition cycle.

Prior to the antiretroviral era, palliative care was a predominant feature in mitigating the suffering of advanced AIDS patients (Shorthill and DeMarco 2017). The universal rollout of ART dramatically increased life expectancy and significantly improved the quality of life for PLWHA. HIV has since been re-characterised from a life-threatening illness to a chronic condition. In recent years, a 48% decline in global AIDS-related deaths was reported, from 1.9 million in 2005 to 1.0 million in 2016 (UNAIDS 2017). This has consequently led to an increase in the number of older people living with HIV. Middle-aged and older people living with HIV increasingly report episodes of frailty, which increases the likelihood of not being able to purchase and prepare healthy meals, ultimately contributing to food insecurity and undernutrition (Willig et al. 2016). Within an older HIV population, considerably higher levels of morbidity are observed compared to their HIV-negative counterparts (Guaraldi et al. 2011). Included among the list of morbidities are chronic kidney disease, type 2 diabetes, cardiovascular disease, hypertension, cirrhosis, osteoporosis and cancers (Willig et al. 2016). As a result, the need for palliative care has dramatically increased to manage the rise in non-communicable diseases (Herce et al. 2014). Yet in low-to-middle-income countries (LMICs), access to healthcare in general is limited, and access to palliative care is even more limited. Sub-Saharan Africa has the highest disease burden, yet only 5% of people in need of palliative care services receive it (Herce et al. 2014).

Food supplementation has proven to be an integral part of palliative care for PLWHA by improving health and nutritional status as well as quality of life. It has been implemented at clinic and community levels and involves therapeutic and supplementary feeding alongside regular nutritional assessment to monitor improvement. A qualitative study reported that in addition to physical care and integration into health services, the need for financial and nutritional support was also important to participants (Mkwinda and Lekalakala-Mokgele 2016). This provides an indication of the need for further incorporation of nutrition rehabilitation in the palliative care approach (Nakawesi et al. 2014).

FOOD SUPPLEMENTATION

A therapeutic food is a specially formulated dietary supplement aimed at providing nutritional benefit to the user. Therapeutic foods are traditionally developed for the treatment of severe acute malnutrition (SAM) (USAID 2016).

Ready-to-use therapeutic foods (RUTFs) have a higher caloric density compared to regular foods and provide an adequate source of nutrients necessary for recovery (UNICEF 2013). They also have a shelf-life of up to two years and do not require refrigeration, which is ideal for distribution in emergencies and other resource-limited settings. As RUTFs are not water based, there is little risk of bacterial contamination. Although widely used, it was initially developed to support infant and young child feeding (IYCF) (UNICEF 2013) (Figure 28.2).

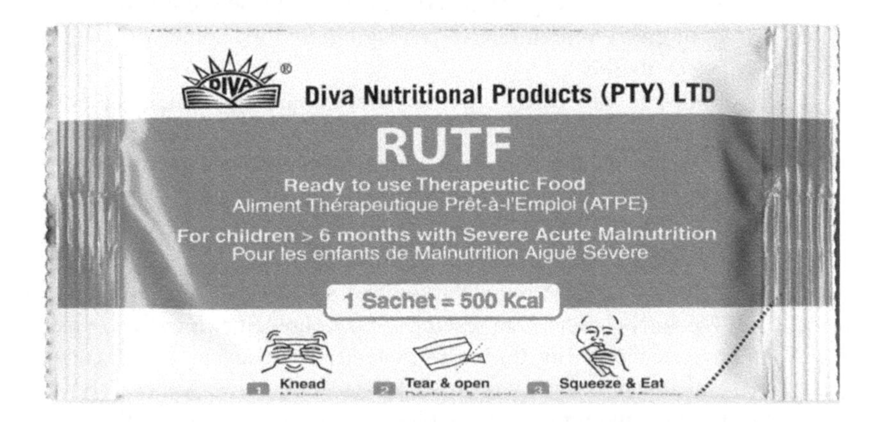

FIGURE 28.2 Ready-to-use therapeutic food supplement available in Zambia.

A very popular brand of RUTF is Plumpy'Nut; launched in 1996 by the therapeutic food manufacturer Nutriset. Plumpy'Nut is an energy-dense, micronutrient-fortified peanut butter and milk powder mix (Table 28.1). It was developed specifically for the nutritional rehabilitation of severely acute malnourished children aged six months and older, but it is also used as a food supplement for PLWHA (Nutriset 2016). Several studies conducted in countries with a triple burden of HIV, food insecurity and undernutrition have shown the effectiveness of Plumpy'Nut in (1) reversing micronutrient deficiencies, (2) causing weight gain and (3) improving ART adherence (Audain et al. 2015).

For instance, in Senegal, 65 PLWHA were randomly allocated either standard hospital diet supplemented with 100 g Plumpy'Nut per day for nine weeks or a standard hospital diet alone. Supplementation met energy (2147 kcal) and zinc (10.4 mg) requirements. After nine weeks, significant increases in body weight (11%) and fat-free mass (11.8%) were observed in the RUTF group but not in the control group. Fat-free mass gain was higher among patients receiving ART compared to those without ART. There was also a significant decrease in anemia prevalence (Diouf et al. 2016).

Lipid-based nutrient supplements (LNS) are another RUTF that has shown to be effective against weight loss in PLWHA, particularly in pregnant and lactating women (Kayira et al. 2012). Examples of LNS manufactured by Nutriset include "Plumpy'Sup," "Plumpy'Doz," "Plumpy'Soy" and "Plumpy'Mum," all of which are formulated to meet the nutritional needs of different vulnerable populations (Nutriset 2016). Each LNS consists of peanut paste, vegetable oil, dry skimmed milk, dry whey, dextrin-maltose, sugar and a micronutrient premix (Kayira et al. 2012). The key difference between an LNS such as Plumpy'Sup and Plumpy'Nut lies in their energy, nutrient and essential fatty acid composition. An intervention study involving LNS supplementation among breastfeeding women in Malawi observed a reduction in weight loss for both women who were receiving ART and women who were treatment naïve compared to the control group (Kayira et al. 2012).

Although technically not a RUTF as it requires preparation, corn-soya blend (CSB) is one of the most commonly administered therapeutic foods. The CSB supplement consists of heat-treated maize and soya beans, with a vitamin and mineral premix (World Food Programme [WFP] 2010). It is typically mixed with water and flour and served as a porridge, biscuit or paste (WHO 2008). While proving beneficial in improving both nutritional status and adherence to treatment in PLWHA, some studies have shown CSB to be less effective than RUTF in this regard (Audain et al. 2015).

Despite its effectiveness, administering and ensuring adherence to therapeutic food supplements can prove problematic among PLWHA. Factors including taste, suitability for the local context, treatment and disease side effects and improper use appear to be notable for supplementation uptake and adherence (Brown et al. 2015; Dibari et al. 2012; Rodas-Moya et al. 2017). In Thailand, a qualitative study on the acceptability of therapeutic food supplementation among PLWHA revealed six themes: supplements should (1) reflect local food culture; (2) be convenient and have perceived health benefits; (3) have "softer" sensory characteristics (less intense scent and flavour); (4) have a soft, easy-to-swallow texture; (5) have attractive packaging; and (6) come with support from peer counsellors (Rodas-Moya et al. 2017).

A Kenyan study revealed factors including taste, diet monotony, clinical side effects of HIV, sharing with household members and mixing with other foods as hindrances that prevented half the study population from maintaining their daily consumption of RUTF. The study also revealed that staff administering the RUTF were not adequately trained in therapeutic diet counselling (Dibari et al. 2012).

In Vietnam, a study was conducted to determine the acceptability of a locally produced therapeutic food and imported food supplement (Plumpy'Nut) among 80 HIV-positive children (aged three to seven years) and 80 HIV-positive adults. One serving of both supplements each provided 500 kcal of energy per day. To improve acceptability, the local supplement was developed as a compressed bar to mimic a popular Vietnamese snack (Brown et al. 2015; Nga et al. 2013). Although both supplements led to significant weight gains in children and adults, findings indicated that the local supplement was preferred and consumed more in children and adults (Brown et al. 2015).

TABLE 28.1
Nutrient Composition of Plumpy'Nut Ready-to-Use Therapeutic Foods (RUTF)

	For 100 g Plumpy'Nut		For 92 g (serving size)		For 100 g Plumpy'Nut		
	Min	Max			Min	Max	
Energy (kcal)	520	550	500	Iron (mg)	10	14	10.6
Proteins (% of total energy)	10	12	10	Iodine (μg)	70	140	92
Proteins	13	16	12.1	Selenium (μg)	20	40	27.6
Percentage of milk proteins	50% of total proteins	–	>50 of total proteins	Sodium (mg)	–	290	<267
Lipids (% of total energy)	45	60	56	Vitamin A (μg)	800	1200	840
Lipids	26	36	29.9	Vitamin D (μg)	15	20	15
Fatty acid n-6 (% of total energy)	3	10	7 (=4 g)	Vitamin E (mg)	20	40	18.4
Fatty acid n-3 (% of total energy)	0.3	2.5	0.7 (=0.35)	Vitamin C (mg)	50	132	49
Carbohydrates	41	58	45 (36% total energy)	Vitamin B1 (mg)	0.5	1.5	0.55
Fibre content (%)	–	<5	<5	Vitamin B2 (mg)	1.6	3.0	1.66
Moisture (%)	–	2.5	2.5	Vitamin B6	0.6	0.9	0.55
Calcium (mg)	300	500	276	Vitamin B12 (μg)	1.6	3.0	1.7
Phosphorous (mg)	300	500	276	Vitamin K (μg)	15	30	19.3
Potassium (mg)	1100	1400	1022	Biotin (μg)	60	90	60
Magnesium (mg)	80	100	84.6	Folic Acid (μg)	200	400	193
Zinc (mg)	11	14	12.9	Pantothenic Acid (mg)	3	6	2.85
Copper (mg)	1.4	1.8	1.6	Niacin (mg)	5	9	4.88

Source: Adapted with permission from the Plumpy'Nut booklet, Nutriset. 2014. *Plumpy'Nut booklet*, France. Available at: https://docplayer.net/39303490-Nutriset2014-all-rights-reserved.html.
Abbreviations: g, grams; Kcal, kilocalories; mg, milligrams; μg, micrograms.

GUIDELINES: REQUIREMENTS AND RECOMMENDATIONS

According to the United Nations International Children's Emergency Fund (UNICEF) and the WHO, RUTFs must fulfil specific nutrient requirements, including an energy density between 5.2 and 5.5 kcal/g, between 10% and 12% of total energy from protein (with at least 50% derived from milk products), 45%–60% of total energy from lipids and a maximum water content of 2.5% (Tables 28.2 and 28.3) (WHO 2009).

Irrespective of HIV status, WHO recommends therapeutic food supplementation for severely undernourished individuals (body mass index [BMI] <16 kg/m^2) until their BMI becomes stabilized. Such treatment typically lasts approximately three to eight months. Upon initial weight recovery (BMI <18.5 kg/m^2), supplementary feeding with micronutrient fortified blended flours is usually recommended, subject to availability. For severely wasted and underweight children, it is recommended that 200 kilocalories (kcal) per kilogram (kg) be given per day until they reach their target weight; which is typically around 6–10 weeks (Sunguya et al. 2012). In infants, apart from water and breastmilk, the RUTF should be their only food source during rehabilitation.

It is generally recommended that PLWHA meet their nutrient requirements from their available food supply. However, provided their diet is inadequate, therapeutic food supplementation can prove beneficial given its high energy density and micronutrient content. The energy requirements for non-pregnant PLWHA typically range between 10% and 30% higher than an HIV-negative individual and may be even higher if the person is undernourished or has an opportunistic infection (WHO 2008). In addition, an increased protein intake of 1.5–2.0 g/kg of body weight is needed to build lean mass, and between 1.0 and 1.4 g/kg is needed for lean mass preservation (Willig et al. 2016).

ETHICAL ISSUES

Randomised control trials (RCTs) involving the use of a "treatment" group and a "control" group provide important information for determining the efficacy of an intervention. Yet assessing the efficacy of a food supplement in a food-insecure population using a RCT poses a significant ethical dilemma. For instance, if all participants are HIV positive and uniformly food insecure, is it ethical to administer a food supplement to one group and not the other? Given the high risk of mortality involved, many investigators choose not to include a control group, or rather do a comparative study and assess the efficacy of one food supplement over another (Audain et al. 2015; Swaminathan et al. 2010).

TABLE 28.2
Recipe for Ready-to-Use Therapeutic Foods (RUTF)

Component	Weight (%)
Full-fat milk	30
Sugar	28
Peanut butter	25
Vegetable oil	25
Mineral-vitamin mix	1.6

Source: Adapted with permission from *Guidelines for an Integrated Approach to the Nutritional Care of HIV-Infected Children (6 Months–14 years)* World Health Organization (WHO). 2009. *Guidelines for an Integrated Approach to the Nutritional Care of HIV-Infected Children (6 Months–14 years).* WHO, Geneva. Available at: https://www.who.int/nutrition/publications/hivaids/9789241597524/en/

TABLE 28.3
Nutritional Composition of Ready-to-Use Therapeutic Foods (RUTF)

Component	Amount
Sodium (mg)	290
Potassium (mg)	110–1400
Calcium (mg/100 g)	300–600
Magnesium (mg/100 g)	80–140
Phosphorus (excluding phytate) (mg/100 g)	300–600
Iron (mg/100 g)	10–14
Zinc (mg/100 g)	11–14
Copper (mg/100 g)	1.4–1.8
Selenium (μg/100 g)	20–40
Iodine (μg/100 g)	70–140
Vitamin A (mg/100 g)	0.8–1.1
Vitamin D (μg/100 g)	15–20
Vitamin E (mg/100 g)	20
Vitamin K (μg/100 g)	15–30
Vitamin B1 (mg/100 g)	0.5
Vitamin B2 (mg/100 g)	1.6
Vitamin B6 (mg/100 g)	0.6
Vitamin B12 (μg/100 g)	1.6
Vitamin C (mg/100 g)	50
Folic acid (μg/100 g)	200
Niacin (mg/100 g)	5
Pantothenic acid (mg/100 g)	3
Biotin (μg/100 g)	60
n-6 fatty acids (% of total energy)	3–10
n-3 fatty acids (% of total energy)	0.3–2.5
Energy (Kcal/100 g)	520–550
Protein (% of total energy)	10–12
Lipids (% of total energy)	45–60
Moisture content (%)	2.5

Source: Adapted with permission from *Guidelines for an Integrated Approach to the Nutritional Care of HIV-Infected Children (6 Months–14 years)* World Health Organization (WHO). 2009. *Guidelines for an Integrated Approach to the Nutritional Care of HIV-Infected Children (6 Months–14 years)*. WHO, Geneva. Available at: https://www.who.int/nutrition/publications/hivaids/9789241597524/en/.

Abbreviations: g, grams; Kcal, kilocalories; mg, milligrams; μg, micrograms.

A study in South India attempted to overcome this ethical hurdle by conducting a nonrandomized comparison with participants from different sites and providing the supplement to everyone enrolled at the end of the study. This required the use of a mixed-model analysis to control for the differences in baseline characteristics of enrolling participants. Still, for the duration of the study, one group received a daily macronutrient supplement, while the other group received just standard care. This led to the supplement group experiencing significant increases in body weight, BMI, mid-upper arm circumference, fat-free mass, and body cell mass compared to the control group, and the control group experiencing a decline in CD4+ count. However, after adjusting for baseline differences, it was found that anthropometric and clinical differences between the two groups were not statistically significant; hence, the study design made the supplement appear to provide no real benefit (Swaminathan et al. 2010).

In infants and young children, food supplementation can raise its own ethical concerns. Exclusive breastfeeding is known to be largely superior to any type of replacement feeding, even in the presence of HIV infection. Administering formula feeding, even with a formula of high nutritional value, can be problematic due to high cost, lack of clean water for mixing or stigma attached to women who do not breastfeed (WHO 2011). Even babies who are HIV positive are encouraged to breastfeed and slowly introduce small quantities of nutrient-rich foods. When suitable, ART is provided during pregnancy and lactation, which minimizes the risk of transmitting HIV via breastmilk (WHO 2011). Any infant formula, regardless of whether it was developed to treat SAM or HIV symptoms, should be regulated by a board or committee prior to it reaching the market. Parents should be made aware of the false marketing claims made by replacement feeding producers (Tiwari et al. 2016).

LIMITATIONS TO FOOD SUPPLEMENTATION

It is a widely accepted fact that food supplementation in isolation is not a sustainable initiative. In most cases in LMICs, food supplements (e.g., Plumpy'Nut) are produced outside of the affected area and imported with help from donor funding. Several ingredients included in even locally prepared therapeutic foods, such as the micronutrient premixes, are either imported or donated by the WFP (Audain et al. 2015).

It is therefore necessary to approach food supplementation as part of a long-term food security intervention. This could involve the investment in 100% locally produced therapeutic foods. In Malawi, a locally produced supplement was shown to cause weight gain, improve physical activity and increase treatment adherence in HIV-positive adults, the majority of whom were at WHO clinical stage IV of the disease. In addition, the local supplement was more affordable than the CSB being donated by the WFP (Bahwere et al. 2009).

Nutritional concerns among PLWHA are exacerbated by high levels of food insecurity. In countries facing a triple burden of HIV, food insecurity and undernutrition, food supplementation can promote the nutritional recovery of undernourished HIV patients. However, it does not address key underlying food insecurity issues, including a lack of regular access to food of adequate nutritional quality (Yager et al. 2011).

Household food insecurity in LMICs needs to be addressed within the context of the ongoing HIV epidemic to ensure a sustainable impact on improving nutritional status (Aberman et al. 2014; Yager et al. 2011). This could involve the promotion of social protection initiatives that provide support for vulnerable households to improve access to safe and nutritious food to help meet daily nutrient requirements. Therefore, priority should eventually be shifted from short-term food supplementation to a more longer-term dietary management of HIV.

KEY FACTS: LINKING FOOD SUPPLEMENTATION AND PALLIATIVE CARE IN HIV

- Approximately half of adults and children living with HIV had access to antiretroviral therapy in 2015.
- Undernourished people living with HIV are between two and six times more likely to die within the first six months of initiating antiretroviral therapy.
- The most recent definition of palliative care focuses on the provision of care as early as possible along the course of the chronic illness.
- Therapeutic food supplements are traditionally developed for the treatment of severe acute malnutrition.
- Ready-to-use therapeutic food provides an adequate source of nutrients necessary for AIDS recovery.

SUMMARY POINTS

- Despite a global decline in the number of new infections, a significant proportion of individuals are becoming infected each day, and the global HIV prevalence remains high, especially in Sub-Saharan Africa.
- Antiretroviral therapy can help combat factors that lead to undernutrition. In its absence, the risk of people living with HIV and AIDS becoming undernourished is increased. Insufficient food consumption can also lead to undernutrition. Undernutrition then weakens the immune system, causing an increase in opportunistic infections and furthering the progression of HIV.
- Food insecurity is a contributing factor to HIV-associated wasting, as well as a primary reason for a lack of adherence to antiretroviral therapy. This is the key argument for food supplementation to be integrated into HIV palliative care.
- HIV infection causes damage to the epithelial barrier of the gastrointestinal tract. The resulting immune activation produces reactive species, which further degrades the intestinal lining.
- Higher levels of morbidity are observed among older people living with HIV and AIDS compared to their HIV-negative counterparts, which emphasises the need for increased palliative care to manage the rise in non-communicable disease burden.
- The World Health Organization recommends therapeutic food supplementation for individuals with a body mass index of less than 16 kg/m^2, irrespective of their HIV status. For severely wasted and underweight children, 200 kilocalories (kcal) per kilogram (kg) is recommended until their target weight is reached.
- Ready-to-eat therapeutic foods must fulfil specific nutrient requirements, including an energy density between 5.2 and 5.5 kcal/g, between 10% and 12% of total energy from protein (with at least 50% derived from milk products), 45%–60% of total energy from lipids and a maximum water content of 2.5%.
- Among people living with HIV and AIDS, supplementation aims to not only treat undernutrition but also reduce mortality and improve antiretroviral therapy adherence.
- Assessing the efficacy of a food supplement using randomised control trials poses an ethical dilemma, given the nature of the control group not receiving any supplementation. If the trial involves severely undernourished individuals, this could result in a higher mortality rate within the control group that receives supplementation.
- Exclusive breastfeeding is recommended for infants younger than six months, followed by a slow introduction to nutrient-rich foods. Formula feeding can be problematic due to high cost, lack of clean water or stigma attached to women who do not breastfeed.
- Current food supplementation is not sustainable, as most supplements are imported with help from donor funding. Food supplementation should be part of a long-term food security intervention. This could involve the promotion of social protection initiatives that provide support for vulnerable households to improve/increase access to safe and nutritious food to help meet daily nutrient requirements. Priority should shift from short-term food supplementation to a more longer-term dietary management of HIV.

LIST OF ABBREVIATIONS

AIDS	Acquired Immune Deficiency Syndrome
ART	Antiretroviral Therapy
BMI	Body Mass Index
CSB	Corn-Soya Blend
g	gram
GI	Gastrointestinal

HIV	Human Immunodeficiency Virus
IYCF	Infant and Young Child Feeding
kcal	kilocalories
kg	kilogram
LMICs	Low-to-Middle-Income Countries
LNS	Lipid Nutrient Supplement
m	metre
PEPFAR	President's Emergency Plan for AIDS Relief
PLWHA	Persons Living with HIV/AIDS
RCT	Randomized Controlled Trial
RUTF	Ready-to-Eat Therapeutic Food
SAM	Severe Acute Malnutrition
UNAIDS	Joint United Nations Programme on HIV/AIDS
UNICEF	United Nations Children's Fund
USAID	United States Agency for International Development
WFP	World Food Programme
WHO	World Health Organization

REFERENCES

Aberman, N.-L., Rawat, R., Drimie, S., Claros, J.M., Kadiyala, S. 2014. Food security and nutrition interventions in response to the AIDS epidemic: Assessing global action and evidence. *AIDS Behav.* 18, 554–565.

Audain, K.A., Zotor, F.B., Amuna, P., Ellahi, B. 2015. Food supplementation among HIV-infected adults in Sub-Saharan Africa: Impact on treatment adherence and weight gain. *Proc. Nutr. Soc. FirstView* 1–9.

Bahwere, P., Sadler, K., Collins, S. 2009. Acceptability and effectiveness of chickpea sesame-based ready-to-use therapeutic food in malnourished HIV-positive adults. *Patient Prefer. Adherence* 3, 67–75.

Brown, M., Nga, T.T., Hoang, M.-A., Maalouf-Manasseh, Z., Hammond, W., Thuc, T.M.L., Minh, T.H.N., Hop, T.L., Berger, J., Wieringa, F.T. 2015. Acceptability of two ready-to-use therapeutic foods by HIV-positive patients in vietnam. *Food Nutr. Bull.* 36, 102–110.

Colecraft, E. 2008. HIV/AIDS: Nutritional implications and impact on human development. *P. Nutr. Soc.* 67(1), 109–113. doi:10.1017/S002966510800609.

Dibari, F., Bahwere, P., Le Gall, I., Guerrero, S., Mwaniki, D., Seal, A. 2012. A qualitative investigation of adherence to nutritional therapy in malnourished adult AIDS patients in Kenya. *Public Health Nutr.* 15, 316–323.

Diouf, A., Badiane, A., Manga, N.M., Idohou-Dossou, N., Sow, P.S., Wade, S. 2016. Daily consumption of ready-to-use peanut-based therapeutic food increased fat free mass, improved anemic status but has no impact on the zinc status of people living with HIV/AIDS: A randomized controlled trial. *BMC Public Health* 16.

Guaraldi, G., Orlando, G., Zona, S., Menozzi, M., Carli, F., Garlassi, E., Berti, A., Rossi, E., Roverato, A., Palella, F. 2011. Premature age-related comorbidities among HIV-infected persons compared with the general population. *Clin. Infect. Dis. Off. Publ. Infect. Dis. Soc. Am.* 53, 1120–1126.

Herce, M.E., Flick, R.J. 2015. Integrating HIV and palliative care: Ending the false dichotomy. *Lancet HIV* 2, e310–311.

Herce, M.E., Elmore, S.N., Kalanga, N., Keck, J.W., Wroe, E.B., Phiri, A., Mayfield, A. et al. 2014. Assessing and responding to palliative care needs in rural Sub-Saharan Africa: Results from a model intervention and situation analysis in Malawi. *PLOS ONE* 9(10), e110457.

Kayira, D., Bentley, M.E., Wiener, J., Mkhomawanthu, C., King, C.C., Chitsulo, P., Chigwenembe, M. et al. 2012. A lipid-based nutrient supplement mitigates weight loss among HIV-infected women in a factorial randomized trial to prevent mother-to-child transmission during exclusive breastfeeding1234. *Am. J. Clin. Nutr.* 95, 759–765.

Mkwinda, E., Lekalakala-Mokgele, E. 2016. Palliative care needs in Malawi: Care received by people living with HIV. *Curationis* 39, 1664.

Nakawesi, J., Kasirye, I., Kavuma, D., Muziru, B., Businge, A., Naluwooza, J., Kabunga, G. et al. 2014. Palliative care needs of HIV exposed and infected children admitted to the inpatient paediatric unit in Uganda. *Ecancermedicalscience* 8, 489.

Nga, T.T., Nguyen, M., Mathisen, R., Hoa, D.T., Minh, N.H., Berger, J., Wieringa, F.T. 2013. Acceptability and impact on anthropometry of a locally developed Ready-to-use therapeutic food in pre-school children in Vietnam. *Nutr. J.* 12, 120.

Nutriset. 2014. *Plumpy'Nut booklet*, France. Available at: https://docplayer.net/39303490-Nutriset2014-all-rights-reserved.html

Nutriset. 2016. From Treatment to the Prevention of Malnutrition. Nutriset. Available at: https://www.nutriset.fr/en/from-treatment-to-prevention-of-malnutrition

Rodas-Moya, S., Pengnonyang, S., Kodish, S., de Pee, S., Phanuphak, P. 2017. Psychosocial factors influencing preferences for food and nutritional supplements among people living with HIV in Bangkok, Thailand. *Appetite* 108, 498–505.

Shorthill, J., DeMarco, R.F. 2017. The relevance of palliative care in HIV and aging. *Interdiscip. Top. Gerontol. Geriatr.* 42, 222–233.

Singer, A.W., Weiser, S.D., McCoy, S.I. 2015. Does food insecurity undermine adherence to antiretroviral therapy? A systematic review. *AIDS Behav.* 19, 1510–1526.

Sunguya, B.F., Poudel, K.C., Mlunde, L.B., Otsuka, K., Yasuoka, J., Urassa, D.P., Mkopi, N.P., Jimba, M. 2012. Ready to use therapeutic foods (RUTF) improves undernutrition among ART-treated, HIV-positive children in Dar es Salaam, Tanzania. *Nutr. J.* 11, 60.

Suttajit, M. 2007. Advances in nutrition support for quality of life in HIV/AIDS. *Asia Pac. J. Clin. Nutr.* 16, 318–322.

Swaminathan, S., Padmapriyadarsini, C., Yoojin, L., Sukumar, B., Iliayas, S., Karthipriya, J., Sakthivel, R. et al. 2010. Nutritional supplementation in HIV-infected individuals in South India: A prospective interventional study. *Clin. Infect. Dis.* 51, 51–57.

Tiwari, S., Bharadva, K., Yadav, B., Malik, S., Gangal, P., Banapurmath, C.R., Zaka-Ur-Rab, Z., Deshmukh, U., Visheshkumar, Agrawal, R.K. 2016. Infant and young child feeding guidelines, 2016. *Indian Pediatr.* 53, 703–713.

UNAIDS. 2017. UNAIDS Data 2017. Joint United Nations programme on HIV/AIDS (UNAIDS) Available at: http://www.unaids.org/sites/default/files/media_asset/20170720_Data_book_2017_en.pdf

UNICEF. 2013. Ready-To-Use Therapeutic Food for Children with Severe Acute Malnutrition. Position Paper, No. 1, June 2013. United Nations Children's Fund. Available at: https://www.unicef.org/media/files/Position_Paper_Ready-to-use_therapeutic_food_for_children_with_severe_acute_malnutrition__June_2013.pdf

USAID. 2015. Multi-Sectoral Nutrition Strategy 2014- 2025. Technical Brief: Nutrition, Food Security and HIV. Available at: https://www.usaid.gov/sites/default/files/documents/1864/nutrition-food-security-HIV-AIDS-508-revFeb17.pdf

USAID. 2016. Ready-To-Use Therapeutic Food Commodity Fact Sheet. Emergency Food, RUTF Spread Pouch-150/92 G 110170. Available at: https://2012-2017.usaid.gov/what-we-do/agriculture-and-food-security/food-assistance/resources/ready-use-therapeutic-food

World Food Programme (WFP). 2010. Technical Specifications for the manufacture of: Corn Soya Blend for Young Children and Adults. August 2010. WFP. Available at: https://documents.wfp.org/stellent/groups/public/documents/manual_guide_proced/wfp251133.pdf

World Health Organization (WHO). 1990. *Cancer Pain Relief and Palliative Care, WHO Technical Report Series 804, Publication 1100804.* WHO, Geneva. Available at: http://apps.who.int/iris/bitstream/10665/39524/1/WHO_TRS_804.pdf

World Health Organization (WHO). 2008. *Essential Prevention and Care Interventions for Adults and Adolescents Living with HIV in Resource Limited Settings.* WHO, Geneva. Available at: http://www.who.int/hiv/pub/toolkits/Essential%20Prevention%20and%20Care%20interventions%20Jan%2008.pdf

World Health Organization (WHO). 2009. *Guidelines for an Integrated Approach to the Nutritional Care of HIV-Infected Children (6 Months–14 years).* WHO, Geneva. Available at: https://www.who.int/nutrition/publications/hivaids/9789241597524/en/

World Health Organization (WHO). 2011. *Nutritional Care for HIV-Infected Children April 2011.* WHO, Geneva. Available at: http://www.who.int/elena/titles/bbc/nutrition_hiv_children/en/

World Health Organization (WHO). 2017. *WHO Definition of Palliative Care.* WHO, Geneva. Available at: http://www.who.int/cancer/palliative/definition/en/

Willig, A.L., Overton, E.T., Saag, M.S. 2016. The silent epidemic – Frailty and aging with HIV. *Total Patient Care HIV HCV* 1, 6–17.

Yager, J.E., Kadiyala, S., Weiser, S.D. 2011. HIV/AIDS, food supplementation and livelihood programs in Uganda: A way forward? *PLOS ONE* 6. https://doi.org/10.1371/journal.pone.0026117

29 Palliative Care of Gastroparesis

Sofia Lakhdar and Andrew Ukleja

CONTENTS

INTRODUCTION

Gastroparesis (GP) is a chronic debilitating disorder that is defined as a delayed gastric emptying in the absence of mechanical obstruction (Camilleri 2016). Although it is primarily an idiopathic disorder, it can result from systemic conditions, such as diabetes mellitus, as well as post-surgical complications (e.g., vagotomy, pyloroplasty, fundoplication). Iatrogenic GP develops secondary to inadvertent vagal nerve entrapment or damage during surgery. Idiopathic GP is the most common form of GP, prevalent in young and middle-aged women with a subset of cases developed after an infectious process, most likely viral illness. In collagen vascular diseases and Parkinson disease, GP is secondary to autonomic neuropathy (Soykan et al. 1998). GP may also be induced by several medications that slow gastric motility such as narcotics, glucagon-like peptide 1 agonists and levodopa (Lembo et al. 2016; Schey et al. 2016).

GP is a relatively common and complex condition that is encountered in the gastroenterology practice. The age-adjusted prevalence of GP has been estimated to be 9.6 for men and 37.8 for women per 100,000 in a community-based study (Jung et al. 2009). The age-adjusted incidence of GP was 2.4 per 100,000 person-years for men and 9.8 per 100,000 person-years for women (Jung et al. 2009). While many patients with GP have mild symptoms, some patients present with debilitating symptoms, which include unrelenting nausea, vomiting, early satiety, bloating, postprandial fullness and abdominal pain.

Once a patient develops protracted nausea and vomiting, providing adequate nutrition and hydration can present a challenge for the clinician. Refractory symptoms may lead to malnutrition and weight loss as a result of poor oral intake (Bharadwaj et al. 2016). Therefore, the evaluation of nutritional status and early treatment of malnutrition are essential in the management of refractory GP. Severe vomiting, abdominal pain and malnutrition impact a patient's quality of life (Lacy et al. 2018). This is associated with increased emergency room visits, hospitalizations and subsequent increased healthcare costs (Bharadwaj et al. 2016). While nausea and vomiting are cardinal symptoms of GP, abdominal pain is common and often severe. Those patients who experience severe pain tend to develop an aversion to food and this potentiates the risk of malnutrition. Overall, a thorough understanding of the disease process of GP is essential in order to prevent malnutrition and improve overall quality of life.

PATHOPHYSIOLOGY

The pathophysiology behind GP is still not well understood but encompasses abnormalities in the autonomic nervous system, enteric neurons and smooth muscle cells. Following a meal, the emptying of gastric contents depends on well-coordinated mechanisms involving the motor and myoelectric properties of the different regions of the stomach (Camilleri 2007; Parkman 2017). Gastric filling and emptying are divided into three important events, which include fundic relaxation in response to food ingestion, antral phasic contractions and trituration of large food particles, and finally pyloric relaxation allowing food particles to propagate through the upper gastrointestinal (GI) tract. Gastric contractions are generated by the pacemaker cells, interstitial cells of Cajal (ICC), which are found in the body of the stomach and are regulated by neurohormonal input (Parkman 2015). Gastric motor dysfunction occurs when there is a disturbance at the cellular and neuronal levels, which include loss of interstitial cells of Cajal, loss of neuronal nitric oxide synthase, enteric neuronal degeneration (visceral neuropathy) and smooth muscle disease (myopathy) related to collagen diseases (Parkman 2017). Autonomic neuropathy due to hyperglycemia is commonly encountered in diabetic GP (DGP). Patients with DGP develop neuropathy that affects the interstitial cells of Cajal. However, diabetic patients develop abnormalities at various levels of gastric motility including postprandial gastric accommodation and contractions as well as antral motor function (Ordog et al. 2000). Pain medications such as opiods slow gastric motility and contribute to delayed gastric empting (Jeong et al. 2012).

DIAGNOSIS

A diagnosis of GP is made after a thorough clinical evaluation, detailed patient history and tests assessing the rate of gastric emptying. Initial tests, such as an upper endoscopy or barium study, may first be performed to rule out other causes such as obstruction of the upper GI tract. It is recommended, according the American Gastroenterological Association, that patients with GP should be evaluated for the presence of diabetes mellitus, thyroid dysfunction, neurological disease and autoimmune disorders. History of prior gastric or bariatric surgery should be obtained.

At present, gastric emptying rate is often assessed by gastric scintigraphy. This modality has been widely used and accepted as the "gold standard" for the diagnosis of GP (Abell et al. 2008). Conventionally, the test is performed after ingestion of a bland meal such as eggs or egg substitute that contains a small amount of radioactive isotope. An external camera scans the abdomen and measures the rate of gastric emptying at one, two, three and four hours after the meal was ingested. Greater than 60% of the meal retained at two hours and/or greater than 10% of the meal retention within the stomach at four hours is consistent with the diagnosis of GP.

The SmartPill (Medtronic, Minneapolis, Minnesota) is also used in specialized outpatient centers and provides a simple, painless method to collect data from the GI tract (Kuo et al. 2008). A small electronic device in the form of a capsule is swallowed by the patient, and moves through the entire digestive tract while sending information to a receiver worn by the patient. The recorded information and images provide a detailed record of the gastric emptying time, colonic transit time, whole gut transit time as well as the pressure, pH and temperature as it passes through the entire GI tract. Typically, the SmartPill moves through the stomach in less than four hours, small intestine for less than six hours and large intestine for less than 59 hours. Unfortunately, the SmartPill has limitations and should not be used in cases of intestinal strictures, in those with Crohn disease with stricture or in patients with cardiac pacemakers.

The gastric emptying breath test (GEBT) is a newer non-invasive test to aid in the diagnosis of GP (Bruno et al. 2013). The GEBT allows clinicians to assess how fast the stomach empties solids by measuring carbon dioxide in a patient's breath. The test is conducted over a four-hour period after an overnight fast. After a baseline breath test is conducted, the patient eats a special test meal that includes scrambled eggs with *Spirulina platensis*, a protein enriched with carbon-13, which is measured in breath samples. This test has been validated and utilized mainly in the outpatient setting.

POTENTIAL COMPLICATIONS OF GASTROPARESIS

Patients with GP may experience secondary gastrointestinal disorders, which include gastroesophageal reflux disease (GERD), gastric bezoars and small intestinal bacterial overgrowth (SIBO) (Hasler 2007). Patients with GP have an increased tendency to acid reflux due to impaired stomach contractility and prolonged retention of gastric contents. Furthermore, reflux is exacerbated due to increased gastric distension resulting in relaxation of the lower esophageal sphincter (LES) (Bharadwaj et al. 2016). Acid-suppressive treatment should be strongly considered in those patients. Another complication is the increased risk of developing gastric bezoars. The incidence of bezoar formation determined by barium study was around 6% in GP patients (Levin et al. 2008). Bezoar formation occurs due to the lack of antral-pyloric grinding mechanism and the absence of major motor complexes. Upper endoscopy is required to confirm a definitive diagnosis.

Finally, there has been a correlation between GP and SIBO. In health, peristalsis and normal gastric acid production prevent the colonization of bacteria. It has been shown that an impairment of either would contribute to the colonization of bacteria within the small intestine. Many patients with GP are treated with acid-suppressive medication to reduce reflux symptoms. This resultant hypochlorhydria predisposes this specific subgroup to development of SIBO. Bacterial colonization in the small bowel results in mucosal inflammation, which further results in impaired nutrients absorption (Zaidel and Lin 2003). Patients with SIBO present with symptoms that mimic GP which include gas, bloating, abdominal distension, nausea, diarrhea and decline in nutritional status. It is imperative that patients with GP should be evaluated for concurrent SIBO (Reddymasu and Mccallum 2010). Treatment for SIBO includes a course of antibiotics such as metronidazole, ciprofloxacin, amoxicillin/clavulanate or rifaximin for 7–14 days.

NUTRITIONAL ASPECTS OF GASTROPARESIS

Patients with GP are at a significant risk of nutritional deficiencies. Maintenance of nutrition is essential in GP patients. Approximately 64% of patients with GP were found to have a calorie-deficient diet (Papasavas et al. 2014). Caloric intake was inversely proportional to higher symptom scores (bloating, abdominal fullness, constipation). Patients often develop food aversion secondary to the associated vomiting and abdominal pain. This can lead to common mineral and vitamin deficiencies such as iron, fat-soluble vitamins, thiamine and folate. An initial nutritional assessment should be considered in refractory GP to prevent malnutrition and associated morbidity (Parkman et al. 2011). It has been demonstrated that patients who were experiencing prolonged gastric emptying had severe nutritional deficiencies (Ogorek et al. 1991). Patients at moderate risk of malnutrition require early diet modification to help attenuate symptoms. High-risk patients require a more aggressive approach and nutritional interventions, which include enteral (EN) or parenteral nutrition (PN).

ORAL NUTRITIONAL SUPPORT

The provision of nutrition by the oral route is preferred initially. A target weight goal should be defined. In case of failure to gain weight or further weight loss, EN support should be initiated. Certain dietary modifications are currently suggested by the American College of Gastroenterology (ACG) such as the recommendation of eating more frequent and smaller meals, and having four to six small meals per day (Camilleri et al. 2013) (Table 29.1). Meals should also be composed of low fat content, and soluble fiber is preferred. The reasoning behind this is based on the observation that fat molecules delay gastric emptying and fibers require antral contractility for digestion, of which patients with GP are lacking. Replacing solid food with liquid-based meals should also be encouraged, especially in patients who cannot tolerate a solid diet (Homko et al. 2015). Well-tolerated and not-tolerated types of food are shown in Table 29.2 (Olausson et al. 2014; Wytiaz et al. 2015).

TABLE 29.1
Basic Diet Recommendations for Patients with Gastroparesis

- Eat small meals/avoid large meals
- Eat six or more meals a day
- Chew food well
- Avoid high-fiber foods
- Liquid food preferred over solids
- Pureed or ground food preferred over solids
- Eat high-protein foods
- Sit up after eating for one hour after finishing meal
- Consider short walk after meals

TABLE 29.2
Examples of Foods Having Effects on Symptoms in Gastroparesis

Food Provoking Symptoms	Food Improving or Not Provoking Symptoms
Orange juice	Saltine crackers
Salsa	Jell-O
Broccoli	Graham crackers
Lettuce	
Coffee	Ginger ale
Onions	Gluten-free foods
Tomato juice	Sweet potatoes
Cabbage	Potatoes
Oranges	Tea
Pepper	Clear soup
Pizza	White rice
Sausage	Popsicles
Fried chicken	Applesauce
Bacon	Pretzels
Roast beef	White fish
High fat solid meal	Salmon

TABLE 29.3
Indications for Nutritional Support

Severe weight loss greater than 5%–10% of usual body weight during three to six months
Repeated emergency room visits or hospitalizations for refractory gastroparesis requiring IV hydration/electrolyte replacement or IV-promotility medication
Overall poor quality of life

EN or PN should be considered in patients who continue to present with symptoms despite dietary modifications and pharmacotherapy. Patients with severe GP and significant weight loss greater than 10% of body weight should be started on nutritional support (Table 29.3).

ENTERAL NUTRITION

EN is used in specific patients who fit predefined criteria. Tube placement for enteral access is dependent on several aspects, which include patient/physician preference, duration of EN therapy, and whether the patient is able to tolerate endoscopy or surgery for tube placement. Different routes of enteral access are available, and to date no study has demonstrated an overall superiority of one procedure over the other. These include nasogastric tube, nasoduodenal or nasojejunal tube, gastrostomy, percutaneous gastrostomy with jejunal extension (PEG-J) or jejunal tube through PEG (JET-PEG), direct jejunostomy, and dual gastrostomy and jejunostomy (Maple et al. 2005). Using both gastric and jejunal access has an advantage by the ability to perform gastric decompression, which may significantly reduce symptoms of GP and in parallel jejunal feeding, allowing a patient's nutritional status to improve (Pitt et al. 1985). Unfortunately, a dual G-J system is often a failure, because of J-tube proximal migration and the need for the tube reposition or exchange. Patients often suffer from leakage at the tube site. The tubes are not preferred by the patients for cosmetic reasons.

PARENTERAL NUTRITION

PN may also be used in certain circumstances, especially short term. However, it is rarely used to reverse malnutrition in patients with GP. PN is used in patients who are unable to tolerate EN or oral feeds in a setting of acute illness and preoperatively. PN has been used in patients with GP and evidence of a generalized dysmotility syndrome, which is commonly seen in systemic sclerosis or low visceral myopathy (Warner and Jeejeebhoy 1985).

TREATMENT OPTIONS

Once GP is diagnosed, a tailored and systemic approach is required for the management of GP and its associated malnutrition. In general, oral nutrition, vitamin supplementation, pharmacologic treatments and surgical considerations are imperative in reducing symptoms, improving gastric emptying and preventing malnutrition-associated morbidity.

Management of Hyperglycemia

Hyperglycemia in diabetic GP should be addressed as GP has a deleterious effect on diabetic patients and their glycemic control. Glycosylated hemoglobin levels should be evaluated, and elevated blood glucose levels must be corrected. Episodes of acute hyperglycemia have been shown to exacerbate symptoms of GP by delaying gastric emptying (Jebbink et al. 1994). In diabetic patients, pharmacologic agents used to control hyperglycemia should be cautiously selected as Pramlintide and some glucagon-like peptide-1 analogues delay gastric emptying and should be avoided (Camilleri

2007). Instead, other agents may be used such as dipeptidyl peptidase-4 inhibitors (e.g., Sitagliptin), which do not affect the rate of gastric emptying (Camilleri 2007).

Prokinetics

In conjunction with the dietary modifications mentioned previously, the use of pharmacologic promotility agents (prokinetics) such as metoclopramide, domperidone and erythromycin may be used to improve symptoms and rate of gastric emptying. Metoclopramide is used as a first-line agent and has both prokinetic and anti-nausea properties. However, this medication should be used cautiously because of its potential risks and side effects of QT prolongation and extra-pyramidal manifestations (Sarosiek et al. 2016). The drug is available for use as oral, intravenous and rectal formulations. Domperidone, a dopamine antagonist, is the preferred drug if metoclopramide is not tolerated. It does not cross the blood-brain barrier so does not have neurological side effects, but has potential for cardiac toxicity. Domperidone has a quite potent anti-emetic effect. Domperidone has been shown to be effective in approximately 70% patients in a recent single-center study, but 40% of patients had significant adverse effects, and 12% of patients had to discontinue the therapy (Schey et al. 2016). This drug is not approved by the U.S. Food and Drug Administration but has been used under the investigational new drug (IND) program. Domperidone is available in many countries outside the United States.

Erythromycin, a macrolide antibiotic, has been used with mixed results in GP. It is a motilin receptor agonist that mimics the action of motilin on GI tract smooth muscles (Acosta and Camilleri 2015). Erythromycin has been demonstrated to be effective in improving gastric emptying in GP patients. Erythromycin is more effective when given intravenously rather than orally. It is effective at low doses of 75–250 mg daily. Two main concerns with erythromycin use are loss of effectiveness over time because of downregulation of the motilin receptors, and potential for antimicrobial resistance. Adverse effects of erythromycin include abdominal pain, ototoxicity and QT interval prolongation. In refractory cases of GP, erythromycin can be combined with metoclopramide. Cisapride, increased gastric emptying of both solids and liquids, has been shown to have significant drug-drug interactions. It was withdrawn from markets in the United States and other countries due to the risk of serious cardiac events.

Table 29.4 lists available prokinetic agents.

New prokinetic drugs are in the pipeline with the promise of being as effective as approved drugs, but with less adverse effects (Chedid and Camilleri 2017; Sanger and Pasricha 2017) (Table 29.5). Potential novel drugs include ghrelin agonists with prokinetic activity in GP. Relamorelin has been shown to improve symptoms and gastric emptying in diabetic GP patients. An additional benefit of ghrelin agonists is appetite stimulation. Alternative therapeutic options are available and should be tailored according to symptoms as well as underlying pathophysiology.

TABLE 29.4
Medications with Prokinetic Properties in Gastroparesis

Medication	Mechanism of Action (Dosage)	Side Effects
Metoclopramide	• Dopamine D_2 receptor antagonist • 5-HT_4 receptor agonist • 5-HT_3 receptor antagonist (5–20 mg qid)	Tardive dyskinesia Tremor Black Box warning 2009
Domperidone	Peripheral dopamine D_2 receptor antagonist (10–20 mg qid)	QT prolongation
Erythromycin Azithromycin	Motilin receptor agonist (50–250 mg qid)	QT prolongation Tachyphylaxis
Bethanechol	Muscarinic receptor agonist (25 mg qid)	
Pyridostigmine	Acetylcholinesterase inhibitor (30–60 mg tid)	

TABLE 29.5
Drugs under Investigation for Gastroparesis

Prokinetic Class	Under Investigation
Dopamine receptor antagonists	• Itropride • Levosulpride
Motilin receptor agonist	• **Camicinal (GSK962040)** • RQ-00201894.119
Serotonin 5-HT4 agonist	• **Velusetrag, Prucalopride, Renzapride,** Mosapride, Naronapride, YKP10811
Ghrelin agonist	• **Relamorelin (RM-131)** • TZP-101, TZP-102 • EX-1314
Cholinesterase inhibitor	• Acotiamide • Itropride

Antiemetics

It is important to aggressively control symptoms of nausea and vomiting (Navas et al. 2017). In addition to the prokinetics, the antiemetic agents are offered to improve nausea and vomiting associated with GP. Antiemetic agents can provide symptomatic relief in GP patients. These drugs can be administered orally or parenterally, and some of them rectally (antihistamines, phenothiazines). Scopolamine and granisetron have been used as transdermal patches with good success. The 5-hydroxytryptamine 3 (5-HT3) antagonists such as ondansetron, granisetron and dolasetron, are very powerful drugs, but their cost may be a limiting factor. Phenothiazine derivatives (promethazine, prochlorperazine) and antihistamines (meclizine, cyclizine, dimenhydrinate) have been used with mixed results in GP. These medications have potential for drug interactions including cardiac toxicity (QT prolongation), electrolyte abnormalities, dizziness and psychomotor disturbances. Dronabinol (marinol) is a cannabis derivative with proven antiemetic effect in nausea and vomiting associated with chemotherapy. Marinol (5–10 mg dose, two to three times daily) may improve nausea and vomiting in GP patients. In addition, it can stimulate appetite and help patients gain weight. However, Marinol has serious central nervous system side effects such as anxiety, dizziness, drowsiness, euphoria, hallucinations and seizure, which may limit its use.

Other Drug Therapies

Tricyclic antidepressants (TCAs), selective serotonin and norepinephrine reuptake inhibitors (SSRIs, SNRIs) have been shown to be effective in functional dyspepsia (Sarosiek et al. 2016). These drugs may be beneficial for nausea, pain control and neuromodulation in GP patients. The TCAs (amitriptyline, desipramine and nortriptyline) at low doses seem to be effective for controlling nausea and abdominal pain and are well tolerated (Hasler 2015). However, a low dose of nortriptyline was shown recently to have no effect on overall symptoms in idiopathic GP (Parkman et al. 2013). Most adverse effects are anticholinergic, and associated rather with higher doses of the TCAs. They cannot be used concomitantly with monoamine oxidase (MAO) inhibitors because of risk of "serotonin syndrome." SSRIs (citalopram, duloxetine, fluoxetine, mirtazapine, paroxetine and venlafaxine) have been shown to help with anxiety, chronic pain, depression, early satiety and weight loss and may potentially improve quality of life (Tack and Carbone 2017). In a recent study, mirtazapine at dose 15 mg showed to improve nausea and vomiting after two and four weeks of treatment in 24 patients with GP (Malamood et al. 2017). However, adverse effects were seen in 46.7% of patients. All classes of medications used for gastroparesis are shown in Table 29.6.

TABLE 29.6
Drug Classes for Gastroparesis

Prokinetics
- Dopamine antagonists
- Motilin agonists

Anti-emetics
- Antihistamines, anticholinergics
- Dopamine and serotonin antagonists
- Antineurokininergics
- Cannabinoids
- Benzodiazepines

Other
- Antidepressants
- Antipsychotics

Complementary and alternative medicines such as acupuncture, electroacupuncture and abdominal massage became attractive alternatives for the management of GI symptoms (Gupta and Lee 2016). Acupuncture has often been used for treatment of GI symptoms, including those of GP, mainly in Asian countries. The typical acupuncture points to alleviate GI symptoms include the Neiguan (PC6) and the Zusanli (ST36) (Sarosiek et al. 2017). In a recent meta-analysis of 14 randomized controlled trials, acupuncture improved dyspeptic symptoms such as nausea, vomiting, gastric fullness and loss of appetite in diabetic GP patients compared with the control group (Yang et al. 2013). However, most studies had rather small sample size and high risk of bias. Therefore, there is a need for high-quality randomized trials, but until than acupuncture as a minimally invasive therapy may be utilized because of safety and a few adverse effects (Liu et al. 2015).

When conservative measures fail to control the debilitating symptoms in GP, which embodies a significant therapeutic challenge, more aggressive approaches are warranted. Methods such as intrapyloric botulinum toxin injections, placement of jejunostomy tube or gastric electrical stimulation have been explored and may be considered in these patients.

Intrapyloric Botulinum Toxin Injection

Botulinum toxin A (BTX) is a nerve-blocking agent that has been demonstrated to be effective in a limited number of retrospective studies. Two small randomized placebo controlled trials failed to show benefit of BTX intrapyloric injections in GP based on lack of improvement in GP cardinal symptom index and gastric emptying rate (Arts et al. 2007; Friedenberg et al. 2008). The pylorospasm contributing to dysregulated and uncoordinated emptying may be better controlled with the intrapyloric injection of botulinum toxin. It was suggested that a reduction of pyloric pressure by BTX injection into the pylorus may facilitate an improvement in gastric emptying and relieve symptoms associated with GP (Ukleja et al. 2015). Further research of Botox use is warranted given the limited number of published studies and suboptimal results with standard drug therapy.

Surgical Interventions

GP patients who continue to experience debilitating symptoms despite medical therapy may benefit from surgical intervention. One type of surgery is gastric electrical stimulator placement, which has been shown to demonstrate improvement in symptoms especially of nausea and vomiting relief. Gastric electric stimulation (GES) is acting centrally via afferent vagus nerve stimulation. Evidence suggests that a low-energy high-frequency GES activates the vagal afferent pathways to influence the central control mechanisms for nausea and vomiting. A GES delivers high-frequency low-amplitude waves to gastric muscle and has a potent anti-emetic effect in refractory GP (Abell et al. 2003). This device entrains gastric myoelectric activity through the electrodes that are implanted in the musculature of the gastric wall. The evidence in support of GES is limited and heterogeneous in quality (Lal et al. 2015). Some results may be related to patient selection. The systematic analysis of the effect of GES in GP produced mixed results and raised concern about the benefits of GES. While open-label studies of GES were associated with clinical improvement, controlled trials for GP reported no significant improvement in symptoms (Levinthal and Bielefeldt 2017). The GES effect on gastric emptying rate has not been consistently associated with improvement. In a single-center retrospective study of 151 patients with refractory GP, GES improved symptoms in 7% of patients while 43% of patients had moderate improvement (Heckert et al. 2016). The study also revealed that the response was better in diabetics than in nondiabetic patients. Significant improvement was seen in appetite and early satiety as well as in controlling symptoms of nausea. GES has also been reported to improve quality of life (Tang and Friedenberg 2011). The major complication associated with GES is the risk of device infection. Approximately 10% of GES require removal. Laparoscopic GES implantation can be combined with pyloromyotomy. A recent study showed that a combination of GES and pyloroplasty significantly accelerated gastric emptying and improved symptoms of GP (Davis et al. 2017). In addition, laparoscopic pyloromyotomy alone has been shown recently to be beneficial in regard to symptoms improvement and gastric emptying rate in GP (Mancini et al. 2015).

Another surgery to relieve symptoms of GP is a gastric bypass. This surgery was shown to be effective for obese diabetic patients (Papasavas et al. 2014). Some patients may require subtotal gastrectomy as a treatment choice for refractory GP (Jones and Maganti 2003).

Endoscopic Intervention: Gastric Per-Oral Endoscopic Myotomy or Per-Oral Endoscopic Pyloromyotomy

Gastric per-oral endoscopic myotomy (G-POEM) is a novel non-surgical method of correcting suspected pylorospasm, which may be contributing to a delay in gastric emptying (Gonzalez et al. 2017). A few small studies showed clinically significant improvement in GP symptoms and gastric emptying rate suggesting that G-POEM is an important and less invasive option for selected patients with refractory GP (Khashab et al. 2017; Lembo et al. 2016). In the future, we anticipate that this technique may become very popular because of proven safety and effective control of symptoms of GP.

In severe cases of refractory GP, a feeding tube in jejunal position should be considered, particularly in cases where diet and pharmacologic interventions have not been as effective and the person is losing weight or is requiring frequent hospitalizations for malnutrition and dehydration. The direct delivery of nutrients into the jejunum via a feeding tube may be the sole method of nutritional support in severe cases of GP. However, jejunostomy tube is usually considered as a temporary measure and has been associated with need for frequent replacements and tube leakage. In addition, gastric tube placement for venting can be offered to relieve nausea and vomiting as a palliative option. (See Table 29.7 for non-drug therapies for GP.)

TABLE 29.7
Non-Drug Interventions

Non-Drug Interventions
Botox injections
J-tube feeding
G-tube for decompression
Gastric electric stimulation
Gastric per-oral endoscopic myotomy
Surgery: Roux-en-Y gastric bypass, gastric resection, pyloroplasty

PRACTICAL METHODS/GUIDELINES

Table 29.8 presents an algorithm for the treatment of GP.

ETHICAL ISSUES

In patients with terminal disease, a decision has to be made regarding the benefits of interventions and issues related to quality of life. Many patients with terminal disease have been taking pain medications, which may cause worsening of GP symptoms as a result of drug effects on gastrointestinal motility. In patients with advanced or terminal disease, aggressive therapy may not be warranted. Patient autonomy should be protected.

KEY FACTS

- Malnutrition is a common finding in patients with gastroparesis.
- Accurate nutrition assessment is vital in the initial evaluation of patients with GP.
- Patients with GP also experience other associated conditions including gastroesophageal reflux disease, gastric bezoars, and small bowel bacterial overgrowth.
- GP is associated with poor quality of life, increased emergency room visits and hospitalizations.
- Diet modification is the first step in management of gastroparesis.
- Symptom control is essential part of therapy for gastroparesis.
- Surgical considerations are given in cases of refractory gastroparesis to medical therapy.

TABLE 29.8
Proposed Algorithm for Treatment of Gastroparesis

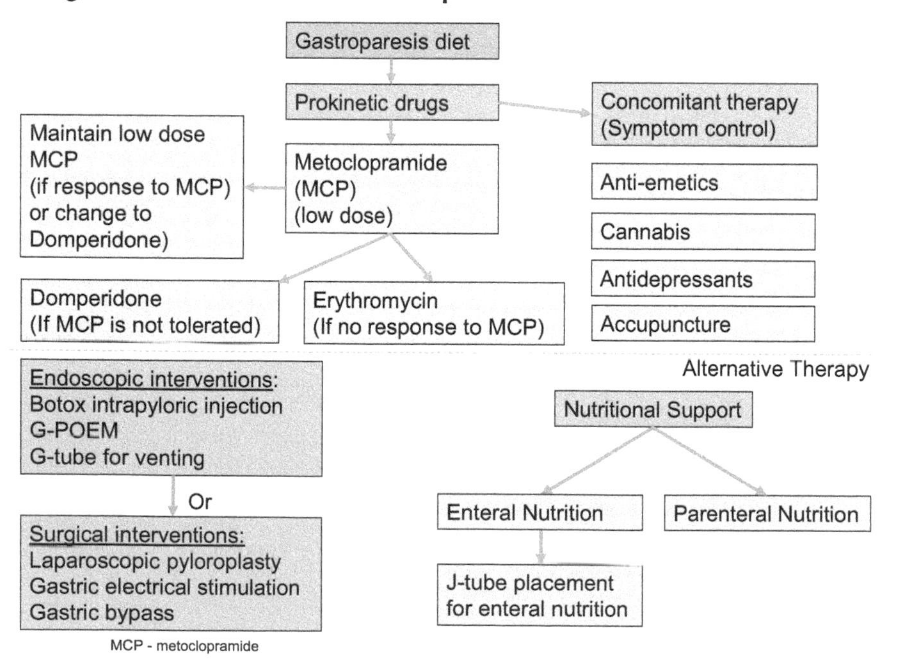

SUMMARY POINTS

- Gastroparesis can be very debilitating and can impact the patient's quality of life resulting in significant medical problems, most notably malnutrition.
- Accurate nutrition assessment is vital in the initial evaluation of a patient with gastroparesis, as malnutrition contributes to significant morbidity and mortality in this patient population.
- Providing nutritional support, treating nutrient deficiencies and maintaining glucose control are essential to alleviate symptoms and improve overall quality of life.
- Drug therapies are often not effective, and adverse effects are a common obstacle in their applications.
- Surgical interventions may be considered in refractory gastroparesis, but the associated risks need to be discussed.
- A novel endoscopic intervention, gastric per-oral endoscopic myotomy, may be a procedure of choice in the near future.

LIST OF ABBREVIATIONS

EN	Enteral Nutrition
GP	Gastroparesis
GEBT	Gastric Emptying Breath Test
GERD	Gastroesophageal Reflux Disease
PN	Parenteral Nutrition
SIBO	Small Intestinal Bacterial Overgrowth

REFERENCES

Abell, T. L., M. Camilleri, K. Donohoe, W. L. Hasler, H. C. Lin, A. H. Maurer, R. W. Mccallum et al. Consensus Recommendations for Gastric Emptying Scintigraphy: A Joint Report of the American Neurogastroenterology and Motility Society and the Society of Nuclear Medicine. *Journal of Nuclear Medicine Technology* 36, no. 1, 2008: 44–54.

Abell, T., R. Mccallum, M. Hocking, K. Koch, H. Abrahamsson, I. Leblanc, G. Lindberg, J. Konturek, T. Nowak, E. M. m. Quigley, G. Tougas, and W. Starkebaum. Gastric Electrical Stimulation for Medically Refractory Gastroparesis. *Gastroenterology* 125, no. 2, 2003: 421–28.

Acosta, A. and M. Camilleri. Prokinetics in Gastroparesis. *Gastroenterology Clinics of North America* 44, no. 1, 2015: 97–111.

Arts, J., L. Holvoet, P. Caenepeel, R. Bisschops, D. Sifrim, K. Verbeke, J. Janssens, and J. Tack. Clinical Trial: A Randomized-Controlled Crossover Study of Intrapyloric Injection of Botulinum Toxin in Gastroparesis. *Alimentary Pharmacology and Therapeutics* 26, no. 9, 2007: 1251–258.

Bharadwaj, S., K. Meka, P. Tandon, A. Rathur, J. M. Rivas, H. Vallabh, A. Jevenn, J. Guirguis, I. Sunesara, A. Nischnick, and A. Ukleja. Management of Gastroparesis-Associated Malnutrition. *Journal of Digestive Diseases* 17, no. 5 2016: 285–94.

Bruno, G., L. R. Lopetuso, L. Laterza, V. Gerardi, V. Petito, A. Gasbarrini, V. Ojetti, and F. Scaldaferri. 13C-octanoic Acid Breath Test to Study Gastric Emptying Time. *Euro Rev Med Pharmacol Sci Suppl* 2 2013: 59–64.

Camilleri, M. Diabetic Gastroparesis. *New England Journal of Medicine* 356, no. 8, 2007: 820–29.

Camilleri, M. Functional Dyspepsia and Gastroparesis. *Digestive Diseases* 34, no. 5, 2016: 491–99.

Camilleri, M., H. P. Parkman, M. A. Shafi, T. L. Abell, and L. Gerson. Clinical Guideline: Management of Gastroparesis. *American Journal of Gastroenterology* 108, no. 1, 2013: 18–37.

Chedid, V. and M. Camilleri. Relamorelin for the Treatment of Gastrointestinal Motility Disorders. *Expert Opinion on Investigational Drugs* 26, no. 10, October 31, 2017: 1189–197.

Davis, B. R., I. Sarosiek, M. Bashashati, B. Alvarado, and R. W. Mccallum. The Long-Term Efficacy and Safety of Pyloroplasty Combined with Gastric Electrical Stimulation Therapy in Gastroparesis. *Journal of Gastrointestinal Surgery* 21, no. 2, 2017: 222–27.

Friedenberg, F. K., A. Palit, H. P. Parkman, A. Hanlon, and D. B. Nelson. Botulinum Toxin A for the Treatment of Delayed Gastric Emptying. *American Journal of Gastroenterology* 103, no. 2, 2008: 416–23.

Gonzalez, J. M., A. Benezech, V. Vitton, and M. Barthet. G-POEM with Antro-pyloromyotomy for the Treatment of Refractory Gastroparesis: Mid-term Follow-up and Factors Predicting Outcome. *Alimentary Pharmacology and Therapeutics* 46, no. 3, 2017: 364–70.

Gupta, E. and L. A. Lee. Diet and Complementary Medicine for Chronic Unexplained Nausea and Vomiting and Gastroparesis. *Current Treatment Options in Gastroenterology* 14, no. 4, 2016: 401–09.

Hasler, W. L. Gastroparesis: Symptoms, Evaluation, and Treatment. *Gastroenterology Clinics of North America* 36, no. 3, 2007: 619–47.

Hasler, W. L. Symptomatic Management for Gastroparesis. *Gastroenterology Clinics of North America* 44, no. 1, 2015: 113–26.

Heckert, J., A. Sankineni, W. B. Hughes, S. Harbison, and H. Parkman. Gastric Electric Stimulation for Refractory Gastroparesis: A Prospective Analysis of 151 Patients at a Single Center. *Digestive Diseases and Sciences* 61, no. 1, 2016: 168–75.

Homko, C. J., F. Duffy, F. K. Friedenberg, G. Boden, and H. P. Parkman. Effect of Dietary Fat and Food Consistency on Gastroparesis Symptoms in Patients with Gastroparesis. *Neurogastroenterology and Motility* 27, no. 4, 2015: 501–8.

Jebbink, R. J. A., M. Samsom, P. P. M. Bruijs, B. Bravenboer, L. M. A. Akkermans, G. P. Vanberge-Henegouwen, and A. J. P. M. Smout. Hyperglycemia Induces Abnormalities of Gastric Myoelectrical Activity in Patients with Type I Diabetes Mellitus. *Gastroenterology* 107, no. 5, 1994: 1390–397.

Jeong, I. D., M. Camilleri, A. Shin, J. Iturrino, A. Boldingh, I. Busciglio, D. Burton, M. Ryks, D. Rhoten, and A. R. Zinsmeister. A Randomised, Placebo-Controlled Trial Comparing the Effects of Tapentadol and Oxycodone on Gastrointestinal and Colonic Transit in Healthy Humans. *Alimentary Pharmacology and Therapeutics*, 35, 2012: 1088–96.

Jones, M. P. and K. Maganti. A Systematic Review of Surgical Therapy for Gastroparesis. *American Journal of Gastroenterology* 98, no. 10, 2003: 2122–129.

Jung, H.-k., R. S. Choung, G. Richard Locke, C. D. Schleck, A. R. Zinsmeister, L. A. Szarka, B. Mullan, and N. J. Talley. The Incidence, Prevalence, and Outcomes of Patients with Gastroparesis in Olmsted County, Minnesota, from 1996 to 2006. *Gastroenterology* 136, no. 4, 2009: 1225–233.

Khashab, M. A., S. Ngamruengphong, D. Carr-Locke, A. Bapaye, P. C. Benias, S. Serouya, S. Dorwat et al. Gastric Per-Oral Endoscopic Myotomy for Refractory Gastroparesis: Results from the First Multicenter Study on Endoscopic Pyloromyotomy (with Video). *Gastrointestinal Endoscopy* 85, no. 1, 2017: 123–28.

Kuo, B., R. W. Mccallum, K. L. Koch, M. D. Sitrin, J. M. Wo, W. D. Chey, W. L. Hasler et al. Comparison of Gastric Emptying of a Nondigestible Capsule to a Radio-Labelled Meal in Healthy and Gastroparetic Subjects. *Alimentary Pharmacology and Therapeutics* 27, no. 2, 2008: 186–96.

Lacy, B. E., M. D. Crowell, C. Mathis, D. Bauer, and L. J. Heinberg. Gastroparesis: Quality of Life and Health Care Utilization. *Journal of Clinical Gastroenterology* 52, no. 1, 2018: 20–24.

Lal, N., S. Livemore, D. Dunne, and I. Khan. Gastric Electrical Stimulation with the Enterra System: A Systematic Review. *Gastroenterology Research and Practice* 2015 2015: 1–9.

Lembo, A., M. Camilleri, R. Mccallum, R. Sastre, C. Breton, S. Spence, J. White, M. Currie, K. Gottesdiener, and E. Stoner. Relamorelin Reduces Vomiting Frequency and Severity and Accelerates Gastric Emptying in Adults with Diabetic Gastroparesis. *Gastroenterology* 151, no. 1, 2016.

Levin, A. A., M. S. Levine, S. E. Rubesin, and I. Laufer. An 8-Year Review of Barium Studies in the Diagnosis of Gastroparesis. *Clinical Radiology* 63, no. 4, 2008: 407–14.

Levinthal, D. J. and K. Bielefeldt. Systematic Review and Meta-Analysis: Gastric Electrical Stimulation for Gastroparesis. *Autonomic Neuroscience* 202 2017: 45–55.

Liu, H., B. Yu, M. Zhang, K. Liu, F-C. Wang, and X-Y. Gao. Treatment of Diabetic Gastroparesis by Complementary and Alternative Medicines. *Medicines* 2, no. 3, 2015: 212–19.

Malamood, M., A. Roberts, R. Kataria, H. Parkman, and R. Schey. Mirtazapine for Symptom Control in Refractory Gastroparesis. *Drug Design, Development and Therapy* 11, 2017: 1035–041.

Mancini, S. A., J. L. Angelo, F. H. Philp, and K. F. Farah. Pyloroplasty for Refractory Gastroparesis. *Am Sure* 81, no. 7, 2015: 738–46.

Maple, J. T., B. T. Petersen, T. H. Baron, C. J. Gostout, L. M. Wong Kee Song, and N. S. Buttar. Direct Percutaneous Endoscopic Jejunostomy: Outcomes in 307 Consecutive Attempts. *American Journal of Gastroenterology* 100, no. 12, 2005: 2681–688.

Navas, C. M., N. K. Patel, and B. E. Lacy. Gastroparesis: Medical and Therapeutic Advances. *Digestive Diseases and Sciences* 62, no. 9, 2017: 2231–240.

Ogorek, C. P., L. Davidson, R. S. Fisher, and B. Kreveski. Idiopathic Gastroparesis Is Associated with a Multiplicity of Severe Dietary Deficiencies. *American Journal of Gastroenterology* 86 1991: 423–28.

Olausson, E. A., S. Störsrud, H. Grundin, M. Isaksson, S. Attvall, and M. Simrén. A Small Particle Size Diet Reduces Upper Gastrointestinal Symptoms in Patients With Diabetic Gastroparesis: A Randomized Controlled Trial. *American Journal of Gastroenterology* 109, no. 3, 2014: 375–85.

Ordog, T., I. Takayama, W. K. Cheung, S. M. Ward, and K. M. Sanders. Remodeling of Networks of Interstitial Cells of Cajal in a Murine Model of Diabetic Gastroparesis. *Diabetes* 49, no. 10, 2000: 1731–739.

Papasavas, P. K., J. S. Ng, A. M. Stone, O. A. Ajayi, K. P. Muddasani, and D. S. Tishler. Gastric Bypass Surgery as Treatment of Recalcitrant Gastroparesis. *Surgery for Obesity and Related Diseases* 10, no. 5, 2014: 795–99.

Parkman, H. P. Idiopathic Gastroparesis. *Gastroenterology Clinics of North America* 44, no. 1, 2015: 59–68.

Parkman, H. P. Upper GI Disorders: Pathophysiology and Current Therapeutic Approaches. *Gastrointestinal Pharmacology Handbook of Experimental Pharmacology* 2017, 17–37.

Parkman, H. P., K. P. Yates, W. L. Hasler, L. Nguyan, P. J. Pasricha, W. J. Snape, G. Farrugia et al. Dietary Intake and Nutritional Deficiencies in Patients with Diabetic or Idiopathic Gastroparesis. *Gastroenterology* 141, no. 2, 2011.

Parkman, H. P., M. L. Van Natta, T. L. Abell, R. W. Mccallum, I. Sarosiek, L. Nguyen, W. J. Snape et al. Effect of Nortriptyline on Symptoms of Idiopathic Gastroparesis. *JAMA* 310, no. 24, 2013: 2640.

Pitt, H. A., L. L Mann, W. E Berquist, M. E Ament, E. W Fonkalsrud, and L. DenBesten. Chronic Intestinal Pseudo-obstruction. Management with Total Parenteral Nutrition and a Venting Enterostomy. *Archives of Surgery* 120, no. 5, 1985: 614–18.

Reddymasu, S. C. and R. W. Mccallum. Small Intestinal Bacterial Overgrowth in Gastroparesis: Are There Any Predictors? *Journal of Clinical Gastroenterology* 44, no. 1, 2010.

Sanger, G. J. and P. J. Pasricha. Investigational Drug Therapies for the Treatment of Gastroparesis. *Expert Opinion on Investigational Drugs* 26, no. 3, 2017: 331–42.

Sarosiek, I., G. Song, Y. Sun, H. Sandoval, S. Sands, J. Chen, and R. W. Mccallum. Central and Peripheral Effects of Transcutaneous Acupuncture Treatment for Nausea in Patients with Diabetic Gastroparesis. *Journal of Neurogastroenterology and Motility* 23, no. 2, 2017: 245–53.

Sarosiek, I., M. Bashashati, and R. W. Mccallum. Safety of Treatment for Gastroparesis. *Expert Opinion on Drug Safety* 15, no. 7, 2016: 937–45.

Schey, R., M. Saadi, D. Midani, A. C. Roberts, R. Parupalli, and H. P. Parkman. Domperidone to Treat Symptoms of Gastroparesis: Benefits and Side Effects from a Large Single-Center Cohort. *Digestive Diseases and Sciences* 61, no. 12, 2016: 3545–551.

Soykan, I., I. Sarosiek, B. Sivri, and R. W. Mccallum. Demographic, Clinical Characteristics, Psychological Profiles, Treatment and Follow-up of Gastroparesis. *Digestive Diseases and Sciences* 114, 1998: 2398–404.

Tack, J. and F. Carbone. Functional Dyspepsia and Gastroparesis. *Current Opinion in Gastroenterology* 33, no. 6, 2017: 446–54.

Tang, D. M. and F. K. Friedenberg. Gastroparesis: Approach, Diagnostic Evaluation, and Management. *Disease-a-Month* 57, no. 2, 2011: 74–101.

Ukleja, A., K. Tandon, K. Shah, and A. Alvarez. Endoscopic Botox Injections in Therapy of Refractory Gastroparesis. *World Journal of Gastrointestinal Endoscopy* 7, no. 8, 2015: 790–98.

Warner, E. and K. N. Jeejeebhoy. Successful Management of Chronic Intestinal Pseudo-Obstruction with Home Parenteral Nutrition. *Journal of Parenteral and Enteral Nutrition* 9, no. 2, 1985: 173–78.

Wytiaz, V., C. Homko, F. Duffy, R. Schey, and H. P. Parkman. Foods Provoking and Alleviating Symptoms in Gastroparesis: Patient Experiences. *Digestive Diseases and Sciences* 60, no. 4, 2015: 1052–58.

Yang, M., X. Li, S. Liu, Z. Li, M. Xue, D. Gao, X. Li, and S. Yang. Meta-Analysis of Acupuncture for Relieving Non-organic Dyspeptic Symptoms Suggestive of Diabetic Gastroparesis. *BMC Complementary and Alternative Medicine* 13, no. 1, 2013.

Zaidel, O. and HC Lin. Uninvited Guests: The Impact of Small Intestinal Bacterial Overgrowth on Nutritional Status. *Practical Gastroenterology* 27, no. 7, 2003: 27.

30 Role of Palliative Care in Severe and Enduring Eating Disorders

Patricia Westmoreland and Philip S. Mehler

CONTENTS

INTRODUCTION

Anorexia nervosa (AN) has the highest mortality of any psychiatric illness. Although 40% of patients recover, 20% continue to have some symptoms; another 20% are chronically ill, requiring frequent hospitalizations; and 20% of individuals die from the illness (Steinhausen 2002). Historically, it has been noted that the longer an individual has suffered from an eating disorder, the lower the chance of full weight restoration and recovery. However, a recent study provides basis for optimism. Although only one-third of individuals with AN recovered within the first decade of follow-up, at 22 years, two-thirds of patients with AN had recovered (Eddy et al. 2016). The author of this study noted, "Our findings that recovery remains possible even after long-term illness argue for active treatment rather than palliative care for most patients" (Eddy et al. 2016).

Although the majority of patients with eating disorders have the propensity to recover fully, the notion that recovery may be less likely at a certain point for a small group of patients has led to the concept of severe and enduring eating disorders (SEEDs). Individuals with SEEDs are a subgroup of patients whose illness is chronic but not necessarily imminently life-threatening. These individuals are often profoundly underweight (with a body mass index [BMI] < 13) and physically disabled. Individuals with SEEDs typically exhibit the physical sequelae of a long-standing eating disorder including osteoporosis, renal failure, bowel dysfunction and cognitive dysfunction. They require the regular attention of a multi-disciplinary team (Robinson 2009; Hay and Touyz 2015).

Managing individuals with SEEDs requires a shift from focusing on cure to careful consideration as to what is the best possible approach for each individual. Many such individuals do not wish to pursue treatment designed to return them to a normal body weight despite this approach conferring an optimal prognosis (Lund et al. 2014; Steinhausen et al. 2009). This traditional method of treatment is frequently intolerable for patients who have already endured multiple (and lengthy) hospitalizations only to once again relapse. A harm reduction model is one way of working towards maintaining some level of functioning outside the hospital. This approach includes restoring weight to a minimally acceptable level to reduce the risk of imminent death, although the individual may have to return for short hospital stays when he or she falls below that weight or electrolytes become abnormal.

For individuals with SEEDs who cannot tolerate remaining at a minimal weight, palliative care may be considered. Palliative care involves managing pain and other problematic symptoms with the goal of optimizing the individual's quality of life, even though the medical burden of that individual's eating disorder may soon lead to deterioration and death.

The topic of futility is of considerable debate with regard to psychiatric illnesses. There is also a distinction between allowing an individual to refuse nutrition and hence end his or her life (futility), providing the means with which to assist that person in ending his or her life (physician-assisted death) and actually administering the medicine that leads to death (euthanasia).

This chapter focuses on palliative care, futility and physician-assisted suicide and euthanasia.

PALLIATIVE CARE

The goal of palliation is to reduce suffering through comfort care, including identification and treatment of comorbid conditions and the management of pain. Palliative care (symptomatic relief from mental or physical pain) is not synonymous with hospice care, but these terms are frequently used interchangeably (Geppert 2015). Palliative care does not necessarily mean giving up, but instead optimizing care for the chronically ill individual by decreasing physical and psychic pain (Trachsel et al. 2015). SEED patients who undergo palliative care are those for whom any further treatment (be it with the goal of normalizing weight, or achieving weight sufficient for harm reduction) is unlikely to resolve or decrease their illness and suffering. The goal is to be comfortable during the remainder of their life, albeit a shortened life. Patients who elect to undergo palliative care often have untreatable comorbidities, for example, severe major depressive disorder that does not respond to treatment or severe intractable medical comorbidities (e.g., renal failure, severe osteoporosis). Symptomatic relief includes analgesics for pain associated with osteoporosis and stress fractures, wound care for decubitus ulcers, psychotropic medications to reduce anxiety symptoms, depression and perseverative thinking, and to improve sleep. Palliative care may take place in the patient's home, a hospital, a skilled nursing unit or a hospice care unit.

ETHICAL ISSUES: FUTILITY, PHYSICIAN-ASSISTED DEATH AND EUTHANASIA

FUTILITY

The concept of futility has sparked a contentious debate as it pertains to eating disorders. There is a lack of clarity as to what is meant by the term *end stage* as it applies to an eating disorder. The study by Eddy et al. demonstrated that cure is possible for individuals with AN even after 20 years of illness (Eddy et al. 2016). In addition, medical complications of AN are treatable, even in their most severe forms (Westmoreland et al. 2016). Compounding these issues is the concern as to whether patients with severe eating disorders have the capacity to make decisions regarding their care.

Decisional capacity is an individual's ability to understand information regarding his or her condition, reason through the information needed in order to make a decision regarding his or her care, appreciate the consequences of the decision he or she makes and communicate his or her choice (Appelbaum and Grisso 1988). It is questionable whether individuals with severe eating disorders have the capacity to decide that further treatment is futile when the core symptom of their illness is a cognitive distortion resulting in their refusal to believe that starving themselves is life threatening. There is a threshold in starvation-related states in which individuals exhibit a decline in cognition because of chemical changes in their brains (Matusek et al. 2010). This was well demonstrated in the Minnesota study when a group of volunteer males, starved to well below ideal body weight, developed behaviors around food synonymous with those seen in individuals whose starved state is a result of an eating disorder (Keyes et al. 1950).

Individuals with severe eating disorders are often deemed to lack capacity. Since cognitive distortions and incapacity generally lessen with weight gain, treatment providers feel obligated to treat patients so that their cognitive distortions resolve, and their decision-making is no longer impaired (Geppert 2015). For individuals who are not competent to refuse treatment and who meet criteria for danger to self and/or grave disability, involuntary treatment can be a useful modality in treating life-threatening eating disorders (Westmoreland and Mehler 2016, 2017). Individuals who are treated on an involuntary basis are frequently the most severely and chronically ill, and who therefore face the greatest risk of death. However, although their clinical condition meets the burden of proof required for certification (i.e., they *can* be certified), this does not necessarily mean these patients *should* be certified (Westmoreland et al. 2017). Patients who have been ill for a long period of time may not ultimately benefit from inpatient treatment with the goal of full weight restoration, and there may well be a point at which this type of treatment (even if mandated) is futile (Ward et al. 2015). Despite incapacity regarding decision-making, individuals with SEEDs do have lengthy experience regarding their illness and their quality of life and are capable of determining whether that quality of life justifies continued attempts at active treatment, harm reduction, or palliative or hospice care. Determining the best course of action for an individual with SEEDs means balancing the ethical principles of autonomy, beneficence, non-maleficence, justice and duty to protect. There is inherent subjectivity in weighing these principles. Physicians should reflect on their own personal biases, invite other stakeholders into the decision-making process and explain the reason behind the decision they ultimately make (Matusek et al. 2010). Treatment providers should also be cognizant that the right decision may vary at different times during treatment. Plans should be made when a patient is well and has capacity, for the time that this patient no longer has capacity (psychiatric advance directives).

In the following two cases, individuals with SEEDs were permitted to refuse treatment, which led to their death. O'Neill et al. (1994) reported on a 24-year-old female in the United Kingdom who had suffered from AN for over seven years, was hospitalized 11 times over five years, and had been treated with naso-gastric feeding. At the time of her hospice admission, she was severely underweight and suffering from pressure sores, urinary incontinence and multiple fractures. A week after admission to the hospice unit, she developed delirium and died. While the decision to admit this patient to hospice care was a joint decision involving the psychiatric consultant, hospice director, the patient's family and the patient herself, her decision-making capacity does not appear to have been evaluated prior to the decision to admit her to hospice (O'Neill et al. 1994). Following this case report, Ramsey and Treasure (1996) noted members of the Royal College of Psychiatrists special interest group on eating disorders voiced minimal support for hospice/terminal care for individuals with AN. They disagreed that this individual's illness was incurable, and questioned the failure to try a full range of treatment options.

A case in the United States also outlined futility in treating an individual with chronic AN. According to the treatment team of a 30-year-old patient, forcing her into involuntary treatment or waiting for her to voluntarily engage in treatment were unlikely to cure her eating disorder or afford her a reasonable quality of life (Lopez et al. 2010). Despite the initiation of hospice care, she was reluctant to discuss end-of-life issues and insisted she would not die, nor did she want to die. She died three weeks after admission to a hospice care unit. Despite questions about her capacity, her treatment team noted that even if she had been declared legally incompetent regarding decision-making, "Then what?" They suggested that patients with a poor prognosis who face a terminal course should be given the more humane choice of hospice care versus being forced into a treatment stay that has questionable benefit (Lopez et al. 2010).

In a 2012 case series, two patients who also chose to succumb to their illness were noted to have decision-making capacity when they elected to pursue end-of-life care (Campbell and Aulisio 2012). The patients in this study were older than those described by O'Neill et al. (1994) and Lopez et al.

(2010), had longer periods of failed treatments and their refusals of life-sustaining care had been consistent over a long period of time.

Several cases from the United Kingdom argue opposing sides of the futility debate as it pertains to SEEDs. In *Local Authority vs. E (2012)*, a patient with a severe and chronic AN had previously executed advance directives refusing compulsory feeding. Her parents and physicians argued she was comparatively well when she executed the directives. The judge opined that Ms. E currently suffered from similar cognitive distortions at the time of the hearing as she did at the time she executed the directives, and ruled that the value of life trumps the presumption that further treatment will fail, and ordered that Ms. E be treated – involuntarily force fed.

Two years later, in *NHS Foundation Trust vs. Ms. X (2014)*, Ms. X, who had suffered from AN for 14 years, opposed being force fed. The judge ruled in her favor, despite Ms. X lacking decision-making capacity. The judge opined that forced feeding against her wishes was inhumane, and interfered with her autonomy. The judge noted that while forced feeding (resulting in weight gain) can be mandated, psychological treatment cannot be forced (McKenzie 2015). However, this line of reasoning ignored that weight gain significantly predicts outcome, although it is unclear exactly how weight gain changes cognition and prepares the individuals to tolerate weight restoration (Lund et al. 2014; Steinhausen et al. 2009).

In *Re. Miss W*, W (age 28) had suffered from a severe and enduring eating disorder for 20 years with multiple admission, amounting to 10 years spent in inpatient care. Two proposals were considered (1) for Miss W to be re-fed through a nasogastric tube under sedation, involving her being rendered unconscious for six months and (2) discharge to her parents' home with a community support program. This was predicated on the recognition that her condition was not treatable, and acute treatment was no longer recommended. The judge opined that Miss W's discharge to the community was the "least worst option" (*Re. Miss W. 2016*), but noted, regarding "circumstances as they now exist and for so long as they continue," Miss W would not be readmitted if her health were further to deteriorate. If, however, a significant period of time passed, accompanied by signs that her thinking and behavior were amenable to change, she could seek readmission.

In 2016, a court in the United States also ruled that a woman with severe AN had the right to refuse forced feeding. A 29-year-old woman, identified as "A.G.," had been assigned a guardian by the state who had obtained a court order for surgical placement of a gastrostomy tube in order to forcibly feed A.G. She experienced refeeding syndrome and heart failure and removed the tube (*In the Matter of A.G. 2016*). A.G. did not want further treatment. The guardian sought an order allowing A.G. to enter palliative care. The medical staff and members of the bioethics committee at the treating institution concluded A.G. was capable of making her own medical decisions. The State of New Jersey objected, arguing that A.G. was not capable of making informed decisions about her treatment. Judge Paul Armstrong opined A.G.'s testimony was "forthright, responsive, knowing, intelligent, voluntary, steadfast and credible," and A.G. understood that death was a possible outcome (*In the Matter of A.G. 2016*). The court recognized her right to live free from medical intervention. The court did not rule on her competency but adopted a paradigm of cooperative spirit of the patient, parents, treatment team and ethics committee of the hospital. A.G. died within several months of the court decision. The American Academy of Eating Disorders responded to the A.G. case noting that, "Despite the potentially fatal consequences of these illnesses, full recovery from an eating disorder at any age can be possible"; however, "a role for palliative care is recognized" (American Academy of Eating Disorders 2016).

Physician-Assisted Death and Euthanasia

Physician-assisted death is legal in several European countries as well as in Canada and some states in the United States. At least three European countries currently allow active euthanasia (in which a physician administers a lethal dose of medication to a patient). In the United States, laws that allow physicians to prescribe medications intended to end an individual's life do not allow euthanasia.

Laws regarding physician-assisted death in the United States are limited to terminal medical conditions (patients who are expected to survive less than six months and for whom there is no known cure for their condition) and preclude psychiatric conditions. The Netherlands, Belgium and Switzerland have expanded criteria for physician-assisted death (and euthanasia) to include patients experiencing "irremediable suffering, whatever the cause" (Appelbaum 2017). This has made it permissible for patients suffering from psychiatric illness to request physician-assisted death (and, if available in that country, euthanasia).

In Canada, medical assistance in dying (MAID) has also been extended to individuals with psychiatric illness. The Canadian Supreme Court ruled that physician-assisted death could not be prohibited for a competent adult who (1) consents to the termination of life and (2) has a grievous and irremediable medical condition that causes enduring suffering that is intolerable to that individual, and demonstrates that a condition is irremediable; an individual is *not* required to accept a treatment that he or she finds unacceptable (*Carter v. Canada 2015*).

In 2016, E.F., an individual with a conversion disorder, sought, and was granted medical assistance in dying on the basis of her mental disorder which caused intractable muscle spasms resulting in severe pain. She also suffered from digestive dysfunction, resulting in her being unable to eat. She had lost significant weight and muscle mass and could not ambulate. E.F.'s quality of life was described as "non-existent" (*Canada [Alberta] v E.F. 2016*). Although the government challenged that she met criteria for MAID, the court granted her request, and she died within weeks. The Canadian law has since been modified and requires "an advanced state of irreversible decline" and that death be reasonably foreseeable (*Statutes of Canada 2016*). The American Psychiatric Association has adopted a position statement opposing physician-assisted death for mental disorder noting that a psychiatrist should not prescribe or administer a medication to a person who is not terminally ill for the purpose of causing death (APA 2016).

Laws regarding physician-assisted suicide and euthanasia as they pertain to psychiatric patients have not existed for sufficient time to assess the long-term consequences of these laws. However, there already appear to be some alarming trends. In the Netherlands, two people requested death for mental disorders in 2010, and by 2015 the number had grown to 56 (Boztas 2016). Two recent retrospective studies, one from the Netherlands and the other from Belgium, have uncovered another troubling pattern with regard to the demographics of individuals requesting physician-assisted death. In both studies, over half the individuals requesting death for psychiatric concerns had a personality disorder diagnosis (Kim et al. 2016; Thienpont et al. 2015). In addition, although treatment-resistant depression was responsible for the majority of death requests in individuals requesting relief from intractable mental suffering, between 10% and 15% of cases in the Netherlands (2011–2014) involved diagnoses of anxiety and post-traumatic stress disorder and 3% were due to eating disorders (Kim et al. 2016). Approximately 70% were female and under 70 years old, and personality disorders, as well as a propensity for social isolation and loneliness, were pervasive in that sample (Kim et al. 2016). There is concern about these demographics (female, under 70 years old, diagnosed with a personality disorder, depressed and socially isolated) noting that they closely approximate individuals with chronic AN (Wall 2017). A news report regarding recent cases in Europe involving individuals with AN highlights concerns about which treatments have been tried prior to the individuals being approved for euthanasia (Independent.co.uk 2016; Liveaction 2013). The prevailing thought is that individuals do not have to try any treatment modality they find unacceptable, making the determination of what type of condition is (or is not) curable a highly subjective determination. This is especially relevant with regard to eating disorders where the adequacy of prior treatment trials, and periods of remission, can be hard to define, and are at times not remembered by patients and their loved ones. In other medical settings, it has been found that the presence of depression is associated with the rejection of treatment even in situations with a good medical prognosis (Lee and Ganzini 1992).

GUIDELINES REGARDING EATING DISORDERS AND FUTILITY

Some eating disorder professionals oppose palliative and end-of-life care, citing concern regarding a "slippery slope" argument that would make all patients with SEEDs inherently eligible for end-of-life care. Proponents of this view note when the illness itself compromises a patient's ability to make a fully competent decision, overriding a patient's autonomy may be justified under the doctrine of paternalism in an effort to save that patient's life and return him or her to a state where she or he can make an informed and competent decision. There is justifiable reluctance on the part of eating disorder professionals to undertake any treatment that bears little hope of advancing a patient's quality of life, directly opposes the wishes of that patient and family, and simply extends a life of suffering, even if the patient has diminished capacity. Yet, physicians are understandably also reluctant to give up hope. These two opposing forces should be balanced by a careful assessment of each individual's circumstances so that patients are not forced into an intolerable living situation merely because they are deemed to lack capacity. Indeed, even if that patient does not have decision-making capacity, he or she is still likely capable of appraising his or her suffering (Kendall 2014; Yager 2015). Futility should therefore be considered on a case-by-case basis, and applied when considering a particular treatment intervention, at a particular time, for a particular patient.

Frameworks that balance a patient's wishes with concerns about that patient's impaired decision-making capacity and refusal of further treatment have been proposed. Draper proposed respecting the autonomy of the individual if that individual had been affected for eight or more years, not forcibly treating those who have been force fed on previous occasions, respecting the wishes of individuals who have insight into the effect AN has had on their lives, and not permitting individuals to make decisions about their care when they are close to death (Draper 2000).

Another framework denoted that before decisions regarding further episodes of care are made, (1) the patient should be competent (i.e., ideally between episodes); (2) the individual must know that refusing nutrition will lead to death; (3) the individual's decision to die must be based on a realistic assessment of current quality of life, and the low probability that treatment will succeed; and (4) the individual must be consistent in communicating his or her desires (McKinney 2015).

APPLICATION TO OTHER AREAS OF TERMINAL OR PALLIATIVE CARE

Eating disorders are a *forme fruste* of medical and psychiatric illness. They are particularly complex in that, in their most severe form, individuals are so cognitively affected as to frequently lose the capacity to make further decisions regarding their care. Although the medical sequelae of an eating disorder are sufficiently severe so as to rival the physical consequences of a chronic, degenerative and terminal physical condition, they have their roots in a mental disorder and should be evaluated as such in terms of the individual's capacity to refuse life-saving treatment. However, it should also be recognized that the burden of having a severe, long-term condition that profoundly affects quality of life and engenders both physical and mental suffering may rival the pain experienced by any individual whose source of suffering has its roots in a medical condition (such as cancer or a degenerative disorder). Therefore, efforts should be made to undertake a thorough evaluation of each individual and his or her circumstances and suffering, including an assessment of the utility of further active treatment, and the psychological impact of such treatment, even if such an individual were deemed to lack capacity. Conversely, such principles should be readily utilized when evaluating an individual whose terminal condition had its roots in a physical (rather than psychological) illness. Physical illnesses may progress to affect the brain just as much as a condition that is primarily psychiatric in origin. Care should be taken to document an individual's wishes while he or she still has capacity (advance directives) and assess capacity when there is concern regarding this. Just as for SEEDs, a willingness to explore and assess an individual's suffering and the emotional and physical costs of an illness (capacity aside) should always be in place.

SUMMARY POINTS

- Ethical decisions in individuals with severe and enduring eating disorders are "fraught with ambiguity and complexity because there are no clear cut decisions" (Matusek et al. 2010).
- Each case must be considered individually. It is important to realistically assess each patient's capacity for recovery or ability to engage in a harm reduction or palliative care model. At the same time, one must remain in touch with the wishes of the patient, the patient's family and the patient's treatment team.
- Futility is controversial, but it may be of expanding relevance for a small set of patients with AN whose illness is severe and enduring.
- Arriving at that decision should only be as a result of an extensive decision-making process. However, failure to consider this as an option for patients with a severe and enduring eating disorder perpetuates the stigma of mental illness as separate from physical illness.
- The roles of physician-assisted death and euthanasia are emerging topics in mental health which cannot merely be ignored.
- Individuals with severe and enduring eating disorders may broach these topics, and the law may well be shaped by their advocating to live – or die – on their own terms.

KEY FACTS: SEVERE AND ENDURING EATING DISORDERS AND PALLIATIVE CARE

- Recovery is possible for the majority of patients with an eating disorder.
- Treatment options for severe and enduring eating disorder include harm reduction and palliative care.
- There is a question of futility for individuals with severe and enduring eating disorders.
- Frequently there is incapacity of individuals with severe and enduring eating disorder to refuse treatment.
- Capacity is perhaps not the ultimate deciding factor in allowing an individual with severe and enduring eating disorder to refuse further treatment.
- Physician-assisted death and euthanasia are burgeoning topics for individuals with severe and enduring eating disorders.

LIST OF ABBREVIATIONS

AN	Anorexia Nervosa
BMI	Body-Mass Index
BN	Bulimia Nervosa
SEEDs	Severe and Enduring Eating Disorders

REFERENCES

Academy for Eating Disorders. 2016. The Academy for Eating Disorders advocates for early intervention and specialized care for eating disorders in response to Morristown, NJ ruling. *Newswise.* https://www.newswise.com/articles/the-academy-for-eating-disorders-advocates-for-early-intervention-and-specialized-care-for-eating-disorders-treatment-in-response-to-morristown-nj-ruling

American Psychiatric Association (APA). December 2016. Position Statement on Medical Euthanasia. Approved by the Board of Trustees. https://psychiatry.org/psychiatrists/search-directories-databases/policy-finder

Appelbaum P. 2017. Should mental disorders be a basis for physician-assisted death? *Psychiatric Services* 68(4): 315–317.

Appelbaum PS, Grisso T. 1988. Assessing patients' capacities to consent to treatment. *N Engl J Med* 319: 1635–1638.

Boztas S. Netherlands sees sharp increase in people choosing euthanasia due to "mental health problems". *The Telegraph*, May 11, 2016. http://www.telegraph.co.uk/news/2016/05/11/netherlands-sees-sharp-increase-in-people-choosing-euthanasia-du/
Campbell AT, Aulisio MP. 2012. The stigma of "mental illness": End stage anorexia and treatment refusal. *Int J Eat Disord* 45: 627–634.
Canada (Attorney General) v EF. 2016. ABCA 155.
Carter v Canada (Attorney General). 2015. 1 SCR 331.
Draper H. 2000. Anorexia nervosa and respecting a refusal of life-prolonging therapy: A limited justification. *Bioethics* 14(2): 120–133.
Eddy KT, Tabri N, Thomas JJ et al. 2016. Recovery from anorexia nervosa and bulimia nervosa at 22-year follow-up. *J Clin Psychiatry* 78(2): 184–189.
Fiano C. 2013. Belgian woman suffering from anorexia euthanized. Liveaction.org
Geppert CMA. 2015. Futility in chronic anorexia nervosa: A concept whose time has not yet come. *Am J Bioethics* 15(7): 34–43.
Hay P, Touyz S. 2015. Treatment of patients with severe and enduring eating disorders. *Current Opin Psych* 28: 473–477.
In the Matter of A.G. 2016.
Keyes A, Brozec J, Henschel A, Nichelsen O, Taylor HL. 1950. *The Biology of Human Starvation*. Vols. 1 and 2. University of Minnesota Press, Minneapolis.
Kendall S. 2014. Anorexia nervosa: The diagnosis. *Bioethical Inquiry* 11: 31–40.
Kim SYH, De Vries RG, Peteet JR. 2016. Euthanasia and assisted suicide of patients with psychiatric disorders in the Netherlands, 2011 to 2014. *JAMA Psychiatry* 73: 362–368.
Lee MA, Ganzini L. 1992. Depression in the elderly: Effects on patient attitudes to life sustaining therapy. *J Am Geriatr Soc* 13(2): 21–26.
Local Authority v E. 2012. EWHC 1639.
Lopez A, Yager J, Feinstein RE. 2010. Medical futility and psychiatry: Palliative care and hospice care as a last resort in the treatment of refractory anorexia nervosa. *Int J Eat Disord* 43: 372–377.
Lund BC, Hernandez ER, Yates WR, Mitchell JR. 2014. Rate of inpatient weight restoration predicts outcome in anorexia nervosa. *Int J Eat Disord* 42: 301–305.
Matusek JA, O'Dougherty Wright M. 2010. Ethical dilemmas in treating clients with eating disorders: A review and application of an integrative ethical decision-making model. *Eur Eat Disorders Rev* 18: 434–452.
McKenzie R. 2015. Ms. X: A promising new view of anorexia nervosa, futility, and end-of-life decisions in a very recent English case. *Am J Bioethics* 15(7): 57–58.
McKinney C. 2015. Is resistance (n) ever futile? A response to "Futility in chronic anorexia nervosa: A concept whose time has not yet come" by Cynthia Geppert. *Am J Bioethics* 15(7): 53–54.
NHS Foundation Trust v. Ms. X. 2014. EWCOP 35.
O'Neill J, Crowther T, Sampson G, Anorexia nervosa. 1994. Palliative care of terminal psychiatric disease. *Am J Hospice and Palliative Care* 11(6): 36–38.
Payton M. Sex abuse victim in her 20 s allowed by doctors to choose euthanasia due to incurable PTSD. Independent.co.uk, 2016.
Ramsey R, Treasure J. 1996. Treating anorexia nervosa: psychiatrists have mixed views on the use of terminal care for anorexia nervosa. *BMJ* 312(20): 182.
Re. Miss W. 2016. EWCOP 13.
Robinson P. 2009. *Severe and Enduring Eating Disorder (SEED). Management of Complex Presentations of Anorexia and Bulimia Nervosa.* John Wiley and Sons, Chichester, UK.
Statutes of Canada. 2016. Chapter 3, An Act to Amend the Criminal Code and to Make Related Amendments to Other Acts (Medical Assistance in Dying), June 16.
Steinhausen HC. 2002. The outcome of anorexia nervosa in the 20th century. *American Journal of Psychiatry* 159(8): 1284–1293.
Steinhausen HC, Grigoroiu-Serbanescu M, Boyadjieva S et al. 2009. The relevance of body weight in medium-term to long-term course of adolescent anorexia nervosa. Findings from a multi-site study. *Int J Eat Disord* 42: 19–25.
Thienpont L, Verhofstadt M, Van Loon T et al. 2015. Euthanasia requests, procedures and outcomes for 100 Belgian patients suffering from psychiatric disorders: A retrospective, descriptive study. *BMJ open* 5: e007454.
Trachsel M, Wild V, Biller-Andorno N, Krones T. 2015. Compulsory treatment in chronic anorexia nervosa by all means? Searching for a middle ground between a curative and palliative approach. *AJOB* 15(7): 55–56.
Wall BW. 2017. The competency paradox in somatic disease. *J Am Acad Psychiatry Law* 45: 426–428.

Ward A, Ramsay R, Russell, Treasure J. 2015. Follow-up mortality study of compulsorily treated patients with anorexia nervosa. *Int J Eat Disord* 48: 860–865.

Westmoreland P, Johnson C, Stafford M, Martinez R, Mehler PS. 2017. Involuntary treatment of patients with life-threatening anorexia nervosa. *J Am Acad Psychiatry Law* 45: 419–425.

Westmoreland P, Krantz MJ, Mehler PS. 2016. Medical complications of anorexia nervosa and bulimia nervosa. *Am J Med* 129(1): 30–37.

Westmoreland P, Mehler PS. 2016. Caring for patients with severe and enduring eating disorders (SEED): Certification, harm reduction, palliative care, and the question of futility. *J Psychiatr Pract* 22(4).

Westmoreland P, Mehler PS. 2017. Ethical and medico-legal considerations in treating patients with eating disorders. In: Mehler PS, Andersen AE (eds); *Eating Disorders: A Guide to Medical Care and Complications*. John Hopkins University Press, Baltimore MD.

Yager J. 2015. The futility of arguing about medical futility in anorexia nervosa: The question is how you would handle highly specific circumstances. *Am J Bioethics* 15(7): 47–50.

31 End-of-Life Decisions in Persons with Neurodevelopmental Disorders

Michela Uberti, Giuseppe Chiodelli, Giovanni Miselli, Roberto Cavagnola, Francesco Fioriti, Mauro Leoni, Maria Laura Galli, Giovanni Michelini, and Serafino Corti

CONTENTS

INTRODUCTION

During the twentieth century, there was a changing about the idea of mental retardation (neurodevelopmental disorder [NDDs]); it became an existential condition determined by an interaction between individual functioning and his contest instead to be considered an incurable disease. The definition of this condition also evolved in the course of time following this paradigm shift. The most recent definition of NDDs (American Psychiatric Association, 2013) comprises intellectual disabilities and autism spectrum disorders, the main causes of cognitive impairment in children and adults.

At the beginning of 1900, the definition of mental deficiency meant that "the person affected was unable to carry out his social roles" (Tredgold, 1908). The ideas of dependency and dangerousness, not curability, were prevalent, and the people with NDDs were segregated into isolated institutes. In the 1940s, the *American Journal of Mental Deficiency* defined mental retardation as "a condition characterized by a lack of social skills during all life derived from an arrest of neurocognitive development. The origin of the neurocognitive disorders could be acquired or hereditary and it is not possible to treat this condition" (Doll, 1941). The medical approach was prevalent, and the attention was addressed to physical health and basic needs. In 1969, B. Nirje, the director of the Swedish Association for Retarded Children, promoted the Normalization Principles, "related to a cluster of ideas, methods, and experiences put into practice that let the mentally retarded to obtain an existence as close to the normal as possible" (Nirje, 1969). The revolutionary concept was that everything in a person's life has developmental potential; normalization improves human relationship and understanding, whereas isolation and segregation foster ignorance and prejudice. It means that one of the main rights of people with NDDs is the opportunity to have their choices, wishes and desires taken into consideration and respected.

The Normalization Principle determined an important step forward for people affected by NDDs, and now the attention is focused on the need to guarantee everyone equal opportunities and rights.

This revolutionary vision developed new models of care based on a quality-of-life (QoL) perspective.

QUALITY OF LIFE AND SELF-DETERMINATION

QoL is based on a general feeling of well-being, positive social involvement and opportunities to achieve personal potential.

The success of the QoL concept brought the World Health Organization (WHO) to promote a Quality of Life Group to develop further the concept of QoL and its instruments (WHO, 1995, 1997). In 2002 the publication of the article "Conceptualization, Measurement and Application of Quality of Life for Persons with Intellectual Disabilities: Report of an International Panel of Experts" (Shalock et al., 2002) identified eight domains of QoL that became the actual referent model. The eight domains are as follows:

- *Emotional well-being*: Safety, stable and predictable environments, positive feedback
- *Interpersonal relations*: Affiliations, affection, intimacy, friendships, interactions
- *Material well-being*: Ownership, possessions, employment
- *Personal development*: New skills, purposive activities, assistive technology
- *Physical well-being*: Healthcare, mobility, wellness, nutrition
- *Self-determination*: Choices, personal control, decisions, personal goals
- *Social inclusion*: Natural supports, integrated environments
- *Rights*: Privacy, ownership, due process, barrier free environments

The QoL model proposes an ecological vision of NDDs that is seen as an existential condition related to health condition, personal factors, and social and cultural contexts.

This new model of care enables people with NDDs to become protagonists of their life. They can chose experiences based on their own values and preferences.

This allowed a new concept to be known: self-determination.

The idea of self-determination became central for people with NDDs.

Researchers including Michael Wehmeyer highlighted how it can be very difficult to promote self-determination when there are limits to the number and type of activities that people with NDDs can perform independently (Wehmeyer and Schwartz, 1998). So it becomes a priority to give people with NDDs more opportunities to make choices and express preferences in their daily lives. The scientific research also demonstrates that choice-making opportunity is a strong predictor of self-determination.

But if we improve decision-making opportunities in many aspects of their lives, what happens when we talk about health and end-of-life decisions?

There are beliefs that still prevent the possibility of choice on healthcare decisions for people with NDDs. The most common beliefs are as follows:

- People with NDDs are unable to make decisions.
- They refuse treatments because they do not understand their utility and so the wishes of people with NDDs, especially those with severe/profound intellectual disability, are often not taken into consideration when decisions about potentially burdensome medical interventions are concerned (Bekkema et al., 2014).

- Sometimes carers are reluctant to disclose information about end of life, fearing that the persons with NDDs might become upset and unable to cope (Tuffrey-Wijne and McEnhill 2008).
- There is inequity in healthcare provisions for people with NDDs with a lack of end-of-life care planning.
- Staff lacks experience in caring for people with NDDs (Cook and Lennox, 2000; Tuffrey-Wijne, 2007; Dunkley and Sales, 2014).

COMMUNICATION PROBLEMS

Communication is one of the biggest barriers: communication problems can impede timely diagnosis and symptoms assessment; they can cause the carers to fail in letting people with NDDs grasp what has been said. A study reports that communication difficulties are a major obstacle in providing palliative care among this population (Tuffrey-Wijne and McEnhill, 2008). Cogher (2005) provided the following definition: "Communication occurs when two or more people correctly interpret each other's language and/or behavior." People with NDDs have communication problems due to both a lack of comprehension and a lack of verbal and social skills, which affects assessment and prevents providing psychological support. They can also have difficulties expressing their needs due to a limited vocabulary and lack of sentence-formulation skills. They can express pain and discomfort with challenging behaviors because of their incapacity to use verbal or non-verbal language.

Professionals can also face problems understanding people with NDDs due to their inability to interpret needs such as pain or any kind of discomfort. Professionals also express their concerns about the difficulty for people with NDDs to understand their health problems and, consequently, the therapeutic opportunities (Murphy, 2006). Researchers demonstrate that quality of care is linked to the communication skills between people with NDDs and professionals (Tuffrey-Wijne and McEnhill, 2008). However, there is still a lack of knowledge and skills by professionals in meeting the health needs of people with NDDs. Care staff should be competent and appropriately skilled, and it becomes a priority to provide training on communication based on both verbal and non-verbal language. In people with NDDs a non-verbal component of communication could be very important; Argyle (1988) said that non-verbal communication is five times more influential than verbal communication. Non-verbal aspects include facial expressions, gestures, interpersonal spacing and posture. The difficulty faced by professionals in comprehending these components could be a big barrier to understanding needs and wishes of people with NDDs (Regnard et al., 2007).

EXPERIENCE OF FONDAZIONE SOSPIRO

Fondazione Sospiro is a residential facility with 19 small centres for about 400 people with NDDs; the average age of the patients is 50 years (standard deviation [SD] = 11.99; range 18–90 years). The number of males is double that of females. About half of this population needs a high level of support in a QoL perspective.

The principal diagnosis is NDD, with intellectual disability and autism spectrum disorder, and the gravity of the cognitive disability goes from mild to profound, with a progressive increase of support needed in every aspect of daily life.

The increase of the average age exposes people with NDDs to chronic, degenerative and malignant illness that are usually referred to in old age, such as dementia or heart failure or some type of cancer (Coppus, 2013; De Vreese et al., 2009). One of the aims of the research group of Fondazione Sospiro is the application of the QoL model in palliative care and end-of-life decisions.

Working in this direction, our professional carers face daily difficulties in guaranteeing choices and wishes of people with Intellectual Disability in every domain of QoL. One of the most important challenges is to support people with NDDs to improve their awareness about their health condition. The difficulties become stronger when a degenerative and incurable illness is diagnosed. It is not easy to communicate bad news to everyone, but trying to inform people with NDDs about their illness involves all of the problems previously described.

One of the difficulties that our research group often meets concerns the inadequacy of our organization to provide palliative care. One of the beliefs of professional carers is that care of people at the end of life requires specialized equipment usually available only in hospitals.

Another worry is the lack of experience and competence of the professionals to provide palliative care.

We are facing these issues by organizing specialized training on palliative needs for all of the professionals working in Fondazione Sospiro. Our goals are to improve professionals' awareness of palliative needs and care in residential facilities and focus on the needs of people at the end of life including every domain of QoL. A central point that has been stressed is the importance of having the possibility of choosing the place where to have palliative care and also where to die.

The training program of Fondazione Sospiro now provides staff members with annual courses about end-of-life decisions and needs.

The second crucial problem we are facing is how to support people with NDDs in making decisions about health and palliative care.

The main questions our group raised were as follows:

- How can we improve their communicative skills?
- Which are the available instruments to reach this goal?
- How can we guarantee the respect of their choices and rights?

The answers to these questions require a multidisciplinary approach in order to provide clinical, emotional and functional support focused on communication, wishes and values, allowing people with NDDs and their family to understand health problems and make decisions about palliative care and end-of-life choices in a QoL perspective.

The third issue was the involvement of fellows, friends and staff members in the palliative care, by providing them with a complete knowledge of diagnosis and prognosis and the related choices.

The working group is composed of a physician for medical needs, a nurse for health practices aspects, an educator and a psychologist for emotional and spiritual needs.

GUIDELINES

Our research group identified five steps to support people in making decisions regarding end-of-life choices.

First Step

The first step is related to an accurate diagnosis that defines health status and life expectancy, based on the identification of all therapeutic opportunities and their risks and advantages.

In 1997 the Oviedo Convention, the Convention on Human Rights and Biomedicine, stipulated that everyone has the right to be informed about his or her health, and only after having provided full and complete information, can a person express his or her own choice about his or her health (Oviedo Convention, 1997).

Human dignity and the person's right to maintain his integrity are recognized in the Charter of Fundamental Rights of the European Union (the "Charter," 2014). In particular, the Charter requires that "any intervention in the field of biology and medicine cannot be performed without free and informed consent. People not able to make decisions and give consent should have a legal representative. His duty is to guarantee the respect of values and wishes of his protected."

Based on these principles, physicians and nurses must be capable of giving people with NDDs and their family all the available information about their health problems and the therapeutic opportunities.

Furthermore, psychologist and professional educators provide to assess individual's values and preferences (Di Paola, 2016).

Second Step

A meeting with the Heads of Disability Department and the Medical Equipe is necessary to share information about the person and his or her illness. During the meeting, the team defines and highlights the events related to the illness and how to build up the interview based on the comprehension skills of the person.

Third Step

The third step is based on the assessment of verbal and non-verbal skills that are necessary to build up an interview. The goal is to develop a way to increase awareness of the health condition of the individual with NDD, providing information such as diagnosis, prognosis, available treatment and QoL issues. The adopted language is fitted on the skills and cultural background of the person, to allow the person to fully understand every possible choice and make decisions with respect to his or her values. It is also possible to use pictures or images in order to support the person in making decisions. It is important to pay particular attention to selecting the images: for example, someone affected by a medium up to a severe degree of intellectual disability could have some difficulties correctly interpreting figurative images such as pictures. But, using photos could be too cruel or disturbing for some people.

The interview starts by explaining to an individual why it is necessary to talk about his or her health condition. It is very important to describe in the most understandable and clear way every symptom and its complications. The interviewer can repeat all of the information and verify with some questions the real comprehension and then the efficacy of conversation, if necessary. Once the person has showed a full comprehension of his or her illness, the interviewer starts to describe all of the therapeutic opportunities, focusing on symptoms previously identified. For example, in case of heart failure we can consider breathlessness, feet and legs edema, oliguria and the therapy necessary to treat every symptom.

An example could be: "If you happen to be short of breath, would you accept oxygen therapy? Oxygen can help you to breathe well and so you can perform some of your favourite activities. But an oxygen machine could be noisy and the mask could impede you from speaking or eating."

Arguments about funeral and memorial services are discussed during the interview.

During the interview, a psychologist or an educator who knows the person well, verifies the capacity of the interviewed to understand everything, as well as his or her ability to pay attention. It is possible to take some breaks to allow the person to restore himself or herself. The interview is filmed to review it and verify if the carrying out method was properly chosen. After about six months, it is possible to repeat the interview to confirm or change previous decisions.

Fourth Step

After the interview, the team organizes a second meeting with the department director and the medical director. Family and legal tutor, if present, become involved in this meeting.

The aim is to explain to them the procedure, as well as seek feedback, sharing and supporting their own end-of-life choices.

At this occasion the research group provides information on how to draw up a formal document based on the defined "advance directive."

An advance directive is a written statement of wishes, preferences and choices regarding end-of-life care decisions; it is a road map for future healthcare.

Fifth Step

When an advanced directive is available, the working group shares it with the staff and eventually also with the people living with the subject.

Physicians and nurses give indications for an everyday routine, while the services coordinator properly advises how to change the routine and the working plan in order to satisfy the needs and wishes of people at the end of their life.

CONCLUSIONS

During the last two years, the application of this model in end-of-life care allowed the professional staff to define a project of care that truly respects the values and wishes of the person who is dying.

As a result of international studies and research, the Fondazione Sospiro's working group has developed a serious and evidence-based endeavor to give people suffering from NDDs the opportunity to become the protagonist in every aspect of their life.

Dame Cicely Saunders introduced the concept of total pain such as "physical, emotional and social pain and the spiritual need for security, meaning and self-worth" (Saunders, 1975).

According to the QoL model this holistic approach considers all aspects that characterize everybody's life. Terminal care cannot avoid considering the cultural and social background of a person at the end of his or her life.

Work on the assessment of values and preferences is really necessary to develop a plan of care that regards every aspect of palliative care.

There is still a lot of work to be done, such as carrying on the research of a model of communication measured to suit capacities and abilities of people with NDDs.

A good communication level must be guaranteed between the staff members, the specialists on palliative care and the families. It is essential to share all of the information on the end-of-life choices to protect the rights and the decisions of the people with NDDs.

At one time, when providing QoL in terminal illness, it was not possible to apply every step of the aforesaid model of care. Bad communication regarding the real health condition and the prognosis of the illness from physicians and nurses to other members of the staff and family led to a lack of knowledge about the need for supports necessary to promote QoL.

Working to support people with NDDs in their lifespan in guaranteeing their self-determination is one of the most important aims of scientific research. A recent study demonstrated that European National Palliative Guidelines do not consider the needs of people with NDDs (Samson et al., 2015).

Developing a way to tailor the communication of bad news and end of life to the real skills of people with NDDs should be a priority in medical care, to give them the opportunity to make every day of their life full of sense and dignity.

KEY FACTS

- NDDs are actually seen as an existential condition instead of a non-curable illness.
- This evolution determined the development of the rights of this population and the implementation of the possibility of choice in everyday activity.
- With an increase in average, people with NDDs meet the health problems that characterize middle and advanced age and it becomes necessary to support them in end-of-life decisions with the implementation of a guideline in decision-making in palliative care by professionals trained in the care of this population.

SUMMARY POINTS

- The principle of self-determination highlights the empowerment of people with NDDs in most aspects of their life.
- These persons are capable of expressing their values and wishes so as to reach a better quality of life.
- Unfortunately, when it is necessary to talk to people with NDDs about illness and healthcare, it becomes very difficult to face issues such as giving bad news, explaining the therapeutic opportunities and explaining the nature of the palliative care.
- Improving the awareness of people with NDDs highlights their capacity of expression, comprehension and communications with professionals, and at the same time allows them to achieve a better quality of life.

Important aspects to be considered are:

1. The concept of NDDs
2. Thc paradigm of quality of life
3. Supporting self-determination in NDDs
4. Supporting end-of-life decision-making in people with NDDs
5. Guaranteeing dignity in quality of life

LIST OF ABBREVIATIONS

NDD Neurodevelopmental Disorders
QoL Quality of Life

REFERENCES

American Psychiatric Association. 2013. *Diagnostic and Statistical Manual of Mental Disorders*, Fifth Edition. American Psychiatric Association, Washington, DC.

Argyle, S. 1988. *Bodily Communication*. Methuen, London.

Bekkema, N., De Veer, A.J.E., Wagemans, A.M.A., Hertogh, C.M.P.M., Francke, A.L. 2014. Decision making about medical intervention in the end-of-life care of people with intellectual disability. A national survey of the considerations and beliefs of GPs, ID physicians and care staff. *Patient Education and Counseling* 96 (2): 204–209.

Cogher, L. 2005. Communication and people with learning disabilities. In: Grant, G., Goward, P., Richardson, M., Ramcharam, P. (eds). *Learning Disability: A Life Circle Approach to Valuing People*. Open University Press, Maidenhead, pp. 260–284.

Cook, A., Lennox, N. 2000. General practice registrars' care of people with intellectual disabilities. *Journal of Intellectual Developmental Disability* 25 (1): 69–77.

Coppus, A.M.W. 2013. People with intellectual disability: What do we know about adulthood and life expectancy? *Developmental and Disabilities Research Reviews* 18 (1): 6–16.

Council of Europe. Convention for the Protection of Human Rights and of the Human Being with regard to the Application of Biology and Medicine (Convention on Human Rights and Biomedicine or the Oviedo Convention) (CETS n. 164), adopted in Oviedo on April 4. 1997. Entered into force on December 1, 1999.

De Vreese, L.P., Mantesso, U., De Bastiani, E., Gomiero, T. 2009. *La nuova longevità nella Disabilità Intellettiva*. Liguori Editore, Napoli.

Di Paola, L.S. 2016. Introduzione alle procedure di valutazione delle preferenze delle persone con Disabilità Intellettiva e dello Sviluppo. *Giornale Italiano dei Disturbi del Neurosviluppo* 1 (1): 11–20.

Doll, E. 1941. The essentials of an inclusive concept of mental deficiency. *American Journal of Mental Deficiency* 46: 214–229.

Dunkley, S., Sales, R. 2014. The challenges of providing palliative care for people with intellectual disabilities: A literature review. *International Journal of Palliative Nursing* 20 (6): 279–284.

European Commission. 2014. Charter of Fundamental Rights of the European Union.

Murphy, J. 2006. Perceptions of communication between people with communication disability and general practice staff. *Health Expects* 9 (1): 49–59.

Nirje, B. 1969. The normalization principle and its human management implications. In: Kugel, R.B., Wolfensberger, W. (eds). *Changing Patterns in Residential Services for the Mentally Retarded*, Chapter 7. President's Committee on Mental Retardation, Washington DC, pp. 179–195.

Regnard, C., Reynolds, J., Watson, B., Matthews, D., Gibson, L., Clarke, C. 2007. Understanding distress in people with severe communication difficulties: Developing and assessing the Disability Distress Assessment Tool (DisDat). *Journal of Intellectual Disability Research* 51 (4): 277–292.

Samson, E.L., van der Steen, J.T., Pautex, S., Svartzman, P., Sacchi, V., Van den Block, L., Van den Noorgate, N. 2015. European palliative care guidelines: How well do they meet the needs of people with impaired cognition? *British Medical Journal Supportive and Palliative Care* 5: 301–305.

Saunders, C. 1975. *The Care of the Dying Patient and His Family*. London Medical Group: documentation in medical ethics (5).

Shalock, R.L., Brown, I.R., Cummings, R.A., Felce, D., Matikka, L., Keith, K.D., Parmenter, T. 2002. Conceptualization, measurement, and application of quality of life for persons with intellectual disabilities: Report of an international panel of experts. *Mental Retardation* 40 (6): 457–470.

Tredgold, A.F. 1908. *Mental Deficiency*. University of California.

Tuffrey-Wijne, I., McEnhill, L. 2008. Communication difficulties and intellectual disabilities in end-of-life care. *International Journal of Palliative Nursing* 14 (4): 189–194.

Tuffrey-Wijne, I., McEnhill, L., Curfs, L., Hollins, S. 2007. Palliative care provision for people with intellectual disabilities: Interviews with specialist palliative care providers in London. *Palliative Medicine* 21 (6): 493–499.

Wehmeyer, M., Schwartz, M. 1998. The relationship between self-determination and quality of life for adults with mental retardation. *Education and Training in Mental Retardation and Developmental Disabilities* 33 (1): 3–12.

WHO. 1995. The definition of quality of life and development of international quality of life assessment instruments. *Social Science and Medicine* 41: 1403–1409.

World Health Organization. 1997. *Measuring Quality of Life: The World Health Organization Quality of Life Instruments*. Author, Geneva.

32 Appetite-Stimulant Use in the Palliative Care of Cystic Fibrosis

Samya Z. Nasr and Aarti Shakkottai

CONTENTS

INTRODUCTION

Cystic fibrosis (CF) is a chronic, life-shortening disease that affects approximately 30,000 patients in the United States (Table 32.1). The nutritional goal for CF is to achieve normal growth and development. Evidence has shown that lung function is associated with nutritional status in CF and that nutritional status is an independent predictor of survival (McColley et al. 2017). However, 10% of CF patients are ≤10th percentile for weight and ≤5th percentile for height (CF Foundation Patient Registry 2015). In a recent study, 40% of CF patients were not meeting the minimum energy requirements (Calvo-Lerma et al. 2017). Good nutritional status is dependent on the consumption of adequate nutrients, which is driven by complex, inter-related factors such as physical hunger, appetite, food-related behaviors, emotions, knowledge and beliefs (Table 32.2). Patients with CF have chronic respiratory infections which affect their appetite. They also have a high resting energy expenditure. Malabsorption from pancreatic insufficiency is also an issue for most CF patients. They consequently have higher than normal caloric requirements. Ultimately, achieving good nutritional status is dependent on the consumption of adequate nutrients, which is driven by complex, inter-related factors such as physical hunger, appetite, food-related behaviors, emotions, knowledge and beliefs (Table 32.2).

Diagnosing the cause of an individual's malnutrition requires careful, multidisciplinary history taking, physical examination and overall patient/ family assessment (Table 32.3). Broadly, some of the

TABLE 32.1
Key Facts of Cystic Fibrosis (CF)

1. Cystic figrosis was first described in 1938 by Dr. Dorothy Anderson.
2. It is an autosomal recessive disease that affects Caucasians more than other ethnic groups.
3. It primarily affects the lungs, pancreas, digestive tract and sweat glands.
4. It results in gradual deterioration of lung function, fat malabsorption, nutrition deficiency and failure to thrive.
5. Median age of survival is over 42 years.
6. Patients have a higher caloric requirement in order to maintain normal weight gain and growth.
7. Good nutritional status has been associated with better lung function and lower morbidity and mortality.

factors that could lead to malnutrition in a patient with CF include decreased appetite, malabsorption, metabolic changes such as intestinal inflammation, liver disease or insulin resistance and increased energy expenditure.

Appetite stimulants (AS), although efficacious in treating malnutrition in CF, should be prescribed if decreased food intake secondary to inadequate appetite is the principal cause of the malnutrition and all other contributing factors have been assessed, ruled-out or treated (Chinuck et al. 2007, 2014).

APPETITE STIMULANTS

Megestrol Acetate

Megestrol acetate (MA) (Megace) is a synthetic, orally active derivative of progesterone. One of the side effects of MA is appetite stimulation and weight gain. The mechanism of action has not been established. It has been postulated that the effect is partly mediated by neuropeptide Y, a potent central appetite stimulant. Another speculation of its mechanism of action is that it is a potent inducer of adipocyte differentiation in 3T3-L1 cells *in vitro*, raising the possibility that it stimulates the conversion of fibroblasts to adipocytes, thereby blocking or reversing the effect of

TABLE 32.2
Issues Contributing to Poor Appetite or Poor Food Intake

Cystic Fibrosis (CF) Related		Can Occur in People with Cystic Fibrosis	
Acute illness, pulmonary exacerbation, inflammation, increased cytokines	Poor gastric emptying and/or gastroesophageal reflux	Depression, anxiety, stress or sadness	Eating disorder or disordered eating behaviors
DIOS (distal intestinal obstructive syndrome) or constipation leading to abdominal pain and nausea	Nasal polyps which may impair taste or the ability to eat and breathe comfortably at the same time	Inflammatory bowel disease	Appetite neuro-transmitter abnormality (ghrelin, peptide Y, leptin, insulin)
Avoidance of foods mistakenly thought to be "bad" for CF ("carbohydrates causing CF-related diabetes," "fats causing abdominal pain," "milk/milk products causing secretions" etc.).	Sinusitis which may be associated with pain with chewing, or altered taste	Medications (some antidepressants or attention deficit hyperactivity disorder [ADHD] medications)	Economic or access issues
Burden of therapies on time and energy to prepare and eat nutritious foods		Abdominal pain, bloating or other symptoms of malabsorption	

Source: Adapted from Nasr SZ, Drury D. *Pediatr Pulmonol.* 2008;43(3):209–219.

TABLE 32.3
Workup Strategies for Malnutrition in Cystic Fibrosis

	Symptoms	Information, Tests and Possible Intervention Strategies
Appetite	Decreased food intake	Diet history, food records History of events leading to poor appetite: • Temporal onset • Symptoms at the time of onset • Emotional/social/financial coexisting issues • Behavioral issues around eating Observe mealtime interactions
	Early satiety	Gastric motility study
	Avoidance of high-energy foods	Body satisfaction, desired body weight, eating attitudes, purging behaviors (i.e., non-compliance to enzymes to lose weight)
Absorption/ digestion	Abdominal pain Gas Bloating Frequent, foul stools Visible oil loss	72-hour fecal fat coefficient of dietary fat intake Enzyme history: • List of foods or beverages with which enzymes are not taken • Information on when and how enzymes are taken • Reported compliance to prescribed enzymes Low intestinal pH resulting in poor enzyme bioactivity: • Good compliance to enzymes reported and observed • Enzyme dose 1000–2500 IU lipase/kg/meal • Minimal response to enzyme dose adjustments in recent past • Acid suppression or acid blocker therapies may be beneficial
	Stool mass palpitated	Abdominal x-ray; DIOS history
	Refractory symptoms	Rule out other gastrointestinal processes common in CF: bacterial overgrowth, constipation, intussusceptions, CF-related liver disease, and/or the co-existence of lactose intolerance, celiac disease, etc.
Metabolism	Growth failure or unintentional weight loss	Oral glucose tolerance test to rule out glucosuric energy losses
	Increased respiratory symptoms leading to elevated energy requirements	Aggressive respiratory and physiotherapies
	Use of systemic and/or inhaled corticosteroids	Linear height more affected than body weight or body mass index; bone age delay
	Hyponatremia	Recurrent hyponatremia or hyponatremic dehydration

Source: Adapted from Nasr SZ, Drury D. *Pediatr Pulmonol.* 2008;43(3):209–219.

tumor necrosis factor on lipocyte differentiation (Loprinzi et al. 1992). It has been used successfully as an appetite stimulant in adult patients with cancer and acquired immunodeficiency syndrome (AIDS) (Strang 1997).

MA has been used in CF to treat anorexia and weight loss (Eubanks et al. 2002; Marchand et al. 2000; Nasr et al. 1999). In a case report, four patients, ages 10–18.5 years, with severe CF lung disease, anorexia and weight loss received MA at a dose of 400–800 mg daily for a duration of 6–15 months. Patients' appetite improved, with an increase in mean weight for age percentile from less than 5th to 25th after six months of therapy. Quality of life improved also (Nasr et al. 1999). Side effects were not reported in this report. A randomized, double-blind, placebo-controlled, crossover study of MA in 12 malnourished children with CF was conducted over a 12-week period, followed by a 12-week washout, then the alternative treatment. The age range was 21 months–10.4 years, the dose was 10 mg/kg/day. Weight Z-score, body fat and lean body mass (LBM) increased, and pulmonary function improved in patients given MA. There was little change in linear growth during MA therapy. Side effects included glucosuria, insomnia, hyperactivity and irritability (Marchand et al. 2000). There were abnormalities in glycemic control (Marchand et al. 2000). Another randomized, double-blind, placebo-controlled study was conducted on 17 CF patients age six years and above. MA dose used was 7.5–15 mg/kg/day. The study duration was six months. The treatment group had significant increase in weight-for-age Z-score and reached 100% of their ideal body weight within three months of therapy. Weight gain included both fat and fat-free mass as measured by dual-energy X-ray absorptiometry (DXA). Pulmonary function improved in the treatment group. Reversible adrenal suppression was observed in most patients who received MA. Some patients suffered from insomnia and moodiness while on MA (Eubanks et al. 2002). MA was also reported to cause testicular failure and Cushing syndrome, both of which appear to be reversible (Eubanks et al. 2002).

Cyproheptadine Hydrochloride

Cyproheptadine hydrochloride (CH) (Periactin) is a first-generation antihistamine that is both histamine and serotonin antagonist. It has a secondary effect of appetite stimulation. The mechanism of action is unknown, but it is not due to hypoglycemic-induced hyperphagia, as evidenced by normal glucose tolerance testing and normal insulin levels. Also, it is not due to an increase in endogenous growth hormone (GH). CH has been used as an appetite stimulant in asthma, tuberculosis, HIV and cancer (Homnick et al. 2004; Homnick et al. 2005). A 12-week, randomized, double-blind, controlled study of CH versus placebo was conducted in 18 CF patients (mean age of 15 years). The dose was 4 mg QID over a three-month period. Sixteen patients completed the study. Subjects in the CH group showed significant increase in weight, height, body mass index (BMI) percentiles, ideal body weight/height, weight for age Z-scores and fat and fat-free mass compared to the placebo group. There were no differences in antibiotic use or spirometric measures between the two groups. Transient mild sedation occurred in the CH group (Homnick et al. 2004).

A follow-up study was conducted to evaluate the long-term use of CH (Homnick et al. 2005). Sixteen CF patients enrolled and 12 completed a nine-month open-label trial following the completion of the double-blind study. Subjects who switched from placebo to CH demonstrated significant weight gain over three to six months. Those who continued CH maintained the weight they gained. There were some improvements, not statistically significant, in selected spirometric measures and side effects continued to be mild. Of note, self-reported adherence to CH during the study was variable and ranged from twice daily to four times a day use (Homnick et al. 2005).

Dronobinal (Marinol)

Dronabinol (Marinol) is an oral form of Δ-9-tetrahydrocannabinol dissolved in sesame oil in soft gelatin capsules. It is the principal psychoactive substance present in marijuana. It is utilized as an alternative to smoked marijuana for AIDS wasting syndrome and nausea following chemotherapy. An important gap in the knowledge base about dronabinol has been an accurate assessment of its abuse potential. Several studies cite the use of marijuana for treatment of cancer-related anorexia, nausea, vomiting, pain and mood disorders. There is no evidence of abuse or diversion of dronabinol. There is no street market or value for dronabinol. Furthermore, it does not provide effects that are considered desirable in a drug of abuse – the onset of action is slow and the effects are dysphoric and unappealing (Calhoun et al. 1998).

A long-term study of dronabinol was conducted in 94 late-stage AIDS patients who had previously participated in a six-week double-blind placebo-controlled study. The long-term use of dronabinol resulted in consistent increase in appetite with trends toward weight stabilization and modest weight gain. In addition, the data from this study suggested that it may be administered long-term in this patient population without development of tolerance to the therapeutic effect. Few patients developed adverse events including anxiety, confusion, euphoria and somnolence (Beal et al. 1997).

It has been proposed to administer dronabinol to adolescent and adult CF patients to alleviate malnutrition and help treat wasting (Fride 2002). It was utilized in 11 CF patients with severe nutritional deficiencies who had failed conventional interventions such as nutritional counseling and high-calorie supplements. Patients receiving dronabinol had a significant improvement in weight during the treatment period ($P = 0.03$). Side effects were euphoria, hallucinations and lethargy. All side effects responded to dose reduction. No patients stopped the medication due to side effects (Anstead et al. 2003).

Antipsychotic/Antidepressant Agents

Antipsychotic Drugs

Excessive body-weight gain (BWG) is a common side effect of some typical and atypical antipsychotic drugs (APDs). Weight gain is linked to a decreased metabolic rate, increased caloric intake and decreased physical activity. It is generally believed that there are multiple mechanisms by which APDs induce weight gain, but their precise nature remains unknown. Weight gain may be a multifactorial process, involving serotonergic, histaminergic and/or adrenergic neuro-transmission. APDs achieve their therapeutic effects by modulating the activity of these neural pathways. It might also be due to the blockade of certain receptors, for example 5-HT2c, that modulate appetite and body weight. APDs vary in their propensity to cause weight change. The largest weight gains are associated with clozapine and olanzapine, and the smallest with quetiapine and ziprasidone. Risperidone is associated with modest weight gain that is not dose related. Clozapine and olanzapine appear to display a high propensity to induce glucose dysregulation and dyslipidemia. Insulin secretion is preserved and thus high serum insulin levels are observed which leads to peripheral insulin resistance, and ultimately, glucose intolerance and type 2 diabetes mellitus (DM). Sudden BWG, insulin resistance, increased appetite and related endocrine changes also may be involved in the development of glucose intolerance and dyslipidemia in predisposed individuals. Patients' blood glucose and lipids should be monitored before treatment and at regular intervals (Baptista et al. 2002).

The use of olanzapine in an 18-year-old female with CF and severe body dysmorphism led to a significant increase in body weight. This observation led to an open-label trial of low-dose olanzapine in a group of 12 adults with severe CF disease who had been losing weight despite maximal conventional therapy. When compared to baseline, change in BMI after six months of therapy was statistically significant ($P = 0.01$, Wilcoxon sign-rank test) (Ross et al. 2005).

Antidepressants

Psychological functioning is being increasingly assessed in both children and adults with CF. One study of 67 CF patients between the ages of 18 and 30 years revealed symptoms of depression in approximately 33% of the participants (Knudsen et al. 2016). It was associated with poor treatment adherence (Knudsen et al. 2016) which has been associated with lower body mass index (BMI), higher healthcare costs and worsening disease severity (Shakkottai et al. 2015; Nasr et al. 2013). Antidepressants have been used, in addition to other psychosocial interventions, to treat depression in CF patients (Elgudin et al. 2004).

Antidepressants have been used as appetite stimulants, given that their side-effect profile includes appetite dysregulation. Antidepressants with non-adrenergic and specific serotonergic effects have been shown to block the 5HT2C serotonin receptor. Blockage of this receptor may lead to an increase in appetite. These drugs also block the 5-HT3 serotonin receptor, which is implicated in promoting nausea and occasional emesis. These two symptoms are usually associated with decreased appetite and failure to gain adequate weight in patients with severe CF disease (Boas et al. 2000).

Mirtazapine (Remeron) is a noradrenergic and specific serotonergic antidepressant (NaSSA) that has been used as an appetite stimulant in CF. It also has an antihistamine effect. It is well tolerated and is superior to most antidepressants in its anti-anxiolytic effects, sleep improvement and gastrointestinal side effects. Its main side effect is weight gain (Boas et al. 2000; Sykes et al. 2006).

Mirtazapine has been used as an appetite stimulant in two studies of malnourished CF patients (Boas et al. 2000; Sykes et al. 2006). The first study was a pilot study of five patients age 14–19 years with mean forced expiratory volume (FEV1) of 41.4% with growth failure. All subjects demonstrated an increase in weight (5.8 kg, $P < 0.01$), body fat (13.9–21.8 kg, $P < 0.01$) and weight gain velocity (–3.9 before starting treatment versus 27.4 kg/year after treatment, $P < 0.05$). Subjects reported mild sedation, dry mouth, increased thirst and increased appetite but did not feel these symptoms justified stopping the medication (Boas et al. 2000). The second study was a retrospective study. Six patients were enrolled. Age range was 10–17 years at the start of therapy. Duration of therapy ranged from 8 to 28 months. All patients had an increase in BMI percentile for age (mean 10.3%, median 8% and range 2%–25%). Adverse effects were limited to somnolence (Sykes et al. 2006).

Recombinant Human Growth Hormone (rhGH)

Human growth hormone is a single polypeptide chain composed of 191 amino acids (molecular weight 22 KD) and coded on chromosome 17. It is secreted in a pulsatile fashion by the somatotrophs of the anterior pituitary gland. It stimulates the production of insulin-like growth factor (IGF-1) in the liver and other organs (muscle, bone and adipose tissue) (Windisch et al. 1998; Thaker et al. 2015) and promotes protein synthesis and fat utilization and decreases glucose oxidation.

Recombinant growth hormone (rhGH) or somatotropin has been approved by the U.S. Food and Drug Administration (FDA) for treating AIDS-associated wasting. It has also been used in the posttraumatic state to reduce nitrogen loss. The nitrogen retention induced by GH is associated with increased whole-body protein synthesis and LBM as well.

The recommended dosage of rhGH is 4–6 mg administered by subcutaneous injection daily. It is significantly more expensive than other appetite stimulants. The adverse effects associated with rhGH therapy include headache, nausea, fever, vomiting, intracranial hypertension (pseudotumor cerebri), moderate-severe edema, arthralgias, carpal tunnel syndrome, gynecomastia, insulin resistance and glucose intolerance. Nonetheless, treatment has generally been well tolerated. In children, using rhGH for long-term replacement can lead to irreversible adverse effects such as slipped capital femoral epiphysis, acromegaly and leukemia (Windisch et al. 1998).

Studies in patients with CF have documented a delay in pubertal maturation. However, there is a poor correlation between weight gain and linear growth, suggesting that nutritional supplementation alone may not be the best means for improving short stature in CF (Hardin 2002).

Although individuals with CF have normal spontaneous and stimulated GH levels, they have been shown to have low levels of GH effector proteins such as insulin-like growth factor 1 (IGF-1) suggesting that the growth failure in CF may be due to a relative insensitivity to GH (Thaker et al. 2015). Inflammatory markers such as IL-1,IL-6 and TNF-α have also been shown to decrease levels of IGF-1 and could therefore be contributing to the growth abnormalities seen in CF. There is a positive linear correlation between IGF-1 levels and height ($r = 0.66$, $p < 0.0001$) and weight ($r = 0.61$, $p < 0.0001$) in CF (Switzer et al. 2009).

Several studies have documented the safety and efficacy of GH in improving growth and clinical status in CF patients (Hardin et al. 2001; Hardin et al. 2006; Hardin et al. 2005a,b; Schnabel et al. 2007; Stalvey et al. 2012). GH has been resulting in significantly greater height, height velocity, weight, weight velocity and change in lean tissue mass. There was significant improvement in delta forced vital capacity (FVC) during the studies. There was an improvement in respiratory muscle strength. Hospitalizations and outpatient intravenous antibiotic courses significantly decreased. A multicenter, randomized controlled cross-over trial of 61 prepubertal CF patients, conducted over a two-year period showed significantly greater gains in height, weight, lean mass and bone mineral content in those receiving GH (Hardin et al. 2006). After cessation of daily GH injections, the positive effects on height and weight velocity were sustained (Hardin et al. 2006).

GH has been shown to enhance nutrition and growth in CF children receiving enteral nutrition and has shown to safely improve height, weight, bone mineralization and clinical status in pubertal adolescents with CF (Hardin et al. 2005a,b).

Another multicenter, randomized, placebo-controlled, double-blind trial that included 63 CF children (bone age 8–18 years) showed significant improvement in height, growth velocity and IGF-1 levels among those treated with GH (Schnabel et al. 2007).

Open-label, controlled clinical trial of rhGH in 68 prepubertal children ≤14 years of age and with CF showed significant improvement in height, weight and lean body mass in the rhGH group. There was also a significantly greater increase in the FVC in the treatment group. There were significant differences in FEV1 after adjusting for baseline disease severity (Stalvey et al. 2012).

Anabolic Androgenic Steroids

Since anabolic androgenic steroids (AAS) are derivatives or structural modifications of the parent steroid hormone, testosterone, they exhibit both anabolic and androgenic activities. Their anabolic effects include promotion of protein synthesis, nitrogen retention and skeletal muscle growth, while their androgenic effects include the development and maintenance of primary and secondary sexual characteristics in males and male-pattern baldness, deepened voice, clitoromegaly and growth of facial hair in females.

Oxandrolone has marked anabolic activity and few androgenic effects (ratio 10:1), as compared to testosterone and methyl-testosterone. It cannot be aromatized to estrogen, thereby minimizing estrogen-dependent advancement of bone age, particularly in children who are still growing (Varness et al. 2009). Oxandrolone is the only AAS that is FDA approved for restitution of weight loss after severe trauma, extensive surgery or chronic infections. It is also approved for use in malnutrition due to alcoholic cirrhosis, and Duchene's or Becker's muscular dystrophy. Statistically significant improvements have been reported in the areas of body composition, recovery, muscle strength and function. Oxandrolone has been used in acute catabolic disorders (e.g., burn injury and acute multiple trauma) and in chronic catabolic disorders such as chronic obstructive pulmonary disease (COPD), and Crohn's disease. It has also been used in wasting associated with HIV/AIDS. Adverse effects include hepatic dysfunction (increased transaminase levels) and androgenic effects (alopecia, hirsutism, deep voice and clitoromegaly in girls and women) (Orr and Singh 2004).

Prednisone has been studied in CF patients with mild-moderate pulmonary disease to assess its effect on the pulmonary inflammatory process (Auerbach et al. 1985). The study was a four-year, double-blind, placebo-controlled trial of alternate-day prednisone (2 mg/kg) in 45 CF patients. The patients in the prednisone group showed better growth and pulmonary function and less morbidity compared with those in the placebo group. No complications were reported. Because of this observation, the U.S. Cystic Fibrosis Foundation sponsored a multicenter, double-blind, placebo-controlled trial of alternate-day prednisone at a dose of 2 mg/kg (high dose), 1 mg/kg (low-dose), or placebo every other day for four years. Two hundred eighty-five patients from 15 CF centers were enrolled in the study from 1986 to 1987. An interim safety analysis was done with mean duration in the study of 33.9 months for the high-dose, 35.3 months for the low-dose, and 36.8 months for the placebo groups. This analysis revealed increased frequency of cataracts, growth retardation and glucose abnormalities among patients in the high-dose group.

In view of these results, it was recommended by the study ombudsman and a special advisory panel that the study drug be discontinued for all patients in the high-dose prednisone group. At the end of the study, there was significant improvement in the 1 mg group compared to placebo in FVC ($P < 0.025$) in patients colonized with *Pseudomonas aeruginosa* at baseline (Eigen et al. 1995). In addition, there was significant improvement in predicted forced expiratory volume in 1 second (FEV_1) in the 1 mg/kg group compared to placebo ($P < 0.02$) and reduction in serum IgG concentrations (1 mg/kg versus placebo, $P < 0.007$; 2 mg/kg versus placebo, $P < 0.003$). From six months onward, height Z-scores fell in the 2 mg/kg group compared to placebo ($P < 0.001$). For the 1 mg/kg group, height Z-scores were lower at 24 months. An excess of abnormalities in glucose metabolism was seen in the 2 mg/kg group compared with the placebo group ($P < 0.005$) (Eigen et al. 1995).

APPLICATIONS TO OTHER AREAS OF TERMINAL OR PALLIATIVE CARE

Weight loss and malnutrition occur frequently in other terminal diseases, and as with CF, it is important to identify and correct any underlying issues before initiating drug therapy aimed solely at increasing appetite and/or promoting weight gain. Much of the data on the use of appetite stimulants originate in diseases other than CF (Beal et al. 1997; Loprinzi et al. 1992; Strang 1997; Windisch et al. 1998). Megestrol has been shown to increase appetite, decrease nausea and improve general sense of well-being in cancer patients and AIDS patients (Loprinzi et al. 1992; Strang 1997). The stimulatory effects of cyproheptadine on appetite were originally reported in asthmatic patients who were prescribed the drug for its antihistamine properties (Lavenstein et al. 1962). Today, cyproheptadine is used less as an antihistamine and more as an appetite stimulant (Homnick et al. 2004). The cannabanoids have been used for anorexia, nausea, vomiting, pain and mood elevation in cancer patients since the 1970s even though a legal pharmaceutical formulation was not available until the 1980s (Calhoun et al. 1998). While dronabinol is only FDA approved for use in anorexia in AIDS patients and for treating nausea and vomiting due to cancer chemotherapy, it has been applied off-label to other illnesses like CF (Beal et al. 1997; Fride 2002; Anstead et al. 2003). Recombinant human growth hormone has been used in AIDS-associated wasting and in the posttraumatic states. However, it is not widely studied in other terminal illnesses. Anabolic steroids have been widely utilized in many other chronic diseases. Anorexia and weight issues are not unique to CF patients, and most of the agents used in CF for appetite stimulation have been shown to be useful in other terminal illnesses.

GUIDELINES

Please see Table 32.3 for workup strategies and guidelines.

ETHICAL ISSUES

The ethical issues surrounding the use of appetite stimulants in CF are minimal. The biggest concern is that for most of these drugs the appetite stimulation is frequently a side effect rather than the effect they are indicated for and FDA approved for. For example, Cyproheptadine is indicated for use as an antihistamine; the antidepressants are indicated for depression and related mood disorders and antipsychotics are indicated for psychiatric illness. While the suspension form of Megestrol is approved for use in AIDS-induced anorexia, cachexia and weight loss, the tablet form is only indicated for palliative treatment in breast or endometrial cancer, which was the originally studied use.

Second, no medication is without the potential for adverse effects. Megestrol can cause reversible adrenal suppression/failure, testicular failure and impotence (Loprinzi et al. 1992; Eubanks et al. 2002; Marchand et al. 2000). Dronabinol has the potential for abuse; however, to date there is minimal evidence of abuse or diversion and it is not thought to possess any street value (Calhoun et al. 1998). Antipsychotics may cause insulin resistance, glucose dysregulation and dyslipidemia (Baptista et al. 2002; Ross et al. 2005). Additionally, there may be a social stigma that surrounds use of these agents. It is important to discuss the potential adverse effects of these agents with patients and families so they can participate in the risk versus benefit decision to start any of these agents.

KEY FACTS

- Appetite stimulants are helpful in improving weight gain.
- Improving weight gain can lead to improvement of quality of life.
- Improving weight gain can lead to improved survival.

SUMMARY POINTS

- Appetite stimulants can help increase caloric intake and improve weight gain.
- Table 32.4 shows a summary of appetite stimulants discussed.
- Etiology of weight loss should be identified and addressed before appetite stimulants can be offered.
- Choice of appetite stimulant should be made according to the physician's experience, patient age and preference, severity of disease and side effects.
- Table 32.5 shows an algorithm of workup and intervention for patients with cystic fibrosis.

LIST OF ABBREVIATIONS

AAS Anabolic Androgenic Steroids
APDs Antipsychotic Drugs
BMI Body-Mass Index
BWG Body-Weight Gain
CF Cystic Fibrosis
CH Cyproheptadine Hydrochloride
LBM Lean Body Mass
MA Megestrol Acetate
rhGH Recombinant Human Growth Hormone

TABLE 32.4
Summary of Appetite Stimulants in Cystic Fibrosis

Drug	Dosage	Side Effects
Megestrol acetate (MA)	400–800 mg/day or 7.5–15 mg/kg/day orally	Glucosuria, insomnia, hyperactivity, irritability, reversible adrenal suppression
Cyproheptadine hydrochloride (CH)	4 mg BID–QID or 0.5 mg/kg/day orally	Transient mild sedation
Dronabinal (Marinol)	2.5 mg qd–5 mg BID, PO	Anxiety, confusion, euphoria, somnolence
		Antipsychotic
Olanzapine	5–20 mg qd orally	Liver dysfunction, sleepiness, hyperglycemia
Risperidone	0.5–5 mg qd orally	Glucose dysregulation, dyslipidemia
		Antidepressants
Mirtazapine (Remeron)	15 mg qd orally	Mild sedation, dry mouth somnolence
Recombinant human growth hormone (rhGh)	4 – qd mg SC injection	Mild edema, arthralgia, carpal tunnel syndrome, gynecomastia, insulin resistance, glucose intolerance. In children, slipped capital femoral epiphysis acromegaly, leukemia
		Anabolic Androgenic Steroids (AASs)
Oxandrolone	0.1 mg/kg/day BID, orally	Hepatic dysfunction, androgenic effects in females (alopecia, hirsutism, deep voice, clitormegaly), development of primary and secondary sexual features in males

Source: Adapted from Nasr SZ, Drury D. *Pediatr Pulmonol.* 2008;43(3):209–219.

TABLE 32.5
Algorithm for Cystic Fibrosis Patients at Nutritional Risk (Body Mass Index Percentile ≤25% or Poor Weight Gain for Three Months)

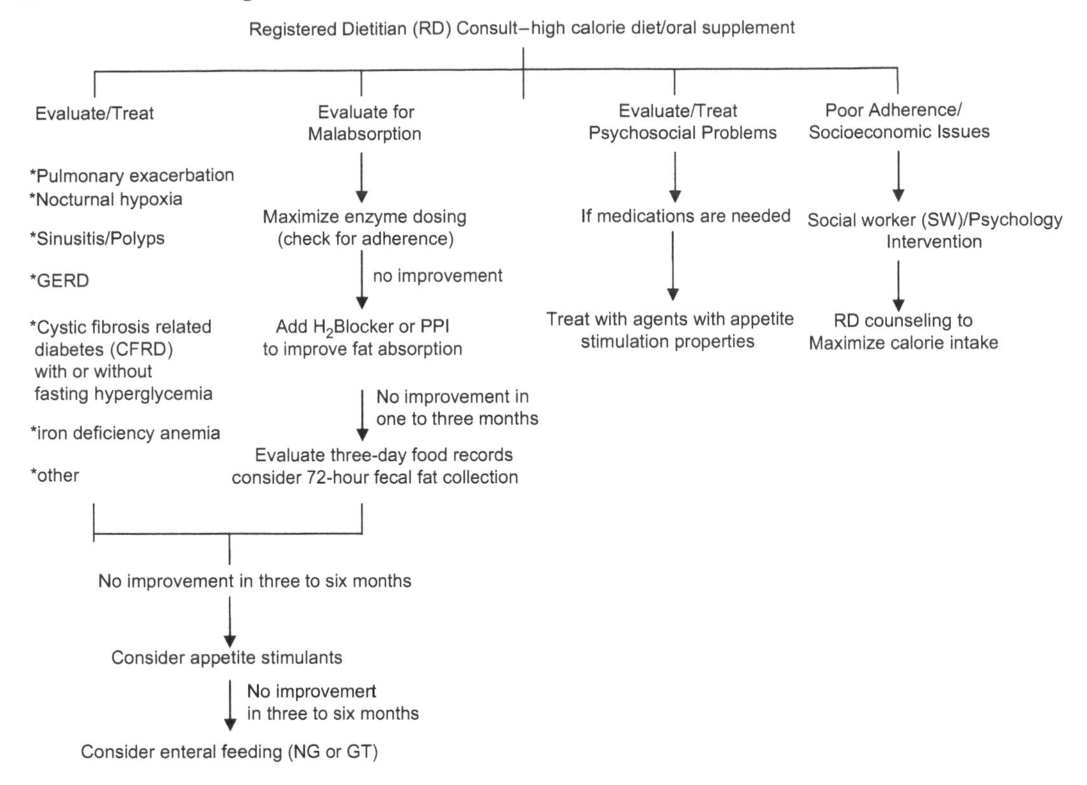

Source: Adapted from "Appetite Stimulants Use in Cystic Fibrosis." *Pediatric Pulmonology*. 2008;43:200–219.

REFERENCES

Anstead MI, Kuhn RJ, Martyn D, Craigmyle L, Kanga JF. Dronabinol, an effective and safe appetite stimulant in cystic fibrosis. *Pediatr Pulmonol*. 2003;36:343.

Auerbach HS, Williams M, Kirkpatrick JA, Colten HR. Alternate-day prednisone reduces morbidity and improves pulmonary function in cystic fibrosis. *Lancet*. 1985;2:686–688.

Baptista T, Kin NMKNY, Beaulieu S, de Baptista EA. Obesity and related metabolic abnormalities during antipsychotic drug administration: mechanisms, management and research perspectives. *Pharmacopsychiatry*. 2002;35:205–219.

Beal JE, Olson R, Lefkowitz L et al. Long-term efficacy and safety of dronabinol for acquired immunodeficiency syndrome-associated anorexia. *J Pain Symptom Manage*. 1997;14:7–14.

Boas SR, McColley SA, Danduran MJ, Young J. The role of mirtazapine as an appetite stimulant in malnourished individuals with CF. *Ped Pulmonol*. 2000;30:325.

Calhoun SR, Galloway GP, Smith DE. Abuse potential of dronabinol (Marinol®). *J Psychoactive Drugs*. 1998;30:187–195.

Calvo-Lerma J, Hulst JM, Asseiceira I et al.; MyCyFAPP Project. Nutritional status, nutrient intake and use of enzyme supplements in paediatric patients with cystic fibrosis: A European multicentre study with reference to current guidelines. *J Cyst Fibros*. 2017;16(4):510–518.

Chinuck R, Dewar J, Baldwin DR, Hendron E. Appetite stimulants for people with cystic fibrosis. *Cochrane Database Syst Rev*. 2014;(7):CD008190.

Chinuck RS, Fortnum H, Baldwin DR. Appetite stimulants in cystic fibrosis: A systematic review. *J Hum Nutr Diet*. 2007;20(6):526–537.

Cystic Fibrosis Foundation Patient Registry. 2015. Annual Data Report. Bethesda, Maryland. ©2016 Cystic Fibrosis Foundation.

Eigen H, Rosenstein BJ, FitzSimmons S, Schidlow DV. A multicenter study of alternate-day prednisone therapy in patients with cystic fibrosis. Cystic fibrosis foundation prednisone trial group. *J Pediatr*. 1995;126:515–523.

Elgudin L, Kishan S, Howe D. Depression in children and adolescents with cystic fibrosis: Case studies. *Int J Psychiatry Med*. 2004;34:391–397.

Eubanks V, Koppersmith N, Wooldridge N et al. Effects of megestrol acetate on weight gain, body composition, and pulmonary function in patients with cystic fibrosis. *J Pediatr*. 2002;140:439–444.

Fride E. Cannabinoids and cystic fibrosis: A novel approach to etiology and therapy. *J Cannabis Ther*. 2002;2:59–71.

Hardin DS. Growth problems and growth hormone treatment in children with cystic fibrosis. *J Pediatr Endocrinol Metabolism*. 2002;15:731–735.

Hardin DS, Adams-Huet B, Brown D et al. Growth hormone treatment improves growth and clinical status in prepubertal children with cystic fibrosis: Results of a multicenter randomized controlled trial. *J Clin Endocrinol Metab*. 2006;91:4925–4929.

Hardin DS, Ellis KJ, Dyson M, Rice J, McConnell R, Seilheimer DK. Growth hormone improves clinical status in prepubertal children with cystic fibrosis: Results of a randomized controlled trial. *J Pediatr*. 2001;139(5):636–642.

Hardin DS, Ferkol T, Ahn C, Dreimane D, Dyson M, Morse M, Prestidge C, Rice J, Seilheimer DK. A retrospective study of growth hormone use in adolescents with cystic fibrosis. *Clin Endocrinol (Oxf)*. 2005a May;62(5):560–566.

Hardin DS, Rice J, Ahn C et al. Growth hormone treatment enhances nutrition and growth in children with cystic fibrosis receiving enteral nutrition. *J Pediatr*. 2005b;146:324–328.

Homnick DN, Homnick BD, Reeves AJ, Marks JH, Pimentel RS, Bonnema SK. Cyproheptadine is an effective appetite stimulant in cystic fibrosis. *Pediatr Pulmonol*. 2004;38(2):129–134.

Homnick DN, Marks JH, Hare KL, Bonnema SK. Long-term trial of cyproheptadine as an appetite stimulant in cystic fibrosis. *Pediatr Pulmonol*. 2005;40:251–256.

Knudsen KB, Pressler T, Mortensen LH, Jarden M, Skov M, Quittner AL, Katzenstein T, Boisen KA. Associations between adherence, depressive symptoms and health-related quality of life in young adults with cystic fibrosis. *Springerplus*. 2016;5(1):1216.

Lavenstein AF, Dacaney EP, Lasagna L, Van Metre TE. Effect of cyproheptadine on asthmatic children. *JAMA*. 1962;180:912–916.

Loprinzi CL, Johnson PA, Jensen M. Megestrol acetate for anorexia and cachexia. *Oncology*. 1992;49:46–49.

Marchand V, Baker SS, Stark TJ, Baker RD. Randomized, double-blind, placebo-controlled pilot trial of megestrol acetate in malnourished children with cystic fibrosis. *J Pediatr Gastroenterol Nutr*. 2000;31:264–269.

McColley SA, Schechter MS, Morgan WJ, Pasta DJ, Craib ML, Konstan MW. Risk factors for mortality before age 18 years in cystic fibrosis. *Pediatr Pulmonol*. 2017;52(7):909–915.

Nasr SZ, Chou W, Villa KF, Chang E, Broder MS. Adherence to dornase alfa treatment among commercially insured patients with cystic fibrosis. *J Med Econ*. 2013;16(6):801–808.

Nasr SZ, Drury D. Appetite stimulants use in cystic fibrosis. *Pediatr Pulmonol*. 2008;43(3):209–219.

Nasr SZ, Hurwitz ME, Brown RW, Elghoroury M, Rosen D. Treatment of anorexia and weight loss with megestrol acetate in patients with cystic fibrosis. *Pediatr Pulmonol*. 1999;28:380–382.

Orr R, Singh MF. The anabolic androgenic steroid oxandrolone in the treatment of wasting and catabolic disorders. *Drugs*. 2004;64:725–750.

Ross E, Davidson S, Sriram S et al. Weight gain associated with low dose olanzapine therapy in severely underweight adults with cystic fibrosis. *Pediatr Pulmonol*. 2005;40:350.

Schnabel D, Grasemann C, Staab D, Wollmann H, Ratjen F. A multicenter, randomized, double-blind, placebo-controlled trial to evaluate the metabolic and respiratory effects of growth hormone in children with cystic fibrosis. *Pediatrics*. 2007;e1230–e1238.

Shakkottai A, Kidwell KM, Townsend M, Nasr SZ. A five-year retrospective analysis of adherence in cystic fibrosis. *Pediatr Pulmonol*. 2015;50(12):1224–1229.

Stalvey MS, Anbar RD, Konstan MW, Jacobs JR, Bakker B, Lippe B, Geller DE. A multi-center controlled trial of growth hormone treatment in children with cystic fibrosis. *Pediatr Pulmonol*. 2012;47(3):252–263.

Strang P. The effect of megestrol acetate on anorexia, weight loss and cachexia in cancer and AIDS patients. *Anticanc Res.* 1997;17:657–662.
Switzer M, Rice J, Rice M, Hardin DS. Insulin-like growth factor-I levels predict weight, height and protein catabolism in children and adolescents with cystic fibrosis. *J Pediatr Endocrinol Metab.* 2009;22(5):417–424.
Sykes R, Kittel F, Marcus M, Tarter E, Schroth M. Mirtazapine for appetite stimulation in children with cystic fibrosis. *Ped Pulmonol.* 2006;40:389.
Thaker V, Haagensen AL, Carter B, Fedorowicz Z, Houston BW. Recombinant growth hormone therapy for cystic fibrosis in children and young adults. *Cochrane Database Syst Rev.* 2015 May 20;(5):CD008901.
Varness T, Seffrood EE, Connor EL, Rock MJ, Allen DB. Oxandrolone improves height velocity and BMI in patients with cystic fibrosis. *Int J Pediatr Endocrinol.* 2009;2009:826895.
Windisch PA, Papatheofanis FJ, Matuszewski KA. Recombinant human growth hormone for AIDS-associated wasting. *Ann Pharmacother.* 1998;32:437–445.

33 Use of Cannabinoids in Palliative Nutrition Care

Kelay E. Trentham

CONTENTS

INTRODUCTION

Cannabis and cannabinoids are used as both traditional remedies and modern medicinal therapies to manage a number of nutrition-related issues including nausea, vomiting, anorexia and weight loss as well as pain and inflammatory conditions. While many healthcare providers are familiar with legal cannabinoid-based pharmaceuticals, they may be less familiar with whole cannabis-based products. As patient interest in medical cannabis increases, healthcare providers who possess a working knowledge of cannabis' efficacy, methods of administration, pharmacokinetics, contraindications and adverse effects will be best equipped to educate and assist patients in making informed decisions about its use. In addition, employment of bioethics principles can help provide a framework for a productive and appropriate discussion about this often controversial means of pain and symptom management.

While cannabis is thought to be one of the oldest plants cultivated for fiber making, ca. 4000 BCE (Duvall 2015), the earliest recorded mention of its use as medicine appears to be ca. 1700 BCE in ancient Egypt (Russo 2007). Cannabis was included in China's first pharmacopeia in first century BCE (Duvall 2015). Sir William O'Shaughnessy is credited with bringing cannabis to modern Western medicine when, in 1840, he described its analgesic, sedative, anti-inflammatory, anti-spasmodic and anti-convulsant effects and its use in palliating a patient's end-stage rabies symptoms (Aggarwal 2016). For some time, cannabis was included in the United States Pharmacopeia, but was counted as a controlled substance in the 1925 International Opium convention and banned in the United States in 1938 (Duvall 2015). Interest in access to the whole cannabis plant for medicinal purposes, rather than only government-approved pharmaceutical cannabinoid medicines, has burgeoned in the United States with more than half of U.S. districts passing medical use laws since the late 1990s (Procon.org 2017). Cannabis possession, whether for recreational or medicinal purposes, remains illegal in most countries with only a small number of countries having widely legalized medical use to date (Duvall 2015).

CANNABINOIDS AND THE ENDOCANNABINOID SYSTEM

Cannabis Sativa L is a species of the *Cannabaceae* family thought to have as many as four distinct genetic subspecies: *C. sativa, C. indica, C. ruderalis* and *C. afghanica* (Piomelli and Russo 2016). Although in folklore some have used the terms *indica* and *sativa* to describe differences in cannabinoid content and therefore physiologic effects, they have more formally been used to indicate differences in plant morphology and use (*indica:* fiber/seed, *sativa:* psychoactive effects) (Backes 2014, Duvall 2015). Decades of interbreeding and hybridization have resulted in a wide variety of cannabis chemotypes termed, chemovars; as a result, plants have varying levels of physiologically and psychologically active compounds. Thus, it is suggested that a given chemovar's effects instead be described upon correlation of its biochemical analysis with its observed effects on patients (Piomelli and Russo 2016).

Understanding what makes cannabis unique requires knowledge of the human-endocannabinoid system. This system is composed of cannabinoid receptors, endogenously produced cannabinoids (endocannabinoids) and the enzymes responsible for their synthesis and deactivation (Vermuri and Makriyannis 2015). The primary cannabinoid receptors, termed CB1 and CB2, exhibit different distribution patterns with CB1 present primarily in the nervous system and CB2 present primarily in peripheral and immune tissues (Battista et al. 2012). Via interaction with these receptors, endocannabinoids exert effects on various physiological processes including immune, metabolic, hormonal and cognitive and behavioral functions, to name a few (Battista et al. 2012). Phytocannabinoids are plant-derived substances that interact with the endocannabinoid system and/or share similar chemical structure to cannabinoids (Gertsch et al. 2010). The cannabis plant contains over 120 phytocannabinoids, as well as terpenoids, both of which exert a wide variety of physiologic effects and account for interest in its medicinal use (Russo 2011; Morales et al. 2017). It is thought that synergistic effects of cannabis' phytocannabinoids and terpenoids may be responsible for the belief that use of the whole plant is more effective than use of individual synthesized or extracted cannabinoids for desired medicinal effects. This concept of cannabis synergism has been termed "the entourage effect" (Russo 2011).

CANNABINOID AND TERPENOID EFFECTS

Of the 120-plus phytocannabinoids, only a small number have been well researched. Table 33.1 lists the most abundant and commonly studied phytocannabinoids and noted physiologic effects of cannabinoids. The most widely known cannabinoids are Δ-9-tetrahydrocannabinol (THC) and cannabidiol (CBD). Noted therapeutic properties of THC include analgesic, anti-emetic, anti-inflammatory, anti-spasmodic, orexigenic and sedative effects (Russo and Guy 2006). Noted therapeutic properties of CBD include analgesia, anti-convulsant, antipsychotic, anxiolytic and anti-emetic effects. When used concurrently with THC (from 2:1 to 1:2 of THC to CBD), CBD reduces the undesirable effects of THC such as anxiety, sedation and tachycardia (Russo and Guy 2006). Cannabinoid medicines include synthetic or semi-synthetic single-molecule pharmaceuticals, liquid cannabis extracts and whole cannabis, also referred to as a phytocannabinoid dense botanical (Aggarwal et al. 2009). Table 33.2 summarizes the various types of cannabinoid medicines, their active compounds and clinical usage status. Dronabinol and nabilone are prescribed to manage chemotherapy-induced nausea and vomiting; dronabinol is also used for anorexia accompanied by weight loss in AIDS patients. Nabiximols is prescribed for muscle spasticity in multiple sclerosis and pain in advanced cancer, while Epidiolex is prescribed for treating certain refractory seizure syndromes (Vemuri and Makriyannis 2015; US Food and Drug Administration 2018). Availability of both prescription and non-prescription forms of cannabis will vary by country.

Terpenoids, which are the essential oil components of the cannabis plant that give it its characteristic aroma and flavor, have noted physiologic effects (Russo 2011). They are found in many different plants, including several used in and as foods, and have generally recognized as safe

TABLE 33.1
Commonly Studied Cannabinoids and Cannabinoid Physiologic Effects

Cannabinoids	Delta-9-tetrahydrocannabinol (Δ-9-THC or THC)
	Delta-8-tetrahydrocannabinol (Δ-8-THC)
	Cannabinol (CBN)
	Cannabidiol (CBD)
	Cannabigerol (CBG)
	Cannabichromene (CBC)
	Delta-9-tetrahydrocannabivarin (THCV)
	Cannabivarin (CBV)
	Cannabidivarin (CBDV)
	Cannabinodiol (CBND)
	Cannabielsoin (CBE)
	Cannabicyclol (CBL)
	Cannabitriol (CBT)
Physiologic effects	Analgesic
	Anti-anxiety
	Antibiotic
	Anticonvulsant
	Anti-emetic
	Antifungal
	Anti-inflammatory
	Antioxidant (neuroprotective)
	Antispasmodic
	Bronchodilatory
	Cytotoxic (antitumor)
	Muscle relaxant
	Psychoactive
	Sedative

Source: Morales, P. et al. 2017. *Progress in the Chemistry of Organic Natural Products* 103:103–131; Russo, E.B. 2011. *British Journal of Pharmacology* 163:1344–1364.

(GRAS) status in the United States (Russo 2011). Terpenoids found in cannabis include limonene, pinene, myrcene, linalool, ß-caryophyllene, caryophyllene oxide, nerolidol, and phytol (Russo 2011). Their documented pharmacologic activities include analgesia, anti-anxiety, anti-inflammatory, bronchodilation, sedative, anti-convulsant and anti-fungal to name a few (Russo 2011).

EFFICACY OF CANNABIS FOR PALLIATING NUTRITION-RELATED SYMPTOMS

There is evidence that cannabinoids may be effective for palliating nutrition-related symptoms such as anorexia, chemotherapy-induced nausea and vomiting, taste changes and weight loss as well as pain. Available evidence is summarized in Table 33.3 and primarily includes studies of cannabinoid pharmaceuticals. Limitations of these studies include lack of placebo (in some cases), small numbers of test subjects, lack of blinding and retrospectively reviewed data. In most of these studies, cannabinoid dosing is specific in dose and frequency rather than ad lib use based on tolerance and relief of symptoms, the latter of which represents a pattern more typical of persons using whole cannabis products. In addition, studies of single cannabinoids are unlikely to represent the effects of the full spectrum of cannabinoids and terpenoids that are available in whole cannabis

TABLE 33.2
Types of Cannabinoid Medicines

Category	Names (Trade)	Active Compound(s)	Clinical Usage Status
Cannabinoid pharmaceuticals	Dronabinol (Marinol)	Synthetic THC	Prescription
	Nabilone (Cesamet)	Synthetic THC analog	Prescription
	Levonantradol	Synthetic THC analog	Research discontinued
Liquid cannabis extracts	Cannabidiol (Epidiolex)	CBD	Prescription
	Nabiximols (Sativex)	THC and CBD	Prescription
Phytocannabinoid dense botanicals	Whole cannabis and associated products	THC, CBD, other cannabinoids, terpenoids	Legality, availability and product forms vary by country, state or local municipality

Source: Vemuri, V.K. and A. Makriyannis. 2015. Clinical Pharmacology and Therapeautics 97:553–558.
Abbreviations: CBD, cannabidiol; THC, tetrahydrocannabinol.

products. As shown in Table 33.4, an observational study of cancer patients using medical cannabis ad lib showed statistically significant improvements in degree of self-reported anorexia, nausea, vomiting and weight loss (Bar-Sela et al. 2013). Finally, it should be noted that the aforementioned observational study and a number of reviews suggest that cannabinoid pharmaceuticals and whole cannabis alike provide modest to significant relief of cancer and neuropathic pain compared with placebo or active controls (Martín-Sánchez et al. 2009; Lynch and Campbell 2011; Aggarwal 2013;

TABLE 33.3
Studies of Various Cannabinoids for Palliation of Nutrition-Related Issues

Condition	Cannabinoid Type	Study Results	References
Anorexia:			
Cancer	Dronabinol	Less effective than Megestrol (S)	Jatoi et al. (2002)
		Increased appetite versus placebo (S)	Brisbois et al. (2011)
	Whole cannabis extract (THC+CBD versus THC)	No difference	Strasser et al. (2006)
HIV/AIDS	Dronabinol	Increased appetite (S)	Beal et al. (1995)
			DeJesus et al. (2007)
	Dronabinol and cannabis	Increased calorie intake (S)	Haney et al. (2007)
Nausea/vomiting:			
Cancer treatment	Dronabinol	Reduced nausea: >neuroleptics and placebo, =ondansetron (S)	Machado Rocha et al. (2008), Meiri et al. (2011)
HIV/AIDS	Cannabis (smoked)	Reduced nausea: =/> dronabinol	Musty and Rossi (2001)
	Nabiximols	Reduced nausea (S)	Duran et al. (2010)
	Dronabinol	Reduced nausea (S)	Beal et al. (1995)
			DeJesus et al. (2007)
Taste changes (cancer)	Dronabinol	Improved taste (S)	Brisbois et al. (2011)
Weight loss:			
Cancer	Dronabinol	Not effective	Jatoi et al. (2002)
	Nabilone	Not effective	Cote et al. (2016)
HIV/AIDS	Dronabinol	Increased or maintained weight	Beal et al. (1995)
	Dronabinol, cannabis versus placebo	Increased weight (S)	DeJesus et al. (2007)
			Haney et al. (2007)

Abbreviations: CBD, cannabidiol; S, statistical significance; THC, tetrahydrocannabinol.

TABLE 33.4
Observed Effect of Whole Cannabis Use on Cancer Symptom Management

Symptom	Grade	Before Use (% patients)	After Six to Eight Weeks Use (% Patients)
Anorexia	0	32	68
	1–2	65	27
	3–4	3	5
Nausea	0	32	69
	1–2	65	27
	3–4	3	4
Vomiting	0	69	92
	1–2	31	8
Weight loss	0	32	67
	1–2	65	33
	3–4	5	0
Pain	0	19	42
	1–2	31	34
	3–4	51	25

Note: The percentage of patients experiencing cancer-related symptoms by symptom grade prior to and after six to eight weeks of *ad lib* whole cannabis use (Bar-Sela et al. 2013). Symptom grades: 0 = none, 1–2 = minimal, 3–4 = severe.

Bar-Sela et al. 2013; Deshpande et al. 2015; Aviram and Samuelly-Leichtag 2017). Although pain is not often thought of as directly impacting nutrition, the most common side effects of opioid pain medications, constipation and nausea, can cause or contribute to preexisting anorexia and nausea (Ross and Alexander 2001; Wiffen et al. 2017). In a survey of persons substituting cannabis for opioid pain medication, 89% agreed that opioid use results in unwanted side effects including constipation and nausea, and 92% agreed that cannabis side effects were more tolerable than those of opioids (Reiman et al. 2017). Thus, cannabis may effectively both reduce and prevent some nutrition-related issues in the palliative care population.

METHODS OF ADMINISTRATION AND PHARMACOKINETICS

Surveys suggest inhalation methods are the most popular means of administration among active medical cannabis users (Hazekamp et al. 2013; Shiplo et al. 2016). A survey of advanced cancer patients who would consider participating in a cannabis clinical trial indicated a preference for oral delivery (tablets/capsules, 71%) followed by oro-mucosal (mouth spray, 42%) or vaporizer (41%) (Luckett et al. 2016). However, as only 13% of respondents had ever used cannabis, their stated preferences may reflect perception of harm from cannabis inhalation. Most notable differences between these modes of administration include onset, duration of effect(s) and metabolite production. As seen in Table 33.5, lung or oro-mucosal delivery results in shorter time to onset (both) and shorter duration of effect (lung) while oral ingestion incurs greater first-pass metabolism. This results in reduced bioavailability of THC due to its conversion to 11-OH-THC (Grotenhermen 2003). In addition, 11-OH-THC is noted to be a highly potent psychoactive metabolite which penetrates the brain more rapidly and in greater amounts than THC (Lemberger et al. 1973; Grotenhermen 2003). Further, when the two are used in a 1:1 ratio, CBD appears to antagonize unwanted physiologic and psychoactive effects of THC (such as tachycardia, sedation, anxiety, memory impairment),

TABLE 33.5
Cannabis Pharmacokinetics by Route of Administration

Route/Examples	Onset	Duration	Bioavailability	Comments
Lung				
Smoking, Vaporization (Huestis 2007; Grotenhermen 2003; Aggarwal 2013)	Seconds to 10 minutes	2–4 hours	10%–35%	Bioavailability depends on volume inhaled, puff duration, length of breath hold
Oro-mucosal				
Tinctures, sprays, mists (Guy and Robson 2003; MacCallum and Russo 2018)	15–45 minutes	6–8 hours	Highly variable, increases with food intake	Less first-pass metabolism
Gastrointestinal				
Tablets, capsules, edibles (food/liquid/candy) (Grotenhermen 2003; Huestis 2007; Aggarwal 2013; MacCallum and Russo 2018)	1–3 hours	6–8 hours	4%–20%	First-pass metabolism results in 11-OH THC and decreased THC availability
Rectal				
Suppository (Grotenhermen 2003; Huestis 2007)	1–8 hours (to "peak concentration")	Not described	Approximately 2× that of oral	Less first-pass metabolism
Topical				
Creams, salves, patches (Valiveti et al. 2004)	1.4 hours[a]	48 hours[a] (patch)	Not described	CBD/CBN concentrations approximately 10-fold higher

Source: Adapted and updated, with permission, from *The Integrative RDN*, Fall 2017, Vol. 20 Issue 2, the newsletter of the Dietitians in Integrative and Function Medicine, a Dietetic Practice Group of the Academy of Nutrition and Dietetics.

Note: The onset and duration of effect(s) and bioavailability of cannabinoids by physiologic route of administration, including examples of methods of administration as well as additional comments regarding bioavailability and metabolism (Grotenhermen 2003, Guy and Robson 2003, Valiveti et al. 2004, Huestis 2007, Aggarwal 2013, MacCallum and Russo 2018). Data are for THC unless otherwise noted.

Abbreviations: CBD, cannabidiol; CBN, cannabinol;11-OH THC, 11-hydroxy-tetrahydrocannabinol; THC, tetrahydrocannabinol; Δ-8 THC, delta-8-tetrahydrocannabinol.

[a] Δ-8 THC in an animal model.

while also providing analgesic, anti-emetic, anxiolytic and anti-psychotic effects independently or synergistically with other cannabinoids (Russo and Guy 2006). Attenuation of THC's psychoactive effects is suggested to be due to CBD's ability to block the conversion of THC to 11-OH-THC (Russo and Guy 2006). Thus, patients who wish to minimize psychoactive effects might be directed to consider oro-mucosally delivered cannabinoid products that allow for delivery of THC and CBD in near equal amounts.

ADVERSE EFFECTS, CONTRAINDICATIONS, DRUG INTERACTIONS AND PRECAUTIONS

As with any medication or herbal product, a discussion of cannabis use should include adverse effects, contraindications, drug interactions and appropriate precautions. Commonly noted short-term adverse effects include anxiety; confusion; disorientation; dizziness; drowsiness; euphoria; fatigue; hallucination; hypotension; impaired memory, learning and psychomotor speed; loss of balance; nausea; psychosis; somnolence; tachycardia; vomiting; and visual disturbances (Deshpande et al. 2015; Whiting et al. 2015; Aviram and Samuelly-Leichtag 2017). Allergy to any form of

TABLE 33.6
Suggested Contraindications and Precautions for Medical Cannabis Use

Contraindication or Precaution	Rationale	References
	Contraindication	
Severe cardio-pulmonary disease	Potential for hypotension, hypertension, syncope, tachycardia, angina, myocardial infarction, cardiomyopathy, cardiac death	Health Canada (2013), Sachs et al. (2015)
Respiratory insufficiency (asthma, COPD)	Potential for acute increase in inflammation and airway resistance, destruction of lung tissue, chronic bronchitis and lung tissue inflammation, increased emphysema risk (smoked cannabis)	Sachs et al. (2015)
Severe hepatic or renal disease	Increased risk of steatosis; limited data on renal effects	Health Canada (2013)
Personal history of psychiatric disorders; family history of schizophrenia	Association between cannabis use and psychosis, schizophrenia	Kahan et al. (2014)
	Precaution	
Substance abuse disorder	Increased risk of cannabis use disorder	Kahan et al. (2014)
Active psychiatric disorder (anxiety, depression, mania)	Risk for exacerbation of psychiatric disorders, suicidality in context of mental health disorder	Sachs et al. (2015)
Concurrent use of high doses of opiates, benzodiazepines, psychoactive drugs and alcohol	Increased or synergistic central nervous system depressant or psychoactive effects	Health Canada (2013)

medicinal cannabinoid or its vehicle is a clear contraindication to use. Cannabis is also not indicated during pregnancy and breastfeeding or for those intending to become pregnant (Health Canada 2013). Some suggested contraindications and precautions and their associated rationales are presented in Table 33.6. Anticipated or reported cannabis-drug interactions are listed in Table 33.7. Finally, additional risks include exposure to microbial or fungal contamination, such as *Aspergillus* from smoked cannabis, or to solvents and unapproved pesticides, such as isopentane and paclobutrazol found in cannabinoid concentrates, and inaccurate content labeling leading to difficulty with dose titration (Raber et al. 2015; Ruchlemer et al. 2015; Vandrey et al. 2015).

APPLICATIONS TO OTHER AREAS OF TERMINAL OR PALLIATIVE CARE

As previously discussed, there is public interest in the medicinal use of whole cannabis and cannabis-based products for various maladies. Specifically, it is often of interest as an alternative to opioids for pain management (Reiman et al. 2017). Similarly, some people may prefer it to other conventional treatments when it is thought that cannabis would have fewer or more tolerable side effects. It has been suggested that in addition to managing nausea, anorexia and pain, cannabis may also have favorable effects on anxiety, depression and insomnia for some and thus be quite useful in palliative or terminal care settings (Abrams and Guzman 2015).

CONSIDERING CANNABINOIDS FOR PALLIATIVE CARE: GUIDELINES

When to consider cannabis for symptom management depends on many factors, including, especially, whether or not it is legally available for use. Where available, cannabinoid pharmaceuticals such as dronabinol, nabilone or nabiximols may be readily employed for patients who have failed other, more conventional, therapies. Since it is not without controversy or complication, it is often suggested

TABLE 33.7
Reported or Expected Cannabis-Drug Interactions

Effect (Reported or Expected)	Drug
Cannabis increases effects of drug: (Reported)	Alcohol
	CNS depressants
Cannabinoids increase bioavailability of drug: (Expected)	Carbamazepine
	Phenobarbital
	Phenytoin
	Primidone
	Rifampin
	Rifabutin
	Troglitazone
Drug increases concentration of:	
THC (Reported)	Ketoconazole
THC (Expected)	Amiodarone
	Boceprevir
	Cimetidine
	Clarithromycin
	Cyclosporine
	Cotrimoxizole
	Diltiazem
	Erythromycin
	Fluconazole
	Fluoxetine
	Fluvoxamine
	Itraconazole
	Isoniazid
	Metronidazole
	Ritonavir
	Voriconazole
	Verapamil
CBD (Reported)	Ketoconazole
CBD (Expected)	Cimetidine
Drug decreases concentration of THC: (Reported)	Rifampin

Source: Health Canada. 2013. Information for health care professionals: Cannabis (marihuana, marijuana) and the cannabinoids. https://www.canada.ca/en/health-canada/services/drugs-health-products/medical-use-marijuana/information-medical-practitioners/information-health-care-professionals-cannabis-marihuana-marijuana-cannabinoids.html (accessed January 13, 2018); Horn, J.R. and P.D. Hansten. 2014. Drug interactions with marijuana. Pharmacy Times. December 2014. http://www.pharmacytimes.com/publications/issue/2014/december2014/drug-interactions-with-marijuana

Abbreviations: CBD, cannabidiol; CNS, central nervous system; THC, tetrahydrocannabinol.

that customary pharmaceutical treatments be tried without success prior to the employment of non-prescription cannabis-based products. It is worth noting that, especially in areas where medical cannabis laws enable relatively easy access to whole cannabis products, patients may elect to try cannabis in place of conventional treatments with or without the support or knowledge of their healthcare provider. Whether actively recommending medical cannabis or discussing a patient's interest in it, it is important that healthcare providers engage in the discussion and provide patients with education and guidelines.

ETHICAL ISSUES

Opinions vary as to whether providers should recommend or discuss medical cannabis with patients. In one survey, 46% of practicing physicians said cannabis should not be recommended at all, and cited concerns about liability and licensure, lack of evidence, practice policy, and news media as influencing their decision not to recommend it (Konrad and Reid 2013). Conversely, although a majority of medical students believe that cannabis can cause physical and mental harm, 74% believe that physicians should recommend it as a medical therapy (Chan et al. 2017). Physicians and other healthcare providers have an ethical responsibility to support patients' autonomy, to minimize risk of patient harm and to act in the patient's best interest. At a minimum, providers should familiarize themselves with current available evidence of cannabis' potential benefits and burdens. Provided local laws do not prohibit it, providers should be open to having a dialogue with patients interested in medical cannabis for symptom management. In some situations, practicing beneficence and respecting autonomy may mean setting aside personal bias and supporting a patient's decision to try cannabis when other means of symptom management have failed. To help patients avoid harm, it is critical that healthcare providers be able to provide patients with accurate information regarding any information relevant to the individual's situation, including pharmacokinetics of preferred administration route, adverse reactions, contraindications and applicable local laws. Minimizing harm could also mean discouraging cannabis use when, in the informed provider's judgement, the risks of using cannabis outweigh its potential benefits. In areas where medical cannabis is easily accessed, patients should have access to adequate education so that they can make an informed decision about its use. Finally, because context is critical, the unique circumstances of each individual patient should be carefully considered by the advising healthcare provider or team.

KEY FACTS: DISCUSSIONS REGARDING CANNABINOIDS FOR PALLIATIVE CARE

- Consider cannabinoids after trials of more conventional treatments are unsuccessful.
- Advise that cannabinoids are contraindicated for persons with cannabinoid allergy, severe cardio-pulmonary disease, respiratory insufficiency (smoked cannabis), severe hepatic or renal disease, personal history of psychiatric disorders or family history of schizophrenia, or for those who are pregnant, breastfeeding or attempting to conceive.
- Counsel patients who desire gastrointestinal administration (tablets, capsules, food/liquid) regarding longer time to onset of effect(s) and longer duration of effect(s) as well as greater first-pass metabolism of tetrahydrocannabinol to 11-hydroxy-tetrahydrocannabinol, which is itself a very potent psychoactive compound.
- Suggest oro-mucosal delivery of whole cannabis–based products to cannabis naïve patients due to shorter onset of effect and less first-pass metabolism.
- Counsel patients using inhaled whole cannabis products of the risk of exacerbation of pulmonary conditions and exposure to contaminants (*aspergillus* in whole cannabis, solvents or pesticides in concentrates).
- Advise that concurrent use of cannabidiol with tetrahydrocannabinol may reduce unwanted psychological and physiological reactions to tetrahydrocannabinol.
- Educate patients as to the limitations of non-pharmaceutical cannabis products including limited or lack of regulation for product quality, purity and accuracy of product content labeling.
- Evaluate for and counsel regarding actual or potential cannabis-drug interactions, including that the use of cannabis concurrently with opiates, benzodiazepines, psychoactive drugs and alcohol may increase central nervous system depressant or psychoactive effects of these drugs.

SUMMARY POINTS

- Cannabinoids are naturally occurring and synthetic compounds which interact with the body's internal cannabinoid receptors producing various physiological effects.
- Noted therapeutic properties of cannabinoids include analgesic, anti-emetic, anti-convulsant, anti-anxiety, anti-spasmodic, anti-inflammatory and sedative effects.
- The phytocannabinoids tetrahydrocannabinol and cannabidiol are the most widely known, though not the only, active constituents of interest in cannabis-based medicines and products.
- There is some evidence that cannabinoids may aid in palliation of anorexia, nausea and vomiting, pain, taste changes, and weight loss.
- Tetrahydrocannabinol is of interest for its potential anti-emetic, analgesic, anxiolytic, gustatory and antispasmodic effects, but also may also induce undesirable psychoactive and physiologic effects.
- Cannabidiol is of interest for its anti-emetic, analgesic and anti-anxiety effects; is devoid of psychoactive effects; and mitigates some of tetrahydrocannabinol's undesirable effects.
- Noted adverse effects of cannabinoids include anxiety, confusion, dizziness, hypotension, impaired memory, paranoia, visual disturbances and tachycardia.
- Whether cannabinoid pharmaceuticals are prescribed or whole cannabis products are suggested may depend on known benefits versus burdens as well as what is legally available to the patient.
- Healthcare providers have a responsibility to provide patients with education regarding cannabis' efficacy, pharmacokinetics, adverse effects, contraindications, actual or potential drug interactions and any other relevant benefits or risks of its use (including local laws and legal risks).
- Providers should consider each patient's unique situation when providing advice regarding medical cannabis use.

LIST OF ABBREVIATIONS

11-OH-THC	11-Hydroxy-Tetrahydrocannabinol
CB1	Cannabinoid Receptor 1
CB2	Cannabinoid Receptor 2
CBD	Cannabidiol
CNS	Central Nervous System
GRAS	Generally Recognized as Safe
THC	Tetrahydrocannabinol

REFERENCES

Abrams, D. and M. Guzman. 2015. Cannabis in cancer care. *Clinical Pharmacology and Therapeutics* 97:575–587.

Aggarwal, S. et al. 2009. Medicinal use of cannabis in the United States: Historical perspectives, current trends, and future directions. *Journal of Opioid Management* 5:153–168.

Aggarwal, S. 2016. Use of cannabinoids in cancer care: Palliative care. *Current Oncology* 23:S33–S36.

Aggarwal, S.K. 2013. Cannabinergic pain medicine: A concise clinical primer and survey of randomized-controlled trial results. *Clinical Journal of Pain* 29:162–171.

Aviram, J. and G. Samuelly-Leichtag. 2017. Efficacy of cannabis-based medicines for pain management: A systematic review and meta-analysis of randomized controlled trials. *Pain Physician* 20:E755–E796.

Backes, M. 2014. *Cannabis pharmacy*. New York: Blackdog & Leventhal.

Bar-Sela, G. et al. 2013. The medical necessity for medicinal cannabis: Prospective, observational study evaluating the treatment in cancer patients on supportive or palliative care. *Evidence Based Complementary and Alternative Medicine* 2013:1–8.

Battista, N. et al. 2012. The endocannabinoid system: An overview. *Frontiers in Behavioral Neuroscience* 6:1–7.

Beal, J.E. et al. 1995. Dronabinol as a treatment for anorexia associated weight loss for people with AIDS. *Journal of Pain and Symptom Management* 10:89–97.

Brisbois, T.D. et al. 2011. Delta-9-tetrahydrocannabinol may palliate altered chemosensory perception in cancer patients: Results of a randomized, double-blind, placebo-controlled pilot trial. *Annals of Oncology* 22:2086–2093.

Chan, E. et al. 2017. Colorado medical students' attitudes and beliefs about medical marijuana. *Journal of General Internal Medicine* 32:458–463.

Cote, M. et al. 2016. Improving quality of life with nabilone during radiotherapy treatments for head and neck cancers: A randomized double-blind placebo-controlled trial. *Annals of Otology, Rhinology and Laryngology* 125:317–324.

DeJesus, E. et al. 2007. THC improves appetite and reverses weight loss in AIDS patients. *Journal of the International Association of Physicians in AIDS Care* 6: 95–100.

Deshpande, A. et al. 2015. Efficacy and adverse effects of medical marijuana for chronic noncancer pain: Systematic review of randomized controlled trials. *Canadian Family Physician* 61:e372–e381.

Duran, M. et al. 2010. Preliminary efficacy and safety of an oromucosal standardized cannabis extract in chemotherapy-induced nausea and vomiting. *British Journal of Clinical Pharmacology* 70:656–663.

Duvall, C. 2015. *Cannabis (Botanical)*. London: Reaktion Books Co.

Gertsch, J. et al. 2010. Phytocannabinoids beyond the *Cannabis* plant—Do they exist? *British Journal of Pharmacology* 160:523–529.

Grotenhermen, F. 2003. Pharmacokinetics and pharmacodynamics of cannabinoids. *Clinical Pharmacokinetics* 42:327–360.

Guy, G.W. and P.J. Robson. 2003. A Phase I, open label, four-way crossover study to compare the pharmacokinetic profiles of a single dose of 20 mg of a cannabis based medicine extract (CBME) administered on 3 different areas of the buccal mucosa and to investigate the pharmacokinetics of CBME per oral in healthy male and female volunteers (GWPK0112). *Journal of Cannabis Therapeutics.* 3:79–120.

Haney, M. et al. 2007. Dronabinol and marijuana in HIV-positive marijuana smokers. *Journal of Acquired Immune Deficiency Syndrome* 45:545–554.

Hazekamp, A. et al. 2013. The medicinal use of cannabis and cannabinoids – An international cross-sectional survey on administration forms. *Journal of Psychoactive Drugs* 45:199–210.

Health Canada. 2013. Information for health care professionals: Cannabis (marihuana, marijuana) and the cannabinoids. https://www.canada.ca/en/health-canada/services/drugs-health-products/medical-use-marijuana/information-medical-practitioners/information-health-care-professionals-cannabis-marihuana-marijuana-cannabinoids.html (accessed January 13, 2018).

Horn, J.R. and P.D. Hansten. 2014. Drug interactions with marijuana. *Pharmacy Times.* December 2014. http://www.pharmacytimes.com/publications/issue/2014/december2014/drug-interactions-with-marijuana

Huestis, M.A. 2007. Human cannabinoid pharmacokinetics. *Chemistry and Biodiversity* 4:1770–1804.

Jatoi, A. et al. 2002. Dronabinol versus megestrol acetate versus combination therapy for cancer-associated anorexia: A North Central Cancer Treatment Group study. *Journal of Clinical Oncology* 20:567–573.

Kahan, M. et al. 2014. Prescribing smoked cannabis for chronic noncancer pain: Preliminary recommendations. *Canadian Family Physician* 60:1083–1090.

Kondrad, E. and A. Reid. 2013. Colorado family physicians' attitudes towards medical marijuana. *Journal of the Americal Board of Family Medicine* 26:52–60.

Lemberger, L. et al. 1973. Comparitive pharmacology of Δ-9-tetrahydrocannabinol and its metabolite, 11-OH-Δ-9-tetrahydrocannabinol. *Journal of Clinical Investigation* 52:2411–2417.

Luckett, T. et al. 2016. Clinical trials of medicinal cannabis for appetite-related symptoms from advanced cancer: A survey of preferences, attitudes and beliefs among patients willing to consider participation. *Internal Medicine Journal* 46:1269–1275.

Lynch, M.E. and F. Campbell. 2011. Cannabinoids for treatment of chronic non-cancer pain; a systematic review of randomized trials. *British Journal of Clinical Pharmacology* 72:735–744.

MacCallum, C.A. and E. Russo. 2018. Practical considerations in medical cannabis administration and dosing. *European Journal of Internal Medicine* 49:12–19.

Machado Rocha, F.C. et al. 2008. Therapeutic use of *Cannabis sativa* on chemotherapy-induced nausea and vomiting among cancer patients: Systematic review and meta-analysis. *European Journal of Cancer Care* 17:431–443.

Martín-Sánchez, E. et al. 2009. Systematic review and meta-analysis of cannabis treatment for chronic pain. *Pain Medicine* 10:1353–1368.

Meiri, E. et al. 2011. Efficacy of dronabinol alone and in combination with ondansetron versus ondansetron alone for delayed chemotherapy-induced nausea and vomiting. *Current Medical and Research Opinion* 23:533–43.

Morales, P. et al. 2017. Molecular targets of the phytocannabinoids – A complex picture. *Progress in the Chemistry of Organic Natural Products* 103:103–131.

Musty R.E. and R. Rossi. 2001. Effects of smoked cannabis and oral Δ 9-tetrahydrocannabinol on nausea and emesis after cancer chemotherapy: A review of state clinical trials. *Journal of Cannabis Therapeutics* 1:29–43.

Piomelli, D. and E.B. Russo. 2016. The *Cannabis sativa* versus *Cannabis indica* debate: An interview with Ethan Russo, MD. *Cannabis and Cannabinoid Research* 1:44–46.

Procon.org. November 30, 2017. 29 legal medical marijuana states and DC. http://medicalmarijuana.procon.org/view.resource.php?resourceID=000881. (accessed December 6, 2017).

Raber, J.C. et al. 2015. Understanding dabs: Contamination concerns of cannabis concentrates and cannabinoid transfer during the act of dabbing. *Journal of Toxicological Sciences* 40:797–803.

Reiman, A. et al. 2017. Cannabis as a substitute for opioid-based pain medication: Patient self-report. *Cannabis and Cannabinoid Research* 2:160–166.

Ross, D.D. and C.S. Alexander. 2001. Management of common symptoms in terminally ill patients: Part I. *American Family Physician* 64:807–814.

Ruchlemer, R. et al. 2015. Inhaled medicinal cannabis and the immunocompromised patient. *Supportive Care in Cancer* 23:819–822.

Russo, E. 2007. History of cannabis and its preparation in saga, science, and sobriquet. *Chemistry and Biodiversity* 4:1614–1648.

Russo, E. and G.W. Guy. 2006. A tale of two cannabinoids: The therapeutic rationale for combining tetrahydrocannabinol and cannabidiol. *Medical Hypotheses* 66:234–246.

Russo, E.B. 2011. Taming THC: Potential cannabis synergy and phytocannabinoid-terpenoid entourage effects. *British Journal of Pharmacology* 163:1344–1364.

Sachs, J. et al. 2015. Safety and toxicology of cannabinoids. *Neurotherapeutics* 12:735–746.

Shiplo, S. et al. 2016. Medical cannabis us in Canada: Vapourization and modes of delivery. *Harm Reduction Journal* 13:30–39.

Strasser, F. et al. 2006. Comparison of orally administered cannabis extract and Δ-9-tetrahydrocannabinol in treating patients with cancer-related anorexia-cachexia syndrome: A multicenter, phase III, randomized, double-blind, placebo-controlled clinical trial from the Cannabis-In-Cachexia-Study-Group. *Journal of Clinical Oncology* 24:3394–3400.

U.S. Food and Drug Administration. 2018. FDA approves first drug comprised of an active ingredient derived from marijuana to treat rare, severe forms of epilepsy. https://www.fda.gov/newsevents/newsroom/pressannouncements/ucm611046.htm (accessed March 26, 2019).

Valiveti, S. et al. 2004. Transdermal delivery of the synthetic cannabinoid WIN 55,212-2: *In vitro/in vivo* correlation. *Pharmaceutical Research* 21:1137–1145.

Vandrey, R. et al. 2015. Cannabinoid dose and label accuracy in edible medical cannabis products. *Journal of the American Medical Association* 313:2491–2493.

Vemuri, V.K. and A. Makriyannis. 2015. Medicinal chemistry of cannabinoids. *Clinical Pharmacology and Therapeautics* 97:553–558.

Whiting, P.F. et al. 2015. Cannabinoids for medical use: A systematic review and meta-analysis. *Journal of the American Medical Association* 313:2456–2473.

Wiffen, P.J. et al. 2017. Opioids for cancer pain – An overview of Cochrane reviews. *Cochrane Database of Systematic Reviews* 7:1–4.

Section VI

Case Study and Resources

34 Case Study
Refractory Cancer Cachexia

David Blum

CONTENT

CASE STUDY

Mr. B, 54 years old, a farmer from a rural area in Switzerland, with a long history of smoking was previously diagnosed with squamous cell carcinoma G3 Carcinoma of the Tonsil pT2 pN2b (4/24) M0 and treated with tonsillectomy, radical neck dissection and received additional radiotherapy with 60 Gray. After a first recurrence a year later he received salvage surgery, but was lost to follow-up thereafter.

Two years later he presented himself with voice changes, and mood changes as well. Additionally he suffered from severe fatigue, which prevented him from working on his farm. A second recurrence was diagnosed by a biopsy from the epipharynx.

In a positron emission tomography (PET) scan, a 4 cm tumor para-retropharyngeal left was seen, furthermore metastases in the lung right (12 mm) and pleura (2.5 × 2 cm) were diagnosed.

The case was discussed at the tumor board, and there was consensus that surgery or reirradiation were not options. And the evaluation of chemotherapy or immunotherapy was proposed. The patient declined a specific tumor therapy but asked for a consultation with the palliative care team.

The patient is attending the palliative care outpatient clinic, and is accompanied by his wife and daughter, a former nurse. As part of the comprehensive assessment at first consultation a systematic symptom assessment is performed and the following scores were obtained: Pain 6/10, Fatigue 3/10, Nausea 4/10, Depression 2/10, Anxiety 4/10, Drowsiness 1/10, Anorexia 5/10, Dyspnea 2/10, well-being 4/10; Minimum 1. Maximum 10.

Physical functioning was rated with a Karnofsky performance status of 70% and cognition was not impaired. Concerning illness understanding was the patient fully aware of his situation: he noticed recurrence a while ago but did not want medical treatment again, and delayed the visit at his general practitioner (GP) as long as possible.

Since he presented with severe pain, an analgesic therapy was initiated, with a nonsteroidal antirheumatic and an opioid, in addition with a prokinetic antiemetic agent and laxative therapy.

The patient presented with involuntary weight loss 8 kg (12%)/1 month, for example, 68 kg–60 kg and clinically with a loss of muscle mass. Nutritional assessment was performed by a nutritionist. Measured dietary intake was (averaged over two days): 1600 kcal/d (6700 kJ/d) (60% of requirements approximately 9300 kJ/d, 56 g protein (80%)/day) In the patient-generated subjective global assessment (PG-SGA) the score was B 14 which equals moderately or suspected malnutrition with significant nutrition impact symptoms affecting dietary intake. Therefore cachexia syndrome was diagnosed with the following secondary nutritional impact symptoms: pain, xerostomia, dysphagia, dental problems and constipation.

In consequence, in nutritional counselling the advice to increase energy and protein content and use moist and soft textured foods with extra sauces, encouraging nourishing foods and supplements was given. Pharmacotherapy with prokinetics and laxativa was already initiated. Counselling in psycho-oncology was performed where topics such as double awareness, legacy and end-of-life preparation were mentioned. The patient and his spouse reported discussions at the family table around food and appetite. The changing body image was bothering the family. The patient and his spouse are intensively discussing the current situation and sometimes quarrel over food. Mr. B wishes for more physical strength and would like to work in the garden. Furthermore, he wants to spend more time with his family. Two adult children live in the village nearby.

In a follow-up consultation, pain control was achieved. Nausea and constipation disappeared with the initiated medication, but fatigue was still present. Concerning nutrition, the patient was able increase his energy and protein intake almost up to the requirements.

As a next step, in order to treat fatigue and maintain physical function, exercise counselling was performed. But rather than exercising, the patient preferred to work with his cattle.

With established symptom control, almost sufficient nutritional intake, moderate activity due to physical work on the farm, understanding of his spouse for mood and appetite changes the patient achieved a decent quality of life for around four months. He was able to hold his weight and activity even though a tumour progression was detectable due to a palpable growing lymph node above the clavicle. Meanwhile, he rented out his farm and started to keep sheep in his garden.

He attended palliative outpatient clinic on a monthly basis. In the last consultation, a clear decline in performance status was observed. The patient declined further diagnostic or therapeutic measures.

There was consensus that cachexia reached the refractory state now, and attempts to increase nutritional intake or physical activity were no longer helpful. The focus was now on palliation. A home care team was organised. One day his wife called to inform us that the patient is now completely bedbound, but without severe other symptoms. The patient died three weeks later in the presence of his family.

His wife came for a bereavement talk two months later. She was still very sad, but grateful as well that her husband was able to be prepared for his death and spend his last weeks at home.

35 Recommended Resources for Diet and Nutrition in Palliative Care

Rajkumar Rajendram, Vinood B. Patel, and Victor R. Preedy

CONTENTS

INTRODUCTION

Palliative care is the holistic treatment of patients with life-threatening illnesses whose conditions cannot be cured [1]. This approach improves the quality of life of patients and their families facing the end-of-life problems associated with terminal illness. The duality of palliative care reaffirms life while recognising dying as "normal." It aims to provide the best possible quality of life for patients and their families by relieving suffering. To achieve this, palliative care focuses on the prevention and treatment of symptoms such as pain and nausea as well as other physical, psychosocial and spiritual problems [1]. There are many misconceptions about palliative care, so it is important to be clear that it neither hastens nor postpones death.

Food and eating are fundamental aspects of daily living. Besides clear effects on morbidity and mortality, diet and nutrition profoundly impact quality of life [2,3]. For example, many social pastimes occur around meals [2,3]. Cachexia is defined as anorexia, weight loss, weakness and fatigue [3]. It reduces performance status and quality of life [3,4]. Cachexia is very common in patients who require palliative care [2,4]. It is extremely distressing for patients and their families [2]. Nutritional support alone cannot reverse cachexia [4]. Indeed, it is truly devastating that cachexia is often refractory to any therapeutic intervention [4].

So, while terminally ill patients must receive food and beverages, the focus of their provision should be to improve quality of life and relieve symptoms rather than strive to reduce morbidity and mortality in vain. However, this simplistic statement disguises the plethora of clinical, ethical and moral dilemmas surrounding diet and nutrition in palliative care [4,5]. Furthermore, these dilemmas are often increased with advances in the understanding of cachexia and the availability of novel nutritional therapies. However, an analysis of the available literature shows that compared to some other fields, the available literature in peer-reviewed journals is relatively sparse. For example, a rudimentary analysis of published works on diet and nutrition shows that, in the past five years, there have been 26 times more research papers on infants than on palliative care. Furthermore, there have been 80 times more diet and nutrition papers on obesity, and 32 more on cancer, compared to palliative care. Nevertheless, there has been an approximate 400% increase in the number of papers on diet and nutrition in palliative care over the past 20 years.

For those new to the field, it is difficult to know which of the myriad of available sources are reliable. To assist colleagues who are interested in understanding more about diet and nutrition in palliative care, we have therefore produced expert-led tables containing reliable, up-to-date resources on diet and nutrition in palliative care in this chapter. The experts who assisted with the compilation of these tables of resources are acknowledged.

Tables 35.1 through 35.4 list the most up-to-date information on the regulatory bodies and professional societies (Table 35.1), journals on diet and nutrition in palliative care (Table 35.2), books (Table 35.3) and other online resources (Table 35.4) that are relevant to an evidence-based approach to diet and nutrition in palliative care.

TABLE 35.1
Regulatory Bodies, Professional Societies and Organisations

Academy of Nutrition and Dietetics www.eatright.org
African Palliative Care Association www.africanpalliativecare.org
American Academy of Hospice and Palliative Medicine www.aahpm.org
American Society for Parenteral and Enteral Nutrition www.nutritioncare.org
Asia Pacific Hospice Palliative Care Community www.aphn.org
Association for Paediatric Palliative Medicine www.appm.org.uk
British Dietetic Association (BDA) Paediatric Specialist Group www.bda.uk.com/regionsgroups/groups/paediatric/home
Canadian Association of Medical and Surgical Nurses https://medsurgnurse.ca/education-corner/end-of-life-care-and-artificial-nutrition
Canadian Cancer Society www.cancer.ca/en/cancer-information/cancer-journey/living-with-cancer/nutrition-for-people-with-cancer/?region=on
Canadian Hospice Palliative Care Association www.chpca.net
Canadian Society of Palliative Care Physicians www.cspcp.ca
Centre for Palliative Care www.centreforpallcare.org/page/41/resources
eHospice https://ehospice.com/
European Association for Palliative Care www.eapcnet.eu
Get Palliative Care www.getpalliativecare.org
Hospice Foundation of Taiwan www.hospice.org.tw
Hospice Palliative Care Ontario www.hpco.ca
International Association for Hospice and Palliative Care www.hospicecare.com
International Association for the Study of Pain www.iasp-pain.org
Italian Association of Medical Oncology www.aiom.it
Italian Society of Artificial Nutrition and Metabolism (SINPE) www.sinpe.org

(*Continued*)

TABLE 35.1 (*Continued*)
Regulatory Bodies, Professional Societies and Organisations

Japanese Society for Palliative Medicine
www.jspm.ne.jp/jspm_eng/index.html
Japanese Society for Pharmaceutical Palliative Care and Sciences
http://jpps.umin.jp
National Comprehensive Cancer Network
www.nccn.org
National Hospice and Palliative Care Organization
www.nhpco.org
Pallium Canada
pallium.ca
Palliative Care Research Society
www.pcrs.org.uk
Royal College of Paediatrics and Child Health
www.rcpch.ac.uk
The Society for the Promotion of Hospice Care
www.hospicecare.org.hk
Together for Short Lives
www.togetherforshortlives.org.uk
World Health Organization
www.who.int
Worldwide Hospice Palliative Care Alliance
www.thewhpca.org

Note: These are regulatory bodies, professional societies and organisations involved with diet and nutrition in palliative care or other aspects associated with palliative care such as pain control. Some appear in languages other than English, but online translations are useful in extracting information from such sites. At the time of preparing this table, all of the above links were viable, but it is not uncommon for web addresses to change.

TABLE 35.2
Journals Relevant to Palliative Care and Diet and Nutrition in Palliative Care

Section A

Journals Relevant to Palliative Care
Journal of Pain and Symptom Management
Journal of Palliative Medicine
American Journal of Hospice and Palliative Medicine
Palliative Medicine
International Journal of Palliative Nursing
Supportive Care in Cancer
BMC Palliative Care
Palliative and Supportive Care
BMJ Supportive and Palliative Care
Indian Journal of Palliative Care
Journal of Hospice and Palliative Nursing
Medecine Palliative
Annals of Palliative Medicine
European Journal of Palliative Care

(*Continued*)

TABLE 35.2 (*Continued*)
Journals Relevant to Palliative Care and Diet and Nutrition in Palliative Care

Journal of Clinical
Medicina Paliativa
Progress in Palliative Care
Journal of Oncology Practice
Journal of Palliative Care
Current Opinion in Supportive and Palliative Care
PLOS ONE
BMJ Online
Lancet Oncology
JAMA Internal Medicine
Psycho Oncology

Section B

Journals Relevant to Diet and Nutrition in Palliative Care

Journal of Pain and Symptom Management
Supportive Care in Cancer
Journal of Palliative Medicine
American Journal of Hospice and Palliative Medicine
BMC Palliative Care
Palliative Medicine
Annals of Palliative Medicine
Clinical Nutrition
Pediatrics
Current Opinion in Supportive and Palliative Care
Journal of Parenteral and Enteral Nutrition
Nursing Standard Royal College of Nursing Great Britain
BMJ Case Reports
BMJ Open
BMJ Supportive and Palliative Care
Indian Journal of Palliative Care
International Journal of Palliative Nursing
Nutrition
Nutrition and Cancer
Nutrition in Clinical Practice
PLOS ONE
World Journal of Gastroenterology
Cancer
Clinical Journal of the American Society of Nephrology
Cochrane Database of Systematic Reviews

Note: These are journals publishing original research and review articles related to palliative care (*Section A*) or diet and nutrition in palliative care (*Section B*). Included in this list are the top 25 journals that have published the largest number of articles over the past five years. See also *Nature Medicine* (www.nature.com/nm); *New England Journal of Medicine* (www.nejm.org); PLOS ONE (https://journals. plos.org/plosone). Note that some journals in *Section B* have only published about one paper per year.

TABLE 35.3
Relevant Books

Academy of Nutrition and Dietetics Pocket Guide to Enteral Nutrition, 2nd ed. Charney P, Malone A. Academy of Nutrition and Dietetics, 2013.
Academy of Nutrition and Dietetics Pocket Guide to the Nutrition Care Process and Cancer. Grant B. Academy of Nutrition and Dietetics, 2015.
Cannabis: A Complete Guide. Small E. CRC Press, 2016.
Cannabis: From Pariah to Prescription. Russo E. The Haworth Press, 2003.
Cannabis Pharmacy. Backes M. Blackdog & Leventhal, 2014.
Chronic Relief: A Guide to Cannabis for the Terminally and Chronically Ill. Whiteley N. Alivio, 2016.
Clinical Nutrition for Oncology Patients. Roberts M. Jones and Bartlett, 2010.
Diet and Nutrition in Palliative Care: A Guide for Clients and Carers. Adelaide Hills Community Health Service. Government of South Australia, 2012.
Follow the Child. Langton-Gilks S. Jessica Kingsley Publishers, 2018.
Handbook of Cannabis Therapeutics: From Bench to Bedside. Russo E, Grotenhermen F. The Haworth Press, 2006.
Nutrition Care of the Older Adult: A Handbook for Nutrition Throughout the Continuum of Care, 3rd ed. Niedert KC, Carlson MP (Editors). Academy of Nutrition and Dietetics, 2016.
Oncology Nutrition for Clinical Practice. Leser M, Ledesma N, Bergerson S, Trujillo E (Editors), Oncology Nutrition Dietetic Practice Group, 2013.
Oxford Textbook of Palliative Care for Children. Goldman A, Hain R, Liben S. Oxford University Press, 2012.
Palliative Care in Pediatric Oncology. Wolfe J, Jones BL, Kreicbergs U, Jankovic M. Springer, 2018.
Palliative Care Nursing, Principles and Evidence for Practice. Walshe C, Preston N, Johnston B. Open University Press, 2018.

Note: These are books on diet and nutrition in palliative care recommended by the experts and practitioners contributing to this book.

TABLE 35.4
Relevant Online Resources and Information on Diet and Nutrition in Palliative Care

Association of Paediatric Palliative Medicine Master Formulary 4th edition 2017
https://www.appm.org.uk/guidelines-resources/appm-master-formulary/
Basic Symptom Control in Paediatric Palliative Care, The Rainbows Children's Hospice Guidelines
www.togetherforshortlives.org.uk/wp-content/uploads/2018/01/ProRes-Symptom-Control-Manual.pdf
British Columbian Cancer Agency
www.bccancer.bc.ca/our-services/services/library/recommended-websites/living-with-cancer-websites/nutrition-for-people-with-cancer-websites
International Association for Cannabinoid Medicines
http://www.cannabis-med.org/?lng=en
Japan Association for Percutaneous Trans-Esophageal Gastro-tubing (PTEG)
www.pteg.jp/index.html (Japanese only)
Maryland Cancer Collaborative
c.ymcdn.com/sites/ www.hnmd.org/resource/resmgr/MCC_Palliative_Care_Resource.pdf
New Brunswick Hospice Palliative Care Association
www.nbhpca-aspnb.ca/education/…congres/…/nutrition_in_palliative_care.pdf
Patients Out of Time
www.medicalcannabis.com
Videos on advance care planning (Chinese)
www.youtube.com/watch?v=roy-pIUIkPc&t=11s
www.youtube.com/watch?v=3y-Dd9Tk6MA&t=9s
www.youtube.com/watch?v=BzFJ9n8Tf5k&t=18s

Note: These are other recommended internet resources relevant to diet and nutrition in palliative care. While some are in a language other than English, online translations may be useful.

KEY FACTS

- Palliative care is the holistic treatment of patients with life-threatening illnesses whose conditions cannot be cured.
- Food and eating are fundamental aspects of daily living.
- Cachexia is very common in patients who require palliative care.
- Nutritional support alone cannot reverse cachexia.
- The literature on nutrition in palliative care in peer-reviewed journals is relatively sparse.
- There has been an approximate 400% increase in the number of papers on this topic over the past 20 years.

SUMMARY POINTS

- Diet and nutrition in palliative care are under-recognised in modern medicine.
- This chapter lists up-to-date resources on the regulatory bodies, professional bodies, journals, books and websites that are relevant to an evidence-based approach to diet and nutrition in palliative care.
- Analysis of original research shows that there are relatively few papers associated with diet and nutrition in palliative care.

ACKNOWLEDGEMENTS

We would like to thank the following authors for contributing to the development of this resource: Amano K, Audain K, Caccialanza R, Chan H, Chwistek M, Henry B, Koh M, Maetani I, Monturo C, Siraj N, Trentham K and Walshe C.

REFERENCES

1. World Health Organisation. WHO Definition of Palliative Care. www.who.int/cancer/palliative/definition/en (accessed July 26, 2018).
2. Bird A. Perceptions of diet and nutrition in palliative care. *Nature* 2007; 447: 396–8.
3. Morley JE. Cancer and cachexia. *Cur Opin Clin Nutr Metab Care* 2009; 12: 607–10.
4. Fabbro ED, Shalini D, Bruera E. Symptom control in palliative care – Part II: Cachexia/anorexia and fatigue. *J Palliat Med* 2006; 9: 409–21.
5. Ersek M. Artificial nutrition and hydration: Clinical issues. *J Hosp Palliat Nurs* 2003; 5(4): 221–30.

Index

B

C

D

F

G

H

I

N

O

P

Q

R

S

T

U

V

CPSIA information can be obtained
at www.ICGtesting.com
Printed in the USA
LVHW061644240523
46533LV00021B/222

9 780367 727161